BSAVA Manual of Backyard Poultry Medicine and Surgery

T0203391

Editors:

Guy Poland
VetMB BA(cantab)
Redhill, North Somerset, UK

Aidan Raftery
MVB CertZooMed CBiol MRSB MRCVS
Avian and Exotic Animal Clinic,
221 Upper Chorlton Road, Manchester M16 0DE, UK

Published by:

British Small Animal Veterinary Association
Woodrow House, 1 Telford Way,
Waterwells Business Park, Quedgeley,
Gloucester GL2 2AB

A Company Limited by Guarantee in England
Registered Company No. 2837793
Registered as a Charity

The drawings in Figures 2.5, 2.6, 2.8, 2.9, 2.10, 2.12, 2.13, 2.14, 2.15, 2.16, 2.17, 2.18, 2.19, 2.20, 2.21, 2.23, 2.24, 2.25, 10.4, 10.23, 14.1, 14.2, 14.17, 23.9, 23.12, 23.13, 23.14, 23.16, 23.17 and 23.25a were drawn by S.J. Elmhurst BA Hons (www.livingart.org.uk) and are printed with her permission.

A catalogue record for this book is available from the British Library.

ISBN 978 1 905319 43 5

The publishers, editors and contributors cannot take responsibility for information provided on dosages and methods of application of drugs mentioned or referred to in this publication. Details of this kind must be verified in each case by individual users from up to date literature published by the manufacturers or suppliers of those drugs. Veterinary surgeons are reminded that in each case they must follow all appropriate national legislation and regulations (for example, in the United Kingdom, the prescribing cascade) from time to time in force.

Printed in the UK by Cambrian Printers Ltd, Aberystwyth, Ceredigion SY23 3TN
Printed on ECF paper made from sustainable forests

**Save 15% off the digital version of this manual. By purchasing this print edition we are pleased to offer you a reduced price on online access at www.bsavalibrary.com
Enter offer code 15MPB194 on checkout**

Please note the discount only applies to a purchase of the full online version of the *BSAVA Manual of Backyard Poultry Medicine and Surgery* via **www.bsavalibrary.com**. The discount will be taken off the BSAVA member price or full price, depending on your member status. The discount code is for a single purchase of the online version and is for your personal use only. If you do not already have a login for the BSAVA website you will need to register in order to make a purchase.

3890PUBS19

Titles in the BSAVA Manuals series

Manual of Avian Practice: A Foundation Manual
Manual of Backyard Poultry Medicine and Surgery
Manual of Canine & Feline Abdominal Imaging
Manual of Canine & Feline Abdominal Surgery
Manual of Canine & Feline Advanced Veterinary Nursing
Manual of Canine & Feline Anaesthesia and Analgesia
Manual of Canine & Feline Behavioural Medicine
Manual of Canine & Feline Cardiorespiratory Medicine
Manual of Canine & Feline Clinical Pathology
Manual of Canine & Feline Dentistry and Oral Surgery
Manual of Canine & Feline Dermatology
Manual of Canine & Feline Emergency and Critical Care
Manual of Canine & Feline Endocrinology
Manual of Canine & Feline Endoscopy and Endosurgery
Manual of Canine & Feline Fracture Repair and Management
Manual of Canine & Feline Gastroenterology
Manual of Canine & Feline Haematology and Transfusion Medicine
Manual of Canine & Feline Head, Neck and Thoracic Surgery
Manual of Canine & Feline Musculoskeletal Disorders
Manual of Canine & Feline Musculoskeletal Imaging
Manual of Canine & Feline Nephrology and Urology
Manual of Canine & Feline Neurology
Manual of Canine & Feline Oncology
Manual of Canine & Feline Ophthalmology
Manual of Canine & Feline Radiography and Radiology: A Foundation Manual
Manual of Canine & Feline Rehabilitation, Supportive and Palliative Care: Case Studies in Patient Management
Manual of Canine & Feline Reproduction and Neonatology
Manual of Canine & Feline Shelter Medicine: Principles of Health and Welfare in a Multi-animal Environment
Manual of Canine & Feline Surgical Principles: A Foundation Manual
Manual of Canine & Feline Thoracic Imaging
Manual of Canine & Feline Ultrasonography
Manual of Canine & Feline Wound Management and Reconstruction
Manual of Canine Practice: A Foundation Manual
Manual of Exotic Pet and Wildlife Nursing
Manual of Exotic Pets: A Foundation Manual
Manual of Feline Practice: A Foundation Manual
Manual of Ornamental Fish
Manual of Practical Animal Care
Manual of Practical Veterinary Nursing
Manual of Psittacine Birds
Manual of Rabbit Medicine
Manual of Rabbit Surgery, Dentistry and Imaging
Manual of Raptors, Pigeons and Passerine Birds
Manual of Reptiles
Manual of Rodents and Ferrets
Manual of Small Animal Practice Management and Development
Manual of Wildlife Casualties

For further information on these and all BSAVA publications, please visit our website: **www.bsava.com/shop**

Contents

Contributors

John Chitty
BVetMed CertZooMed CBiol MRSB MRCVS
Anton Vets,
Unit 11 Anton Mill Road,
Andover SP10 2NJ, UK

Alison Colville-Hyde
PGCert(Applied Poultry Science)
St David's Poultry Team Ltd,
Nutwell Estate, Lympstone,
Exmouth EX8 5AN, UK

Jan Dixon
BVMS MRCVS
St David's Poultry Team Ltd,
Nutwell Estate, Lympstone,
Exmouth EX8 5AN, UK

Bob Doneley
BVSc FANZCVS(Avian Medicine)
Veterinary Medical Centre,
Building 8156, Main Drive, University of Queensland,
Gatton 4343, Queensland, Australia

Kevin Eatwell
BVSc(Hons) DZooMed DipECZM(Herpetology, Small Mammals)
MRCVS
Royal (Dick) School, Hospital for Small Animals,
Easter Bush Vet Centre, Roslin EH25 9RG, UK

Christine Eckermann-Ross
BS DVM
Avian & Exotic Animal Care,
8711 Fidelity Boulevard, Raleigh,
North Carolina 27617, USA

Neil Forbes
BVetMed DipECZM(Avian) FRCVS
Homer Forbes International,
Woodfield Cottage, Birts Street, Birtsmorton,
Malvern, Worcestershire WR13 6AP, UK

Ursula Heffels-Redmann
DrMedVet (Specialist for Poultry)
Clinic for Birds, Reptiles, Amphibians and Fish,
Justus-Liebig University Giessen,
Frankfurter Str. 91–93,
35392 Giessen, Germany

Helen Hodgkin
BSc(Hons)

Richard Jackson
BVMS(Hons) MRCVS
St David's Poultry Team Ltd,
Nutwell Estate, Lympstone,
Exmouth EX8 5AN, UK

Richard Jones
VSc MSc MRCVS
Avian Vet Services,
Gauntlet Birds of Prey Centre, Manchester Road,
Knutsford, Cheshire WA16 0SX, UK

Michelle Kischinovsky
DVM MRCVS

Maria-Elisabeth Krautwald-Junghanns
ProfDr DrMedVet DipECZM(Avian) ML
Unversität Leipzig, Institute for Avian and Reptilian
Diseases, 04103 Leipzig, Germany

Karin Kreyenbühl
Poultry & Bird Practice,
Rummelring 15, CH-5610 Wohlen AG, Switzerland

Michael Lierz
DrMedVet DZooMed DipECZM(WPH) DipECPVS
Clinic for Birds, Reptiles, Amphibians and Fish,
Justus-Liebig University Giessen,
Frankfurter Str. 91–93,
35392 Giessen, Germany

Ian Mackinson
BSc(Hons) RNutr
Premier Nutrition,
Brereton Business Park, The Levels,
Rugeley, Staffordshire WS15 1RD, UK

Deborah Monks
BVSc(Hons) CertZooMed FANZCVS(Avian Health) DipECZM(Avian)
Brisbane Birds and Exotics Veterinary Service,
191 Cornwall Street, Greenslopes,
Queensland 4120, Australia

Bairbre O'Malley
MVB CertVR MRCVS
Bairbre O'Malley Veterinary Hospital,
Kilmantain Place, Bray, County Wicklow,
A98 PV38, Ireland

Helene Pendl
DrMedVet
Pendl Lab Diagnostic Microscopy,
Untere Roostmatt 7, CH-6300 Zug, Switzerland

Guy Poland
VetMB BA(cantab)
Redhill, North Somerset, UK

Aidan Raftery
MVB CertZooMed CBiol MRSB MRCVS
Avian and Exotic Animal Clinic,
221 Upper Chorlton Road,
Manchester M16 0DE, UK

Drury R. Reavill
DVM DipABVP(Avian, Reptile & Amphibian Practice) DipACVP
Zoo/Exotic Pathology Service,
6020 Rutland Drive, Carmichael CA 95608, USA

Victoria Roberts
BVSc MRCVS
Dorking Breed Club Secretary,
Heather Bank Poultry, Hillings Lane, Menston, Ilkley,
West Yorkshire LS29 6AU, UK

Robert Schmidt
DVM PhD DipACVP
Independent Veterinary Patholology Consultant
specializing in Avian and Exotic Animal Pathology

Sergio Silvetti
DVM CertAVP(ZooMed) MRCVS
Manor Vets, Exotic Animal Medicine and Surgery
Department, 371/373 Hagley Road, Edgbaston,
Birmingham B17 8DL, UK

Steve Smith
BVetMed(Hons) CertZooMed DipECZM(Avian) MRCVS
Tiggywinkles Wildlife Hospital,
Aston Road, Haddenham,
Bucks HP17 8AF, UK

Johanna Storm
Rusu MRCVS
International Zoo Veterinary Group,
Station House, Parkwood Street, Keighley,
West Yorkshire BD21 4NQ, UK

Keith Warner
BVM&S BSc MRCVS

David L. Williams
MA MEd VetMD PhD DipECAWBM CertVOphthal CertWEL
FHEA FRCVS
Department of Veterinary Medicine,
University of Cambridge, Madingley Road,
Cambridge CB3 0ES, UK

Foreword

The *BSAVA Manual of Backyard Poultry Medicine and Surgery* is a much-anticipated addition to the BSAVA's vast range of small and exotic animal titles. This book represents a new subject area and reflects the rise in backyard poultry-keeping. Poultry-keeping is an activity that most people consider 'traditional' and so expect all vets to be able to see and treat their birds, not just 'exotics' practitioners. As such, general small animal practitioners are now frequently being asked to treat poultry, which, I am sure, many would not have anticipated on graduation.

In keeping with BSAVA's forward-looking publications policy, a new subject area sees a new editorial team. The editors are to be congratulated on bringing a fresh approach and producing a genuinely exciting publication that covers not just medicine and surgery, but also husbandry, nutrition and legal issues. The latter part is especially relevant to practitioners unused to prescribing for food-producing animals. To do this they have recruited an impressive range of authors from around the world and from the worlds of exotics and poultry medicine. This symbiotic approach is essential in a new field where conventional poultry medicine knowledge must be complemented by practice-based techniques for working with, what most keepers would consider as, pets.

I am honoured to have been asked to write this foreword in a book I am very much looking forward to using in practice.

John Chitty
BSAVA President 2017/18

Preface

In a world of ever-increasing demand on limited resources, the question of where our food comes from has seldom been so important. In response to this, there has been a resurgence in home grown produce, and an increase in the number of people keeping backyard poultry for a self-sufficient supply of eggs and meat. Not only do backyard poultry produce fresh food, they can teach children a great deal about the role of animals in feeding the human population and they provide fascination and enjoyment for those who keep them. Backyard poultry frequently become an important part of the family and are often seen as much loved pets. There is also a thriving community of poultry keepers interested in the breeding and exhibition of these birds, which are often very beautiful. When a backyard bird becomes ill, therefore, their owner expects access to caring and competent veterinary care, often with an expectation that such care should meet the standard on offer to their dog or cat.

Unfortunately, the veterinary profession has, in places, struggled to live up to this expectation. There are three main reasons for this. First, whilst backyard poultry are considered as pets, their ability to produce safe food (especially in the case of laying chickens) remains a key part of their value to their owners, and this is frequently a source of conflict in treatment terms. Secondly, many practitioners have been unwilling to treat pet poultry due to their lack of knowledge and, thirdly, traditional poultry medicine is geared at treating the flock rather than the individual bird, whilst the knowledge base required to treat pet poultry as individuals is based on treating companion parrots and exhibit birds in zoos. It is the aim of this new BSAVA manual to bring together commercial poultry veterinary surgeons and their flock-based knowledge with companion avian veterinary surgeons and their knowledge of the individual diagnostics, supportive care, medicine and surgery of individual birds, to provide good quality information to help general practitioners provide the level of care to backyard birds that clients expect and deserve. In turn, it is hoped that the help and guidance that this manual provides will make treating backyard poultry more interesting and rewarding, and therefore encourage more practitioners to develop the skills and knowledge to provide a high level of medical care for feathered patients!

Throughout this manual, we have attempted to use evidence-based research, referencing primary research wherever possible. Unfortunately, such research is not always available, and so in many parts of the text we have had to rely upon consensus opinion or expert advice. It is the responsibility of the prescribing veterinary surgeon to use their clinical judgement when following the advice in the manual, and to inform owners of the implications of using drugs off license. We have included information so that practitioners can apply due consideration to the food-producing status of poultry species. All legal regulations followed, including the prescribing cascade, are those in place at the time of publication in the United Kingdom of Great Britain. Users of this manual outside the UK will need to ensure that they are fully versed in the regulations that apply to practice in their region.

We are very proud of the valuable contributions made by all the authors to this manual. We hope that their hard work will provide a useful resource for veterinary practitioners unfamiliar with avian/poultry medicine to deliver improved care for their patients and maybe inspire an interest that they develop further.

Guy Poland and Aidan Raftery
July 2019

Origins and types of poultry

Victoria Roberts

History

Chickens are believed to originate from the red junglefowl (Figure 1.1), a small pheasant from Asia. Early Indian, Chinese and Japanese records show that chickens have been domesticated in Asia for over 4000 years. Pliny in 4 BC described chickens as a source of medicine, whilst another Roman writer, Columella, who died in AD 47, chronicled Dorking-type birds with five toes. When the Romans came to Britain, they seemed surprised to find that the few indigenous fowl were used for cockfighting as well as for food, as they were far keener on maintaining the fighting quality of their troops with good food. Invading forces tended to travel with their fowl, to provide fresh meat, and thus different types of fowl evolved according to the local conditions.

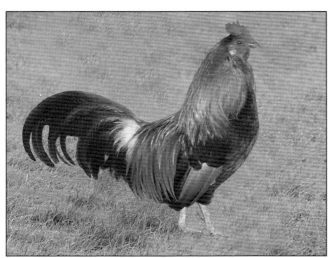

1.1 Red junglefowl (the ancestor of chickens).
(Reproduced from the *BSAVA Manual of Farm Pets*)

Few European authors prior to the 1800s considered the chicken to be anything other than a scavenger that produced the odd egg and meal. The notable exception was the Italian naturalist, Ulisse Aldrovandi. His *On Chickens* (first published in 1598) contains many anatomical illustrations, which are good enough to learn from today, with some of the drawings depicting recognizable breeds. Other records of poultry breeds can be seen in the evocative and beautiful paintings of the 1500s, but it was not until Victorian times that written records on poultry became more common. New World traders increased the genetic pool by bringing fowl back with them. Improved methods of husbandry led to increased egg and meat production, with flocks kept on the edges of towns increasing in size so that the populace could be fed easily. Then, with the coming of the railways, the countryside was 'opened up', thus fast and easy access to urban markets was possible.

A favourite Victorian pastime was cockfighting and many poultry keepers were devastated when the 'sport' was banned in 1849. This affected all walks of life: aristocracy, gentry, traders, publicans, magistrates and schoolboys all took part. Some cockfighting rings went underground (and still maintain their strains of birds and the illegal activity to the present day), but the majority of people turned their energies to the new and rapidly vibrant sport of exhibiting poultry, and thus the great shows were born.

The Victorians did some serious selecting and breeding, with tremendous competition as to who brought a breed to the UK, or who bred or improved a certain line. The books of the time, such as Moubray's *Treatise on Domestic and Ornamental Poultry* (published in 1854), have beautiful and reasonably anatomically correct colour illustrations, which give an indication of the development of the kinds of breeds and species of poultry in those days. Other contemporary titles include Harrison Weir's *Our Poultry*, being the basis for good husbandry, and Edward Brown's *Poultry Breeding and Production*. Then Lewis Wright began amalgamating different texts and his *Book of Poultry* is still in print and popular due to improvements in colour printing.

The first standards for poultry in the UK were produced in 1865 for just a handful of breeds to try and maintain uniformity; it was not until the turn of the century and the importation of breeds from the continent and America that a volume of any size appeared. Internationally, guardians of standards in other countries (e.g. The American Poultry Association, American Livestock Breeds Conservancy, Australian Poultry Societies, German Poultry Association and other European representations; see also Appendix 4) delineate the standards of breeds developed in their respective countries, which should be followed when breeds are brought to different countries. In the UK, each Breed Club delineates the standard for their breed, with The Poultry Club being the overall guardian. Slow changes to standards have been introduced when necessary, but merely altering the standards to suit fashionable judging is not considered acceptable.

Modern books on poultry abound and it is sometimes quite difficult sorting out those written from experience and those just gathering together others' writing, a particular danger being recommendations that are now either illegal or not welfare-friendly. A plethora of specialist poultry magazines providing mainly expert advice are now available for the currently estimated over a million poultry keepers in the UK, with other countries educating and entertaining their poultry keepers in a similar vein, but social media has some catching up to do with accurate information on husbandry and diseases.

In the desire to produce cheap food for a burgeoning human population, poultry keeping was intensified, the main advances being seen in the early 1950s. This meant that flocks were brought indoors to avoid predators, parasites and soil-borne diseases. Hardy pure breeds were originally used to create the ubiquitous broiler and hybrid battery hen, but with selection for egg and meat production, selection for disease resistance was neglected. This problem was probably compounded by the poorly developed nature of poultry medicine at the time, leading to misconceptions about illness and husbandry. Unfortunately, these intensified, sometimes crowded, conditions created the ideal environment for other opportunistic pathogenic bacteria and viruses to emerge, multiply and spread. Many modern poultry diseases can be traced to this intensification, but that is somewhat balanced by the tremendous amount of research then undertaken on diseases, treatment and production, to the benefit not only of poultry but also human medicine.

Breeders of commercial poultry rarely acknowledge their debt to the pure breeds, but are still happy to use a particular trait, such as resistance to a certain disease, to increase the profitability of their commercial birds. This is only possible due to the dedication of fanciers in keeping bloodlines pure over many generations. Since all domestic poultry are heavily selected by humans, it is possible to easily influence their type, characteristics and colour, which is why commercial breeders have made such enormous strides so quickly in being able to produce cheap and plentiful high-protein meat and eggs on demand since the 1950s. Such was the quantity of research undertaken that the feeding of poultry then became a science, and commercially produced, scientifically formulated rations made life much easier for the backyard keeper. There are two main types of commercial chicken (both of which are kept indoors): the meat-producing, very fast-growing broilers; and the egg-laying hens. Smaller scale producers have now developed hardier types of both the high-production meat-producing chickens and egg-laying chickens for outdoor, free-range systems – there is no one chicken type that will produce both meat and eggs successfully commercially.

Backyard poultry keeping went through the doldrums in the 1950s and 1960s, but stalwart breeders kept the nuclei of pure breeds going, fortunately, and there is now a tremendous resurgence in the UK (and worldwide). This has, in part, been fuelled by the 'rescuing' of ex-battery hens, often the first time people have kept small numbers of chickens.

Chickens

Commercial hybrids

An enduring problem with breeding chickens is that, unlike waterfowl, they do not have external genitalia, so sexing the animals is a challenge. However, it was discovered in the 1930s that if a genetically gold male was mated with a genetically silver female, the subsequent chicks were 'sex-linked'. That is, the male and female chicks hatch with different coloured down, with the male colour crossing to the female chicks. Hence, all commercial indoor female hybrids are brown. Strains of hybrids were developed from the 1950s for the battery cage egg industry, to vastly increase production compared with the pure breeds.

Hybrids are available for the backyard keeper in small numbers from specialized distributors. They are uniform in colour, shape and size (Figure 1.2) and examples include Warren, Isa Brown, Hyline and Goldline. They are generally obtained just before laying commences (>20 weeks, point of lay (POL)), to avoid interruption of laying, and are productive for 2–3 years. They are a reasonable price as they are reared in large numbers, influenced by economies of scale. Best production is in excess of 300 eggs per year, each egg taking around 25 hours to be produced.

Ex-battery hens are those commercial hybrids that have come to the end of their (profitable) laying life. As they are kept in temperature-controlled conditions, feather coverage is not good, because the hens do not need the insulation. They are very cheap to purchase and will still lay well for a while. Hundreds of thousands of hens have been rehomed in the past decade in the UK.

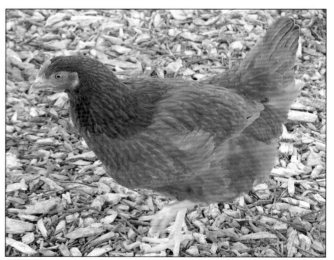

1.2 Commercial brown hybrid chicken.

Outdoor hybrids

The original outdoor hybrid, especially developed for free-range systems with hardiness, good feathering and laying of about 5 years, is the Black Rock (Figure 1.3). There are now several other hybrids available (Figure 1.4), including the Bovans Nera, Calder Ranger, Speckledy (Figure 1.5), Columbian Blacktail, White Star and Blue Belle, which are more productive than pure breeds, hardier than the commercial hybrids and provide different colours of birds and/or eggs. These hens are a little more expensive than the brown hybrids. Best production is 250–275 eggs per year for 4–5 years, each egg taking around 25.5 hours to be produced.

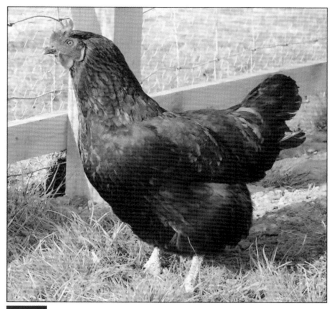

1.3 Black Rock outdoor hybrid chicken.

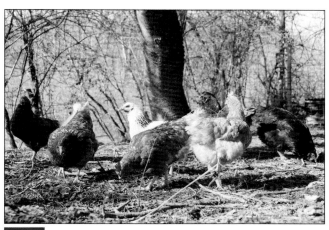

1.4 Young mixed outdoor hybrid chickens.

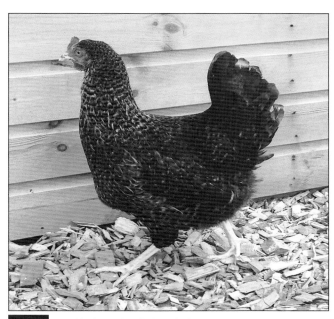

1.5 Speckledy outdoor hybrid chicken.

Pure breeds

Before the innovation of the hybrid, the pure breeds, the traditional breeds of poultry, had been developed in various countries for various purposes. They were the only source of meat- and egg-producing chickens. Commercial flocks consisted of Rhode Island Reds, White Leghorns, White Wyandottes and Light Sussex for eggs, plus Indian Game crossed with White Sussex for meat. There are still some small flocks of the pure breeds being run commercially, ensuring that utility aspects are maintained, because in today's cost-conscious society there are not many who can afford to keep the purely decorative birds.

However, not all useful attributes consist of egg or meat production. The larger, maternal breeds such as the Cochins and Brahmas are valuable as broody hens (i.e. hens that are hormonally determined to incubate eggs) and the foragers such as leghorns and other light breeds help keep insect numbers under control. Pure breeds are also used for exhibiting and have standards for type (shape and size) and colour, with a huge range of different patterns, sizes and feather type seen (see Appendix 4). Pure breeds live and lay eggs for 4–9 years, and on the whole only lay eggs during the longer days. The light breeds will lay the most but can be a bit flighty and nervous. The heavy breeds lay less and eat more, but will produce meat as well. Pure breeds are the most expensive to purchase. Best production is 100–250 eggs per year, depending on the breed and age of the bird, each egg taking up to 26 hours to be produced.

The gene pool of hybrids is necessarily small in the interests of uniformity after many generations of selection. The gene pool of pure breeds varies, depending on how fashionable they are on the show bench, since exhibitors tend to breed closely and sometimes sell on their below standard inbred stock. Too much inbreeding can cause health problems and infertility, but outcrossing can cause breed standard problems if the vendor has not kept good pedigree records. All pure breed poultry can be voluntarily (in the UK) close ringed at about 4 weeks of age (the Poultry Club Ringing Scheme), which identifies the breed, the breeder and the year. In Germany, however, ringing is compulsory for exhibition birds. Rings, of course, may be cut off, so in valuable exhibition breeds, the specific ring number in the UK may also be tattooed under the wing (white tattoo ink is used for black-skinned breeds).

Turkeys

All domestic turkeys are the same species, differing somewhat in size, and come in a wide variety of colours. They originate from America and of the five races, the two which are the ancestors of the ones we have today are the *Meleagris gallopavo gallopavo* (from Mexico; bronze with white tail border) and *Meleagris gallopavo silvestris* (from the eastern seaboard of North America; bronze with brown tail border). The Mexican turkey was developed into the commercial meat bird, plus the paler colours, and the Eastern turkey gave us the red and buff colour series.

Commercial turkeys have been selected for rate of growth and muscle mass, which gives them a very obvious waddling walk (the bronze record being 43.5 kg), but are generally unable to mate naturally. These birds have been termed dimple or broad-breasted and would be the type of turkey seen in supermarkets. The coloured varieties, however, have maintained the wild shape and are termed high-breasted, and are generally very active. Egg production is around 60 per annum.

Waterfowl

Ducks

Domestic ducks, with the exception of the Muscovy duck, are all descended from the lascivious ubiquitous mallard (*Anas platyrhynchos platyrhynchos*; Figure 1.6) and hold the egg-laying record of all poultry: 364 eggs in 365 days, due to the fact that it only takes 24 hours for a duck egg to be produced. The Muscovy duck (*Cairina moschata*; Figure 1.7) has its own niche in meat production, as it is a larger, separate species of perching duck (with sharp claws). Muscovies make very good broody ducks and can also be crossed with mallard types to produce a mule for meat. There are heavy breeds, such as the Silver Appleyard and Saxony, and light breeds, such as the Khaki Campbell and Indian Runner, which lay best. In addition, there are also bantam breeds such as the Call and Black East Indian.

Geese

There are two wild ancestors of geese, the greylag (*Anser anser*; Figure 1.8) and the swan goose (*Anser cygnoides*; Figure 1.9). Most domestic geese are descended from the greylag, with the exception of the African and Chinese breeds, which are descended from the swan goose. Geese are kept as pets, guard animals, for eggs and meat, and as 'lawn mowers' and need substantial areas of grass. However, not all of the breeds will suit all of these purposes, as some of the heavier breeds lay very few eggs. The pure breeds are usually available as young stock in late summer, but some may need to be reserved in advance. It is possible to obtain ordinary mixed breed (utility type) farmyard geese, which can be any colour and pattern but tend to be white, as day-olds or growers (best sexed). Day-old commercial white meat geese are available in late spring.

Ornamental waterfowl

There are a large number of ornamental (wild) waterfowl kept in aviaries or fox-proof fenced enclosures; overhead netting negates the need for pinioning or wing clipping. Ducks, geese and swans can be housed in the same enclosure, as long as there is sufficient shrub and nesting cover, and more than one pond, to avoid bullying.

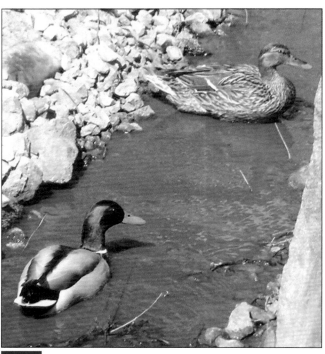

1.6 Mallard duck (the ancestor of most domestic ducks).

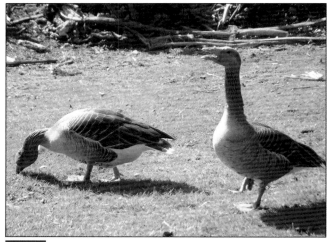

1.8 Greylag goose (the ancestor of most domestic geese).

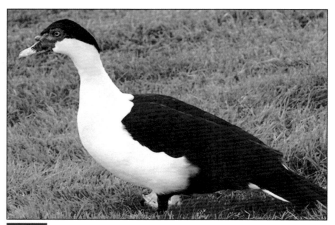

1.7 Muscovy duck.

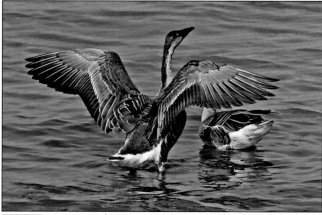

1.9 Swan goose (the ancestor of Chinese and African domestic geese).

Pheasants

There are over 50 species of ornamental pheasant, including the game pheasant, the highly colourful golden pheasant, the flamboyant eared pheasant, the more endangered *Tragopan* spp. and the proud, noisy and spectacular common Indian blue peafowl. Colour mutations in the latter include the Black-shouldered and White peafowl. The wild green peafowl is a different species and is not domesticated.

Most ornamental pheasants are kept as pairs or trios in aviaries. Some species are subject to the Convention on International Trade in Endangered Species (CITES) Appendices, requiring certain conditions for acquisition. Some species of pheasant, such as the grouse spp., the eared pheasant and the tragopans, tame well but most of them, including the partridge, remain nervous and wild, flying upwards at the first sign of perceived danger. Thus, soft netting as an aviary roof is a sensible precaution.

Guinea fowl

There is just one species of guinea fowl (*Numida meleagris*) domesticated in the UK, and these animals are mainly used for meat. Egg production is not particularly good at approximately 50 per year and day-old keets (youngsters) are only available at certain times. Colour mutations include the pearl (dark blue with white spots), fawn (beige with white spots), all fawn, all white, lavender (pale blue with white spots) and lavender and white. Crested guinea fowl (*Guttera pucherani*) are sometimes kept in other countries, but domestication has not progressed with other species such as the royal blue plumaged vulturine guinea fowl (*Acryllium vulturinum*).

References and further reading

Robbins GES (1984) *Partridges, their breeding and management*. World Pheasant Association, Hampshire

Roberts V (1998) *Poultry for Anyone*. Whittet Books, Cambridgeshire

Roberts V (2002) *Ducks, Geese and Turkeys for Anyone*. Whittet Books, Cambridgeshire

Roberts V (2008) *British Poultry Standards*. Wiley-Blackwell, Oxford

Roberts V and Scott Park F (2008) *BSAVA Manual of Farm Pets*. BSAVA Publications, Gloucester

Scott P (1998) *Coloured Key to the Wildfowl of the World*. Wildfowl and Wetlands Trust, Slimbridge

Todd FS (1979) *Waterfowl: Ducks, Geese and Swans of the World*. Sea World Press, California

Chapter 2

Anatomy and physiology

Bairbre O'Malley

External features and integument

Avian skin is very thin and lightweight under the plumage but thicker on the feet and around the beak in order to resist mechanical stress. The epidermis contains keratinocytes which secrete a thin lipid film that helps in the maintenance of the plumage. The dermis is thinner than that of mammals and composed of connective tissue. It contains the feather follicles, smooth muscle and a dense network of nerves and blood vessels. The subcutaneous layer has loose connective tissue and some adipose tissue. In waterfowl this layer is thick to provide insulation, giving a yellow colour to the skin. The skin pigmentation of domestic fowl tends to be yellow, pink or white depending on the breed and the presence of carotenoids in the diet. The Silkie has blue–black skin due to the presence of melanocytes.

There are only two glands in domestic fowl: the aural gland and the uropygial or preen gland. The external ear has aural glands that secrete a waxy material containing masses of desquamated cells. The uropygial gland is a bilobed holocrine gland found at the dorsal base of the tail that produces lipid or sebum and is well developed in waterfowl. It is drained by a pair of ducts which open into a nipple-like papilla dorsocaudally. Sebum produced by this gland and the epidermal cells is spread over the plumage during preening.

The brood patch is an area of skin on the mid-ventral chest between the caudal sternum and the pubic bones. In broody hens, oestrogen causes feather loss in this area and the skin becomes thickened and more vascularized to provide extra warmth for egg incubation. Ducks and geese have no true brood patch, but keep their eggs warm by covering them with down feathers plucked from the breast.

Beak

The beak or bill consists of three layers:

*   A bony base of the premaxilla and mandible
*   A thin vascular dermal layer
*   A heavily keratinized epidermal layer.

The epidermal layer has a very thick stratum corneum that contains hydroxyapatite, calcium, phosphate and keratin. The keratin layer is called the rhamphotheca, with the rhinotheca covering the upper beak and the gnathotheca covering the lower beak.

Combs and wattles

In domestic fowl, the dermis becomes thickened and highly vascularized to form brightly coloured, ornamental outgrowths on the head. The epidermis remains thin, however, making them prone to injury. As the comb and wattle can represent up to 7% of the total body area of the bird, they also play an important role in thermoregulation. The comb is the red projection on the forehead and crown (Figure 2.1), whilst the ricti are triangular folds at the angle of the mouth. The maxillary rictus is roughened externally whilst the mandibular rictus is smooth. The wattles are the folds of skin that hang down from the ventral mandible like a dewlap, whilst the ear lobes are folds of skin that hang ventral to the external ear opening. Ear lobes can be white, red or blue, depending on the breed. (Note: hens with white ear lobes lay eggs with a white shell, as these are genetically linked.)

Many species have a protuberance on the frontal process of the cranium. In some breeds of ducks and geese this fleshy process is called the knob (Figure 2.2). Turkeys have a red distensible fleshy process called a snood (Figure 2.3) as well as caruncles, which are small protuberances on the skin of the head and upper neck. Caruncles are also seen in Muscovy ducks (Figure 2.4). Some species of guinea fowl have a horny process called the helmet or casque, which first appears around 3 months of age and continues to develop for approximately 2 years.

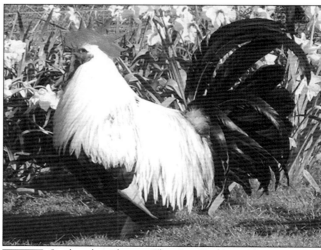

2.1 Comb and wattles on a Silver Grey Dorking cock.
(Reproduced from the *BSAVA Manual of Farm Pets*)

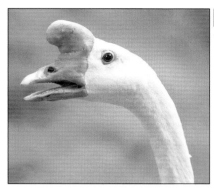

2.2 Knob on a Chinese goose.
(© Fotomicar)

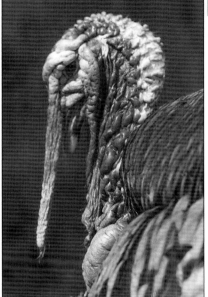

2.3 Snood and caruncles on a turkey.
(© Ezumeimages)

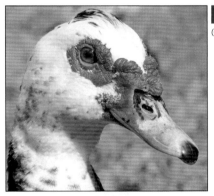

2.4 Caruncles on a Muscovy duck.
(© Rudy Umans)

Podotheca

The podotheca is the distal part of the leg which is non-feathered and covered by scales of keratinized epidermis. The skin on the underside of the foot and digits is thickened in the ventral metatarsophalangeal region with a metatarsal fleshy 'footpad' at each joint. In waterfowl, the skin between the digits is webbed for swimming. The distal phalanx is heavily keratinized into the nail. The dorsal keratin grows faster than the softer ventral keratin, creating the curved shape for perching and grasping. Many male Galliformes (domestic fowl, turkey, guinea fowl, pheasant)

have a keratinized spur with a vascularized osseous core on the caudomedial aspect of the tarsometatarsal region. This elongates by about 1 cm per year, reaching a maximum length of 6 cm. It is small or absent in the majority of female birds, but can be found in older hens.

Feathers

The feathering or plumage of birds can weigh 2–3 times as much as the skeleton. Feathers are arranged in feather tracts called pterylae, of which the domestic fowl has 70. Featherless regions called apteria are also present and may be filled with down. These featherless regions are used for heat dissipation and allow wing and leg movement.

Structure

Feathers are keratinized epidermis derived from specialized follicles set deep in the dermis. The main shaft of the feather is called the rachis (Figure 2.5). It is grooved underneath and ends in a depression called the distal umbilicus. The feather base is called the calamus and ends in the proximal umbilicus, which lies embedded in the feather follicle. The feather vane consists of a sheet of stiff filaments called barbs, which extend at a 45-degree angle on either side from the rachis (Figure 2.6). Each barb contains

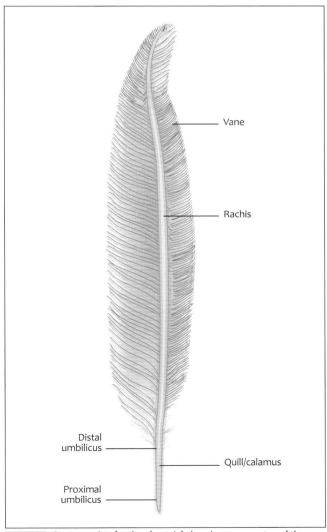

Vane

Rachis

Distal umbilicus

Quill/calamus

Proximal umbilicus

2.5 Contour wing feather (rectrix) showing asymmetry of the vane.

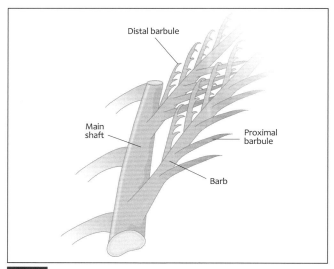

2.6 Barbs, barbules and interlocking hooklets.

fine filaments called barbules. These barbules contain minute hooks, which 'zip' the feathers together creating the smooth appearance required for waterproofing and flight. Birds maintain the plumage by preening, but if there is any structural damage it can only be remedied when the feather is moulted.

Growth

The feather grows from a papilla in the dermis, which projects into the epidermis and has a rich arterial and venous blood supply. Thus, immature feathers will bleed if broken and are called blood feathers (Figure 2.7). Mature feathers have no blood supply. Once the feather is fully formed, germinal activity ceases at the base of the follicle and it enters a resting stage until the next moult. The feather papilla will continue to produce feathers throughout the life of the bird.

Types

There are six main feather types:

- Contour
- Down
- Semiplume
- Hypopenna
- Filoplume
- Bristles.

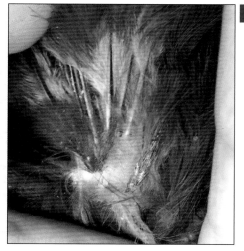

2.7 Blood feathers.

Contour feathers form most of the external plumage and appearance of adult birds. The larger contour feathers are asymmetrical, streamlined for flight and are found on the wings, tail and body surface. The wing feathers (remiges) are divided into primary and secondary feathers. The primary feathers are strongly attached dorsally to the metacarpal and phalangeal bones and are not very moveable. The secondary feathers are attached along the posterior edge of the ulna and have more mobility. The tail feathers (rectrices) are attached to the pygostyle and are used for steering and braking during flight. Covert feathers are smaller contour feathers that form the rest of the external plumage. As they are purely for covering the body and play no role in flight (other than streamlining) they are symmetrical.

Down feathers have a short rachis and non-interlocking barbules, which make them fluffy. These loose barbules trap air next to the skin and provide thermal insulation. In waterfowl they also assist the contour feathers in trapping air and maintaining buoyancy. Down feathers give precocious chicks their downy appearance and also form an insulating layer under the contour feathers in adults. Semiplumes are found alongside feather margins and appear fluffy with a rachis that is longer than the barbs. They aid thermal insulation and increase buoyancy in waterfowl species.

Hypopennae or after feathers have a stiff rachis and almost no barbules. They protrude from the base of the rachis of contour feathers. Filoplumes are bristle-like with a long shaft and a fine tuft of barbs at the tip. They are often found in association with the follicles of contour feathers. Bristles are found at the base of the eyelids, nares and mouth. They have a stiff rachis and a few barbs at the proximal end. It is thought that they have a tactile function, similar to that of mammalian whiskers.

Moulting

Moulting is the replacement of feathers and occurs because the emerging new feather ejects the old feather from its follicle causing it to be shed. Feathers lost prematurely can be replaced immediately or at the next moult. Before the barbs are released they are encased in a feather sheath (pinfeather) which is opened and unfurled by the bird during preening. Birds usually moult in a sequence: the inside primary feathers moult first and the rest of the wing feathers then moult in a staggered manner, so that there is only a small reduction in flight power.

Moulting is triggered by the time of year, light, breeding, nutrition and temperature, and is controlled by thyroidal and gonadal hormones. Adult birds usually moult once a year after breeding when the level of oestrogen and androgen drops. Male ducks and geese moult twice a year. After the breeding season they moult their body feathers over 6–10 weeks but lose all their flight feathers simultaneously, rendering them flightless. As this leaves the birds vulnerable to predation, the new plumage is muted and is called 'eclipse' plumage. Later on in the year or in early spring they undergo another moult to assume the more colourful plumage for sexual display during the mating season. Females usually moult once a year after the young have hatched. This allows them 5–6 weeks to regrow their flight feathers in time to become airborne with their young. Domestic fowl usually moult in the autumn after approximately 50 weeks of egg laying. However, moulting frequency is reduced in chicken and hybrid breeds developed for high egg production.

Moulting is a time of intense physiological pressure for birds. The metabolic rate of a moulting bird has to increase by 15–25% to compensate for the huge drain on energy and protein reserves. Feather loss leads to heat loss so energy intake must be increased, and feather growth increases the demand for protein (especially the amino acids lysine, cysteine and arginine), calcium and iron.

Musculoskeletal system

The skeleton is lightweight for flight but extremely strong with a fused vertebral column and limbs (Figure 2.8). Major bones, such as the humerus, coracoid, pelvic girdle, sternum and vertebrae, are pneumatic with air sacs extending into the medullary cavities. The forelimb is modified to form the wing, whilst the beak and long neck are heavily involved in food prehension.

Skull

The skull is lightweight with a small fused cranium housing the brain and large orbits, which are separated by a thin, bony interorbital septum. The rostral skull contains large honeycomb-like sinuses. Caudally there is a single occipital condyle which articulates with the atlas, enabling birds to rotate their neck to an angle of 180 degrees.

Unlike mammals, the avian upper jaw is extremely mobile relative to the cranium (cranial kinesis; Figure 2.9). An elastic hinge located rostrally allows the bones to bend without disturbing the cranium. This upper jaw movement is either prokinetic or rhynchokinetic. Domestic fowl and Galliformes are prokinetic with small, oval nostrils and the whole upper jaw functions as one unit. Waterfowl are rhynchokinetic (Figure 2.10). They have elongated, slit-like nostrils and only the rostral part of the upper jaw moves.

The upper jaw is formed from the premaxilla, the nasal bone and a small part of the maxilla. The mandible is

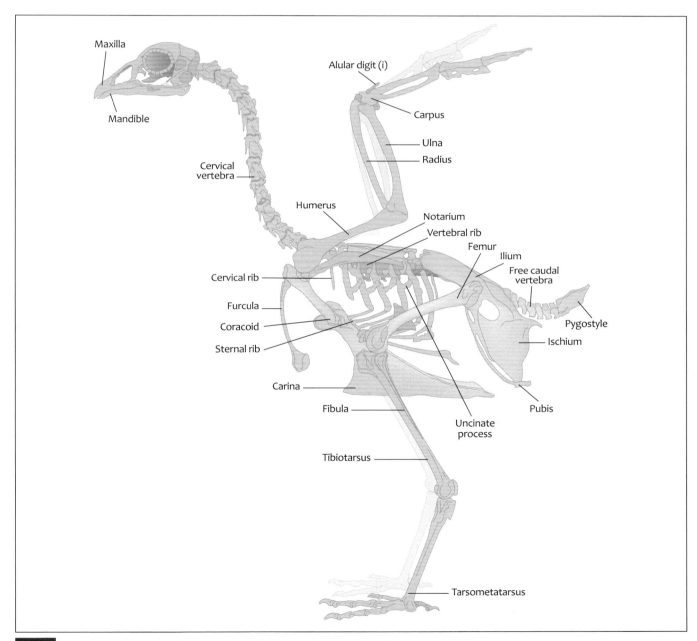

2.8   Skeleton of a chicken (see Figure 2.12 for detailed view of the pectoral girdle and wing).

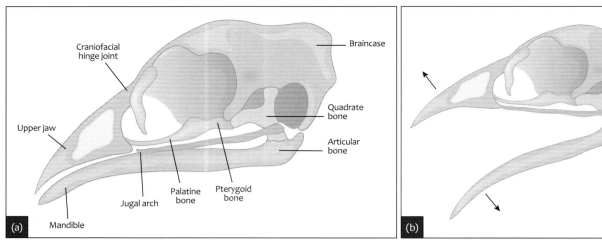

2.9 Cranial kinesis in domestic fowl. (a) Closed-mouth view. (b) Open-mouth view. When the jaw bone is lowered, the quadrate bone pushes the jugal arch and pterygoid–palatine bone rostrally to elevate the upper jaw, facilitating a wide gape.

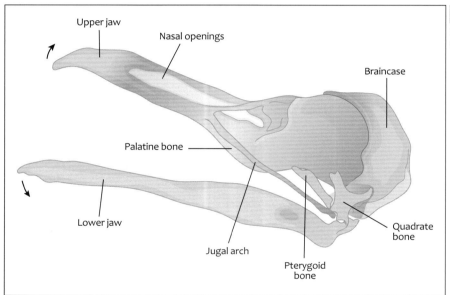

2.10 Rhynchokinesis. In birds such as waterfowl, only the rostral part of the upper jaw moves and the nasal openings are elongated and slit-like.

formed by the fusion of five small bones, which fuse caudally with the articular bone. The dentary bone lies rostrally and forms a fully ossified mandibular symphysis. Caudally the articular bone articulates with the mobile quadrate bone, which is the precursor of the mammalian auditory bones (incus and malleus). The quadrate bone articulates with the cranium and the premaxilla via two thin rod-like bones called the jugal arch (precursor of the zygomatic bone) and the pterygoid–palatine bone. The quadrate bone plays a role in cranial kinesis because when the bird lowers its jaw, it pushes the jugal arch and pterygoid–palatine bone rostrally to elevate the upper jaw, facilitating a wide gape.

Vertebrae

The cervical vertebrae are long, flexible and highly mobile, giving the avian neck the characteristic S-shaped appearance. The number of cervical vertebrae varies from 14–17 in the chicken, turkey and guinea fowl, to 13 in the pheasant (Figure 2.11). The caudal cervical vertebrae have rudimentary ribs, which are the site of attachment for the cervical muscles.

Species	Cervical vertebrae	Thoracic vertebrae	Synsacrum
Chicken	14–17	7 (notarium)	Fused (15–16)
Goose	17–18	9 (notarium)	Fused
Duck	14–15	9 (notarium)	Fused
Pheasant	13	6 (notarium)	Fused (14)

2.11 Number of vertebrae in common species.

Thoracic vertebrae are usually defined as carrying a complete rib. A unique feature of avian ribs is a backward pointing process, the uncinate process, which extends caudodorsally from every rib. These provide a point of attachment for the muscles that extend ventrocaudally to the rib behind. Domestic fowl have seven thoracic vertebrae, whilst ducks and geese have nine. In fowl, usually the last cervical vertebra and first three thoracic vertebrae are fused together into a single vertebra called the notarium. T4 is the only mobile vertebra in the trunk. In broilers this creates a 'weak link' as when ventrally displaced it causes a condition called spondylolisthesis or 'kinky back'.

The synsacrum supports the pelvic girdle (and hence the entire bodyweight of the bird) and is formed by the fusion of caudal thoracic, lumbar, sacral and coccygeal vertebrae. In domestic fowl, the synsacrum contains 15–16 vertebrae. There are only 5–6 free coccygeal vertebrae. The final 4–6 coccygeal vertebrae are fused into one single, flattened upturned bone called the pygostyle, which supports the tail feathers (rectrices).

Sternum

The main feature of the long and narrow sternum is that it has a deep carina or keel for the insertion of the pectoral (flying) muscles. In poor flying birds (such as domestic fowl), the caudal portion of the sternum is perforated. These perforations are lined by fibrous membranes and therefore not ossified.

Pectoral girdle

The pectoral (or thoracic) girdle consists of three bones on each side – the clavicle, coracoid and scapula (Figure 2.12). These bones articulate proximally to form the triosseal foramen, whilst the scapula and coracoid also form a shallow glenoid cavity distally. The clavicles and coracoid bones act to brace the wings. The two clavicles are fused into the furcula (wishbone) for extra strength and have a spring-like action. The coracoid is a short, strong bone which extends out from the sternum like a wing strut. It lies lateral to the jugular veins and subclavian and common carotid arteries, and deep below the cranial edge of the pectoralis muscle. The scapula is a long blade-like bone that lies parallel to the vertebral column and extends as far caudally as the pelvic girdle.

Wings

The wing consists of the humerus, radius and ulna (see Figure 2.12), and is fused distally into a three-fingered manus to provide a strong attachment for the primary flight feathers. The humerus is a short pneumatic bone with a well developed pectoral crest proximally where the

pectoralis muscles insert. The radius and ulna are long bones which lie parallel to one another. The ulna, which lies caudally, is the larger bone. Unlike mammals, the radius and ulna do not twist. The secondary flight feathers insert via ligaments along the caudal aspect of the ulna. The ulnar and radial carpal bones remain separate and attach to the carpometacarpus (fusion of the distal carpal bones and the major and minor metacarpal bones). There are three digits. The first digit (alular) is very mobile and can have one or two phalanges. The major metacarpal bone articulates with the major digit, which has two phalanges. The minor metacarpal bone articulates with the minor digit.

Pelvic girdle

The pelvic girdle slopes backwards and is strongly fused together for perching and activities such as running and swimming. It is formed by fusion of the ischium, pubis and ilium, and is rigidly fused to the synsacrum at the ilium. The pubis is incomplete ventrally, presumably to allow for the passage of eggs. The ventral pelvic girdle has deep bilateral renal fossae to protect the kidneys, nerves and blood vessels. The acetabula are deep and as there are strong femoral attachments, luxation is uncommon. An additional joint between the trochanter of the femur and the anti-trochanter of the ilium enables birds to perch on one leg easily.

Legs

The leg comprises the femur, tibiotarsus, fibula, tarsometatarsus, metatarsal bone and four digits. The femur is a short bone that articulates with the tibiotarsus and patella. It slopes cranioventrally in order to ensure that the feet lie under the bird's centre of gravity. The tibiotarsus is the largest bone and is formed by fusion of the tibia and proximal tarsal bones. The fibula is poorly developed and does not extend beyond the fibular crest. In order to counteract the forces of take-off and landing, the distal limb is strongly fused. The tarsometatarsus is formed by fusion of the second, third and fourth tarsal bones with the

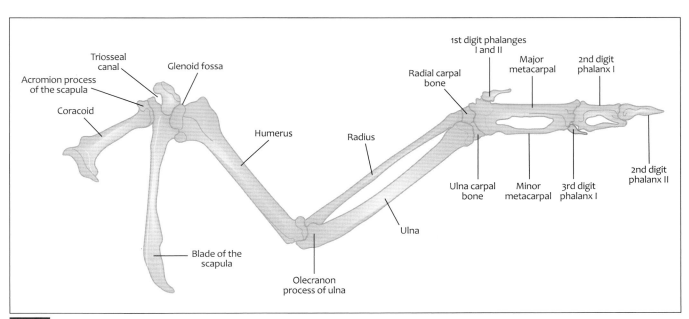

2.12 Ventral view of the pectoral girdle and left wing.

corresponding metatarsal bones. The tibiotarsus forms the equivalent of the hock joint with the tarsometatarsus, and movement here is mainly flexion and extension. The first metatarsal bone lies separately, but is joined to the tarsometatarsus by ligaments and can be mistaken for a phalanx.

Feet

Birds have big feet with four digits that have a varying number of phalanges. The first digit has two phalanges, the second digit has three phalanges, the third digit has four phalanges and the fourth digit has five phalanges. Galliformes are anisodactyl, meaning that they have three toes facing forwards and one toe (digit one) facing backwards (Figure 2.13a), in an adaptation for perching. Ducks and geese are palmate with cranial second, third and fourth digits being webbed (Figure 2.13b). As the feet are adapted for swimming they are unable to grip and the backwards facing digit has no contact with the ground.

Musculature

The highly fused axial skeleton means that birds have very sparse dorsal musculature. Thus, to provide stability for flight, the main muscle mass (up to 20% of bodyweight) is concentrated ventrally at the bird's centre of gravity. The flight muscles comprise the pectoral and supracoracoideus muscles (Figure 2.14). The pectoral muscles extend from the sternum to insert on the medial pectoral crest of the humerus. In most birds these superficial muscles form the main muscle mass as they create the 'down stroke' and are therefore essential for flapping flight. The supracoracoideus muscle is used mainly for take-off and is not necessary whilst in flight. It lies beneath the pectoral muscles and attaches to the ventral sternum. Its tendon runs dorsally through the triosseal canal to insert on the dorsal tubercle of the humerus. This tendon enables the bird to lift its wing for take-off and flight whilst still keeping the main bulk of the muscles ventrally.

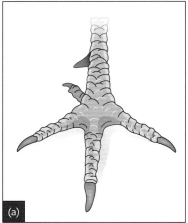

(a)

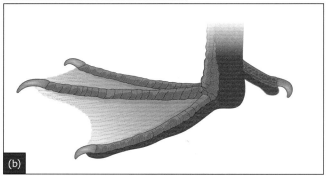

(b)

2.13 (a) Galliformes are anisodactyl. Note the spurs on the caudomedial aspect of the tarsometatarsus. (b) Swimming birds such as ducks and geese are palmate. Note the webbing between the cranial second, third and fourth digits. The capacity to grip is lost and the backward pointing digit loses contact with the ground.

The musculature appears white or red depending on its function and blood supply. Red muscles (e.g. gastrocnemius muscle) contain more of the oxygen-carrying pigment myoglobin than white muscles and have an extensive blood supply. Red muscles are powered by aerobic metabolism and can sustain effort for prolonged periods of time. White muscles are powered by anaerobic metabolism, which is good for rapid contractions (e.g. rapid take-off or short bursts of flapping flight) but tire easily due to the accumulation of lactic acid.

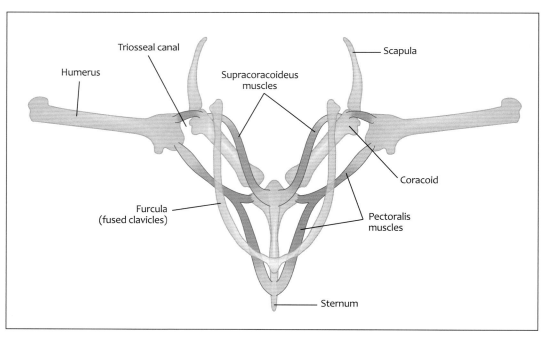

2.14 Ventral origins of the pectoral and supracoracoideus muscles, which allow the heavy musculature to be kept close to the bird's centre of gravity. The supracoracoideus muscle elevates the wings and the pectoral muscles depress the wings.

Humerus

Triosseal canal

Supracoracoideus muscles

Scapula

Coracoid

Furcula (fused clavicles)

Pectoralis muscles

Sternum

Body cavities

The lack of a diaphragm means there is no thorax and abdomen but just one body cavity called the coelom (Figure 2.15). The coelom contains 16 separate cavities: one pericardial cavity, two pleural cavities, eight air sacs (see below) and five peritoneal cavities. The pleural and pericardial cavities resemble those seen in mammals, whilst the peritoneal cavities are unique to birds. These cavities are of significance as they may influence the spread of disease throughout the coelom.

Pericardial and pleural cavities

The right and left pleural cavities are lined ventrally by a peritoneal sheet, the horizontal septum. The pericardial cavity is connected ventrally to the sternum and dorsally to the lung hilus and horizontal septum.

Peritoneal cavities

There is no omentum as seen in mammals. However, there is a double-layered peritoneal sheet called the post-hepatic septum. This septum divides the caudal cavity into three main parts: a middle intestinal cavity and two lateral cavities surrounding the liver. The intestinal cavity lies in the midline and contains the gastrointestinal tract, gonads and left oviduct, each of which lies suspended in its individual mesentery. In the domestic hen, the post-hepatic septum is also the principal peritoneal fat depot. In addition, the septum helps stop the spread of disease by bringing in a healthy blood supply.

Cardiovascular system

Birds have evolved a high performance cardiovascular system for flapping flight. As they have such high aerobic demands the avian heart is 50–100% larger than mammals of a similar size. Birds also have a much higher cardiac output to pump large volumes of blood to the wings, head and flight muscles. This is achieved by a high stroke volume, fast heart rate (resting heart rate of 160–280 beats per minute) and slightly lower peripheral resistance. In addition, birds also have stiffer arteries to improve blood flow and maintain a high blood pressure (ranging from a systolic pressure of 165 mmHg in domestic fowl and ducks to 190 mmHg in turkeys).

The four-chambered heart is attached to the dorsal surface of the sternum, the surrounding air sacs and liver. It lies slightly to the right of the midline and is surrounded by a thin but tough pericardium. Unlike in mammals, the lungs lie dorsal to the heart (not surrounding it) and the liver lobes cover the base of the heart dorsally and laterally. The ascending aorta curves to the right and the cranial and caudal venae cavae enter first into a sinus venosus before entering the right atrium. The right atrioventricular valve is structurally unique to birds in that it has no chordae tendineae and forms only a thick muscular flap of myocardium. With the exception of the left atrioventricular valve, which is tricuspid, the rest of the heart valves are similar to those seen in mammals.

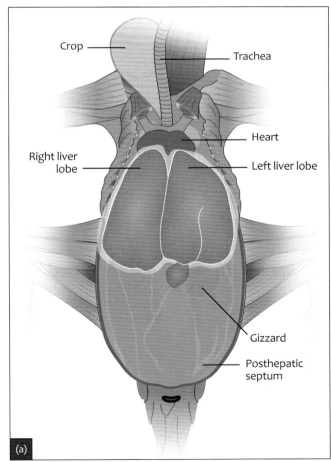
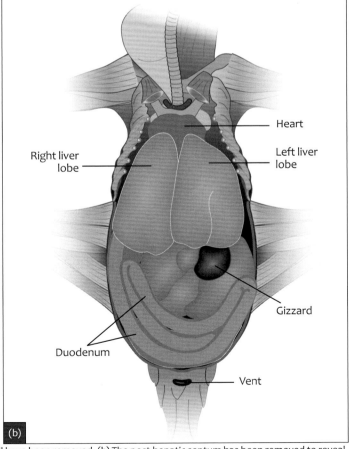

2.15 Ventral view of the coelom. (a) The sternum and abdominal wall have been removed. (b) The post-hepatic septum has been removed to reveal the viscera beneath.

Arterial system

The aortic arch curves to the right and gives rise immediately to the right and left brachiocephalic trunks, which distribute about three-quarters of the cardiac output to the wings, pectoral muscles and head (Figure 2.16). These soon branch into the subclavian arteries, which supply the wings (brachial artery) and flight muscles (pectoral artery), and the carotid arteries, which supply the head. The carotid arteries lie in a groove at the base of the cervical vertebrae and this prevents movements of the flexible neck arresting blood flow to the brain. The pelvic limb is supplied by the external iliac artery and the ischiatic artery, which meets the femoral artery at the stifle to form the popliteal artery. The major avian arteries appear white on gross examination due to the collagen fibres of the tunica adventitia. These fibres produce stiff arteries, which help combat the high avian blood pressure and improve blood flow.

Venous system

The cranial venae cavae are paired and receive blood from the neck and head via the jugular veins and from the wing and breast via the subclavian veins (Figure 2.17). At the angle of the jaw, a jugular anastomosis allows blood to be shunted from the left jugular vein in to the much larger right jugular vein. The venous return from the pelvic limbs and lower body goes through the kidneys via the renal portal

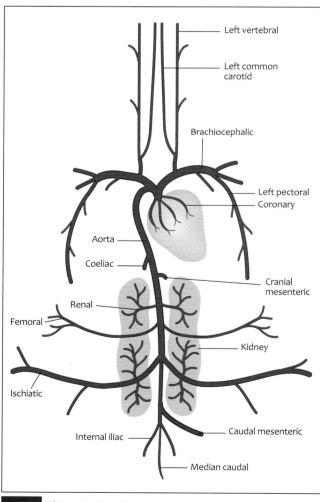

2.16 The major systemic arteries in the bird.

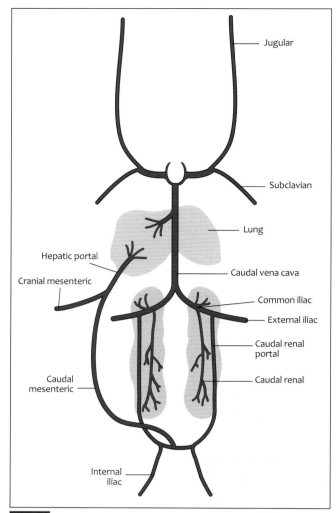

2.17 The major systemic veins in the bird.

vein before reaching the caudal vena cava. The main bulk of the gastrointestinal tract, pancreas and spleen drain into the hepatic portal vein and the liver. Unique to birds is the large caudal mesenteric vein, which drains the hindgut mesentery and connects the hepatic portal vein to the renal portal vein. As blood can flow along this vein in both directions, flow can be switched between the kidneys and the liver (Akester, 1984).

The renal portal vein system is under the control of a unique smooth muscle valve with a rich nerve supply, lying at the junction of the common iliac and renal veins. In emergency situations, high sympathetic activity releases adrenaline (epinephrine), which opens the valve to divert blood away from its normal passage through the kidney to the heart and brain. This can take three routes: via the open valve directly into the caudal vena cava; via the cranial portal vein to the internal vertebral venous plexus; or via the caudal mesenteric vein to the hepatic portal vein and liver.

Respiratory system

The ability to fly means that birds have much higher oxygen demands than mammals. Avian lungs are 10 times more efficient than mammalian lungs in absorbing oxygen due to a number of modifications. They have small fixed lungs, which change little in volume when breathing, and air sacs, which act as bellows but do not participate in gas exchange. This segregation of ventilation and gas exchange helps to increase the total gas exchange surface area by more than 20% compared with mammals. The bellows system also allows more efficient continuous one-way air flow as opposed to the 'in and out' tidal flow of mammals. There is also a much thinner blood–gas barrier and a cross current blood flow. This blood flow at right angles to air flow allows more efficient absorption of oxygen.

Upper respiratory tract

The nasal cavity is compressed laterally and divided medially by a very thin septum. In the domestic fowl and turkey, the nares lie laterally at the base of the beak and have a keratinized flap called the operculum. In some waterfowl, such as the duck, the nasal septum has an opening adjacent to a rostral opening in the nares (nares perviae), allowing communication between both sides of the nasal cavity. Air enters through the nares into the conchae, down through the slit-like choana, across the oropharynx to the glottis.

The nasal conchae are divided into rostral, middle and caudal parts and play a major role in olfaction, filtering and thermoregulation. They are highly vascular, epithelial folds which increase the surface area over which air flows. The caudal nasal concha and nasal cavity communicate with the infraorbital sinus. This is a triangular cavity lying superficially under the skin ventromedial to the orbit. Infection and swelling of this sinus is common in domestic fowl and turkeys.

Lower respiratory tract

Larynx, trachea and syrinx

The larynx or rima glottidis is slit-like and not covered by an epiglottis. It is not involved in sound production. The trachea is long and composed of approximately 120 rigid interlocking rings of cartilage. The long trachea creates air resistance, so the diameter of the larynx and trachea are wider to compensate. To overcome this deadspace, which is 4.5 times that seen in mammals, birds have an increased tidal volume. They also have a much slower and deeper rate of breathing – the respiratory rate of ducks is 65 breaths per minute, for domestic fowl is 30 breaths per minute, for large geese is 17 breaths per minute and for turkeys is 13 breaths per minute.

The syrinx is the 'voice box' in birds and comprises a series of modified tracheobronchial cartilages, two vibrating tympaniform membranes and muscles that vary the membrane tension. The surrounding interclavicular air sac gives the 'voice' resonance by pushing against these membranes. In male ducks, extra resonance is provided by an asymmetrical osseous dilatation on the left side of the syrinx (bulla tympaniformis).

Lungs

The lungs are closely adherent to the ribcage and occupy the craniodorsal part of the body cavity (Figure 2.18). They are bright pink, small and compact with furrow marks from the ribs on the surface. The horizontal septum, a peritoneal sheet, separates the lungs ventrally from the viscera. This septum plays no active role in respiration but passively helps to displace the viscera during breathing.

The primary bronchi run through the whole length of the lungs and terminate in the caudal air sacs. On entering

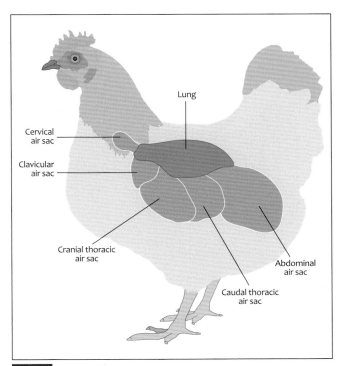

2.18 Location of the lungs and air sacs.

the lungs each bronchus gives rise to 40–50 secondary bronchi. These are divided into four types named according to the area of the lung they supply: mediodorsal, medioventral, laterodorsal and lateroventral. The secondary bronchi terminate in 400–500 tertiary bronchi where blood gas exchange takes place. The tertiary bronchi (called parabronchi) make up the bulk of the lung tissue and can be seen by the naked eye. They lie in close proximity to tiny blood capillaries, giving the lung a highly vascular appearance. They have invaginations called atria that perform gas exchange with tiny air capillaries. The number of tertiary bronchi increase with active flight (the ground dwelling domestic fowl has only 300–500 parabronchi, whilst ducks have approximately 1800 parabronchi).

The tertiary bronchi are divided into paleopulmonic and neopulmonic bronchi. The paleopulmonic bronchi form a parallel series of hundreds of tubes and air flows in the same direction during both inspiration and expiration (Figure 2.19). The neopulmonic bronchi are irregular branched tertiary bronchi and air flow is bi-directional according to the phase of breathing. The domestic fowl has about 20–25% neopulmonic bronchi, whilst in the duck they are less developed and comprise only 10–12%.

Air sacs

The air sacs constitute 80% of the respiratory tract volume and extend from the body cavity into the wing bones, vertebrae and leg bones. They are thin (two cells thick), distensible and transparent sacs, lined with simple squamous epithelium. The air sacs function to create a uni-directional flow of air through the lungs and as they play no role in gas exchange they have little blood supply. They are connected to the secondary bronchi via an opening (ostium), usually located along the ventrolateral border of the lung. The eight air sacs of the domestic fowl comprise one single cervical and clavicular air sac and three pairs of cranial, caudal thoracic and abdominal air sacs. The turkey has seven air sacs – there are no paired caudal thoracic air

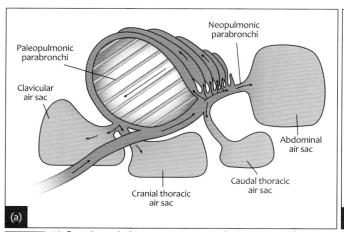

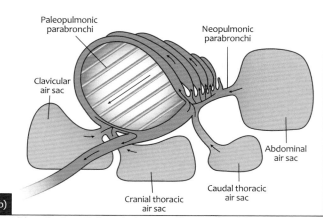

2.19 Air flow through the respiratory tract of a bird during (a) inspiration and (b) expiration. Air flows in the same direction (caudal to cranial) in both phases of respiration.

sacs but there is a combined cervical–clavicular air sac and three pairs of clavicular, cranial thoracic and abdominal air sacs. The air sacs are usually divided into two groups according to their connections to the bronchi. The cranial air sacs (cervical, clavicular and cranial thoracic) connect to the ventral bronchi and the caudal air sacs (caudal thoracic and abdominal) connect to the primary bronchus.

Ventilation

The air sacs act like a bellows to move air through the non-expansile lungs. Both inspiration and expiration require active muscle contractions, and air flow in the paleopulmonic bronchi is always in a caudal to cranial direction. This is controlled by the action of the external and internal intercostal and abdominal muscles. In contrast to mammalian

ventilation, it takes two ventilation cycles to move air completely through the avian respiratory system. The two cycles are identical – it just takes a single bolus of air two breaths before it can be exhaled.

Gastrointestinal system

To facilitate weight reduction for flight, birds have replaced heavy teeth with a crop and gizzard. Consequently, the gastrointestinal system (Figure 2.20) is adapted to process unmasticated food. Food is softened and stored in the crop (ingluvies) before being passed to the gizzard where it is mechanically ground down. Herbivorous birds (such as domestic fowl) also have large caeca to aid cellulose breakdown.

2.20 Lateral view of the domestic hen showing the gastrointestinal and urogenital tracts.

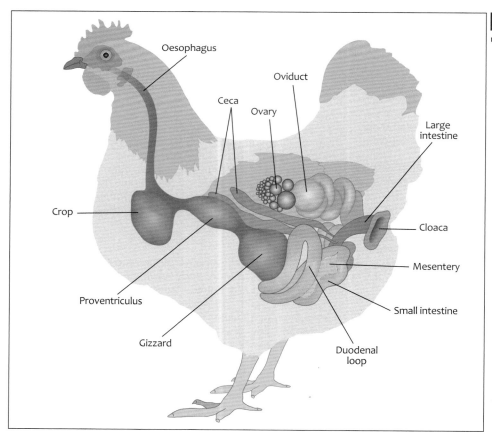

Oropharynx

Birds have no soft palate but instead have a common cavity called the oropharynx. The hard palate is incomplete and contains a median slit called the choana. This closes when food is swallowed to stop it from entering the nasal cavity. Just caudal to the choana lies the infundibular cleft. This is a midline slit-like opening which is the common opening for the auditory tubes (the avian equivalent of the Eustachian tubes).

The oropharynx is lined by stratified squamous epithelium. Keratinized papillae are visible along the roof of the oropharynx, on each side of the choana and around the tongue and larynx. Birds also have lots of salivary glands scattered throughout the oropharynx and the duct openings in the floor and roof are visible with the naked eye. The papillae play an important role in helping the food bolus to pass caudally, lubricated by copious amounts of mucoid saliva.

In Galliformes, the tongue is narrow and pointed, covered by a cornified mucous membrane with backward pointing papillae. It is supported by the hyobranchial (hyoid) apparatus and is non-protrusible. Ducks and geese have a thick, fleshy tongue with a caudal mound called the torus linguae and a shallow median groove dorsally. The rostral border is modified into a scoop with bristles on the lateral margins, which fit into lamellae on the upper and lower beak. During feeding the dorsal groove sucks in water, which is then pressed against the palate and filtered laterally by the bristles, which retain the food particles.

Oesophagus and crop

The oesophagus lies to the right side of the neck and is lined by stratified squamous epithelium with mucous glands to aid the passage of food down the tract. It is much more distensible than in mammals with a dilatation called the crop at the thoracic inlet. In domestic fowl the crop is a large pouch located to the right base of the neck, whilst in ducks and geese the crop is a barely distinguishable fusiform widening. The crop has the same epithelial structure as the oesophagus but no mucous glands and is strongly attached to the underlying skin.

Stomach

The stomach is divided into the glandular proventriculus and the muscular ventriculus (gizzard) (Figure 2.21) separated by an isthmus or intermediate zone. The proventriculus is spindle-shaped and lies to the left of the midline in the craniodorsal coelom. It is covered by the post-hepatic septum and other abdominal organs. It is the glandular portion of the stomach and has many well developed papillae from which the gastric glands open. Its main functions are the production of gastric juices and the propulsion of food into the gizzard. The stomach wall contains epithelial cells, which produce mucus, and oxynticopeptic cells, which produce pepsinogen and hydrochloric acid.

The isthmus opens into the well developed muscular ventriculus. It lies to the left of the midline just caudal to the sternum. This is where food is mechanically broken down aided by the ingestion of small stones or grit. The internal lining of the ventriculus comprises a carbohydrate–protein complex cuticle called koilin, formed by mucosal cell secretions. This protects the epithelium during the grinding process.

Food moves back and forth between the proventriculus and ventriculus by contraction of two thick and two thin

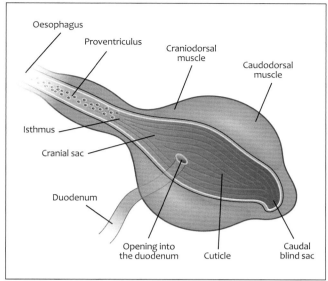

Oesophagus

Proventriculus

Craniodorsal muscle

Caudodorsal muscle

Isthmus

Cranial sac

Duodenum

Opening into the duodenum

Cuticle

Caudal blind sac

2.21 Cross-section of the ventriculus from a granivorous bird showing well developed grinding muscles.

muscular bands arranged to provided rotary and crushing movements. The two thick layers of circular smooth muscle have a high myoglobin content, so appear dark, and are attached to a central tendinous aponeurosis on the left and right. The two thin layers of muscle are paler and form blind sacs cranially and caudally. The opening of the duodenum lies very close to the proventriculus, so food that does not require grinding can bypass the ventriculus completely. The pylorus lies to the right of the ventriculus and is small in the domestic fowl.

Liver and gallbladder

The liver is large with two main lobes that surround the heart and join cranially at the midline. The right liver lobe is larger than the left, with the left liver lobe having a dorsal and ventral part in the domestic fowl and turkey. The gallbladder lies on the visceral surface of the right liver lobe.

Pancreas

The pancreas is pale pink, has three lobes and lies within the anti-mesenteric border of the duodenal loop. It has both endocrine and exocrine functions. It produces the hormones glucagon, insulin and somatostatin, as well as the digestive enzymes amylase, lipase, trypsin and chymotrypsin which help breakdown carbohydrates, fats, proteins and bicarbonate. The pancreatic ducts open into the distal part of the ascending duodenum near the cranial part of the gizzard.

Small intestine

The duodenum is separated from the body wall by the caudal thoracic and abdominal air sacs and as it lies ventrally is clearly visible on post-mortem examination. In the domestic fowl and turkey, the duodenum, jejunum and ileum (Figure 2.22) form a series of short garland-like coils on the right side of the abdominal cavity. In the goose and duck, the duodenum runs to the left and the intestinal loops are more U-shaped. The distal ileum lies dorsal to the duodenum and forms the supraduodenal loop. The boundary between the jejunum and ileum is demarcated

Species	Duodenum (cm)	Jejunum (cm)	Ileum (cm)	Caeca (cm)
Chicken	30	85–120	16	15–25
Duck	22–38	105	15	10–20
Goose	45	165	25	10–20

2.22 Approximate length of the small intestine and caeca in the chicken, duck and goose.

(Data from Koch, 1973)

by the yolk sac remnant (Meckel's diverticulum). This disappears in 50% of chickens but can persist for longer in 80–90% of ducks and geese. The intestinal epithelium has three types of cell: chief cells, which have a brush border to absorb food; goblet cells, which secrete mucus; and endocrine cells, which produce the hormones somatostatin, gastrin and secretin.

Large intestine

The large intestine comprises a short colorectum and well developed caeca. The colorectum is no thicker than the small intestine and resorbs water and electrolytes by anti-peristaltic movements.

Caeca

The caeca are long, paired and dark green and arise from the ileocolic junction. Their main function is to aid the bacterial breakdown of cellulose. The caeca pass cranially at first and then run retrograde with the blind ends lying near the cloaca. The proximal segments have a heavy muscular coat and contain lymphoid tissue (caecal tonsil). The middle parts are thin walled whilst the blind ends are bulbous and have thicker walls.

Food passes down the intestines to the coprodeum (proximal part of the cloaca) but occasionally an unknown mechanism returns the ingesta by retroperistalsis back to the caeca. In the caeca, the long villi absorb any nutrient-rich food and discard the indigestible fraction. A powerful caecal contraction then passes this waste back to the cloaca where it is voided as semi-solid, chocolate brown droppings about once a day.

Cloaca

The cloaca is the common orifice where the digestive and urogenital systems terminate (Figure 2.23). It is a bell-shaped dilatation at the end of the rectum. It lies in the midline in mature male birds, but in mature female birds the enlarged left oviduct pushes it to the right of the midline. The cloaca is divided into three parts:

- The coprodeum is the largest chamber, is lined by villi, and is separated from the urodeum by the coprourodeal fold which prevents faecal contamination during egg laying
- The urodeum or middle component is where the ureters and genital tracts empty into the dorsal and lateral wall, respectively
- The proctodeum ends in the external opening or vent which is controlled by the external anal sphincter. It is a short compartment separated from the urodeum by the uroproctodeal fold. The bursa of Fabricius is located in the dorsal wall.

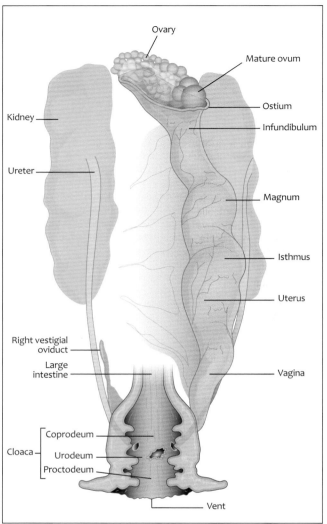

2.23 Cloaca and urogenital tract in a female bird showing the left oviduct and kidneys.

Urinary system

The urinary system consists only of the kidneys and ureters; in keeping with weight reduction, birds have no bladder or urethra. The ureters terminate in the urodeum of the cloaca.

Kidneys

The kidneys are relatively large in the domestic fowl (typically around 7 cm x 2 cm) and extend from the caudal synsacrum cranially as far as the lungs. They lie retroperitoneally and are well protected in the ventral (renal) fossa of the synsacrum. They are roughly divided into cranial, middle and caudal parts by the external iliac and ischiadic branches of the abdominal aorta. The lumbar and sacral plexus nerves also pass through the kidney in this region.

The kidney lacks a distinct cortex and medulla and there is no renal pelvis. The ureter runs along the ventral side of the kidney and branches into collecting ducts, which each drain a lobule. Each lobule can be seen as a small rounded projection (about 1–2 mm in size) and consists of a large area of cortical tissue and a small cone of medullary tissue. The cortical tissue contains both cortical and medullary nephrons, while the medullary cone only contains the loops of Henle, collecting ducts and the capillary network. Cortical nephrons (90%) are like the more primitive reptilian nephron and have no loop of Henle. Medullary nephrons resemble those seen in mammals and play a major role in concentrating urine. Medullary nephrons are located in the cortical region but have their loop of Henle in the medullary region.

Blood supply

The kidney has a dual afferent blood supply – one-third is supplied by the high pressure renal arteries and two-thirds is supplied by the low pressure renal portal veins. The cranial, middle and caudal renal arteries divide into the glomerular arteries, which provide the glomerular filtrate. This is controlled by the state of hydration and the secretion of arginine vasotocin from the posterior pituitary gland. The renal portal vein clears urates from the blood and excretes them via the proximal tubules.

Excretion

Avian urine is semi-solid and viscous and can be separated into a white precipitate (urates) and supernatant fluid (urine). Birds excrete 60% of their nitrogenous waste in the form of chalky white urates. Although the excretion of urates requires far less water than the excretion of other nitrogenous waste, the main benefit of this is for the egg. The developing embryo is able to produce an insoluble (and non-toxic) waste product, leaving the water fraction free to be resorbed. Urine is produced by the glomerular filtrate and 90% is resorbed by the tubules. The major control of urine output is tubular resorption, as in mammals, but avian urine is less concentrated. Uric acid is synthesized in the liver and excreted via the kidney by glomerular filtration (10%) and tubular secretion (90%). In addition, it should be noted that as urates are secreted only by the more primitive cortical nephrons, they are produced independently of urine flow, and so will be seen even in very dehydrated birds.

Reproductive system

The seasonal reproductive cycle of birds is controlled by the hypothalamus, which in spring responds to increasing day length or photoperiod. This stimulates the release of gonadotropin-releasing hormone (GnRH) via the bloodstream to the pituitary gland. The anterior pituitary gland then releases follicle-stimulating hormone (FSH) and luteinizing hormone (LH), which trigger gonadogenesis, ovulation and breeding. After the breeding season, the shortening day length in late summer causes gonad regression and allows time for moulting.

Domestication and selective breeding in poultry has produced birds that have a prolonged reproductive period. Domestic fowl were bred from the red junglefowl, a species that lays eggs indeterminately and can quickly lay more if eggs are lost from the clutch. This characteristic means that they can lay eggs almost daily for 280 days over 50 weeks, followed by a period of moult. The domestic hen reaches sexual maturity at about 16–22 weeks of age and reaches peak egg production about 6–10 weeks after the onset of laying. Eggs are not laid at the same time each day as the ovulation–oviposition cycle of the chicken is approximately 25 hours (range: 24–28 hours). Turkeys and pheasants follow a similar pattern whilst ducks and guinea fowl lay every 24 hours.

Female reproductive tract

The female embryo has two ovaries and oviducts, but only the left one develops, leaving the right ovary and oviduct to regress. However, a persistent right oviduct (visible as a strand of tissue along the ventral side of the caudal vena cava) is a common finding in chickens.

Ovary

The ovary lies caudal to the adrenal gland and near to the cranial tip of the kidney (see Figure 2.23). It is suspended by the mesovarium and consists of a vascular medulla, with nerve fibres and smooth muscle, and a peripheral cortex. It receives its blood supply from a short branch of the left cranial renal artery.

Oviduct

The large oviduct extends from the ovary to the cloaca. In the domestic hen it is approximately 65 cm in length and weighs 75 g, regressing to 15 cm and a weight of 5 g when the bird is not in lay. The oviduct is a massive coiled tube occupying the left dorsocaudal side of the coelomic cavity. It is suspended from the roof of the coelomic cavity by a double-layered sheet of peritoneum, forming a dorsal and ventral ligament that is richly supplied with anastomosing oviductal arteries and veins. The wall of the oviduct consists of a ciliated epithelial lining, glands and smooth muscle. Smooth muscle in the caudal ventral ligament may contribute to egg peristalsis.

The oviduct is divided into five parts:

- Infundibulum (7 cm in length)
- Magnum (30 cm in length) – this is the longest and coiled part of the oviduct and the numerous tubular glands give it a thickened appearance
- Isthmus (8 cm in length) – the folds of the isthmus are less prominent than those of the magnum
- Uterus or shell gland (8 cm in length) – the smooth muscles are thickest in the uterus and vagina
- Vagina (approximately 8 cm in length) – the vagina is separated from the uterus by a vaginal sphincter and has a powerful smooth muscle wall.

Ovulation

FSH stimulates the follicles in the ovary to develop and produce oestrogen from the theca and interstitial cells, as well as progesterone from the granulosa cells. Increasing levels of oestrogen stimulates an LH surge and ovulation. Progesterone continues to be secreted to inhibit further ovulation and stimulate behavioural changes associated with broodiness and incubation. In domestic fowl ovulation usually occurs 30 minutes after an egg has been laid. The left ovary of an actively laying hen resembles a 'bunch of grapes', with thousands of macroscopic and microscopic follicles. These consist of numerous slow-growing follicles and 5–7 rapidly-growing yolk-filled follicles that are arrange hierarchically according to size. Each follicle is suspended by a stalk containing smooth muscle, which has a rich vascular and nerve supply. Protein and lipid synthesized in the liver travel via the ovary to the oocyte (vitellogenesis), where they are made into yolk. Under the influence of LH, the largest follicle (F1) splits to release the primary oocyte. The infundibulum catches the oocyte, facilitated by the abdominal air sac that tightly encloses the ovary. However, if the sequence gets out of sync, oocytes can be lost into the body cavity where they are eventually absorbed (see

Chapter 17 for information on yolk coelomitis). Once ovulation has taken place, the empty follicle (calyx) shrinks and regresses. No corpus luteum remains as there is no developing embryo to maintain.

Fertilization

The funnel of the infundibulum catches the oocyte as it is released from the ovary. As fertilization of the oocyte must take place within 15 minutes of ovulation, it occurs within the funnel of the infundibulum. Sperm, which are deposited in the cloaca, are moved up the oviduct via the action of the cilia and retroperistalsis to the infundibulum.

Egg formation

Fertilization is not a prerequisite for egg formation and development in the bird. Within 15 minutes following release from the ovary, the egg has travelled from the funnel to the tubular or chalaziferous region of the infundibulum, where it is covered by a thin layer of albumen. Passage through the infundibulum takes approximately 15–30 minutes. The egg then moves into the magnum. The glands in this region of the oviduct produce 50% of the albumen, which gives the lumen a milky white colour. As it travels through the magnum, which takes approximately 3 hours, the egg also acquires sodium, calcium and magnesium. The egg then passes into the isthmus. The tubular glands in this region of the oviduct produce the inner and outer shell membranes. A small amount of albumen is also produced in this region. Movement through the isthmus takes about 75 minutes. The egg then passes into the uterus, where it stays for 20 hours. In the uterus the albumen doubles in volume, water is absorbed (plumping effect) and the shell is formed. During the last 15 hours, the highly vascularized uterus rapidly sequesters calcium from the blood, which is used to calcify the eggshell.

Polyostotic hyperostosis: About 10 days prior to laying an egg, the female bird lays down calcium deposits in the medullary cavity of the large bones by increasing absorption from the alimentary tract. The total bone density of the bird increases by around 20% as bony trabeculae are laid down from the endosteum. This is visible radiographically. Parathyroid hormone then mobilizes this calcium depot into ionized calcium, which is used to calcify the eggshell.

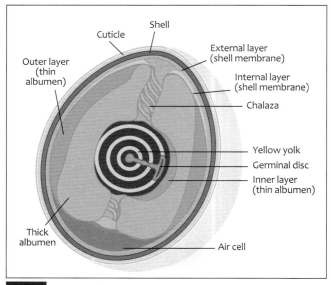

Outer layer
(thin albumen)

Cuticle

Shell

External layer
(shell membrane)

Internal layer
(shell membrane)

Chalaza

Yellow yolk

Germinal disc

Inner layer
(thin albumen)

Thick albumen

Air cell

2.24 The internal structure of the egg.

Egg structure

The egg consists of a germinal disc, yolk, yolk membrane, albumen and shell (Figure 2.24). If the germinal disc is fertilized it is called a blastoderm; if it remains unfertilized it is called a blastodisc. The main source of nutrition for the embryo is the thick, viscous yolk and in the final stages of development it is directly connected to the intestine of the embryo. White yolk comprises mainly protein with some fat, whilst yellow yolk comprises mainly fat with some protein. The yolk membrane forms a barrier between the yolk and the albumen, but is permeable to water and salts.

The albumen is less viscous than the yolk and comprises mainly protein. The albumen is a source of water, which prevents the embryo from drying out and acts like a shock absorber. A thin layer of albumen encloses the yolk membranes and suspends the yolk in the centre of the egg via twisted strands called chalaza. The shell consists of two shell membranes: the testa and the cuticle. The cuticle is the smooth outer layer which is water repellent and acts as a barrier to infection. The testa is the thick, calcified layer which provides the developing embryo with calcium. The testa consists of a matrix of fibres, protein and calcium carbonate. Small flaws between the calcium carbonate crystals form pores which allow the egg to breathe.

Oviposition

During oviposition or egg laying, the uterus contracts whilst the abdominal muscles relax. The egg passes out of the oviduct into the urodeum and is expelled from the vent. The vaginal opening protrudes through the vent in order to minimize contact of the egg with faeces. Passage through the vagina takes only seconds. The rate of oviposition is linked to the rate of ovulation and takes 1–2 hours in the domestic fowl, goose and turkey. It is controlled by prostaglandins, arginine vasotocin and oxytocin, as well as nesting behaviour. For example, hens with access to suitable nesting sites take 1–2 hours to lay their eggs, but in battery hens deprived of suitable sites, nesting behaviour is reduced to just stereotypical pacing for approximately an hour prior to laying.

Male reproductive tract
Testicle, epididymis and vas deferens

The bean-shaped testes are paired and lie near the cranial poles of the kidneys, just caudal to the adrenal glands. Each testis is suspended by a short mesorchium and is surrounded medially by the abdominal air sac. The left testis tends to be larger than the right in immature birds. The resting testes are usually yellow to brown due to lipid accumulation in the interstitial cells. Some breeds such as the Silkie have black testes due to the presence of melanocytes. During the breeding season and under the influence of FSH and LH, the testes of domestic fowl become white and dramatically enlarge to 5 cm in length. Outside of the breeding season, the testes atrophy and shrink to half that size.

The testes consist of seminiferous tubules, which produce sperm, and interstitial cells, which produce androgens, testosterone and androstenedione under the influence of LH. These hormones stimulate the development of secondary sex characteristics including feather coloration, appendages such as the comb and wattles, and courtship behaviours. The epididymis is smaller and less developed than that seen in mammals as sperm maturation occurs in the vas deferens. The tunica albuginea is thin and there is no pampiniform plexus. As birds have no accessory sexual glands, the volume of semen produced is low (e.g. cockerels have an ejaculate of 0.5–1 ml); lymph may contribute to the seminal fluid. In domestic fowl, the epididymis has an appendix which attaches via connective tissue to the ventral part of the adrenal gland (especially on the right side). This is why surgical castration is not always permanent as castrated males can sprout nodules in this area that secrete androgens.

Phallus

Domestic fowl and turkeys have a rudimentary non-protrusible phallus that lies on the ventral lip of the vent. It consists of a small medial tubercle intimately associated on each side with lymphatic folds and vessels. When erect with lymph, the phallus develops a median groove that permits passage of the ejaculate into the everted female oviduct. Anseriformes have a protrusible curved fibrous phallus that conveys semen via a spiral groove. When engorged with lymphatic fluid the phallus erects to a length of 5 cm and is capable of true intromission into the female cloaca. Sperm deposited into the female cloaca can be held in the sperm host glands (spermatic fossulae) at the uterovaginal junction. Sperm can survive for at least 5–11 days in chickens and ducks and 4–6 weeks in turkeys.

Immune system

Birds have both primary and secondary lymphoid organs. The primary organs are the cloacal bursa and thymus. The secondary organs are the spleen, intestinal lymphoid tissue and bone marrow. T lymphocytes develop in the thymus, which reaches a maximum size between 4–17 weeks of age and then begins to involute. The cloacal bursa (bursa of Fabricius) is a dorsal diverticulum in the proctodeum that contains folds of lymphoid tissue and produces B lymphocytes. In Galliformes it is pear-shaped with a thick wall and central cavity, whilst in Anseriformes it is spindle-shaped. In the domestic fowl it reaches a maximum size of 4 g before sexual maturity and begins to involute at about 2–3 months, reducing in size to approximately 0.5 g. Involution is slower in geese, which do not reach sexual maturity until 2 years of age.

Lymphatic vessels are less numerous in birds than in mammals and usually closely follow the blood vessels. Birds do not have lymph nodes but instead have lymphoid nodules scattered throughout the digestive tract, particularly in the oropharynx, caeca and small intestine (Peyer's patches). Ducks and geese have two primitive pairs of spindle-shaped lymph nodes (1–3 cm long): a cervico-thoracic pair near the thyroid gland and a lumbar pair near the kidneys. The spleen lies to the right of the coelom between the proventriculus and the ventriculus. It does not form a significant blood reservoir so is relatively small. It can vary in shape from oval (2 cm diameter) in domestic fowl to triangular in ducks and geese.

Nervous system

The avian brain is smaller than that of mammals and has a poorly developed cerebral cortex. There is a well developed cerebellum for locomotion and large optic lobes for vision. There are 12 pairs of cranial nerves. The brain and spinal cord have three meninges: the dura, arachnoid and pia mater. The spinal cord is the same length as the spinal canal and there is no cauda equina. The spinal cord becomes enlarged at the brachial and lumbar–sacral plexi. Flying birds have a more prominent brachial plexus whilst running birds have a large lumbar plexus.

Sensory organs

Eyes

Birds have excellent vision due to large eyes, well developed optic nerves and large optic lobes in the brain. Most poultry have laterally placed eyes but also have about a 15-degree binocular field of vision. Birds are tetra-chromatic and so have excellent colour vision (i.e. they can see not only the three primary colours red, green and blue, but also the ultraviolet spectrum). There is complete decussation of the optic nerve fibres at the optic chiasma, which means that each eye moves independently and there is no consensual light reflex.

The anterior portion of the eyeball is small and unprotected and covered by the cornea, whilst the posterior part is well protected by a ring of 14–15 scleral ossicles (Figure 2.25). Scleral ossicles are a ring of overlapping bones, which provide strength to the eye and an attachment for the ciliary muscles. The extraocular muscles are less well developed in birds compared with mammals and this is compensated by the ability of birds to rotate their long, flexible necks via the single occipital neck joint. The pupil is round and as the iris contains striated muscle, it cannot be dilated with normal mydriatics. The lens is softer than that seen in mammals.

The retina lacks blood vessels and a tapetum lucidum to prevent shadows and scattering of light and improve visual acuity. The pecten is unique to birds and is believed to supply nutrients to the retina, aid in acid–base balance and facilitate fluid movement within the eye. It is a black, vascular comb-like structure extending from the optic disc into the vitreous body towards the lens. The fundus is usually

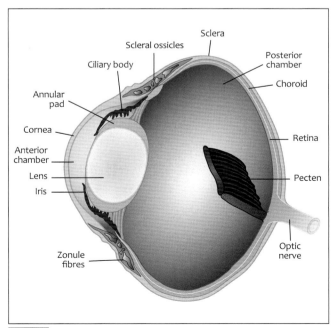

2.25 Cross-section of the avian eye.

grey or reddish. The optic disc is elongated and oval but is mainly obscured by the pecten. The excellent colour vision in domestic fowl is due to the retina having up to 80% cone cells. Being ground dwelling birds they have no actual fovea, but instead have a central area of densely packed cone cells in the retina for greater visual acuity.

Ears

Birds have a short external ear canal but lack a pinna. The ear opening is about 4–5 mm in the domestic fowl and hidden by feathers called ear coverts. The middle ear is the air-filled cavity between the tympanic membrane and inner ear. There is only one bony ossicle called the columella (equivalent of the mammalian stapes), which transmits sound vibrations from the tympanum to the vestibular window of the inner ear. The middle ear is connected to the oropharynx by short, open auditory tubes (see above). The inner ear contains the cochlea, as well as three semicircular canals, the utricle and saccule, which are required for balance.

Olfactory system

Birds do have a sense of smell, although it may not be as highly developed as their vision and hearing. The olfactory system comprises the external nares and the caudal conchae, which are lined with olfactory epithelium and connected to the olfactory bulbs of the brain.

Taste buds

The taste buds lie at the base of the tongue and in the roof and floor of the oropharynx in glandular, non-cornified epithelium. The total number of taste buds in birds is far less than in mammals with domestic fowl having 300 taste buds and mallard ducks having 500, in contrast to the 9000 seen in humans and 17,000 that are present in rabbits.

Organs of touch

Birds have widely distributed mechanoreceptors called Herbst corpuscles located deep in the dermis. These are found on the beak, legs and associated with feather follicles. In the plumage these corpuscles are used to ruffle feathers and help stimulate preening. Waterfowl such as ducks and geese have a beak tip organ, which comprises very sensitive touch receptors. This is located along the edge and tip of the upper beak and helps the bird to search for food underwater.

References and further reading

Akester AR (1984) The cardiovascular system. In: *Physiology and Biochemistry of the Domestic Fowl, Volume 5*, ed. BM Freeman, pp. 172–257. Academic Press, London

Brackenbury JH (1987) Ventilation of the lung–air sac system. In: *Bird Respiration, Volume 1*, ed. TJ Sellar, pp. 39–71. CRC press, Boca Raton

Denbow DM (2000) Gastrointestinal anatomy and physiology. In: *Sturkie's Avian Physiology, 5th edn*, ed. GC Whittow, pp. 299–321. Academic Press, San Diego

Duke GE (1993) Avian digestion. In: *Dukes' Physiology of Domestic Animals, 11th edn, Part iii*, ed. MJ Swenson and WO Reece, pp. 428–437. Cornell University Press, Ithaca

Duncker HR (1979) Coelomic cavities. In: *Form and Function in Birds, Volume 1*, ed. AS King and J McLelland, pp. 39–69. Academic Press, London

Dyce KM, Sack WO and Wensing CJ (2002) Avian anatomy. In: *Textbook of Veterinary Anatomy, 3rd edn*, ed. KM Dyce *et al.*, pp. 799–825. WB Saunders, Philadelphia

Fedde MR (1993) Respiration in birds. In: *Dukes' Physiology of Domestic Animals, 11th edn, Part ii*, ed. MJ Swenson and WO Reece, pp. 294–303. Cornell University Press, Ithaca

Fowler ME (1986) *Zoo and Wildlife Medicine, 2nd edn*. WB Saunders, Philadelphia

Gaunt AS (1987) Phonation. In: *Bird Respiration, Volume 1*, ed. TJ Sellar, pp. 71–97. CRC press, Boca Raton

Gilbert AG (1979) Female genital organs. In: *Form and Function in Birds, Volume 1*, ed. AS King and J McLelland, pp. 237–361. Academic Press, London

Goldstein DL and Skadhauge E (2000) Renal and extrarenal regulation of body fluid composition. In: *Sturkie's Avian Physiology, 5th edn*, ed. GC Whittow, pp. 265–291. Academic Press, San Diego

Gunturkun O (2000) Sensory physiology: vision. In: *Sturkie's Avian Physiology, 5th edn*, ed. GC Whittow, pp. 1–14. Academic Press, San Diego

Hill KJ (1971) The structure of the alimentary tract. In: *Physiology and Biochemistry of the Domestic Fowl, Volume 1*, ed. DJ Bell and BM Freeman, pp. 1–22. Academic Press, London

Hill KJ (1971) The physiology of digestion. In: *Physiology and Biochemistry of the Domestic Fowl, Volume 1*, ed. DJ Bell and BM Freeman, pp. 25–47. Academic Press, London

Hinds DS and Calder WA (1971) Tracheal dead space in the respiration of birds. *Evolution* **25**, 429–440

Hoefer HL, Orosz S and Dorrestein GM (1997) The gastrointestinal tract. In: *Avian Medicine and Surgery*, ed. RB Altman *et al.*, pp. 412–419. WB Saunders, Philadelphia

Hogg DA (1982) Fusions occurring in the post cranial skeleton of the domestic fowl. *Journal of Anatomy* **135(3)**, 501–612

Johnson AL (2000) Reproduction in the female. In: *Sturkie's Avian Physiology, 5th edn*, ed. GC Whittow, pp. 569–596. Academic Press, San Diego

Johnson OW (1979) Urinary organs. In: *Form and Function in Birds, Volume 1*, ed. AS King and J McLelland, pp. 183–237. Academic Press, London

Jukes MG (1983) Control of respiration. In: *Physiology and Biochemistry of the Domestic Fowl, Volume 4*, ed. DJ Bell and BM Freeman, pp. 172–185. Academic Press, London

King AS (1981) Cloaca. In: *Form and Function in Birds, Volume 2*, ed. AS King and J McLelland, pp. 63–107. Academic Press, London

King AS (1981) Phallus. In: *Form and Function in Birds, Volume 2*, ed. AS King and J McLelland, pp. 107–149. Academic Press, London

King AS and McLelland J (1984) *Birds: Their Structure and Function, 2nd edn*. Bailliere Tindall, London

King AS and Molony V (1971) The anatomy of respiration. In: *Physiology and Biochemistry of the Domestic Fowl, Volume 1*, ed. DJ Bell and BM Freeman, pp. 93–169. Academic Press, London

King-Smith PE (1971) Special senses. In: *Physiology and Biochemistry of the Domestic Fowl, Volume 1*, ed. DJ Bell and BM Freeman, pp. 1039–1080. Academic Press, London

Klasing KC (1998) *Comparative Avian Nutrition*. CABI, Oxon

Koch T (1973) Locomotion system. In: *Anatomy of the Chicken and Domestic Birds*, ed. BH Skold and L Devries, pp. 6–65. Iowa State University Press, Iowa

Lake PE (1981) Male genital organs. In: *Form and Function in Birds, Volume 2*, ed. AS King and J McLelland, pp. 1–63. Academic Press, London

Lasiewski RC (1972) Respiratory function of birds. *Avian Biology, Volume II*, ed. DS Farner and JR King, pp. 288–335. Academic Press, New York

Maina JN (1989) The morphometry of the avian lung. In: *Form and Function in Birds, Volume 4*, ed. AS King and J McLelland, pp. 307–368. Academic Press, London

Martin GR (1985) Eye. In: *Form and Function in Birds, Volume 3*, ed. AS King and J McLelland, pp. 311–375. Academic Press, London

Mason JR and Clark L (2000) The chemical senses in birds. In: *Sturkie's Avian Physiology, 5th edn*, ed. GC Whittow, pp. 39–51. Academic Press, San Diego

McLelland J (1979) Digestive system. In: *Form and Function in Birds, Volume 1*, ed. AS King and J McLelland, pp. 69–181. Academic Press, London

McLelland J (1990) *A Colour Atlas of Avian Anatomy*. Wolfe Publishing, Aylesbury

McLelland J and Molony V (1983) Respiration. In: *Physiology and Biochemistry of the Domestic Fowl, Volume 4*, ed. BM Freeman, pp. 63–85. Academic Press, London

Orosz S, Dorrestein GM and Speer BL (1997) Urogenital disorders. In: *Avian Medicine and Surgery*, ed. RB Altman *et al.*, pp. 614–644. WB Saunders, Philadelphia

Payne LN (1984) The lymphoid system. In: *Physiology and Biochemistry of the Domestic Fowl, Volume 5*, ed. BM Freeman, pp. 985–1031. Academic Press, London

Powell FL (2000) Respiration. In: *Sturkie's Avian Physiology, 5th edn*, ed. GC Whittow, pp. 233–259. Academic Press, San Diego

Quesenberry K, Orosz S and Dorrestein GM (1997) Musculoskeletal system. In: *Avian Medicine and Surgery*, ed. RB Altman *et al.*, pp. 517–523. WB Saunders, Philadelphia

Raikow RJ (1985) Locomotor system. In: *Form and Function in Birds, Volume 3*, ed. AS King and J McLelland, pp. 57–149. Academic Press, London

Roberts V and Scott Park F (2008) *BSAVA Manual of Farm Pets*. BSAVA Publications, Gloucester

Rose ME (1981) Lymphatic system. In: *Form and Function in Birds, Volume 2*, ed. AS King and J McLelland, pp. 341–385. Academic Press, London

Scheid P and Piiper J (1971) Direct measurement of the pathway of respired gas in duck lungs. *Respiration Physiology* **11**, 308–314

Scheid P and Piiper J (1972) Cross current gas exchange in avian lungs: Effect of Reversed Parabronchial Air Flow in Ducks. *Respiration Physiology* **16**, 304–312

Scheid P and Piiper J (1987) Gas exchange and transport. In: *Bird Respiration, Volume 1*, ed. TJ Sellar, pp. 97–131. CRC Press, Boca Raton

Schmidt-Nielsen K (1975) Recent advances in avian respiration. *Symposium of the Zoological Society of London*, ed. M Peaker, pp. 33–47. Academic Press, London

Shoemaker VH (1972) Osmoregulation and excretion in birds. *Avian Biology, Volume II*, ed. DS Farner and JR King, pp. 527–551. Academic Press, New York

Siller WG (1983) Structure of the kidney. In: *Physiology and Biochemistry of the Domestic Fowl, Volume 4*, ed. BM Freeman, pp. 91–104. Academic Press, London

Smith FM, West NH and Jones DR (2000) The cardiovascular system. In: *Sturkie's Avian Physiology, 5th edn*, ed. GC Whittow, pp. 141–223. Academic Press, San Diego

Spearman RI (1983) Integumentary system. In: *Physiology and Biochemistry of the Domestic Fowl, Volume 4*, ed. BM Freeman, pp. 211–217. Academic Press, London

Spearman RI and Hardy JA (1985) Integument. In: *Form and Function in Birds, Volume 3*, ed. AS King and J McLelland, pp. 1–57. Academic Press, London

Sykes AH (1971) Formation and composition of urine. In: *Physiology and Biochemistry of the Domestic Fowl, Volume 1*, ed. DJ Bell and BM Freeman, pp. 233–276. Academic Press, London

Taylor TG, Simkiss K and Stringer DA (1971) The skeleton: its structure and metabolism. In: *Physiology and Biochemistry of the Domestic Fowl, Volume 1*, ed. DJ Bell and BM Freeman, pp. 621–639. Academic Press, London

West NH, Lowell Langille B and Jones DR (1979) Cardiovascular system. In: *Form and Function in Birds, Volume 1*, ed. AS King and J McLelland, pp. 235–341. Academic Press, London

Whittow GC (2000) *Sturkie's Avian Physiology, 5th edn*. Academic Press, San Diego

Chapter 3

Behaviour

John Chitty

This chapter mainly discusses the behaviour of the chicken. Other gallinaceous birds and waterfowl are also mentioned where their natural behaviour varies significantly from that of the chicken. The domestic chicken is believed to originate from the red junglefowl (see Chapter 1) and whilst domestication has resulted in a number of physical changes (e.g. altered body shape, increased egg laying and reduced seasonality of laying), fundamental behaviour patterns have basically remained the same. The behavioural problems associated with farmed poultry are well documented, and may also be seen in backyard birds. Behavioural problems tend to stem from keeping methods that do not allow the expression of natural behaviours (see Chapter 19). The prevention of behavioural problems, therefore, requires knowledge of the natural behaviour of birds.

Ontogeny

Chicks are precocial and nidifugous (leave the nest shortly after hatching). Senses are well developed shortly after hatching and there is a rapid imprinting process of the hen and siblings (a synchronous hatch is achieved by means of an initial 'setting' period until all eggs are laid and 'calling out' where in-egg vocalizations of the 'oldest' chick stimulates pipping in the other eggs).

Even though the chicks are able to obtain food for themselves from 2–3 days following hatching (initially nutrition is derived from the internalized yolk sac), these young birds are still dependent on the hen for protection from predators (including other members of the flock), to learn what are appropriate food sources, and for warmth. The hen and clutch will generally separate from the main flock until the chicks are 4–6 weeks old, at which time they are, essentially, independent and adult plumage along with secondary sexual characteristics start to develop. Once mature, females tend to join the flock or move off, depending on the food supply, whilst juvenile males are normally driven away and dispersed by the dominant male.

Senses

Poultry have well developed visual and auditory senses.

- The eyes are positioned on the side of the head and provide an approximately 300-degree field of vision.

Chickens have excellent colour vision and a flicker fusion threshold of >100 Hz. The flicker fusion threshold (or flicker fusion rate) is a concept in the psychophysics of vision. It is defined as the frequency at which an intermittent light stimulus appears to be completely steady to the average observer.
- Chickens have acute hearing and communicate using a range of different sounds (see below).

The beak is extremely sensitive and has a large number of nerve endings in the tip. Chickens have an adequate to good sense of taste. Learning which foods are appropriate is based on visual cues (e.g. size of the food particles) and taste, as well as learned from the hen.

Signalling

Visual

Visual cues are extremely important. Secondary sexual characteristics, such as plumage colour and comb/wattle size, are the most obvious examples of visual cues. Comb size and colour in both males and females are good indicators of health, sex hormone levels and social status.

Vocal

Chickens are a social species and use a wide range of auditory signals (Mench and Keeling, 2001), including:

- Territorial calls
- Warning and predator alarm calls
- Contact calls
- Laying and nesting calls
- Mating calls
- Threat calls
- Submissive calls
- Distress, alarm or fear calls
- Contentment calls
- Food calls.

Some vocalizations appear to have more than one purpose. For example, cockerels may crow in the morning as a territorial call, but will also crow to aggregate the female harem, as an alarm call and as a mating call. Other vocalizations are only evident after sexual maturity (e.g. the soft clucking sounds made by the hen to her chicks).

More solitary gallinaceous birds (e.g. turkeys, peafowl and some pheasants) are less vocal, with the exception of mating and warning calls. Ducks and geese also perform aggregating calls (quacks and honks, respectively) in addition to warning calls (Figure 3.1).

Social structure

Chickens are strongly territorial. The cockerel will form a territory, which it defends from other males using a combination of crowing vocalizations (territorial calls), visual displays and fighting (using its well developed spurs). Within its territory, a cockerel will gather a harem of females (Figure 3.2). These hens tend to stay within the territory, although they can 'drift off' into other territories or be taken over by a new dominant male.

There is a well developed pecking order amongst hens which forms soon after sexual maturity. Interactions between females can be very aggressive, with severe pecks to the head occurring on occasion. Submissive birds will tend to crouch to avert further attack. The presence of a dominant male reduces the severity of these interactions and assists in maintaining a stable pecking order. Once formed the pecking order is quite stable,

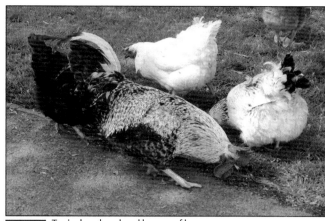

3.2 Typical cockerel and harem of hens. (© J Chitty)

unless there are changes in flock members (e.g. new birds joining an existing flock). Comb/wattle size and colour are good indicators of social position. Hens will leave the flock to brood and rear young. They may feed on the flock periphery once the chicks have hatched, but the hens will not reintegrate with the flock until the chicks are 4–6 weeks old.

Species	Visual signals	Vocalizations	Social structure	Territory	Aggression	Best model for keeping
Turkeys	Males have a gaudy plumage with an elaborate tail display. They also have red wattles in the breeding season (see Figure 3.3)	Males 'gobble' at females in breeding condition	Outside breeding season they exist in single-sex groups. Turkeys become solitary in breeding season as males form territories then seek females. Females nest and rear young on their own, forming a family group in the summer	Only in the breeding season	Male–male aggression in breeding season. Mainly visual display but will fight using spurs	Single male and harem of females
Pheasants	Males have a gaudy plumage and display	Relatively quiet as befits more solitary life. Piercing warning calls	Solitary other than in the breeding season, where males form a territory and gather a female harem. Females nest on their own within territory	Only in the breeding season	As turkeys	Generally kept as a pair year-round, although males may be kept solitary and females introduced in breeding season
Peafowl	Males have a gaudy plumage with an elaborate tail display	Quiet, other than in the breeding season when males utter persistent 'screams'	Solitary	Males are territorial	As turkeys	Single male and harem of 2–3 females
Ducks	Males have a gaudy plumage. Displays vary	Quacking as an aggregating call or hen–chick imprinting call. Warning calls	Generally, a large group with males forming territories in the breeding season. They may either split into pairs or females may disperse on their own to nest	Only in the breeding season	Biting/pecking	Single male and harem of females
Geese	Males display	Softer honks as aggregating calls. Loud honk or hissing as aggression calls	Males form territories and gather harem of females	Only in the breeding season	Biting/pecking and wing beating	Single male and harem of females (see Figure 3.4)

3.1 Natural behaviour of other gallinaceous birds and waterfowl where it differs from that of chickens.

Reproduction

The wild red junglefowl is a seasonal breeder, although seasonality varies according to location and does not always appear related to the number of daylight hours (i.e. light cycle). With domestication, the chicken appears to have become more strongly seasonal, particularly with respect to the light cycle. However, this seasonality is considerably reduced in the commercial laying breeds, which can lay year-round (albeit with some reduction in the winter months).

Cockerels

Cockerels perform both vocal and visual courtship displays – they crow and spread their wing and tail feathers. They also tend to posture by stretching the neck upwards. The turkey stag (Figure 3.3) and peacock have very elaborate visual as well as vocal displays ('gobbling' in the former and 'screaming' in the latter), as they lead relatively solitary lives and only call females into their territories during the breeding season. After the initial mating period, turkey stags become less territorial and actively seek unmated females or those that have lost their first clutch of eggs. In waterfowl, displays are primarily visual and focus on the gaudy male plumage. Some of the courtship displays can be quite elaborate.

Hens

Hens will perform a submission crouch, allowing the male to mate. In commercial flocks, where the hens tend to be more overcrowded, there is some evidence that high-ranking females are less inclined to crouch, meaning that low-ranking hens are mated more often. This situation is counter-intuitive and the reverse of the natural situation: splitting off high-ranking hens into a sub-flock or reducing stocking density will help (Guhl, 1950).

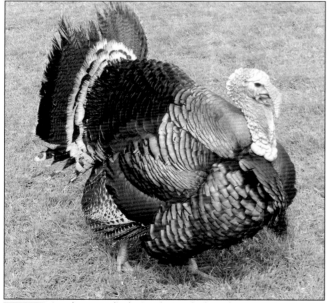

3.3 A turkey stag displaying during the breeding season.
(© J Chitty)

Chicks

As described above, chicks will imprint on the hen (and siblings) soon after hatching. This is stimulated and maintained by visual and vocal cues. Continued auditory cues (e.g. the soft 'pocking' sound) maintain this hen–chick link.

Feeding

Gallinaceous birds are primarily granivorous, but will eat almost any plant material and insects (and even meat or bones if chanced upon) (Figure 3.4). Some birds are very specialized feeders (e.g. Capercaillie), although few of these are maintained in captivity.

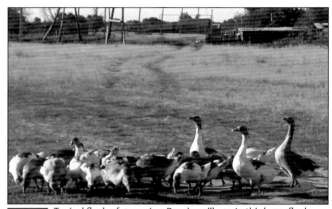

3.4 Typical flock of geese in a Russian village. In this large flock there may be several ganders: one is the dominant male and the others are juveniles and/or subordinates. These are the larger birds 'keeping watch' whilst the females graze.
(© J Chitty)

Grooming

Poultry and waterfowl perform elaborate grooming procedures. Poultry will also dust bathe wherever possible and will often purposefully create a scrape for dustbathing.

Roosting

Poultry tend to roost in trees. Other gallinaceous birds may roost on branches or under bushes, depending on their natural habitat and size/build. Geese and swans tend to roost in the open on flat ground. Depending on the species, ducks may roost in or by water, under bushes or in trees.

References and further reading

Guhl AM (1950) Social dominance and receptivity in the domestic fowl. *Physiological Zoology* **23**, 361–366

McGowan PJK (1994) Phasianidae. In: *Handbook of the Birds of the World: Volume 2*, ed. J del Hoyo *et al.*, pp. 434–553. Lynx Edicions, Barcelona

Mench J and Keeling LJ (2001) The social behaviour of domestic birds. In: *Social Behaviour in Farm Animals*, ed. LJ Keeling and HW Gonyou, pp. 177–210. CABI Publishing, UK

Potts A (2012) *Chicken.* Reaktion Books, London

Scrivener D (2009) *Popular Poultry Breeds.* Crowood Press, Marlborough

Verhoef and Rijs (2003) *The Complete Encyclopaedia of Chickens.* Rebo Publishers, Lisse

Chapter 4

Husbandry

Alison Colville-Hyde and Guy Poland

Understanding the nutritional, physiological and behavioural needs of each poultry species is important in determining day-to-day management, the structure and layout of the housing, and range requirements. Inadequate husbandry will compromise health, welfare and performance in terms of bird growth and egg production. When considering the management and stockmanship requirements of keeping poultry, education and training may be of benefit in some situations. Husbandry must meet the welfare requirements of poultry and take into consideration the Five Freedoms:

* Freedom from thirst and hunger
* Freedom from discomfort
* Freedom from pain, injury or disease
* Freedom to express normal behaviour
* Freedom from fear and distress.

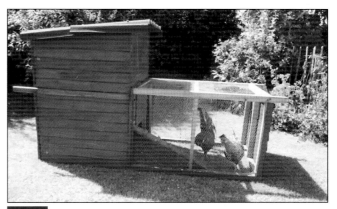

4.1 Small mobile ark.

Housing

Backyard poultry of all types require housing. Housing offers protection from the elements and predators, suitable perching and nesting conditions, cover for feeding and drinking, and a means of containing birds. However, not all types of poultry require all of these things from their accommodation and housing should be carefully designed to meet the needs of its occupants.

Chicken housing

Chickens require access to housing primarily between dusk and dawn as it provides suitable perching in a sheltered and secure environment. It is also important for shelter by day during periods of bad weather. Chicken housing must provide suitable nesting areas for laying and brooding (where desirable) at all times. It is difficult to give exact measurements for the correct size of a chicken house and range area for a small group of birds because every breed (and crossbreed) has variations within the group. However, it is beneficial to give birds as much space as possible, providing they are protected from the weather and safe from predators.

Construction and design

The chicken house should be well ventilated but not draughty (Figures 4.1 to 4.4). This can be achieved by having ventilation holes and windows above the perch

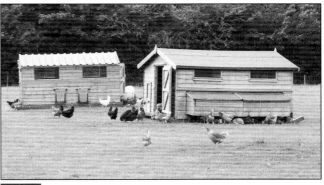

4.2 Field ark for larger flocks.

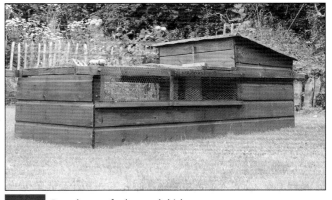

4.3 Broody coop for hen and chicks.

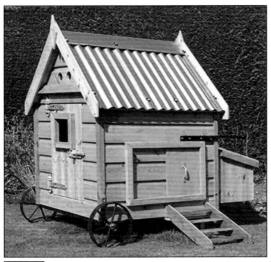

4.4 Poultry house of quality construction.

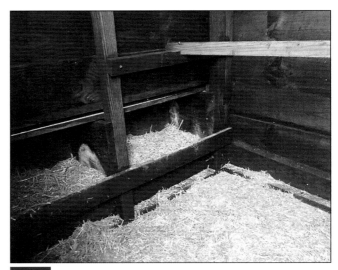

4.6 Perches should be higher than nest boxes.

roosting height. The house should be of sound construction to provide protection from the weather. Insulation can be helpful during periods of hot and cold weather, and housing of a less substantial construction may benefit from being moved into a building during the winter months. All housing should be resistant to predators.

Nest boxes and perches

With regard to laying hens, the provision of perching and nest boxes is essential. Perches, which are important in allowing birds to exhibit roosting behaviour, should be positioned at a height and be of a diameter appropriate for the breed (e.g. high perches are difficult for heavier breeds to access). The bird needs to be able to grip the perch and roost comfortably without suffering damage to its feet from rough edges. Sufficient perching space must be provided to accommodate all of the birds in the house: as a guide 25 cm per bird should be allowed for commercial laying breeds (Figure 4.5). Sufficient space should be available above the perch to allow birds to stand and fully extend their necks.

If perches are lower than nest boxes, birds may roost and defecate in the nests, resulting in dirty eggs (Figure 4.6). Nests must be easily accessible and provide sufficient space to enable birds to exhibit normal nesting behaviour; if this requirement is not met, eggs may be laid on the floor. As a guide, at least one nest should be available for every three hens (Figure 4.7). A lower light intensity

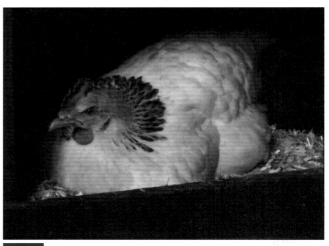

4.7 Hen on a nest.

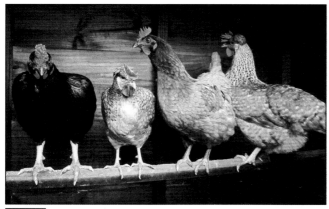

4.5 Chickens on a perch.

within the nest area will encourage birds to lay in this area rather than elsewhere in the house. Placing a china or rubber egg in the nest box will also encourage birds to lay in the boxes. Keeping birds in the house until late morning may reduce the probability of eggs being laid outside.

Range area

If the house does not have an integral run, then birds will benefit from having access to a secure larger area to exercise in and to display natural behaviours (Figure 4.8). Electrified poultry netting is a good compromise if a permanent run is not available. Grass runs are best kept with the grass fairly short as birds can become crop bound when able to consume long fibrous grass. Chickens like to nip off the fresh grass growth and this is easier for them to digest. Mobile houses have the advantage that they can be moved on to new grass regularly, reducing contamination of the pasture. Free draining ground is necessary as worm eggs, *Coccidia* and other potential pathogens can accumulate in wet areas. Shorter grass assists in ultraviolet (UV) rays penetrating the ground to destroy worm eggs, oocysts and other pathogens. The range area also needs to have some shade so that in sunny weather the birds can move out of the heat.

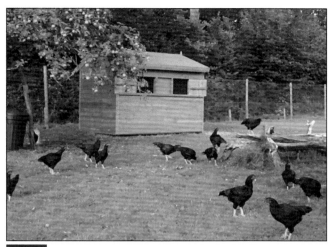

4.8 Secure fenced range area.

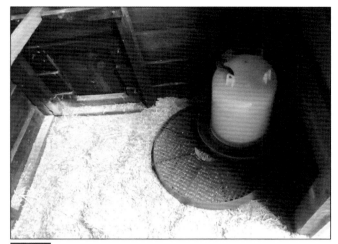

4.10 A drinker on a raised platform.

Drinkers

The design and volume of the drinkers (Figure 4.9) must be such that clean water is available to all birds at all times. Bird size within a flock can vary considerably and thought must be given to the smaller birds which may find it difficult to reach drinkers. Some breeds have particularly large combs and the design of certain drinkers may inhibit their access. Chickens will scratch litter into drinkers if they are not raised sufficiently from the floor. Suspending or placing drinkers on raised platforms will reduce contamination from litter (Figure 4.10). Regular cleaning and disinfection of drinkers and daily replenishment of water will ensure optimum potability and reduce the risk of contamination with potential pathogens. Freezing conditions will necessitate more frequent checking of drinkers.

Feeders

The same principles as for drinkers apply to the design and capacity of feeders for the flock. When in full lay, a commercial free range hen will consume approximately 125 g of food (meal/pellets) per day; bantams require considerably less food, and birds that are not laying eggs frequently also have reduced nutritional requirements (see Chapter 5). Placing feeders within the poultry house may reduce rodents and wild birds accessing the food in the short term, thus reducing wastage and the risk of disease. However, rodents and squirrels will find food if a ready source is continuously available. There are many styles of feeder available (Figure 4.11), but the main consideration is that all birds can access the food, otherwise problems will develop. Treadle feeders are excellent for flocks of six birds or more, as they have a large capacity for food and prevent small wild birds and rodents from helping themselves. The other alternative is to make an enclosure with a mesh or netting to prevent complete access by wild birds and rodents.

Grit: For further information on the use of grit, the reader is referred to Chapter 5.

Kitchen scraps: Kitchen scraps should not be fed to poultry due to the risks of causing intestinal upset and the spread of disease. In the UK, it is illegal to feed kitchen scraps to poultry; however, vegetable material originating outside a kitchen that has not come into contact with material of animal origin can be fed (see Chapters 5 and 26).

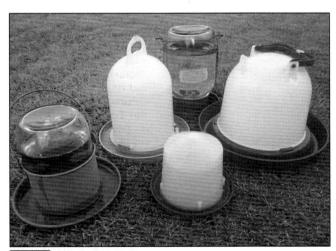

4.9 A selection of drinkers.

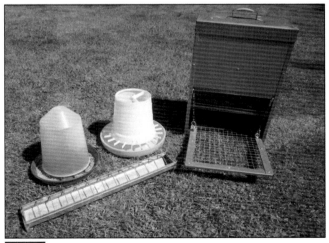

4.11 A selection of feeders. A treadle feeder is shown on the right.

Stocking density

The house must be of a size that allows the birds to move around freely, perch, nest, dust bathe, feed and drink with ease. If the house is too cramped, birds are more likely to develop behavioural problems and diseases are more likely to occur. There will be a pecking order in every poultry house, but if there is not enough room for birds to get away from each other, feather pulling and cannibalistic pecking may develop. In cramped conditions droppings build up quickly, which leads to a high level of ammonia and flies, and consequently leads to a greater potential for respiratory disease and parasite transmission. Overcrowding may also cause a greater incidence of chronic stress since birds may have insufficient room to dust bathe and preen.

Duck and goose housing
Construction and design

Ducks and geese have specific housing requirements as they need to be able to walk into safe night accommodation without injuring themselves. Unlike chickens, which roost on perches, most ducks and geese are ground dwellers. A pop hole and wide ramp are important for ducks to easily access the house. The width and height of the pop hole are dependent on the breed (e.g. Aylesbury ducks are wide and Indian Runner ducks are tall).

The house must be of an appropriate height for the breed; adequate headroom is important so that the birds are not uncomfortable (e.g. Indian Runner ducks need a house that is 50 cm higher than the height at which they naturally stand). As a guide, the floor area of the house for small breeds needs to be 30 cm by 30 cm per bird, for medium sized breeds needs to be 45 cm by 45 cm per bird and for large breeds needs to be upwards of 60 cm by 60 cm per bird.

Ducks must be trained to use their night accommodation, otherwise they will not know to use it. One way to familiarize ducks with their new house is to erect a small run around the house and keep them in the confines of the house and run before letting them out further afield. Ducks are generally suspicious of anything new, so it is important to ensure that they know where their house is and that it can be shut at night.

Nesting

Ducks lay eggs in floor nests, which should be provided.

Range area

Foraging is very important for waterfowl, so they should be provided with a range area large enough for them to exhibit this behaviour. Geese require more space than many duck breeds to allow them to exercise sufficiently. Waterfowl have a requirement to access water for bathing. Ponds should be deep enough to allow ducks to submerse their heads. The pond should be relatively easy to drain to allow it to be cleaned and have water circulation systems equipped with filters to help keep the water fresh. Slatted plastic or wooden decking around the pond will also reduce mess. Ducks will benefit from access to larger areas of water in which to swim.

Drinkers

Ponds provide a source of drinking water for ducks and geese. However, additional drinkers may be required. Waterfowl find it easier to drink from wide troughs or bell drinkers and these are preferable to nipple drinkers, although the latter may be less messy.

Feeders

Waterfowl require feeders of sufficient width and depth to allow them to shovel up food with their bills without hitting the sides of the container. Sufficient trough space should be provided to allow birds to feed without competition; a width of 15 cm per bird is a useful guide.

Turkey housing
Construction and design

Turkeys are less reliant on housing than chickens, although shelter is still required, primarily in the form of a covered roost area. Raised perches should be provided covered by a roof. Sides should be provided on the structure during the winter months, bad weather and in exposed areas. The housing should be sited in an area that is predator proof, or should itself have predator proof wire mesh or solid sides. Turkeys may also be provided with shelter inside larger buildings, as long as perches are provided.

Range area

Access to pasture is required for turkeys since grazing is an important behaviour and source of food. A relatively large area is needed, which should be surrounded by predator resistant fencing that is high enough to prevent the birds from escaping.

Drinkers

A wide range of commercial systems is available for different turkey life stages, many of which are based on plumbed-in installations and nipple drinkers. Nipples are usually red to attract the birds to them. Whilst these systems provide an efficient supply of fresh water and tend to minimize spillage, they are often not practical in a backyard setting. Other drinkers used should be refilled daily and cleaned regularly. Raised drinkers will reduce faecal contamination. Drinkers should allow enough space for all birds to drink without competition.

Feeders

Turkeys have similar requirements to chickens in terms of feeders, although more space and capacity for food per bird will be needed.

Pheasant housing
Construction and design

The high likelihood of escape, the non-indigenous status of many species and, on occasion, the high conservation value of ornamental pheasants mean that they are best suited to restricted enclosures. Whilst small houses, such as an ark and run (similar to that for chickens), can be used, permanent aviaries are a better option.

Ornamental pheasants are best kept in male–female pairs or a trio consisting of one male and two females. Multiple cocks will compete for females, which may lead to fighting. Ornamental pheasants benefit from more space in comparison to game pheasants since they are usually more flighty and may have more extravagant plumage that is vulnerable to damage. An enclosure measuring 3 m by 2 m with a shelter measuring 1 m by 2 m is recommended as a minimum for small species. Larger breeds may require double this space. It is helpful if the enclosures are high enough for a person to stand up in.

Doors allowing entry to the enclosure should be designed in such a way as to minimize the risk of birds escaping – a double gated arrangement can facilitate this. The bottom 30 cm of the enclosure should be boarded to reduce stress to the birds by blocking their view of birds in other enclosures and passing potential predators such as dogs and cats. Extending the wire mesh on the sides of the enclosure to below ground level will reduce the risk of rodents burrowing into the aviary. For this purpose, wire mesh is more resistant to pests but soft netting represents less risk to the pheasants in the event of them ascending rapidly when frightened. The aviary should be sited so as to be sheltered from the prevailing wind but should not be shaded from the sun to the extent that it is continuously in the dark.

The base of the enclosure can be earth or grass, but in either case should be planted with vegetation to provide cover for the birds for seclusion and shelter from the elements. Pheasants will often walk up and down the edges of the enclosure, causing excessive erosion in these areas. A strip of sand along the edges can help to mitigate the effects of this behaviour. Sand is also a useful substrate for the shelter part of the enclosure as faeces can be easily removed.

Perches

Pheasants require high perches in the shelter area. Perches with a cross-section of 50 mm by 50 mm with rounded edges are appropriate for most species.

Drinkers and feeders

A wide range of feeders and drinkers are appropriate. These should be raised from the floor to reduce contamination and cleaned regularly. Fresh water should always be provided. Drinkers must be checked more often during cold weather to ensure that the water is not frozen.

Peafowl housing

Peafowl can be managed in a number of ways. They may be kept entirely free range. This allows the birds great freedom to express their natural behaviour but requires a large range, renders the birds vulnerable to predation and extreme weather, and may inhibit management of breeding. Alternatively, peafowl can be intermittently or permanently confined to a shelter and aviary.

Construction and design

A peafowl aviary must be large, particularly when adult males are kept. A minimum height of 1.8 m and width of 3 m is recommended to accommodate the male train. The minimum length of the aviary is dependent on the number of birds but would typically start at 6 m for a trio of peafowl. The aviary must be covered with a wire mesh due to the flight risk of the birds (Figure 4.12). The use of glass is not recommended in the aviary due to the risk of the bird not seeing it and flying into it. It is beneficial to provide some shade for the birds in the aviary and a windbreak to allow males to display their trains.

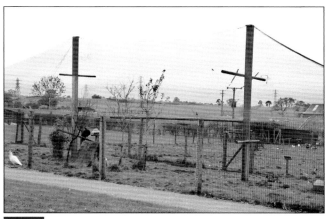

4.12 Peafowl aviary with a netting roof to prevent escape.

Nest boxes and perches

Perches should be provided in the shelter. These should be 1.2 m to 1.5 m off the ground. Perches should be a minimum of 0.9 m from the wall of the shelter in order to accommodate the train of the male. Wooden board perches (typically 5 cm by 10 cm) are recommended over round perches due to the risk of frostbite in the winter. There are reports of peafowl keepers using heated perches during cold weather. It has been suggested that perches should be removed when a peahen is in lay since she may attempt to lay on the perch, commonly resulting in a broken egg. Free range peahens will lay in hollow depressions lined with grass. These can be provided in the aviary and lined with straw or hay. Peahens tend to lay every other day during the laying season and usually in the evening.

Drinkers

The drinker must be of sufficient size for the age of bird to allow them to scoop up the water with their beaks. Access to fresh water is required at all times and the usual precautions are needed to prevent freezing in the winter.

Feeders

Sufficient trough space should be provided for the number of birds being kept when mash or pellet food is provided. A deep trough is useful for reducing waste since peafowl will attempt to scratch the food out. Free range birds will graze on vegetation and insects. Peafowl kept in aviaries may require the provision of additional 'greens' scattered in the enclosure.

Guinea fowl housing

Guinea fowl are relatively hardy birds, particularly with regard to heat stress, and are often kept free range in tropical climates.

Construction and design

Guinea fowl are perching birds, so the housing should provide perches. Low level lighting inside the house will have a calming influence on the birds, although it has been reported that guinea fowl may be reluctant to enter a poorly lit house. Guinea fowl require more training than other types of poultry to get them to use the housing provided, so feeding the birds inside the house at night may encourage them to return to their shelter.

Range area

Guinea fowl display strong foraging behaviour so a suitable range area is important. It should be noted that a 1.5–2 m fence may be insufficient to keep the birds in the enclosure unless their wings have been clipped or pinioned.

Feeders

Guinea fowl often cause a lot of food wastage due to the tearing motion of the head during feeding, which can be reduced by providing deep feeders.

Fundamentals of management

Species- and age-specific flocks

The mixing of numerous poultry species is a common mistake in backyard flocks. Different types of poultry have different nutritional and environmental needs and it is difficult to accommodate these varying needs within the same area. Keeping some combinations of poultry species together may also increase the risk of disease; for example, histomoniasis ('blackhead') in turkeys is transmitted largely via an intestinal nematode (*Heterakis*) carried by chickens.

Mixing birds of different ages can also cause problems since younger birds may be challenged with diseases endemic in the older flock. For this reason most commercial poultry sites operate an 'all-in, all-out' system. Thus, to avoid these problems in a backyard setting, it may be advisable to rear birds of different age groups separately. It should also be noted that birds newly introduced from an outside source may be at risk from diseases endemic in the existing flock. In addition, new birds have the potential to introduce infectious diseases into the flock to which the existing birds are naïve, with possibly serious consequences.

Individual and flock health

Poultry keepers must monitor their birds closely for signs of disease. Simple observation of all birds in the flock at least once daily is essential, with a closer examination required for birds showing any signs of abnormality. Regular screening and treatment (as required) for endoparasites and ectoparasites assists in having healthy, contented birds. Feeding the correct ration for the species, age and purpose of the birds will ensure that they receive the essential nutrients for optimum health. Husbandry, nutrition (see Chapter 5) and preventive healthcare (see Chapter 7) are all closely related.

Investigation and treatment of deformed and infirm birds is required. On occasion, it may be necessary to euthanase birds and, ideally, this should be accompanied by a postmortem examination (see Chapters 10 and 25). Diseased or infirm birds are vulnerable to attack from other members of the flock, potentially causing significant welfare issues. Separating the bullied bird for a time may help, but if it has not been successfully treated when it is reintroduced to the flock, the bullying usually recommences.

Handling

Handling of poultry (Figure 4.13) is essential for good husbandry (see Chapter 6 for further information).

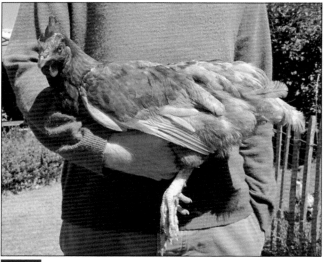

4.13 Handling a bird.

Food treats

Many poultry keepers enjoy hand-feeding or scattering corn and other treats for their birds. However, if not fed in moderation these treats will affect the overall nutritional balance provided to the bird (especially in terms of calcium and phosphorus) and also predispose to obesity. Maize, in particular, has a high calorific value. The increased availability of chicken treats in pet stores is likely to contribute to the incidence of obesity. Obesity will adversely affect the mobility of the bird and egg production, and may lead to orthopaedic problems. The reader is referred to Chapter 5 for information on nutrition and Chapter 8 for details on body condition scoring.

Hygiene

Implementing a hygiene protocol will lower the risk of the spread of disease as cleaning and disinfecting the house, feeders, drinkers and range reduces the build-up of pathogens. As part of a daily cleaning routine, droppings should be removed from the bedding (particularly under the perches and in the nest boxes). This helps to keep the litter fresh and prevents eggs from becoming dirty. Fresh bedding enables birds to scratch and dust bathe, keeping them content and their feathers in good condition. A more extensive cleaning and disinfection protocol should be undertaken seasonally.

- Remove all dry litter and then using a brush sweep out any loose dust and cobwebs.
- Remove any caked-on faeces with a scraper.
- Soak the house in a detergent and then wash out using a power washer or hosepipe. Ensure that all the crevices have been washed out to remove any residual dust.
- Once free of organic matter allow to dry and then apply a disinfectant for poultry diseases at the recommended concentration (see http://disinfectants.defra.gov.uk for a list of disinfectants approved by Defra). A garden hand sprayer is appropriate for an even application of disinfectant. It is important that the specified contact time for the particular disinfectant is observed.
- Replace the bedding. Dust extracted wood shavings are a good choice, although there are several alternatives such as rape straw byproduct, flax-based products and chopped hemp. Chopped straw is a

good choice for use in the nest boxes. The use of hay and long straw is not advisable, as hay is prone to mould and can cause crop impaction and long straw is not easy for birds to scratch and dust bathe in.
- Repair the housing as needed to prevent the birds from injuring themselves and to keep out predators.

Husbandry routines

Husbandry routines (such as those described below) are a very useful tool to help poultry keepers maximize the welfare of their birds and reduce the risk of disease.

Daily routine for laying birds
- Let the birds out in the morning.
- Collect the eggs and remove any droppings from the nest boxes.
- Replenish the feeders and replace water in the drinkers; clean if necessary.
- Observe the birds and seek veterinary attention as required.
- Bring in the feeders at night.
- Shut the birds in at night.

Weekly tasks
- Clean and disinfect the feeders and drinkers.
- Replace soiled bedding in the house and nest boxes.
- Move the house on to fresh grass if it is a mobile unit.
- Move the electric fencing if required.
- Mow the grass.
- Implement pest control as required.

Seasonal tasks
- Thoroughly cleanse and disinfect the poultry house and undertake maintenance as necessary.
- Screen birds for endoparasites and treat as necessary (see Chapter 7).
- Screen birds for ectoparasites and treat as necessary (see Chapters 7, 10 and 13).
- Clip the wings of the birds if required (see Chapter 7).

Hatching and rearing

Successful breeding requires careful management, good husbandry and nutrition. Poultry intended for breeding need to be fed a breeder ration suited to the species. Males and females should be kept in ratios appropriate for their species and breed; a male working too many females will become exhausted and potentially infertile. Fertility rates decline in older birds and parasite burdens and unsuitable housing may also contribute to poor hatches. Buying in birds and hatching eggs from markets or breed shows (Figures 4.14 and 4.15) increases the risk of introducing disease into a flock, either by direct contact, faecal contamination or through the fertile egg.

Natural rearing

Although the process cannot be manipulated to the same extent as artificial incubation and brooding, natural rearing can provide a non-labour intensive route to breeding. A broody bird is one that has entered a hormonal state, which causes changes in behaviour and physiology with

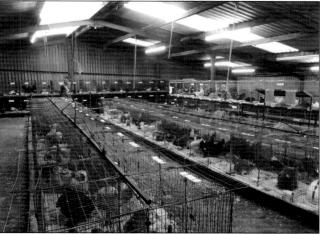

4.14 The disease status of birds bought at markets and breed shows is unknown.

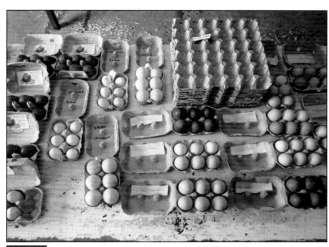

4.15 Hatching eggs for sale.

the sole purpose of hatching and brooding young. The female loses feathers on her ventrum to form the 'brood patch'. She then sits on the clutch of eggs for the duration of incubation, turning them at regular intervals. The bird will incubate any eggs that are of an appropriate size and so can be used to hatch eggs from conspecifics or even other species (e.g. broody silky hens have traditionally been used to incubate falcon eggs).

Broody birds will benefit from a secluded nest and having food and water within easy reach. The nest is safest close to ground level to prevent any unfortunate accidents when the chicks are hatching out. For chickens, a small coop is ideal as it affords the hen and chicks safety and privacy if she is to raise them (see Figure 4.3). The hen will need to leave the nest from time to time, but these periods will be brief, and unless she is quite young and/or flighty, the hen is not likely to abandon the nest unless she has cause to do so (e.g. due to a predator attack). For those poultry species that are kept in small groups (e.g. ornamental pheasants), the female is likely to brood in a nesting area within the normal enclosure.

Once the eggs have hatched, the female will continue to provide warmth for the chicks until they are able to withstand the normal environment by themselves. It is important that water provided for the dam does not pose a drowning risk to the chicks – stones placed in the drinker can be useful to reduce the depth of the water. Chick crumbs should also be made available. For the first 24–48 hours, the chicks receive nutrition from their yolk sacs. During this time, the chicks learn to eat by copying each other and the female.

Artificial rearing
Principles of breeding
General:
- Use birds true to type/breed, in peak health and free of disease.
- Use sexually mature male birds.
- Ensure that the male:female ratio is correct.
- Feed the correct ration to optimize fertility and egg and shell quality.
- Keep nest boxes clean at all times.

Collection and storage of eggs:
- Handle eggs wearing disposable gloves (or have very clean, dry hands).
- Handle eggs with care and use clean egg boxes for transportation.
- Collect eggs frequently and write the date laid in pencil on to each egg.
- Use clean eggs that are perfectly formed; faeces and dirt may cause bacterial contamination of the egg (Figure 4.16).
- Incubate eggs within 10 days of being laid otherwise hatchability will be markedly reduced.
- If being stored, keep eggs at a temperature of 12–15°C and 75–85% relative humidity.
- Store eggs on clean egg trays.

Artificial incubation: Artificial incubators are available in many different designs (Figure 4.17). The two main features that differ are:

- Temperature control – incubators can heat eggs with still air, with circulating air or with contact heat plates
- Turning – some incubators require eggs to be turned manually, although many modern machines will automatically turn eggs.

Due to design differences, the temperature and humidity of the incubator should be set to the manufacturer's recommendations for the species being hatched, and only one species of egg should be incubated at a time.

- Clean and disinfect the incubator between hatches to avoid the transmission of pathogens.
- Place the incubator in a draught-free area on a level surface.
- Ensure that the incubator is heated up in advance to stabilize at the correct temperature for the species.
- Bring eggs to room temperature just before placing them in the incubator to avoid temperature shocks.
- Depending on the design of the incubator, it may be helpful to mark eggs with a cross on one side before placing them in the incubator, to check that they are being turned.
- Fill the incubator to capacity.
- Temperature fluctuations, particularly at the high end, can harm the developing embryo, so ensure that the incubator ventilation holes are clear of obstructions to allow excess heat to escape. It can be useful to put a temperature and humidity monitor into the incubator to ensure that the temperature is correct at the level of the eggs.

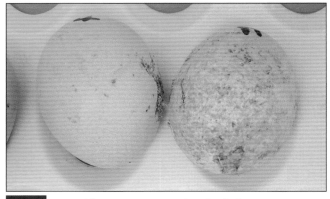

4.16 Dirt and faeces on eggs can infect the chicks.

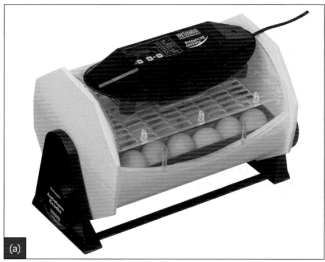

(a)

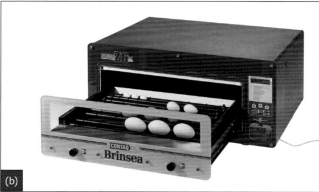

(b)

4.17 Different models of incubator have different design features. (a) A moving air incubator with humidity control and a tilting tray mechanism to turn eggs. (b) A contact and moving air incubator with humidity control and a roller mechanism for turning eggs. (Courtesy of Brinsea Products Ltd)

- Candle eggs between 5 and 7 days from the onset of incubation to check fertility. Clear eggs should be discarded.
- Keep incubation records, including dates, number and source of eggs and incubator settings used.

The incubation periods of different poultry species are listed in Figure 4.18. However, these periods may vary by a day or two, especially if the temperature or relative humidity in the incubator is not set correctly. Eggs should be candled again at this stage to check for any signs of life.

Species	Incubation period
Hybrid laying chicken	21 days (20 days in bantams)
Turkey	28 days[a]
Duck (mallard)	23–29 days[b]
Duck (Muscovy)	35 days[b]
Goose	30–35 days
Pheasant (common)	22–24 days[b]
Guinea fowl	29 days[a]
Peafowl (Indian)	29 days[a]

4.18 Incubation times for different species.
([a] Data from AnAge Database of Animal Ageing and Longevity; [b] Data from Carpenter, 2012)

Digital egg monitors, which use infrared to detect the heartbeat (including heart rate) of the embryo as early as 5 days from the onset of incubation, are a useful alternative to candling, especially when the egg is strongly coloured or has a thick shell.

Hatching

This is the period of time from when the chick starts to make its way out of the egg, to actually emerging and drying off. This process usually takes 3 days from start to finish. Therefore, 3 days before the calculated hatch date, the incubator needs to have the turning mechanism switched off. At 18 days the chick starts 'pipping' its way through the internal membrane into the air cell (known as the internal pip) and takes its first breath. Chicks can be heard at this stage as they will begin to cheep. When hatching eggs under a broody hen, she will communicate with the chicks at this stage, encouraging them to hatch. The chick has a tooth-like projection on the upper beak called the egg tooth, which it uses to work its way out of the egg. The chick will cut through half of the circumference of the shell using the egg tooth, and then use its legs and feet to push away the shell and emerge out of the egg. The egg tooth can be seen after hatching, but will only remain for a day or so before dropping off.

The incubator door should be kept closed, particularly during the final days of incubation in order not to disrupt the hatching environment by altering the temperature and relative humidity. The yolk supplies the chick with nutrients from the onset of incubation to the first 2–3 days post-hatching. Chicks that are unable to hatch on their own may have deformities or other conditions, so consideration should be given as to whether to assist hatching. Dampening the opening on the surface of the egg with a warm fine spray of water or cloth may help (see Chapter 17 for further information).

Drying-off period

Newly hatched chicks are wet (Figure 4.19) and should remain in the incubator until completely dry, allowing them to have a rest in a controlled environment. It is particularly important during this period that the umbilical seal dries in order to prevent any pathogens from entering the chick. Dead and deformed chicks along with their shells should be removed from the incubator; deformed chicks should be euthanased. Chicks are ready to leave the incubator once thoroughly dry; they will also become noticeably active, quite vocal and start pecking at things. The chicks can then be transferred to the brooding area.

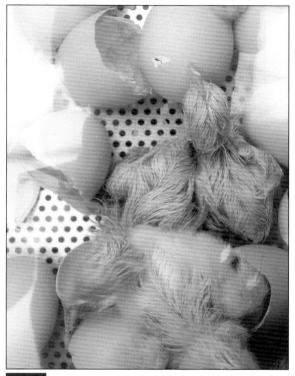

4.19 Newly hatched wet chicks.

Brooding

Brooding is the period of time that the chick relies on human intervention (for heat, food and water) or, with natural rearing, the time the dam is tending to the chick. During this period, chicks are unable to regulate their body temperature. Brooding normally takes 3 weeks, but depends on the environmental temperature. It is important that the brooding phase is carried out correctly (Figure 4.20), as poor practice will have a detrimental effect on the health of the growing chick and subsequently the adult bird. It is important to recognize the difference between contented and discontented chicks, as this enables evaluation of their needs and environmental adjustments to be made. Chicks should behave as a group – at any one time some should be eating, drinking, playing and resting – and be evenly spread across the floor of the brooding area. Chicks should not be overcrowded as this causes distress

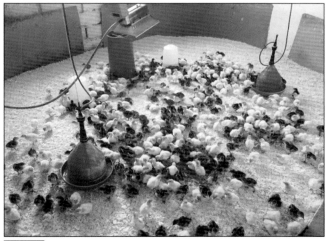

4.20 Good brooding set-up.

and can lead to behavioural problems, such as feather pecking, and disease. Chicks should vocalize a contented chirping sound; they should not be silent or making high-pitched cheeps.

Chick crumb, duck crumb or turkey crumb will need to be provided according to the species. Fresh drinking water must be provided at all times. Use of dust extracted shavings as bedding gives good results as it is hygienic and allows the chicks to dust bathe. It has been shown that levels of feather pecking in older birds are linked to an inability to dust bathe at an early age (Hüber-Eicher and Wechsler, 1997). Fresh bedding should be added when required, and feeders and drinkers should be frequently cleaned. Chicks should not be brooded on a cold floor with no bedding (Figure 4.21).

The temperature of the brooding area should be regulated using heat lamps. The ideal ambient temperature is 32°C, although this may vary depending on the brooding set-up. To set the lamp at the correct temperature hang it over the chicks until they are evenly spread out on the floor underneath it. If the chicks are huddled and piling on top of each other, they are too cold. If the chicks have their beaks open and are moving away from under the heat lamp, they are too warm. Gradually, the chicks will start to display strength and confidence within the brooding pen and with each other. They will be able to spend a little time away from the heat lamp without feeling cold. By day 3, the heat lamp should be raised slightly, lowering the temperature at floor level. Over subsequent days the heat lamp should be raised further, so that the chicks become less reliant on it. The breed of bird and the ambient temperature of the brooding area will determine how quickly the heat source can be removed.

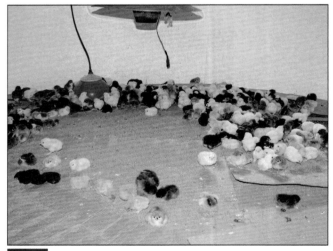

4.21 Poor brooding set-up.

Rearing

The chicks (referred to as poults or growers; Figure 4.22 and 4.23) require a larger growing environment for the rearing period. Different species, as well as the various breeds within a species, have different nutritional and environmental requirements. The three key areas are:

- Provision of an appropriate environment and correct management for the species
- Quality nutrition appropriate to each life stage
- Effective hygiene and disease control.

Term	Life stage, sex or type
Chickens (Gallus gallus domesticus) (collective noun: flock)	
Chick	Young juvenile male or female
Poult, grower	Young bird (all fowl)
Pullet	Female <1 year old
Hen	Female
Cockerel	Male (sometimes used to refer to a young male)
Cock	Male (usually refers to a mature male)
Rooster	Male (American term: usually refers to a mature male)
Broiler	A meat breed bird
Ducks (Anas platyrhynchos domesticus) (collective noun: flock)	
Duckling	Young juvenile male or female
Duck	Male or female. Denotes female alongside use of drake for male
Drake	Male
Turkeys (Meleagris gallapavo) (collective noun: flock or gang)	
Chick	Young juvenile male or female
Poult	Young male or female
Jake	Younger male
Gobbler, tom, stag, cock	Mature male
Hen	Female
Geese (Anser anser domesticus/Anser cygnoides domesticus) (collective noun: flock or gaggle)	
Gosling	Young juvenile male or female
Gander	Male
Goose	Male or female. Denotes female alongside use of gander for male
Guinea fowl (Numida meleagris) (collective noun: rasp)	
Keet	Young juvenile male or female
Hen	Female
Cock	Male
Pheasants (various species) (collective noun: nye)	
Chick	Young juvenile male or female
Hen	Female
Cock	Male
Peafowl (Pavo spp.) (collective noun: muster)	
Peachick	Young juvenile male or female
Peahen	Female
Peacock	Male

4.22 Terms commonly used to describe the different life stages, sex and type of poultry. Usage of these terms is variable and therefore this list cannot be considered exhaustive.

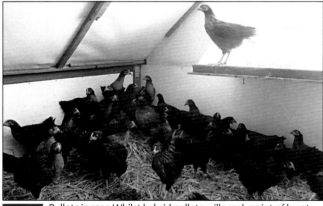

4.23 Pullets in rear. Whilst hybrid pullets will reach point of lay at about 20–24 weeks of age, some pure breeds will not mature until 28–34 weeks of age.

Birds should be reared in their own age group (ideally as hatched) and not mixed with other birds of different ages. It is strongly advised not to mix bantams with large fowl due to the larger birds bullying the smaller ones. It is not advisable to hatch the chicks in small batches and rear them in one mixed group – this is likely to lead to behavioural problems and increase the risk of the spread of disease. Rearing multiple species together is also not recommended as the birds all have different needs.

Feeding: Not only are there differences in the nutritional requirements of different poultry species during rearing, but also differences between the breeds. Typically, traditional breeds grow far slower than commercial breeds. During the first few weeks, the growing chick develops its skeleton, followed by the muscle tissue and sexual organs, and then lays down fat. The speed at which these anatomical developments take place is dependent on the breed.

Figures 4.24 and 4.25 provide guides to feeding ages for commonly available feeds.

Once chickens are on layers pellets, mixed corn can be given as a scratch feed at the end of the day. Many poultry keepers find the reaction of their chickens to corn scratch feed rewarding, but it is very important that mixed corn is fed in moderation to prevent unbalanced nutrition. Layers pellets should be fed at the point of lay to meet the high nutritional requirements of producing eggs, providing calcium for the shell and maintenance of the physiology of the bird.

Environment: If birds are cramped and in a highly populated pen then fighting, feather pulling, cannibalism and disease can become problems. Birds should be provided with enough space inside the house to demonstrate natural behaviours (i.e. scratching the litter, perching, dust bathing) and there should be sufficient feeders and

Species	Approximate age of feeding (weeks)[a]					
	Diet	Starter[b]	Chick[b]	Grower/rearer	Maintenance/holding	Layer/breeder
	Form	Crumbs	Crumbs or meal	Pellets or meal	Pellets	Pellets or meal
Chicken		0–3	4–8	9–16	–	17 onwards
		–	0–10[c]	11–16	–	17 onwards
Duck		0–2	3–5	6–10[d]	11 to POL	POL onwards
		–	0–6[c]	7–10[d]	11 to POL	POL onwards
Goose		–	0–4	5–10/12[d]	11/13 to POL	POL onwards
Turkey		0–4	5–12	13–16[d]	17 to POL	POL onwards
		–	0–12[c]	13–16[d]	17 to POL	POL onwards
Guinea fowl		0–4	5–8	9–16[d]	17 to POL	POL onwards
		–	0–8[c]	9–16[d]	17 to POL	POL onwards
Ornamental pheasant and peafowl		0–4	5–8	9–19	20 to POL	POL onwards
		–	0–8[c]	9–19[d]	20 to POL	POL onwards

4.24 A guide to feeding ages for commonly available poultry feeds for egg-laying birds. [a]Always refer to feed labels for more specific details on age of feeding. [b]These diets typically contain a coccidiostat (ACS), although plain versions are often available and should be used when feeding to non-target species. [c]It is preferable to feed crumbs for the first 2 weeks and then move on to pellets. [d]If a maintenance/holding diet is not available then continue on grower/rearer diet until point of lay. POL = point of lay. Ideally the layer or breeder diet should be introduced 2–4 weeks before the birds start laying.
(Courtesy of I Mackinson)

Species	Approximate age of feeding (weeks)[a]					
	Diet	Starter[b]	Chick[b]	Grower/rearer	Finisher/fattener	Maintenance/holding
	Form	Crumbs	Crumbs or pellets	Pellets	Pellets	Pellets
Chicken		0–2	3–5	6 to end	6 to end	8 onwards[c]
		–	0–5[d]	6 to end	6 to end	8 onwards[c]
Duck		0–2	3–5	6 to end	6 to end	8 onwards[c]
		–	0–5[d]	6 to end	6 to end	8 onwards[c]
Goose[e]		–	0–4[d]	5 to end	5 to end	10/12 onwards
Turkey		0–4	5–12	13 to end	13 to end	20 onwards
		–	0–12[d]	13 to end	13 to end	20 onwards
Guinea fowl		0–4	5–8	9 to end	9 to end	13/14 onwards
		–	0–8[d]	9 to end	9 to end	13/14 onwards
Ornamental pheasant and peafowl		0–4	5–8	9–19	–	20 onwards
		–	0–8[d]	9–19	–	20 onwards

4.25 A guide to feeding ages for commonly available poultry feeds for meat and ornamental birds. [a]Always refer to feed labels for more specific details on age of feeding. [b]These diets typically contain a coccidiostat (ACS), although plain versions are often available and should be used when feeding to non-target species. [c]For adult non-laying ornamental birds introduce a maintenance/holding diet. [d]It is preferable to feed crumbs for the first 2 weeks and then move on to pellets. [e]Geese require access to fresh pasture.
(Courtesy of I Mackinson)

drinkers to give each bird easy access to food and water. Bedding needs to be dry and friable so that it does not get capped by excessive droppings, causing it to become wet and sticky. Birds cannot scratch in the bedding if this happens and this can lead to foot burns and hock marks. Good choices of bedding include chopped straw or dust extracted shavings or a mixture of both. Paper-based bedding (such as newspaper) may not be sufficiently absorbent.

Broiler birds: With broiler (meat) birds, there is typically a greater emphasis on achieving faster growth and higher meat quality whilst minimizing inputs. However, it is important that these aims are not met at the cost of the welfare of the bird. Broilers can be provided with low perches if desired. If the perches are too high, the birds may damage themselves when getting on and off them (e.g. fractures of the keel can occur when jumping off the perch and landing on the ground, and breast blisters can result from rubbing against a sharp perch edge). Commercial broilers, which are very fast growing, are not provided with perches. This aids management of the house. Feed should be withdrawn about 6 hours prior to slaughter, or the night before if the birds are scheduled for slaughter early in the morning. This will prevent contamination of the carcass by food from the crop and also reduce the amount of faecal material within the bird at the time of slaughter.

Acknowledgements

Richard Jackson contributed to the coverage of natural incubation.

References and further reading

Boulianne M, Hunter BD, Physick-Sheard PW, Viel L and Julian RJ (1993) Effect of exercise on cardiac output and other cardiovascular parameters of heavy turkeys and relevance to the sudden death syndrome. *Avian Diseases* **37**, 98–106

Carey JR and Judge DS (2000) *Longevity Records: Life Spans of Mammals, Birds, Amphibians, Reptiles and Fish*. Available from: http://www.demogr.mpg.de/longevityrecords/

Carpenter JW (2012) *Exotic Animal Formulary, 4th edition*. Saunders Elsevier, St Louis

Hüber-Eicher B and Wechsler B (1997) Feather pecking in domestic chicks: its relation to dustbathing and foraging. *Animal Behaviour* **54**, 757–768

McNab BK (1966) An analysis of the body temperatures of birds. *The Condor* **68**, 47–55

Ryser A and Morrison R (1954) Cold resistance in the young Ring-Necked Pheasant. *The Auk* **71**, 253–266

Useful websites

AnAge Database of Animal Ageing and Longevity
http://genomics.senescence.info/species/index.html

Guinea Fowl Production – Poultry and Rabbits Section, Division of Non-Ruminants, Department of Animal Production, Botswana
http://www.gov.bw/Global/MOA/Guinea%20Fowl%20Production.pdf

United Peafowl Association
http://www.unitedpeafowlassociation.org

The World Pheasant Association
http://www.pheasant.org.uk

Chapter 5

Nutrition

Helen Hodgkin and Ian Mackinson

In the wild, poultry consume a wide range of raw materials to satisfy their nutritional requirements and predominantly eat to satisfy their energy requirement. Poultry require a variety of nutrients for maintenance, health, growth, development and reproduction. The level and ratio of nutrients needed differs according to the species, age and productive state of the bird. However, all birds require proteins, carbohydrates, fats, minerals, trace elements, vitamins and water.

Nutrients

Proteins

Protein is needed to satisfy the amino acid requirement of the bird. There are 22 amino acids present in the body and these are categorized as either essential or non-essential. Essential amino acids are those that the bird is unable to synthesize itself and therefore must rely solely on dietary supply. The primary limiting amino acid in poultry is methionine, requirements of which must be met to ensure health and productivity are not compromised. The main factor that determines the protein and amino acid requirements of the bird is its productive state. Growing birds have a high amino acid requirement to enable muscle growth and development, whereas in laying birds lower protein diets will adequately support egg production. Adult birds generally have the lowest protein requirement. The protein content of the diet is known as crude protein, which is calculated by multiplying the nitrogen content by 6.25, and is given as a percentage of the diet.

Carbohydrates

Cereal grains contain high amounts of carbohydrates, typically in the form of starch, and are therefore a major contributor of energy in poultry diets. In the UK, poultry feeds predominately contain wheat as the main cereal source. Some carbohydrates, including the polysaccharides present in the hull, are poorly digested by the bird and increase viscosity of the gut digesta. Commercial diets include exogenous enzymes (xylanases and glucanases) which aid digestion and increase nutrient availability.

Fats and oils

Oils and fats are concentrated sources of energy and provide lipids (fatty acids and their derivatives), which are essential for growth and cell synthesis, as well as vital components of cell membranes. Linoleic acid (C18:2) is considered to be the main essential fatty acid in poultry, deficiencies of which result in loss of membrane function.

Minerals, trace elements and vitamins

Calcium is the most abundant mineral in the body and is required for skeletal development and numerous cellular functions, including the contraction of muscle cells and intracellular signaling. A laying bird requires around two or three times more calcium than a growing bird due to the amount of calcium deposited in the eggshell. In laying birds, the calcium for eggshell formation is supplied both directly from the diet and also through mobilization of skeletal stores. The requirement for calcium in laying birds increases with age, whilst growing birds have the highest requirement in the starter phase to support skeletal development.

Phosphorus is also a major mineral with its main role being as a component of bone. In addition, it is an essential component of numerous organic compounds involved in many vital metabolic pathways. The ratio of calcium to phosphorus in bone is approximately 2:1; it is therefore critical to ensure the correct dietary balance of these minerals to support normal skeletal development in growing birds. In commercial feeds, a phytase enzyme is added to improve the bioavailability of calcium and phosphorus, which are chelated to the anti-nutritive phytate present in plant sources.

Sodium and chloride are both essential to support optimal health and productivity; however, too high a concentration can lead to an osmotic imbalance, increased water consumption and consequently wetter droppings. Trace elements, including iron, manganese, zinc, selenium, copper and iodine are required in small amounts; the latter four are cofactors to enzymes, whilst iron is essential in haemoglobin. Vitamins are categorized as either water-soluble or fat-soluble. Water-soluble vitamins are not stored in the body, whereas fat-soluble vitamins are.

- Water-soluble vitamins (e.g. folic acid, biotin, pantothenic acid, niacin, B1, B2, B6 and B12) primarily act as coenzymes and play an important role in key metabolic processes such as fat, protein and carbohydrate metabolism.
- Fat-soluble vitamins include vitamin A, D3, E and K. Vitamin A is essential for vision and healthy skin. Vitamin D3 regulates calcium and phosphorus absorption and therefore plays a role in bone development. Vitamin E is a known antioxidant. Vitamin K is important for the synthesis of blood coagulation factors.

The required levels of trace elements and vitamins are typically met via the routine addition of premixes during feed manufacture. Water offers an additional route of supplementation, particularly for vitamins, with multivitamin 'tonics' being used strategically during times of stress (e.g. such as disease challenge) when dietary intake may be suboptimal.

Water

Water is the most important chemical in the body and thus an essential nutrient for all animals. *Ad libitum* access to clean water is vital for normal bird activity and optimal health and productivity. Water quality is fundamental and is an often overlooked factor.

> Poorly maintained and unsanitary water containers can be a reservoir for bacteria and viruses that can adversely affect the health and productivity of the bird. Water containers should be regularly cleaned and, if necessary, disinfected with a suitable cleaning solution to help avoid bacterial contamination (see Chapter 4)

Energy

Carbohydrates and fats are the main dietary sources of energy, which is vital for body temperature regulation, maintenance, reproduction, growth and development, and normal activity. The common energy system used in poultry is metabolizable energy (ME), expressed as megajoules per kilogram (MJ/kg) or occasionally in kilocalories per kg (kcal/kg). This is the total amount of energy available to the bird from the feed (i.e. the gross energy minus the energy voided in the faeces and urine). The ME of a raw material or feed is variable due to the varying efficiencies of the digestive tract of the bird, which can be influenced by age, breed, sex and gut microflora.

Nutritional requirements

There is a wealth of published data and guidelines on the nutritional requirements for commercial poultry (chickens and turkeys used for meat and eggs) in scientific publications, reference books and breed company literature. However, when it comes to species such as peafowl and ornamental pheasants, there is a dearth of relevant and reliable sources of information. To overcome this knowledge gap, it is necessary to combine basic principles with existing information from other species and apply this to each phase of the bird's life in order to select suitable feeds and feeding programmes.

Growing birds

Young birds require a higher percentage of protein than adult birds in order to supply the body with the essential amino acids needed for cell replication and growth. Commercial meat birds are usually fed between four and six different feeds to satisfy their requirements throughout each phase of development and to ensure optimal growth. For example, commercial broiler chickens are typically fed starter, grower, finisher and withdrawal feeds over the 5–7 week growing period, whereas turkeys may be fed up to six feeds due to the longer growing period (4–6 months).

During the 'starter' phase (first 2–4 weeks) feeds contain the highest crude protein and calcium content to support initial skeletal development and muscle growth.

For meat birds, feeds following the starter diet have a reduced protein, calcium and phosphorus content, but higher levels of carbohydrates and fats to support growth and increasing maintenance requirements. For laying birds, during the rearing phase (0–16 weeks), the feeds generally have a reduced carbohydrate, fat and protein content due to slower growth rates and length of time to reach sexual maturity (18–20 weeks for commercial layer breeds). Vitamin, mineral and trace element levels in feeds tend to decrease as the bird ages (and increases in bodyweight) due to the higher feed consumption.

Adult laying and breeding birds

Adult laying birds require feed that adequately meets their maintenance requirements plus the demands of egg production. Commercially available layer diets typically contain moderate protein levels (15–17%) and energy (11–11.5 MJ/kg) levels. Calcium levels are significantly higher than those in feeds for growing birds (e.g. 4% *versus* 1%) in order to support eggshell calcification and medullary bone mineralization, which acts as a labile reserve of calcium. The vitamin, mineral and trace element requirements of adult layers remain relatively constant throughout the laying period. For breeding birds, where the intention is to hatch the eggs, an adequate supply of vitamins and trace elements is essential to ensure embryo survival and chick viability. For this reason it is necessary to feed a specific breeder diet because standard layer diets do not provide adequate levels of micronutrients.

Adult non-productive or ornamental birds

Adult birds that are neither growing nor laying require sufficient carbohydrates, fats, proteins, minerals, vitamins and trace elements to support maintenance and normal activity. Maintenance (or holding) diets are typically lower in proteins, carbohydrates and fats compared with feeds for growing and laying birds.

Feeds and feeding
Natural diets

In the wild, poultry are omnivores, scavenging a variety of grains, nuts, leaves and insects. These are all consumed to provide the bird with sufficient nutrients to satisfy their energy requirements for their productive state (e.g. laying birds would naturally eat more grain to provide the energy needed for egg production, than fully grown and non-producing adult birds). Each natural food has a different nutrient composition, thus eating a combination of food sources ensures that a nutrient deficiency in one foodstuff is offset by the nutrients contained within another.

> In general, birds tend to avoid toxic plants due to the bitter taste. Guidance on which plants to avoid is provided by the Poultry Club of Great Britain (www.poultryclub.org/poultry/poisonous-plants-and-toxins). The list includes: rhubarb leaves; rapeseed; yew; laburnum seeds; potato sprouts; sweet pea; ragwort; meadow buttercup; oleander; henbane; moist irises; vetch; clematis; corn cockle; privet; black nightshade; rhododendron; castor bean; common St John's Wort; and some fungi. However, there are often no specific data or references supporting toxicity for many of these plants and their inclusion in the list is based purely on anecdotal evidence

Complete feeds

The nutritional requirements of backyard poultry can be generally satisfied by feeding a commercially available complete feed. Complete feeds are formulated by trained and experienced nutritionists to ensure that they are adequately balanced in all essential nutrients. These feeds undergo numerous quality control checks and analyses, from raw material intake through to finished product, to ensure consistent nutrient composition is achieved.

A compound feed is preferable to home-mixing to ensure that birds receive a balanced and nutritionally adequate diet. It is also advisable to purchase feed that has been supplied by a feed compounder approved under an appropriate assurance scheme (e.g. Universal Feed Assurance Scheme (UFAS) in the UK) who are independently audited to ensure that they meet specific quality and safety standards.

Ingredient composition

The nutritional values of some common feed ingredients are summarized in Figure 5.1.

Cereal grains (mainly wheat; Figure 5.2a) typically contribute >50% of the feed and are selected on the basis of their nutrient composition and relative cost. Grains are primarily added due to the source of energy they provide, but also contribute to the total protein level of the diet. The protein content of cereal grains alone is not enough to meet the bird's requirement, therefore other ingredients are required to increase the overall protein content in the feed. Common protein sources used by UK feed compounders include soya bean meal (Figure 5.2b), extracted rapeseed, extracted sunflower seed, fishmeal and legumes such as peas and beans.

Fats and oils are included in poultry feeds because they provide a very high energy source (see Figure 5.1). Commonly used fats in UK poultry feeds include:

- Vegetable oils (soya, rapeseed, sunflower, maize oil)
- Commercial fat blends (blends of vegetable oils, acid oils and used cooking oils).

Feed additives

Coccidiosis is a common protozoal disease affecting the intestinal tract of birds, leading to enteritis and consequently having an adverse effect on health and productivity. Coccidiosis spreads through contact with contaminated faeces, therefore in commercial practice anticoccidials (often denoted as ACS on feed labels) are included in the feed for growing birds (particularly broilers and turkeys).

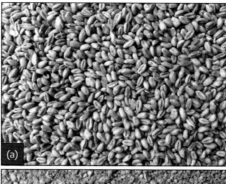
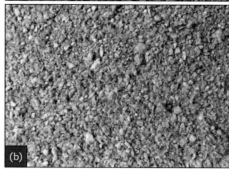

5.2 Key ingredients used in complete poultry feeds. (a) Wheat grains. (b) Extracted and toasted soya bean meal.

Prophylactic use is preferred as infection can occur before clinical signs are seen. Immunity develops over time and thus it is not necessary to use anticoccidials beyond a certain age and in adult birds. Precise instructions regarding the maximum age for feeding anticoccidials and any contraindications are given on the feed label.

> In commercial broiler production, anticoccidials are usually withdrawn before slaughter to meet regulatory requirements. A plain diet can be fed to meat birds prior to slaughter to ensure that the appropriate withdrawal period is adhered to (refer to the feed label for further information)

It is also increasingly common for layer/breeder replacement birds to be vaccinated against the main species of coccidians, thus removing the need to treat the feed. Inclusion of an authorized product in the drinking water may provide an alternative approach for the treatment and control of coccidiosis.

Exogenous enzymes (such as xylanases, glucanases and phytases) are routinely added to poultry feeds, which helps to combat the anti-nutritive effects of raw diets. Permitted yellow and red colourants are normally included in feeds for laying birds to ensure adequate colouring of the egg yolk.

Feed form

Commercial feed is available as meal (also referred to as mash), crumbs and pellets (Figure 5.3). Young growing birds are normally fed crumbs for the first few weeks of life (up to approximately 2–4 weeks of age) because the small particle size ensures they receive an adequate intake of feed. Pellets minimize selection of feed ingredients by the bird and are usually preferred for most backyard flocks as they reduce food wastage, which can attract pests and rodents. Bearded and crested fowl are more suited to pellets to avoid accumulation of mash in their beards or topknots, which could cause their companions to peck and spoil their feathers.

Component	Wheat	Wheat feed	Soya bean meal (Hi-Pro)	Sunflower seed extraction	Soya bean oil	Fishmeal
Crude protein (%)	10.7	15.4	47	28–36	0	66
Energy (MJ/kg)	13	8.5	10.3	6.2–7.5	38.3	12.85
Oil (%)	2.3	4.5	2.6	2.4–2.6	98.5	7.7
Methionine (%)	0.17	0.22	0.65	0.62–0.78	0	1.75

5.1 Nutritional composition of some ingredients used in complete feeds for poultry.
(Data from Premier Atlas, 2014)

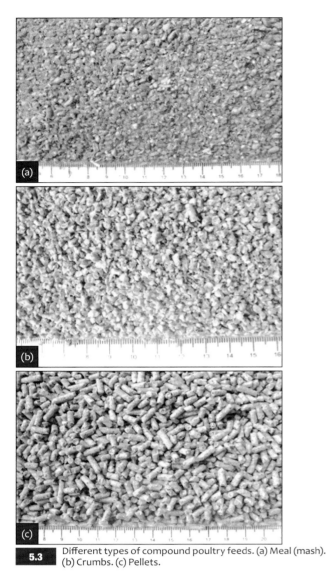

5.3 Different types of compound poultry feeds. (a) Meal (mash). (b) Crumbs. (c) Pellets.

A mash diet offers advantages, depending on the type of bird and the intended use. Feeding a mash diet keeps birds busy for longer, as it is harder to consume large quantities quickly, and thus helps to prevent excess feed consumption. Smaller birds, such as bantams, may struggle to consume standard layer pellets, so offering feed in meal form helps ensure adequate feed intake. Alternatively, smaller pellets which are produced for ornamental breeds can be used.

Feed troughs should be regularly cleaned to remove any build-up of feed and to prevent spoilage.

Commonly available complete feeds

There is a variety of complete poultry feeds available from feed/agricultural merchants, country stores, garden centres, pet shops and via the internet. The most common include:

- Chick or starter crumb (± anticoccidials)
- Grower pellets
- Layers pellets or layers meal
- Breeder pellets.

In addition, it is also possible to source age-specific diets for waterfowl (ducks and geese), turkeys, pheasants and ornamental breeds, as well as specific fattening diets for meat birds.

Feed storage

Feed should be stored in a cool and dry environment, out of direct sunlight and inaccessible to rodents, wild birds and other wild animals. It is essential to ensure the feed stays dry because if the moisture content becomes elevated there is the potential for the growth of mould and the production of mycotoxins, which can be detrimental to the health and production of the bird. Vitamins slowly degrade with time; therefore, feed should be consumed by the specific expiry date on the feed label.

Practical guidance on feeding of complete diets

Ideally feed should be specific for the species and intended use (e.g. turkey feed for turkeys, waterfowl feed for ducks, layers feed for laying chickens). However, it is recognized that there may be a relatively restrictive range of feeds available for the range of backyard poultry covered in this manual. The section below provides some guidance on feeding based on commonly available complete feeds.

> It is advisable to always read the feed label for information on feeding guidelines and to ensure that there are no incompatibilities or contraindications with regard to the intended species

Growing birds: The main diets available are chick (and/or starter) crumbs (protein content typically 18–20%) and grower pellets (protein content typically 15–17%). These are typically designed for feeding to egg-laying chickens during their rearing phase (day 1 to around 16–18 weeks of age). In the absence of species-specific diets, these diets are suitable for feeding to growing chickens (meat-type), ducks, turkeys, geese, guinea fowl, peafowl and ornamental pheasants, although the growth rate may be slower.

- Geese obtain a significant proportion of their nutrients from grazing on grass; therefore, the level of feed supplementation depends on pasture availability.
- Game birds and peafowl have a higher protein requirement than other species, indicated by their natural diet which includes insects and vegetation. Preferably, feeds with protein levels higher than standard chick and grower feeds should be sourced.
- Turkeys also have a higher protein requirement, so using specific turkey feeds will ensure optimal growth rates.

Adult laying birds: The predominant type of feed available is pellets (or meal), which is primarily designed for feeding to laying chickens producing table eggs. The normal age for introduction of this diet is 16–18 weeks of age and the bird will remain on this feed throughout its productive cycle. In the absence of species-specific diets, this diet is suitable for feeding to adult birds of other species where the eggs are for consumption.

- For breeding birds it is necessary to use a suitable breeder feed to ensure optimum hatchability and chick survival.
- If laying free-range geese are being kept then it is advised to supplement their pasture intake with a layer diet to provide the birds with enough vitamins and minerals to support egg production.

Adult non-productive or ornamental birds: If available, it is preferable to provide a holding/maintenance feed to ensure that the minimum requirements for protein, carbohydrates and fats are met and that a balanced supply of vitamins and trace elements is provided. A typical plain poultry grower diet offers a suitable compromise if specific feeds are not available.

Non-processed feeds, whole grains and forage

Complete feeds have been carefully formulated to contain a balance of all essential nutrients. Consumption of any additional sources of feed/forage will very likely lead to an imbalance (and potential deficiency) in the nutrient intake of the bird and have a detrimental effect on health and productivity.

> When using a complete feed, the use of supplementary feed or forage (e.g. whole or mixed grains and vegetables from the garden) should be discouraged to avoid an imbalance in nutrient supply. Young rapidly growing birds and laying birds with a high rate of egg production are particularly susceptible to an imbalance in nutrient supply

However, it is not uncommon for owners to feed backyard poultry a variety of supplementary feeds, including whole grains and kitchen scraps. Thus, where supplementary feeding is practised, it should be limited to a maximum of 10–15% of the bird's daily diet, to minimize the impact on overall nutrient supply.

> In the European Union, the feeding of kitchen scraps is *illegal* and is deemed a potential food safety risk. (The reader is referred to the Animal Health and Plant Agency (https://www.gov.uk/guidance/supplying-and-using-animal-by-products-as-farm-animal-feed) for further information.) Readers in other regions should adhere to local regulations to ensure that both animal health and food safety are maintained

Birds with access to a range or scratch area will exhibit foraging behaviour and, depending on the availability of natural food, this may represent a significant proportion of their daily diet and directly impact daily nutrient intake. The proportion of natural food *versus* complete feed should be considered when investigating problems that may be related to nutritional deficiencies. Access to long grass should be avoided, as should feeding grass clippings, as the crop can become impacted, which may subsequently lead to starvation.

Whilst not essential, supplementary grit may be offered as this helps assist digestion of the feed through the grinding action of the ventriculus. Birds with access to a range will naturally pick up grit. For laying birds, complete feeds contain adequate calcium to support eggshell formation. However, oyster shell may be provided as a supplementary calcium source, either mixed in with the feed (at a rate of up to 2.5 g/kg of feed) or offered in a separate feeder (at a rate of up to 3 g/bird per day).

Feed labels

European Commission (EC) Labelling Regulations (No. 767/2009) specify the precise information that feed compounders are legally obliged to include on all feed labels. A label should be attached to each individual bag of feed (or the accompanying paperwork for bulk deliveries). An example of a feed label is shown in Figure 5.4.

Most sections of the label are self-explanatory, but the following notes provide additional information to assist with interpretation:

5.4 An example of a label for layer pellets. UFAS = Universal Feed Assurance Scheme; VMD = Veterinary Medicines Directorate.

- Analytical constituents:
  - This does not include all of the nutrients within the feed, just those that require declaration
  - All nutrients in this section are covered by permitted tolerances detailed in European Commission Regulation No. 939/2010
  - Crude ash – essentially a measure of the total mineral (organic) content in the feed
  - Crude fibre – predominately comprises cellulose, lignins, pectins and hemicellulose.
- Composition:
  - A list of the ingredients in descending order, including an indication of any genetically modified (GM) derived materials
  - Wheat flour – the by-product from flour milling
  - Soya bean meal (extracted and toasted) – by-product from the extraction of oil (soy oil) from soya beans
  - Sunflower seed extraction – by-product from the extraction of oil from sunflower seeds
  - Calcium carbonate – a source of calcium from limestone
  - Mono calcium phosphate – a source of calcium and phosphorus
  - Sodium chloride – a source of sodium and chloride from salt
  - Sodium bicarbonate – a source of sodium
  - DL methionine and lysine hydrochloride (HCl) – synthetic amino acids.

- Additives:
  - Vitamin A and D3 are compulsory declarations. The declaration of vitamin E is voluntary
  - Trace elements declared as the level of the element added to the feed
  - Antioxidant – included to protect certain ingredients (e.g. vitamins) against oxidative degradation
  - Colourants – included to ensure an acceptable yolk colour is achieved. Lutein and zeaxanthin are 'yellow' xanthophylls, which are commonly derived from marigolds. Capsanthin is a 'red' xanthophyll, typically derived from red peppers.

References and further reading

Leeson S and Summers JD (2001) *Scott's Nutrition of the Chicken, 4th edn.* University Books, Canada

Leeson S and Summers JD (2004) *Commercial Poultry Nutrition, 3rd edn.* Nottingham University Press, Nottingham

National Research Council (1994) *Nutrient Requirements of Poultry, 9th revised edn.* The National Academies Press, Washington

Verhoef E and Rijs A (2003) *The Complete Encyclopedia of Chickens, 2nd edn.* Rebo Publishers, The Netherlands

Useful websites

Premier Nutrition Poultry Technical Services
https://www.premiernutrition.co.uk/poultry/poultry-technical-services

The Department for Environment, Food and Rural Affairs (Defra)
https://www.gov.uk/government/organisations/department-for-environment-food-rural-affairs

The Poultry Club of Great Britain
http://www.poultryclub.org/

Chapter 6

Handling, transportation and hospitalization

Guy Poland and Aidan Raftery

Handling and restraint

Poultry need to be handled for many reasons. The owner may need to handle the birds to move them in or out of housing, for transportation purposes, to examine them for problems and to administer medication. In addition, poultry may be handled for petting or showing purposes (Figure 6.1). For clinical staff, good handling of poultry is essential to enable meaningful examination and for the administration of treatment. Capture, handling and restraint must be carried out in a way that minimizes stress and the risk of injury. It is important to remember that birds caught and handled in a veterinary context may have pathology and the technique used should not put pressure on or exacerbate such problems.

Chickens

Herding chickens into a small area will aid capture and reduce unnecessary stress caused by a lengthy chase. Some hens will crouch when approached, making them easy to pick up. With other birds it may be necessary to place a hand firmly but gently over the dorsum or to place a hand over each wing. Under certain circumstances, it may be more efficient and less stressful to use a net to capture chickens. Birds must be removed carefully from the net to avoid injury.

The ideal way to lift and carry a chicken is to place one hand on the dorsum to prevent the bird from flapping its wings. The other hand is then slid under the ventrum from a cranial direction and one leg held between the little finger and ring finger, with the other leg held between the index finger and thumb. The bird is then lifted and held across the handler's waist (Figure 6.2). Some procedures, such as oral drug administration, can be performed by an assistant whilst the chicken is restrained in this way. For information on restraint for clinical examination, see Chapter 8.

Chickens can also be carried with one hand placed over each wing (Figure 6.3), although care must be taken to ensure that the bird's breathing is not impaired by excessive pressure. Traditionally and commercially, chickens are often held and carried by the shanks; however, this is not recommended in the context of backyard poultry as it is more likely to cause distress, discomfort or injury to the bird. Chickens should never be carried by the neck or wings.

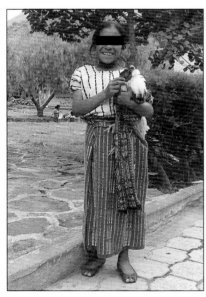

6.1 A young girl on the shores of Lake Atitlan, Guatemala, holding her prize cockerel.

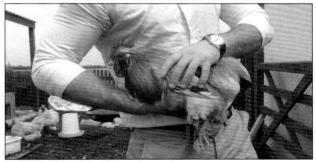

6.2 A bantam cockerel being held with one hand supporting the keel and restraining the legs, and the other hand preventing the wings from being flapped.

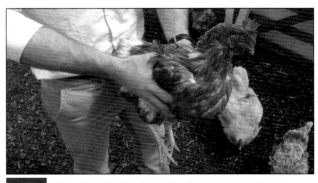

6.3 A hen being held with one hand supporting each wing.

Hens are rarely aggressive towards the handler, but the person handling the bird should always be aware of the possibility of being pecked or scratched, and should not hold the bird too close to their eyes. Some cockerels may be quite aggressive and can cause considerable damage with their well developed spurs. It may be beneficial to wrap an aggressive or flighty chicken in a towel, but care must be taken to ensure that the bird's breathing is not restricted.

Ducks and geese

Ducks and geese should not be caught or handled by their legs due to the risk of injury. It is acceptable to grasp ducks and geese by the neck in order to catch them but, once caught, they should be immediately restrained properly in order to prevent injury. The use of an appropriately designed hook can assist with the capture of ducks and geese, but this should be used with caution.

The bird can be lifted by holding the neck with one hand and wrapping the other arm around the bird's body to support its weight and prevent flapping (Figure 6.4). Care is required to ensure that excessive pressure is not applied when holding the neck, as this may result in tearing of the skin or cause other soft tissue damage. Geese should never be lifted by the neck alone and it is not recommended to lift ducks in this manner.

Ducks and geese can also be restrained, lifted and carried with one hand under the keel and the legs supported between the fingers. When carrying the bird, it may be helpful to tuck the head under the upper arm (Figure 6.5). Geese may also be caught and carried by holding both shoulder joints.

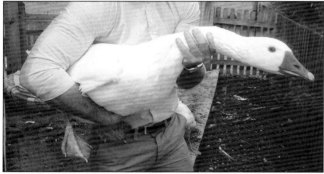

6.4 A goose being held under one arm with the neck restrained with the other hand.

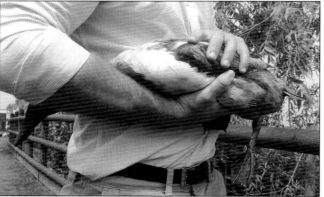

6.5 A duck being supported in a similar manner to the chicken in Figure 6.2, but the head has been placed under the handler's arm to offer further restraint and to calm the duck.

To reduce the risk of biting, it is important to have good control of the head of the goose. Muscovy ducks have sharp claws, so it is advisable to wear thick gloves when handling these birds. A swan bag can be useful to keep geese and large ducks restrained for short periods of time. In addition, ducks are relatively amenable to being walked in groups and this should be considered as an alternative to handling where appropriate (Figure 6.6).

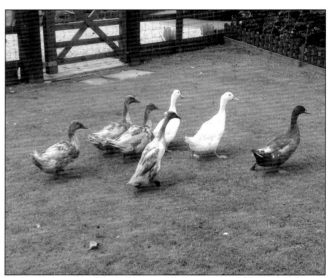

6.6 A group of ducks being herded around a paddock, avoiding the need to handle the birds directly.

Turkeys

Turkeys should be caught and carried by grasping the furthest shoulder in one hand and holding the legs together in the other hand. The turkey should then be lifted and held firmly against the body. Adult turkeys can also be carried by holding both shoulder joints. Young turkeys can be carried with one hand under the keel, supporting the legs between the fingers, and the other hand holding the wings. Turkeys should never be carried by the wings, head, neck, tail or legs.

Guinea fowl

Guinea fowl are captured by placing both hands over the wings. The birds are lifted and carried in a similar way to chickens, with one hand supporting the keel and holding the legs between the fingers and the other hand holding the wings. Guinea fowl are relatively intolerant of handling, and thus a firm grip is required. Guinea fowl should not be carried by the legs.

Ornamental pheasants and peafowl

Ornamental pheasants and peafowl vary considerably in terms of how amenable they are to handling, but are usually flighty and may require netting. As with many species, capture is aided by low light levels. Ornamental pheasants can be caught by placing one hand over each wing. They can be lifted and carried in this manner, or by supporting the keel and legs with one hand and the wings with the other hand. Peafowl are caught in the same manner as ornamental pheasants. They can be carried by wrapping one arm around the body and holding the legs together with the other hand.

Transportation

Most backyard poultry are only transported once from the breeder to their new home. Birds that are bred on the holding may never require transportation. However, some owners may need to transport birds to a veterinary practice and others may wish to show their birds at poultry exhibitions. It is important that birds are transported in a manner that protects them from injury and minimizes stress.

Requirements for transportation

Legislation exists regarding the transportation of all animals, including poultry. Unnecessary suffering must be prevented in all cases, but many specific requirements apply only to transportation for commercial purposes (see Chapter 26). Unless they are being taken to or from a place for veterinary treatment, sick and injured birds should not be transported. Chemical restraint is rarely indicated or appropriate for transporting poultry and is seldom used.

In general terms, the following factors should be considered prior to transportation:

- Container construction
- Space
- Sound, motion and light
- Thermal comfort and ventilation
- Food and water
- Bedding.

Container construction

Containers must be of a suitable construction and material to prevent physical injury and allow good hygiene.

Space

Birds must be provided with enough space during transportation to allow some movement, but this should be limited to reduce the risk of injury. The presence of conspecifics may have a beneficial effect in reducing stress.

Sound, motion and light

The motion of the vehicle should be considered and driving style and routes adapted to minimize excessive movements during transportation. The vehicle should be kept as quiet as possible and birds should not be transported with other animals (such as dogs). Low lighting levels have a calming effect and reduce stress.

Thermal comfort and ventilation

Ventilation and temperature must be controlled to ensure that birds are able to thermoregulate and that carbon dioxide does not build up within the container. Although birds are susceptible to both hyperthermia and hypothermia, overheating is more likely to be encountered, often due to insufficient air flow.

Food and water

The provision of food and water during transportation needs to be considered. This is of greater importance for long distance journeys, where it should be provided either on a continuous basis or at regular intervals. However, it should also be recognized that providing water may not be practical since spillage can cause problems. In the UK,

poultry transport regulations require that food and water are provided after a maximum of 12 hours for adult birds and 24 hours for chicks, provided that the journey is completed within 72 hours of hatching. Where food and/or drink is not provided during transportation, it is essential that it is provided up until the start of the journey and as soon as the birds are unloaded.

Bedding

Bedding should be provided in the container to reduce the risk of the birds damaging their feet and to absorb faeces.

Capture and release

Birds must be captured and released in a calm manner to minimize stress; good handler training can help to achieve this. It is recommended that the flock is herded into a small area before an attempt is made to catch the bird(s) required. If possible, birds should be captured in an environment with low lighting levels, as this will have a calming effect (this is easier for poultry housed in barns). Sufficient time should be allocated to ensure that capture is not undertaken in a hurry, but not completed so far in advance of transportation that the caught bird is left in the container for an extended period of time. Birds should be unloaded and released as soon after transportation as possible.

Contingency planning

Sufficient food and water should be carried for birds being transported in case of unforeseen delays. Where hypothermia or hyperthermia is a particular concern, provision should be made to keep the birds cool or warm (as required) in the case of a vehicle breakdown.

Transporting chickens, guinea fowl and pheasants

Chickens, guinea fowl and pheasants are best transported in solid-sided boxes. The solid sides reduce light levels, which has a calming effect on the birds. There should be a sufficient number of ventilation holes, and top-loading boxes reduce the stress when lifting birds in and out. In hot weather, containers with wire mesh sides or top may be required to allow adequate ventilation. The holes in the mesh should not be large enough to allow the bird to stick its head through, since this would render it vulnerable to injury. Wire mesh floors should not be used since these may cause injury to the feet. Wooden shavings or straw should be used to line the container, to increase the bird's grip during transportation and reduce the risk of foot injury. A suitable substrate will also provide some environmental enrichment and help to reduce the mess from faeces.

Boxes must be of sufficient height to allow the bird to stand upright and wide enough to allow some movement, but not to enable the bird to spread its wings as this may result in injury. Cat carriers are frequently unsuitable as they are often front-loading and not of sufficient height. However, disposable top-loading cardboard pet carriers are often an ideal size and have the advantage of being more hygienic because they are used on a single occasion and then discarded. Wooden boxes, whilst durable, can be difficult to disinfect thoroughly between uses.

Multiple birds can be transported together, which may help to reduce stress levels, but they should be from the same cohort. Individuals vulnerable to pecking (e.g. those with an open wound) are best transported alone. Cockerels should not be transported together in the same container. Particular attention should be paid to the ambient temperature within the box when multiple individuals are carried, since it is likely to rise more quickly. It is important that the boxes are properly secured in the vehicle to prevent excessive movement. If birds from different cohorts are being transported in different containers but within the same vehicle, careful consideration of biosecurity is needed, and boxes should be placed as far apart as possible to reduce the risk of disease transmission.

Hypothermia can be a problem when transporting chicks. This is primarily controlled by using a relatively smaller box with a larger number of chicks to conserve heat. An external heat source may be required. It is usually not appropriate to provide bedding in the container as there is a risk the chicks will eat it.

Commercially, poultry are often transported in modular crate systems. The use of such systems is beyond the scope of this Manual.

Transporting ducks and geese

Ducks and geese can be transported using similar principles to those described above for chickens, but they are more susceptible to overheating due to their thick insulation. Wire mesh cages (with a solid floor) may therefore be more suitable than solid boxes, especially during warmer weather. A water mister can be useful for keeping birds cool, especially in the case of heat stress. Waterfowl can also be transported in large numbers in a suitable low trailer. They can be walked up a ramp into the trailer, which is likely to be less stressful than direct handling. There should be a sufficient number of ducks in the trailer to prevent excessive movement. It is important that there are no sharp edges in the trailer that might cause damage to the duck's feet. Bedding (such as straw) should be used to line the floor of the transportation (Figure 6.7). It is often beneficial to transport ducks that get on well together or bonded geese as a group to reduce stress to the birds.

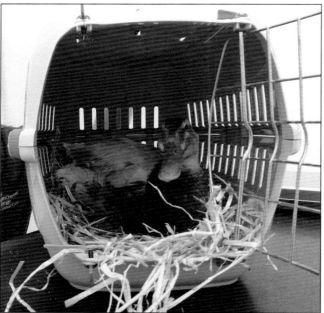

6.7 An example of a suitable front-loading transportation carrier for a duck.

Ducks and geese, like all other poultry, should not be transported loose in the cabin of a car or on the lap of an owner since this presents an unreasonable risk of injury to both the bird and human occupants, as well as of the bird escaping. It would also constitute an unsecured load and may be illegal in many jurisdictions. It is not acceptable to transport ducks and geese with their legs tied. It may be appropriate to use a swan bag (or similar) during transportation, but this should only be used when necessary and it is often not required.

Transporting turkeys

Turkeys can be transported in a similar way to chickens but their larger size and weight may demand sturdier containers. Turkeys may also be transported in low trailers.

Transporting peafowl

Peafowl without a train can be transported in a similar manner to chickens, although a fully grown peahen will require a larger box than an adult chicken. A specially constructed long box is required to transport peacocks with a full train in order to accommodate its whole length. It is also possible to improvise a tail guard where an appropriate transportation box is unavailable.

Additional requirements for ill or injured birds

Ill or injured birds may require additional bedding to support them during transportation. They may also require additional heat sources, especially if they are showing signs of shock, and may be more vulnerable to stress from outside stimuli such as noise.

Hospital facilities

Most of the species covered in this manual are relatively large birds with special hospitalization requirements. Birds should be accommodated away from dogs, cats and other potential predators to minimize stress. The ideal avian ward should have lighting that can be dimmed to provide visual security. However, a similar effect can be achieved by covering the front of the hospital cage. Hospital cages should be of a size that the bird can be captured easily but still large enough that the bird can extend their wings in all directions and turn around without damaging their plumage (Figure 6.8). Species with large tails that are especially vulnerable to damage (e.g. Indian peafowl) should be fitted with tail guards during hospitalization.

Enclosures for waterfowl may be more difficult to provide as the birds should have access to water. In a hospital setting, this can be provided in the form of a large tub or a built-in depression in the floor. Providing the opportunity to swim has many benefits for waterfowl. The minimum depth of the water should allow the bird to submerge its head. Many species need to be able to wet their plumage completely; if for medical reasons this is not advisable, then the bird should be sprayed a minimum of twice daily to promote preening. Thick rubber matting (or equivalent) should be provided as a preventive measure for the heavier birds as pododermatitis can develop if they are hospitalized for more than a very short period of time. Turkeys are also prone to pododermatitis if they stand still for long periods, especially when circulation is compromised by a disease

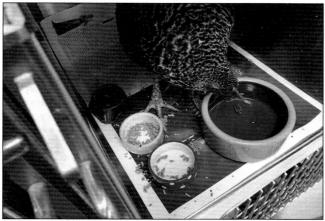

6.8 Accommodation for a chicken in a hospital ward. Note the heavy ceramic bowls which are used to provide food and water.

process. A thermometer and hydrometer should be visible in each enclosure so that the temperature and humidity can be monitored. Hyperthermia is more of a risk than hypothermia when poultry are hospitalized.

The substrate used must have a low risk of being ingested and causing a gastrointestinal obstruction. Hay is contraindicated as it commonly causes crop impactions, especially in chickens. Newspaper should be used as it is safe, clean and any droppings passed can be easily seen.

Appropriate food should be available. If a bird is being fed an unusual diet, then the owner should be asked to provide some of the feed for the hospitalization period. Birds are more likely to eat familiar foods whilst hospitalized. Food is usually provided in heavy ceramic bowls. In some instances, scattering the food on the floor can stimulate feeding behaviour, although this has to be balanced against the risk of faecal contamination of the food. Water should always be available.

The chicks of poultry are precocial and when hospitalized should not be kept alone. The required temperature for the accommodation is dependent upon the age and species of the bird. Chicks are often presented in a collapsed hypothermic and dehydrated state, requiring immediate intensive care (see Chapter 8).

Intensive care unit

Ideally an intensive care unit where the temperature is thermostatically controlled should be available (Figure 6.9). This will facilitate the best treatment for hypothermic collapsed cases. These units often also allow controlled humidity, which can be invaluable.

If an intensive care unit is not available, it may be possible to improvise. It is important to ensure that the correct temperature is not provided at the expense of adequate ventilation. Care must also be taken to ensure that the patient does not become hyperthermic or receive a localized thermal injury from prolonged contact with a moderate heat source such as a hot water bottle or 'hot hands' (latex gloves filled with hot water and used as disposable hot water bottles). These heat sources are most commonly associated with localized thermal injuries in debilitated or anaesthetized animals. This type of injury is not recognized at the time of occurrence but seen a few days later when the cause and effect may not be linked. Any hypothermic bird in contact with a heat source should be monitored every 15–20 minutes until stable. The supporting temperature will need to be reduced as the bird becomes normothermic to avoid hyperthermia. This is especially

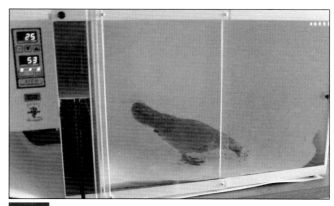

6.9 Intensive care unit.

important if the bird is unable to move or has reduced sensation. Forced air-warming systems are now available in many veterinary practices and can be used with air blankets to provide safe thermal support.

Cages should also be available in which oxygen and/or nebulization can be effectively delivered. These cages are smaller than the normal hospital enclosures, so when they are in use it is even more important to monitor temperatures.

Equipment

Much of the equipment required for avian patients will already be available in a small animal veterinary practice. Listed below are some of the extra items that should be stocked for use with poultry. Many of these items will not be used on a daily basis, but when they are required may be essential.

- A swan bag can be very useful for handling geese or other large birds. If this is not available, a selection of clean towels can be used instead. Covering the head with a breathable towel can have a calming effect by removing stressful stimuli.
- Weighing scales capable of weighing in increments suitable for the sizes of bird seen are essential (see Chapter 8).
- Microcontainers for the collection and processing of blood samples are required for individuals where size imposes limitations on the sample volume that can be collected.
- Endoscopy is a very useful diagnostic technique in birds; however, they can usually be referred for this procedure. In cases of tracheal obstruction, an air sac tube can be placed prior to referral.
- Feeding tubes and needles of different sizes should be available for crop feeding and administering medication by gavage. Orogastric tubes used for canine and feline patients will be suitable for larger birds. Foods suitable for feeding via tube can be very useful; however, normal pelleted rations can be ground down for tube feeding if required. Critical cases may require enteral feeding (see Chapter 8).
- Intraosseous catheters are needed to provide fluid therapy in collapsed birds where vascular access is difficult.
- Uncuffed endotracheal tubes in a range of sizes are required for anaesthesia. Air sac tubes should also be available to manage tracheal obstructions in an emergency. Ventilators are very useful during longer surgical procedures, although manual ventilation can be employed as an alternative. Capnometry and the ability

to measure blood pressure and monitor body temperature greatly improve the safety of anaesthesia. Blood pressure measurement and body temperature monitoring also facilitate better management of critical cases.

Staff training

Staff working in veterinary practices that deal with avian clinical cases should be provided with the appropriate training. Receptionists should have some training in how to recognize cases that need to be seen immediately but if there is any doubt they should hand the call over to a suitably qualifed person for telephone triage and first aid advice (i.e. veterinary surgeon or veterinary nurse with suitable qualifications/experience). They should also be able to provide owners with instructions on the safe transport of birds to the veterinary practice.

Veterinary surgeons (veterinarians) and nurses should be trained in rapid and proficient capture, otherwise handling will be a very stressful experience for the bird, which may have a negative effect on its recovery. Staff must be able to recognize the signs of illness and be capable of providing supportive care in these cases. Veterinary surgeons and support staff should be experienced in resuscitation techniques for birds (see Chapter 8). This is an ongoing process as recommended protocols are subject to change. In addition, veterinary staff may benefit from visiting a specialist avian practice.

A reference library with relevant textbooks and journals should be provided. Joining organizations such as the Association of Avian Veterinarians, attending continuing education courses on avian medicine, and attending conferences where avian medicine topics are presented are also strongly recommended to keep up to date with current best practice.

Chapter 7

Preventive healthcare

Guy Poland

As in other fields of veterinary medicine, strives should be made to move from a reactive healthcare programme to a preventive one. Preventive healthcare strategies ensure maximal welfare as well as saving time and expense in treating avoidable disease. Correct nutrition (see Chapter 5) and good husbandry (see Chapter 4) are essential prerequisites for preventive healthcare. This chapter discusses the implementation of health plans and focuses on vaccination and parasite control in particular. Other considerations covered include wing clipping, pest control, hygiene and biosecurity. See Chapter 4 for more information on hygiene protocols and husbandry routines.

Health plans

A health plan can take many forms, from general written advice to flock-specific verbal or written strategies. By considering and formulating a health plan, poultry keepers will become more in tune with the needs of their flocks. The development of tailored health plans is an excellent opportunity for veterinary surgeons (veterinarians) to offer their clients good quality advice and will help to enhance the client–clinician bond.

A health plan should consider the following areas:

- Housing
- Outdoor ranges
- Feeding and water
- Flock behaviour
- Procedures for introducing new stock
- Hygiene practices
- External disease risks
- Identification of health issues.

As a result of this analysis, appropriate measures should be recommended. Where these measures require a one-off action, a target deadline for completion should be proposed. For regular measures, such as cleaning and disinfection, it is useful to design a routine with daily, weekly, monthly and seasonal jobs. A target date should be set for review of the health plan. The time interval between reviews will vary according to the needs of the flock, but 6-monthly health plan reviews accompanied by a site visit might be appropriate in many cases. This may allow the clinician to ensure that the flock can be legitimately regarded as under their care, which is a key component of responsible prescribing practice.

Vaccination

Vaccination of commercial poultry flocks is commonplace. Morbidity and mortality due to infectious disease can cause significant financial losses, the cost of which will far outweigh that of vaccination programmes. However, vaccination of small flocks is relatively rare due to cost, availability and a lack of planning. Frequently, small flocks contain birds from many different sources, which may be of different vaccination status.

Vaccination should be based on a risk–benefit analysis. Risk is calculated by multiplying the likelihood of an event happening by the severity of such an event. This can be carried out subjectively or on a quantitative basis by assigning a value to categories of risk and severity. For vaccination of poultry, this can be summarized as:

Vaccinate when:

(Likelihood of adverse reactions x severity of adverse reactions) + cost of vaccine + cost of administration + potential production losses

is less than

(Likelihood of disease x severity of disease x value of the bird) + (likelihood and severity of disease in humans).

There may be circumstances where the vaccination of poultry may be prohibited or mandated (e.g. in the case of a national disease outbreak), thus overriding an individual flock risk–benefit analysis.

Figure 7.1 lists the vaccines currently available for the prevention of poultry diseases in the UK. Several preparations may be available for a given disease. Some vaccine preparations are only available on veterinary prescription (POM-V), whilst others may be supplied by a veterinary surgeon, pharmacist or suitably qualified person (POM-VPS).

Vaccines are available through normal veterinary supply chains or direct from manufacturers (with the exception of avian influenza). Unfortunately, most vaccines are only sold in multi-dose packages to administer to large numbers of birds. Such packages (e.g. vials of freeze-dried vaccine) usually need to be administered immediately upon opening. This will lead to a lot of waste in small flocks, making administration uneconomical by commercial standards. However, the cost may still be accessible to owners of backyard poultry. Often breed associations may organize sharing of a vaccine package between several owners. This may be a practical solution in some cases, but attention must be given to correct prescribing procedures and biosecurity.

Disease	Target birds	Typical age	Route of administration	Duration of immunity	Available in combination vaccine	Minimum number of doses
Avian encephalomyelitis virus	Breeder hen progeny	Before lay	In water	12 months in progeny	No	1000
Avian infectious laryngotracheitis	Pre-lay chickens	Growers	Eye drop	One laying period	No	1000
Avian influenza	Chickens, ducks, other bird species	Growers	i.m. or s.c.	12 months	No	1000
Avian pneumovirus	Breeder, broiler and pre-lay chickens	Young chicks then before lay	In water, eye drop or spray	3 weeks or as a primer	Yes	1000
Avian rhinotracheitis virus	Broiler and future layer and breeding chickens	Day-old and/or growers	Eye drop, nasal drop, spray or i.m.	16 weeks or one laying period	Yes	250
Chicken anaemia virus	Broiler-breeder hen progeny	Growers then before lay	i.m. or s.c.	At least 10 weeks	No	500
Escherichia coli	Broiler-breeder hen progeny	Growers then before lay	i.m. or s.c.	First 7 weeks in progeny	No	500
Eimeria spp.	Chickens	Young chicks	In feed, water or spray	40 days to 36 weeks	No	1000
Erysipelas	Turkeys	Twice as growers	s.c.	23 weeks	No	500
Egg drop syndrome virus	Future laying and breeding hens	Before lay	i.m.	One laying period	Yes	1000
Infectious bursal disease virus	Chickens	Eggs, day-old and young growers	s.c., *in ovo*, spray or in water	At least 42 days	Yes	500
Infectious bronchitis virus	Chickens	Day-old onwards	Spray, eye drop, nose drop or in water	6 weeks	Yes	500
Marek's disease[a]	Chickens	Egg, day-old and up to lay	i.m., s.c. or *in ovo*	At least 4 weeks Antibodies persist for 2 years	Yes	1000
Mycoplasma gallisepticum	Future laying chickens	Growers	Spray	24 weeks	No	500
Mycoplasma synoviae	Laying chickens	Growers	Spray	44 weeks	No	500
Newcastle disease virus	Broiler, broiler-breeding and future laying chickens Turkeys	Day-old and young chicks	Spray, eye drop or oral	4–6 weeks	Yes	1000
Ornithobacterium rhinotracheale	Broiler-breeder progeny	Growers then before lay	i.m. or s.c.	43 weeks of lay to give first 14 days in progeny	No	1000
Pasteurella multocida	Future layer and breeder hens, ducks and turkeys	Twice as growers	s.c.	6–16 weeks	No	1000
Reovirus	Adult birds and their progeny	Growers	i.m. or s.c.	Susceptible period in progeny	Yes	1000
Salmonella spp.	Breeding and laying chickens and their progeny	Young chicks and growers then before lay	i.m. or orally	40 weeks; 14 days in progeny	No	500
Turkey rhinotracheitis virus	Turkeys (chickens)	Young chicks then as growers	i.m., spray or eye drop	6–9 weeks or laying period with booster	Yes	500

7.1 Summary of the typical properties of vaccines authorized for use in poultry species in the UK. [a] Some preparations are stored in liquid nitrogen.

Specific instructions for the storage and administration must be followed as per the vaccine datasheet. The reader is referred to Chapter 9 for general advice on different routes of drug administration. In some cases, the administration of a vaccine must take place at an age younger than the age at which an owner would acquire the bird. Indeed, some vaccines are intended to confer immunity to chicks of vaccinated stock via maternally derived antibodies. Where this is the case, it may be appropriate to advise poultry keepers to source vaccinated birds or eggs for hatching. Although many vaccines carry zero withdrawal periods, it is essential to check the market authorization as some do not.

As all vaccines currently available have been developed for the commercial market, the age of administration and duration of immunity are targeted towards production birds with a relatively short productive life span. Backyard poultry flocks often contain birds that live to an older age than commercial birds. Vaccine manufacturers may be able to provide immunity data for older birds and give advice on administration of vaccines to mature or geriatric birds.

Wing clipping

Traditionally, wing clipping is a commonly used technique performed by smallholders. It is employed to prevent poultry birds from flying at heights and distances that would be sufficient for them to escape their range. Usually, wing clipping does not prevent all flight and poultry may still escape if the boundaries are inadequate. The need for wing clipping and the technique used varies between poultry species.

The principles of the 'five freedoms' of animal welfare should be considered prior to recommending or carrying out wing clipping. In particular, animals should have the freedom to express normal behaviour and this freedom may be reduced as a result of wing clipping. Where possible, outdoor enclosures should be designed so that birds with normal wing plumage are unable to escape. This might involve higher fences or even fully enclosed outdoor spaces. Provision of sufficient environmental enrichment, space, shelter, food and water will all reduce the bird's drive to venture beyond its intended range.

Chickens

In practice, wing clipping is not often needed in backyard chicken flocks and should therefore be performed based on need rather than as a routine procedure. It is achieved by clipping the outer primary feathers of one wing to the level of the end of the primary coverts (Figure 7.2). Whilst both wings can be clipped, a unilateral approach is more successful since it makes flight unbalanced. It is important to ensure that there is no blood in the quill (typically following a moult) when the feather is clipped, in order to prevent profuse bleeding. Heavy duty scissors work well. Since feathers do not grow continuously, clipping will only need to be repeated once new feathers have grown after a moult (typically once a year for adults).

Turkeys

Domestic turkeys are typically too large to fly significant distances, although younger and/or smaller turkeys may be able to fly far enough to escape an enclosure. The primary feathers are clipped in the same way as those in chickens, and adult turkeys usually moult once a year. When kept with female turkeys, male turkeys do not require their wings to be clipped since they are unlikely to venture far from the females.

Ducks

A partial clip is usually performed in ducks. This differs from the technique described for chickens in that the outer two primary feathers are left intact. It is recommended to trim only one wing. Blood feathers must be avoided and clipped feathers will be replaced following a moult. It is often stated that moulting occurs twice a year, but in some types of duck it may occur on a yearly basis. Certain breeds are more likely to fly away than others (Figure 7.3). It should be noted that some light breed domestic ducks can flutter over a fence downhill with the help of a strong breeze.

Geese

As with ducks, the requirement to clip the wings of geese partly depends on the breed (see Figure 7.3). The same technique is used in geese as in chickens, and most geese typically moult twice a year (although some geese may only moult once a year).

Guinea fowl

The same technique is used in guinea fowl as in chickens, although it is often reported that guinea fowl can retain a surprising amount of flying ability following the procedure. Trimming of some or all of the secondary flight feathers may be of benefit in difficult cases.

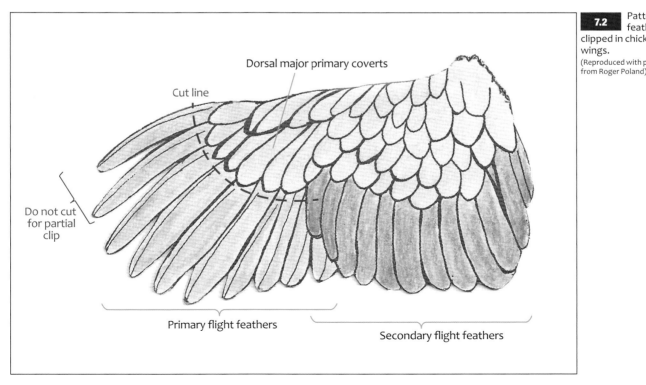

7.2 Pattern of feathers clipped in chicken wings.
(Reproduced with permission from Roger Poland)

Dorsal major primary coverts

Cut line

Do not cut for partial clip

Primary flight feathers

Secondary flight feathers

Duck breeds likely to need wing clipping

• All ornamental or wild ducks (e.g. mallard or any other wildfowl species, native or non-native if these have not already been pinioned)
• Domestic duck breeds such as:
  • Bantam
  • Black East Indian
  • Call
  • Muscovy (especially females)

Duck breeds unlikely to need wing clipping
• Any domestic ducks classified as light or heavy

Goose breeds likely to need wing clipping
• All ornamental or wildfowl (e.g. Canadian goose, greylag goose), or any other wild species, native or non-native if these have not already been pinioned

Goose breeds unlikely to need wing clipping
• Any domestic goose breeds

7.3 Summary of duck and geese breeds that may require wing clipping.
(Courtesy of Victoria Roberts)

Peafowl

Since peafowl typically roost in trees, wing clipping is controversial as it limits their ability to reach suitable perching sites. If wing clipping is desirable, it is recommended to start with a partial clip and to increase the number of primary feathers trimmed incrementally until a suitable balance is achieved between providing the bird with the ability to reach suitable perching sites and limiting its ability to roam.

Ornamental pheasants

Pheasants may have their wings clipped using the same technique as described for chickens. Ornamental pheasants are often kept in an aviary, which negates the need for wing clipping. Pinioning might be considered as an alternative strategy to control the flight of ornamental pheasants; it may be that a one-off pinioning procedure may cause less stress to the bird than repeated capture for wing clipping (see below). Adult pheasants typically moult once a year.

Pinioning

Pinioning is a technique used to restrict permanently the ability of a bird to fly and involves the surgical removal of the distal wing at the level of the fused metacarpal bone. The legality of this procedure varies between regions and in the UK is regarded as an act of veterinary surgery and is illegal in farmed birds. The technique for pinioning is discussed in Chapter 24.

Pest control

The term 'pest' is used to describe an animal that does not typically cause disease directly but instead may be a vector for infectious disease or which may cause destruction to the environment, including housing or feed supplies. Pest species encountered in relation to backyard poultry include rodents, wild birds and insects. Effective control of pests will reduce morbidity and mortality through transmitted diseases, food losses and spoiling, and damage to housing.

Rodents

Rodent species are an important reservoir for infectious disease. In the context of poultry species, they can be a source of *Yersinia pseudotuberculosis*, fowl cholera, avian influenza, *Campylobacter jejuni*, *Salmonella* spp. and infectious bronchitis infection. They can also consume large amounts of poultry feed, steal eggs and cause damage to housing, particularly if it is constructed from wood. Occasionally, rodents may also harm birds directly by biting them.

Rodents can be controlled either by increasing the resistance of housing to infestation and ensuring good husbandry, or by reducing the rodent population. Feed should be stored in a cool, dry place where there are no gaps to allow the entry of rodents. Structures should be inspected regularly for unintended gaps due to broken or loose materials or holes made by rodents, and any such damage should be swiftly repaired. Sheds and hutches that are sited on a concrete plinth are more resistant to rodents tunnelling under them. Any spilt food should be regularly cleared and not allowed to accumulate.

Rodent populations are often controlled through poisoning. In the UK and Europe, anticoagulant rodenticides (such as difenacoum) are most commonly used, whereas in North America, vitamin D-related poisons are more typically employed. Rodent traps that kill rodents using powerful spring-loaded mechanisms or electric shocks, shooting with air rifles or firearms and the use of predators such as cats and terrier breeds of dog may offer an alternative to poisons.

Before any programme of rodent population control is initiated, careful consideration of the ethics of such action is required. Equally, a thorough risk assessment of the effect on non-target species must be carried out. Livestock, pets and, importantly, wildlife may be harmed unintentionally. When using poisons, it is highly recommended that rodenticides be placed in containers that restrict access to anything larger than a rodent. Many rodent control techniques may be restricted or prohibited by local legislation and due consideration must be given to their use.

Wild birds

Wild birds can be an important reservoir for diseases and may be responsible for a significant loss of feed. In particular, wild birds are believed to be a common source of *Trichomonas* spp. and, in the case of an outbreak, avian influenza. In most cases, population control of wild birds is not an acceptable practice, although it may be legal to shoot certain species. The use of bird-scaring devices, such as scarecrows and kites, may be of benefit as long as they do not cause distress to the poultry being protected. The primary control mechanism should be through good husbandry practices and enclosure design. It is essential to use feeders that minimize food spillage and to clear any spilled food regularly. It is essential that water dispensers are cleaned and refilled regularly, in particular to reduce faecal contamination. Where wild birds are problematic, netting can be used over the range to prevent them from entering, and vegetation overhanging the area can be cleared to prevent wild birds from perching above the range and depositing droppings. A solid roof over the poultry range provides better protection and may be required by the local authorities at certain times, such as during an outbreak of avian influenza. See Chapter 4 for examples of suitable poultry housing.

Insects

Non-parasitic insects are not commonly encountered as a problem with backyard poultry in temperate areas such as the UK, but in some parts of the world may be an important cause of food loss and a vector for disease transmission. Well maintained sealed food bins offer protection to food in storage. The use of appropriate insecticides may be required to protect housing.

Predators

Adequate fencing must be provided around poultry in order to reduce the risk of predator attack, particularly from foxes. Ensuring that the door to the house is shut as soon as the birds come in to roost is also essential. Attacks from pet dogs are surprisingly common and adequate precautions should be taken to prevent this from happening.

Beak clipping

Beak clipping has traditionally been regarded as a routine procedure in commercial flocks in order to reduce mutilation as a result of pecking. In many parts of the world, legislation has been introduced to limit the practice (see Chapter 26). This is because cannibalism is now recognized to be largely due to poor husbandry rather than a primary problem. The beak is very well innervated and beak clipping can cause significant discomfort. Without the pressures of intensification, cannibalism should be a rare occurrence in backyard poultry flocks. Routine beak clipping therefore should not be performed in these birds and is not covered in this manual. Where cannibalism is encountered in backyard birds, the underlying cause should be addressed (see Chapter 19) and, if necessary, victimized birds separated from dominant individuals.

Parasite control

Poultry species are vulnerable to a range of endoparasites (protozoan and helminth species) and ectoparasites (insect and arachnid species). Identification of parasites and the diseases associated with them are discussed in the relevant chapters (see Chapters 10, 13 and 16). As with vaccination, preventive control measures for parasitic diseases must take into consideration the costs of treatment and the benefits of prevention.

Endoparasites

Nematodes

Flubendazole and fenbendazole are authorized in poultry. Susceptibility of *Capillaria* spp. may differ between the two drugs, but an unauthorized alternative is rarely, if ever, indicated. Reports of nematode resistance to flubendazole in poultry species appear uncommon. Various herbal alternatives exempt from licensing requirements are available, but the absence of reliable efficacy data means that it is difficult to recommend these preparations at this time. In fact, a small scale study by Squires *et al.* (2012) found a 99.4% reduction in faecal egg counts in birds treated with flubendazole, but only minimal or no reduction in faecal

egg counts in birds treated with a commercially available herbal wormer (not significantly different from the untreated group).

Flubendazole and fenbendazole are administered in feed or in water depending on the preparation (the manufacturer's instructions for dosing should be followed). It is important that when it is administered in feed, the legal implications are considered. For example, in the UK a keeper is only allowed to mix the authorized preparation into the feed if the eggs produced by the treated birds are used solely for private consumption (see Chapter 26 for further information).

Treatment intervals with flubendazole should be based on faecal analysis. The technique used to determine faecal egg counts is described in Chapter 10. A discussion on the diagnosis and treatment for each individual nematode species can be found in Chapter 16. For example, the presence of any *Capillaria* may be considered grounds for treatment due to the pathogenicity of the species. However, for other pathogenic nematodes, only a moderate or heavy faecal egg count or the presence of multiple life stages might be justification for treatment and there is some debate as to when intervention is required.

There are reports of fenbendazole causing toxicity in columbiform birds (Gozalo *et al.*, 2006) and other bird taxa. This has led to concerns about the safety of other benzimidazoles in bird groups and, although there are no published studies reporting such problems with either flubendazole or fenbendazole in poultry species, it would be prudent to limit treatment to where there is good justification.

Coccidia

Coccidia, namely *Eimeria* spp., can be a significant cause of morbidity and mortality (see Chapter 16) and are most devastating when naïve birds are exposed to a high infectious load. Whilst control of coccidiosis in a severe disease outbreak tends to focus on the use of coccicidal drugs, control of endemic coccidiosis is frequently based on cocciostatic drugs. These drugs allow a bird to be exposed to a coccidian in their environment, but by reducing the ability of the protozoans to replication, it gives the bird the opportunity to raise an appropriate immune response. Coccidiostatic drugs, such as decoquinate, diclazuril, halofuginone, lasalocid, maduramicin, monensin, narasin, nicarbazin, robenidine and salinomycin, are mixed into feed by the feed supplier and do not require a veterinary prescription in the UK.

Alternatively, vaccination can be considered. The vaccines available contain live attenuated sporulated oocysts and can be administered to chicks in feed, water or as a course spray (see Figure 7.1). *Eimeria* vaccines are species-specific and host-specific and are rendered ineffective by anticoccidial agents administered during the period of onset of immunity.

Good husbandry and biosecurity will mean that coccidia should not be allowed to build up in significant numbers. This can be achieved by frequent removal of all bedding and the use of an oocidal disinfectant. In some cases, the use of deep litter systems may help to destroy oocysts due to an increase in temperature from decomposition. The use of coccidiostatic drugs and vaccination is rarely needed in backyard poultry flocks.

Histomonas

This protozoal infection causes typhlitis and liver necrosis in turkeys and, increasingly, chickens (a condition often known as 'blackhead'; see Chapter 16). The lifecycle of *Histomonas* involves the nematode *Heterakis gallinarum*, which infects the caeca of chickens (although direct transfer of *Histomonas* through cloacal drinking is possible). Control of histomoniasis, therefore, involves reducing exposure to *Heterakis* eggs. Turkeys and chickens ideally should not share the same ground; however, if this is not possible, an appropriate anthelmintic regime should be implemented in the chickens.

Ectoparasites

The diagnosis of and disease associated with northern fowl mites, red mites and lice in poultry is discussed in Chapters 10, 13 and 21. For flocks where these parasites have not been identified as a problem, specific control measures are not required. However, even in these cases, good preventive care relies upon regular and careful monitoring of the flock for the presence of louse and mite infestations. Keepers should inspect the plumage of their birds regularly for the presence of lice and northern fowl mites, and a regular inspection of the house at night (with a torch) helps to identify red mite infestations. It is important to note that it is common to find lice on healthy birds and in small numbers they may not be of any clinical or practical significance. Holdings with a history of mite and/or severe louse infestations should implement a programme of control to reduce the risk of future problems. In the case of heavy louse infestations, there should also be an investigation to ensure that any predisposing problems are identified and resolved. Red mite control is based on treatment of the environment, particularly the house. Treatment of the birds is neither required nor effective since reinfestation will occur from untreated surroundings. Control of northern fowl mites and lice may require direct treatment of birds, which can be problematic since there are no treatments authorized for this type of use in many regions, including the UK.

Husbandry

Regular replacement of bedding helps to suppress infestations. Wooden structures are particularly associated with red mite infestations; the mites seek refuge in the cracks in the material when not on the birds. It may be that the use of plastic housing can help reduce red mite populations since these structures tend to have less crevices and are easier to clean. Providing access to dust bathing sites is also likely to reduce ectoparasite loads. It is thought that parasite control was an important contributory factor in the evolution of dust bathing behaviour.

Pyrethroids

Permethrin- and pyrethrum-based powders are usually applied directly to the bedding and show residual activity. Whilst previously considered effective against red mites and northern fowl mites, there is increasing evidence of field resistance in both groups (Beugnet *et al.*, 1997; Mullens *et al.*, 2004; Yazwinski *et al.*, 2005; Marangi *et al.* 2009). Although there are no authorized preparations to apply directly to birds, it may be possible to justify the use of certain pyrethroids following the prescribing cascade (see Chapter 26 for further information on the cascade). Careful consideration of drug residues is required (Marangi *et al.*, 2012). It is advisable that poultry keepers are made aware that cats are particularly sensitive to pyrethroid toxicity.

Diatomaceous earth

Diatomaceous earth kills arthropods through desiccation and there is increasing evidence to support its use in poultry. A study by Maurer *et al.* (2009) showed efficacy *in vitro* against red mites. Another study by Mullens *et al.* (2012) showed that two consecutive weekly applications of a liquid preparation to the vent feathers resulted in a significant reduction in northern fowl mite infestations persisting for less than 2 weeks. Bennett *et al.* (2011) reported that dusting birds with diatomaceous earth reduced northern fowl mite numbers. Martin and Mullens (2012) found that birds using dust baths containing sand and diatomaceous earth showed a dramatic reduction in northern fowl mite and louse populations after 1 week, although there was no reduction in birds that did not use the dust baths and populations returned once the dust baths were withdrawn. When applying diatomaceous earth, operators should wear appropriate protective equipment to prevent breathing in the fine powder, which could potentially have respiratory effects.

Direct heat

The use of blow torches to heat treat the surfaces of wooden structures (to kill mites) is also recommended by some, but extreme caution is required to prevent setting fire to the house.

Predatory mites

The predaceous mite species *Androlaelaps casalis* and *Stratiolaelaps scimitus* have been shown to reduce red mite numbers significantly under laboratory conditions (Lesna *et al.*, 2012). Predatory mites that target red mites are commercially available and are indigenous to the UK. It is important that any biological control agent used does not carry any risk to native flora and fauna, so the availability and legality of such products may be restricted in other locations. Other control agents, such as pyrethroids or diatomaceous earth, cannot be used prior to or during administration of predatory mites since they will also harm the predatory mites.

Neem tree seed extract

This naturally derived substance has been shown to be very effective against red mites (e.g. Locher *et al.*, 2010) as well as other arthropods. It is commercially available and is indicated for infestations of red mites, northern fowl mites, tropical fowl mites, scaly leg mites, poultry lice, fleas and ticks. It can be sprayed on the house or applied directly to the birds.

Other control agents

Endectocides authorized for use in other veterinary species (such as fipronil-based sprays and spot-on treatments and cattle pour-on treatments) are often recommended for use in backyard poultry, but this is difficult to justify following the prescribing cascade or even, as is the case with fipronil, not permitted in some regions including the European Union. The use of dichlorvos-based products has been banned in many regions, including the European Union. There are a number of naturally derived powders commercially available for the control of mites; however, published research into their efficacy is currently limited.

There is a detergent-based cleaner available for poultry housing, which is widely reported to decrease red mite infestations significantly by 'cleaning the waxy coating that covers red mites, leading to them dying from dehydration', but controlled studies are lacking to support its efficacy.

Future control methods

Aside from neem tree seed extract, a number of other plant extracts have been studied recently as potential candidates for the control of red mites. Certain extracts have shown toxic effects (eugenol, geraniol and citral at higher concentrations; Sparagano *et al.*, 2013), persistent toxic effects (lavender and thyme oils, Nechita *et al.*, 2015; and carvacrol without thymol, Masoumi *et al.*, 2016) and repellent effects (thyme, oregano and lavender oils, and carvacrol without thymol) against red mites. Pritchard *et al.* (2016) used thyme oil, insecticidal glue and double-sided sticky tape as barriers to impede the movement of mites *in vitro*, and Barimani *et al.* (2016) have shown that carvacrol-filled traps can be used to significantly reduce red mite populations under field conditions. In another field trial, Faghihzadeh *et al.* (2014) demonstrated the successful use of garlic extract for controlling red mites. Some of these extracts may already be marketed in commercial products and may become an important part of future control strategies.

Sulphur dust in dust bags has been trialled successfully by Murillo and Mullens (2016) for the control of northern fowl mites and may offer a future control strategy for this ectoparasite. Future control strategies could also utilize vaccination of poultry with proteins extracted from red mites (Harrington *et al.*, 2009; Bartley *et al.*, 2015) but research is ongoing.

Hygiene and biosecurity

Successful preventive healthcare cannot be achieved without good husbandry (see Chapter 4). Accumulation of faecal material in the house will increase transmission of diseases via the faeco–oral route. Similarly, unclean water troughs and drinkers will act as a conduit for infection, especially due to the high likelihood of faecal contamination from both poultry and pests. Bacteria frequently adhere to one another within a matrix of extracellular material on the surface of drinkers (collectively known as a biofilm), which will not be removed without thorough cleaning and disinfection.

Resistant bacterial and fungal spores, encapsulated virus particles, worm eggs and oocysts can remain viable within the house for days to months and even years. It is therefore important that the house is periodically depopulated, cleaned and disinfected with an appropriate biocidal agent. It is advisable to use disinfectants that have been approved by the regulatory authorities. In the UK, the Department for the Environment, Food and Rural Affairs (Defra) approves disinfectants based on laboratory testing and lists them on its website (http://disinfectants.defra.gov.uk). Not all infectious agents (in particular coccidia) are included in this testing, so the indications on the label for each agent should be taken into account before it is used.

Infectious disease transmission through other fomites (in particular humans and their clothing) must also be carefully considered. Poultry owners should be educated to use appropriate protective clothing, particularly when moving between groups of poultry and even within the same holding. Alternative footwear should be worn or at the very least a disinfectant footbath should be used.

The introduction of new birds to a holding often leads to the precipitation of disease in either the existing population or the new individuals. The two groups are likely to have differing immune statuses based on different exposure to pathogens and vaccination histories, and they may be naïve to agents brought in by the new arrivals or pre-existing in the flock. New arrivals should be isolated for a minimum of 2 weeks and owners should ensure that clothing and equipment does not spread disease between the two groups. Long-term separation of the groups should be considered but where this is not possible the groups should only be mixed after the birds have been observed to be disease-free for at least 2 weeks.

Acknowledgements

Thank you to Dr Sheelagh S. Lloyd for reviewing the prevention of parasitic diseases.

References and further reading

Barimani A, Youssefi MR and Tabari MA (2016) Traps containing carvacrol: a biological approach for the control of *Dermanyssus gallinae*. *Parasitology Research* **115**, 3493–3498

Bartley K, Wright HW, Huntley JF *et al.* (2015) Identification and evaluation of vaccine candidate antigens from the poultry red mite (*Dermanyssus gallinae*). *International Journal for Parasitology* **45**, 819–830

Bennett DC, Yee A, Rhee YJ and Cheng KM (2011) Effect of diatomaceous earth on parasite load, egg production and egg quality of free-range organic laying hens. *Poultry Science* **90**, 1416–1426

Beugnet F, Chauve C, Gauthey M and Beert L (1997) Resistance of the red poultry mite to pyrethroids in France. *Veterinary Record* **140**, 577–579

Faghihzadeh Gorji S, Faghihzadeh Gorji S and Rajabloo M (2014) The field efficacy of garlic extract against *Dermanyssus gallinae* in layer farms of Babol, Iran. *Parasitology Research* **113**, 1209–1213

Gozalo AS, Schwiebert RS and Lawson GW (2006) Mortality associated with fenbendazole administration in pigeons (*Columba livia*). *Journal of the American Association for Laboratory Animal Science* **45(6)**, 63–66

Harrington D, El-Din HM, Guy J, Robinson K and Sparagano O (2009) Characterization of the immune response of domestic fowl following immunization with proteins extracted from *Dermanyssus gallinae*. *Veterinary Parasitology* **160**, 285–294

Lesna I, Sabelis MW, van Niekerk TGCM and Komdeur J (2012) Laboratory tests for controlling poultry red mites (*Dermanyssus gallinae*) with predatory mites in small 'laying hen' cages. *Experimental and Applied Acarology* **58**, 371–383

Locher N, Klimpel S, Abdel-Ghaffar F, Al Rasheid KAS and Mehlhorn H (2010) Light and scanning electron microscopic investigations on MiteStop®-treated poultry red mites. *Parasitology Research* **107**, 433–437

Marangi M, Cafiero MA, Capelli G *et al.* (2009) Evaluation of the poultry red mite, *Dermanyssus gallinae* (Acari: Dermanyssidae) susceptibility to some acaricides in field populations from Italy. *Experimental and Applied Acarology* **48**, 11–18

Marangi M, Morelli V, Pati S *et al.* (2012) Acaricide residues in laying hens naturally infested by red mite *Dermanyssus gallinae*. *PLoS One* **7**, e31795

Martin CD and Mullens BA (2012) Housing and dustbathing effects on northern fowl mites (*Ornithonyssus sylviarum*) and chicken body lice (*Menacanthus stramineus*) on hens. *Medical and Veterinary Entomology* **26**, 323–333

Masoumi F, Youssefi MR and Tabari MA (2016) Combination of carvacrol and thymol against the poultry red mite (*Dermanyssus gallinae*). *Parasitology Research* DOI: 10.1007/s00436-016-5201-4

Maurer V, Perler E and Heckendorn F (2009) *In vitro* efficacies of oils, silicas and plant preparations against the poultry red mite *Dermanyssus gallinae*. *Journal of Experimental and Applied Acarology* **48**, 31–41

Mullens BA, Soto D, Martin CD, Callaham BL and Gerry AC (2012) Northern fowl mite (*Ornithonyssus sylviarum*) control evaluations using liquid formulations of diatomaceous earth, kaolin, sulfur, azadirachtin and *Beauveria bassiana* on caged laying hens. *Journal of Applied Poultry Research* **21**, 111–116

Mullens BA, Velten RK, Hinkle NC, Kuney DR and Szijj CE (2004) Acaricide resistance in Northern fowl mite (*Ornithonyssus sylviarum*) populations on caged layer operations in Southern California. *Poultry Science* **83**, 365–374

Murillo AC and Mullens BA (2016) Sulfur dust bag: a novel technique for ectoparasite control in poultry systems. *Journal of Economic Entomology* DOI: 10.1093/jee/tow146

Nechita IS, Poirel MT, Cozma V and Zenner L (2015) The repellent and persistent toxic effects of essential oils against the poultry red mite, *Dermanyssus gallinae*. *Veterinary Parasitology* **214**, 348–352

Pritchard J, Küster T, George D, Sparagano O and Tomley F (2016) Impeding movement of the poultry red mite, *Dermanyssus gallinae*. *Veterinary Parasitology* **225**, 104–107

Sparagano O, Khallaayoune K, Duvallet G, Nayak S and George D (2013) Comparing terpenes from plant essential oils as pesticides for the poultry red mite (*Dermanyssus gallinae*). *Transboundary and Emerging Diseases* **60**, S2: 150–153

Squires S, Fisher M, Gladstone O *et al.* (2012) Comparative efficacy of flubendazole and a commercially available herbal wormer against natural infections of *Ascaridia galli*, *Heterakis gallinarum* and intestinal *Capillaria* spp. in chickens. *Veterinary Parasitology* **185**, 352–354

Yazwinski TA, Tucker CA, Robins J *et al.* (2005) Effectiveness of various acaricides in the treatment of naturally occurring *Ornithonyssus sylviarum* (northern fowl mite) infestations of chickens. *Journal of Applied Poultry Research* **14**, 265–268

Chapter 8

Clinical examination and emergency treatment

Aidan Raftery and Michelle Kischinovsky

A thorough clinical examination is essential for each patient; however, obtaining a complete history of the bird and its flock is also important to be able to make diagnostic and therapeutic plans. It is crucial for the veterinary clinician to be familiar with the normal parameters for the species presented. True familiarity only comes from examining normal birds; it is recommended that every opportunity is taken to perform a clinical examination and husbandry review of normal birds before clinical cases are accepted.

Information for receptionists

Receptionists in veterinary practices that accept poultry cases need training in recognizing cases that need to be seen immediately, those that can be seen within 24 hours of contact with the surgery (see below) and those that can wait longer to be seen. Receptionists also need to be informed of which veterinary surgeons (veterinarians) within the practice are accepting poultry cases and where to refer if no one is available to deal with the case.

Receptionist telephone triage

Cases that should be seen as soon as possible:
- Injury from a predator
- Profuse blood loss
- Acute respiratory distress
- Unable to stand

Cases that should be seen within 24 hours of contact with the surgery:
- Decrease in food intake
- Change in attitude, personality or behaviour
- Fluffed posture
- Decreased vocalization
- Change in breathing or abnormal respiratory sounds
- Acute enlargement or swelling of any body part
- Regurgitation
- Discharge from eyes, nostrils or mouth
- Decrease or increase in water consumption
- Change in number and appearance of droppings

The receptionist should advise the owner to bring with them a fresh faecal sample, a sample of the food being given (plus the food label which provides the nutritional information), any treatments already being administered and any vitamins, minerals or other supplements being given. If the bird, or another from the flock, has already been seen at another veterinary practice, arrangements should be made to have the medical treatment history available at the time of consultation.

The receptionist must not give medical advice over the telephone; however, emergency first aid instructions are essential in some cases. Any first aid instructions provided should be clear and easy to follow. If there is any doubt, then a veterinary surgeon or nurse with avian medicine qualifications and/or experience should be consulted.

It should be remembered that many birds conceal disease, which means that they are often severely ill by the time they are presented to the veterinary surgeon and likely to need urgent attention.

History

Collecting historical information is often a much lengthier process in avian cases than in canine and feline cases. The time taken to collect the history is a useful period during which to observe the bird before it is handled. The bird's behaviour, awareness of its environment, movement, body conformation and respiratory rate and depth should be noted.

A history form can be given to the client to complete prior to the consultation. This may help save time and allow the veterinary surgeon to determine important areas relevant to the clinical case quickly and explore these in more depth by further questioning. To ensure collection of a thorough history, it is advisable to have a standard list of questions that are covered in a set order. The history can be divided into information about the individual bird, the flock, the environment, the diet provided and the clinical signs (including any historical clinical signs). Obtaining a thorough patient history will help establish a list of differential diagnoses by ruling out conditions that are more commonly seen at a different age, with a different diet or with different husbandry.

Individual bird history

The following should be taken into consideration when obtaining an individual bird's history:

- What species and breed is the bird?
- How old is the bird? Is the hatch date known or is it an estimate?

- Has the bird been sexed? If not, is the sex obvious?
- Record the bird's unique identification (name, passive induced transponder, ring number or any scars that can be used to identify it as an individual)
- How long has the owner had the bird and what age was it at the time it was acquired?
- Where is the bird from (source)? Was it hatched on-site or at another facility? If it was hatched at another facility, is there any information about its source?

Flock history

The following should be taken into consideration when obtaining a flock history:

- What is the source of the flock (e.g. large-scale breeder, dealer, auction, ex-commercial birds, 'rescue' birds or small hobby breeder)? It should be borne in mind that some flocks are sourced as eggs and incubated and hatched on-site
- Was the flock established at one time or have there been many introductions? The timing and source of the latest birds introduced to the flock should be recorded
- Is there a mixture of different species within the flock? Some pathogens can be carried by one species in which they cause reduced or zero pathogenicity but transmitted to a different species in which they cause disease (e.g. histomoniasis is primarily a disease of turkeys but may be carried by chickens, which are more resistant to its pathological effects)
- What is the flock structure? Is a male present? If so, what is the male to female ratio? What is the group size? How do the birds interact and socialize (see Chapter 3)?
- For what purpose are they kept (e.g. as pets, for eggs or meat, or for ornamental display)?
- What is the reproductive history of the flock? Has there been any decrease in egg production? Have any abnormal eggs been produced?
- Have the flight feathers been trimmed or have any of the birds been pinioned?
- What is the vaccination status of the flock? Have some or all of the birds been vaccinated? If so, with what vaccine and at what age?

Environmental history

The environment is an important factor for many conditions. The following should be taken into consideration when obtaining an environmental history:

- Are the birds free ranging or are they in an enclosed run? If they are in an enclosed run, is it covered? What species of wild birds can gain access to the area and to the food? In the case of ducks and geese, is there contact with wild waterfowl?
- For waterfowl, is there a pond available? What is the water quality in the pond? Could toxins (such as lead fishing weights) be present?
- Is there a problem with rodents attracted by the food? How is control of vermin managed?
- Is there contact with neighbouring flocks? What species are in contact?
- What type of housing is provided? What material (wood and plastic are the most common) is it constructed from? Is the size adequate for the birds that use it and, where appropriate, are sufficient nest boxes provided?

- What substrate is used in the housing? What type of surfaces are provided in the external environment? It should be recognized that some surfaces are more likely to result in pododermatitis, whilst others can result in a build-up of potential pathogens (e.g. mycobacteria)
- How often are the house, perches and nest boxes cleaned? What cleaners and disinfectants are used? In the case of a restricted enclosure, is it moved regularly or are the birds rotated around different areas? (For detailed information on housing and the surrounding environment, the reader is referred to Chapter 4.)

Nutritional history

The following should be taken into consideration when obtaining a nutritional history (see also Chapters 4 and 5):

- What diet is fed?
  - Is it appropriate for the species and its lifestage?
  - Are other items being fed (e.g. as treats) which, if eaten disproportionately, would unbalance the diet?
  - What are the food preferences and do the birds get an opportunity to select? (It should be remembered that, if allowed to choose food items, this could result in some birds selecting a deficient diet)
- How is the food stored?
  - Is it in sealed containers? (This is more important for small flocks that would take longer to use a bag of food)
  - Has the food exceeded its expiry date?
  - Are rodents or other animals able to gain access to the food stores?
  - Is it stored in a dry environment? (Occasionally, keepers of small flocks purchase food from open bags in a pet store. This should be discouraged as the expiry date is unknown)
- How is the food dispensed?
  - Are the dispensers used appropriate for the species being fed?
  - Are the dispensers designed to avoid faecal contamination?
- Is grazing available for the species that need it?
  - Is the grass of an appropriate length?
- Is grit provided?
  - What type is offered?
- Is water always on offer?
  - How is water offered?
  - Are the dispensers appropriate for the species?
  - Is the water changed regularly?
  - How are the dispensers kept clean?
- Are vitamins and/or mineral supplements provided?

Medical history

Information should be obtained regarding any previous illness of the individual or of the in-contact birds, even if there was no veterinary treatment. Where there was a veterinary examination, the records should be obtained and the results of any treatments administered noted. Post-mortem results of any deaths can provide important information about diseases endemic in the flock.

Current problem

The following should be taken into consideration when obtaining information about current medical problems:

- Number of birds and the species/breeds affected. Is the problem restricted to one age group or sex of birds?

- Timescale of progression and/or spread to other individuals
- Any changes to the environment or diet occurring prior to the problem
- Have there been any new introductions to the flock or new in-contact animals?
- What clinical signs have been noted by the owner? Have there been any behavioural changes in the flock, including in the apparently healthy birds?
- If there are deaths within the flock then a post-mortem examination is the best route to a rapid diagnosis (see Chapter 25)
- Have any changes in food and water consumption (increase or decrease) been noted? It should be borne in mind that in large flocks small changes may not be noticed. In some cases, increased quantities of grit may be consumed
- Are the affected birds quieter, sleeping more or found further away from others in the flock? Are they fluffed up? Hyperexcitability is sometimes seen, often in association with increased activity. Seizures are occasionally reported
- Coughing, sneezing and head shaking can be associated with pathology of the respiratory system (see Chapter 15). Reports of oculonasal discharge should also raise suspicion for respiratory pathology
- Dysphonia is occasionally reported and may be related to pathology of the syrinx
- Record any changes in the droppings. Ideally, a fresh sample should be presented with the bird. Often what is expelled in the clinic is more liquid than normal due to the stress of travel and handling.

Weighing and body condition scoring

Every bird presented for clinical examination should be weighed and its weight recorded (Figure 8.1). Bodyweight is often a good indicator of response to treatment. A historical bodyweight can be very useful for comparison with the current bodyweight. Often the easiest way to obtain an accurate bodyweight is to place the transport container with the bird still inside directly on the scales. The bird can then be removed and the container weighed again, and the difference calculated. Larger birds that arrive wrapped in a towel or bag can be placed directly on

Score	Pectoral musculature	Keel	Nutritional condition
0	Little muscle cover with concave profile	Prominent ridge	Cachectic
1	Little muscle cover but flat in profile	Keel palpable above muscles	Skinny
2	Moderately developed muscle cover with convex profile	Keel level or just above muscle	Optimal
3	Well developed bulging muscle cover	Muscles over keel	Overweight
4	Convex profile of keel area	Fat tissue extending up over the keel and pectoral muscles	Obese

8.2 Body condition scoring for laying hens. The pectoral musculature should be palpated and determined whether it is convex or concave. The protuberance of the keel should be graded.

the scales and the weight of the bag subtracted later. Birds weighing <1 kg should be weighed to the nearest gram; birds weighing <10 kg should be weighed to the nearest 10 g.

Body condition scoring is not an exact science. The most commonly used parameters are the size of the pectoral musculature and protuberance of the keel (Figure 8.2). However, there are significant differences between species, breeds and individuals. The clinician should become familiar at least with the average body condition of the most commonly presented bird group at the practice.

Clinical examination

It may be beneficial for clients presenting a new animal to complete a history/husbandry questionnaire that can be reviewed prior to the examination. As there are many different breeds with unique characteristics, it is essential to be familiar with common species and breed differences, presenting sexual dimorphisms and age-dependent appearances, as well as normal biological and physiological values (Figure 8.3). It is only possible to detect the abnormal when one is familiar with the normal.

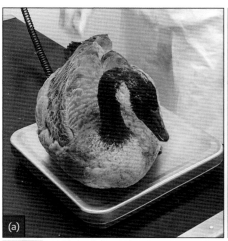
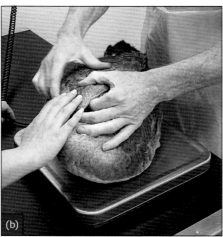
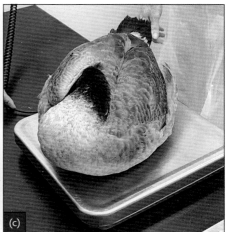

8.1 (a–c) Weighing a goose. Placing the head under the wing often has a calming effect and allows enough time to obtain an accurate weight.

Species	Lifespan (years)	Typical adult bodyweight (kg)	Body temperature (°C)	Heart rate (beats per minute)[a]	Respiratory rate (breaths per minute)[a]	Sexual maturity
Hybrid laying chicken	3–8	1.8 (F)	40.5–43	220–360[4]	12–37[4]	22–24 weeks
Turkey	Up to 12[2b]	Up to 20	40.5–43	93–163[4]	28–49[4]	1 year
Duck (mallard)	10–15[1]	1.1 (F)[1] 1.26 (M)[1]	40.5–43	180–230[1]	30–95[1]	1 year[1]
Duck (Muscovy)	10–15[1]	1.1–1.5[1]	40.5–43	180–230[1]	30–95[1]	1 year[1]
Goose	Up to 31[2]	Up to 10	40.5–43	–	17	2–3 years
Pheasant	10–18[1]	1.15[1]	40.5–43	–	–	1 year[1]
Guinea fowl	10–15[3]	1.3[3]	40.5–43	–	–	6 months
Peafowl (Indian)	Up to 20[1]	4.2[3]	40.5–43	–	–	2 years[3]

8.3 Biological and physiological values for poultry species. These figures should be used as a guide only due to limited published studies, breed variation and physiological and environmental influences. [a] There is a relationship between avian bodyweight and heart rate and respiratory rate, which should be considered when assessing these parameters. [b] Record is for wild type in captivity.
(Data from: [1] Carpenter, 2012; [2] Carey and Judge, 2000; [3] AnAge Database of Animal Ageing and Longevity; [4] Greenacre and Morishita, 2014)

Prior to the clinical examination, a visual assessment of the patient should be undertaken. At a distance, the wings, head and body posture, and breathing pattern (rate and depth) should be observed. Locomotion should also be evaluated. The general level of consciousness of the bird should be assessed (i.e. is the bird alert and interested in its surroundings, is it sleepy or in a stupor and requiring strong stimuli to arouse it?). It should be noted that these characteristics may change when the patient is handled. A bird should be bright, alert and responsive, holding its head upright and its wings tightly against the body.

If severe dyspnoea is present or develops once the examination has commenced, the assessment should be gentle and brief. Prior to a full clinical examination it may be necessary to hospitalize the patient in a dimly lit, quiet room. Supplemental oxygen should be provided if the patient is dyspnoeic. A brief clinical examination should include the following:

- Check for bleeding
- Observation of the breathing pattern
- Check for discharges
- Check vent and whether pasting of droppings around the vent is present
- Assess stance, gait, wing and head posture
- Assess overall feather condition
- Check for abdominal swelling.

Restraint for examination

When lifting the bird for examination, as a general rule one should reach over the back of the bird with both hands to hold the wings against its body. To restrain the bird, the handler should reach under the keel of the bird and place a finger between its legs, then gently scoop the bird up so it is leaning on their arm with its neck restrained under the handler's armpit (Figure 8.4).

The technique may vary depending on the size of the bird and it is important to bear in mind that not all birds are used to being handled; therefore, necessary precautions should be taken. Some species have sharp spurs and/or toenails, which may harm the handler (Figure 8.5). Other species are very large and through their sheer size, strength and powerful wing flap can inflict significant injuries to the handler, owner or the bird itself. It is not advised to restrain a bird by its wings or to carry it upside down by its legs as this may lead to fractures or muscle and soft tissue injury. Holding the bird upside down can cause regurgitation and possibly subsequent aspiration pneumonia.

Gloves, a large towel or an assistant may be required to complete the physical examination. In some cases, darkening the room may reduce the bird's stress levels, making it easier to catch, restrain and examine the animal. Chemical restraint should not be necessary for examination of backyard poultry and waterfowl. For further information on the capture and restraint of poultry, see Chapter 6.

Routine examination

A routine examination should be methodical and systematic. Assistance from a member of staff who is trained in handling birds minimizes stress during the examination. It should be noted that pheasants and peafowl tend to be

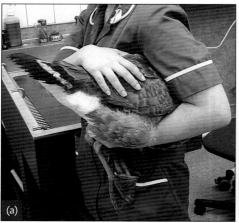
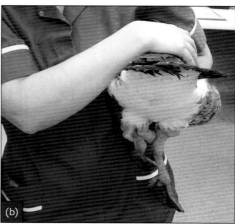

8.4 (a, b) Safe restraint technique for examination of poultry.

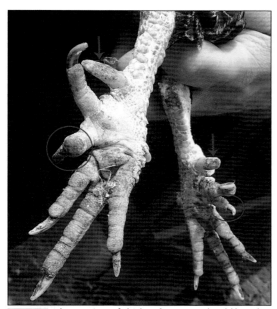

8.5 Plantar view of chicken feet. Care should be taken when handling birds as many species have sharp spurs (arrowed) and toenails, which can be harmful. On occasion, additional toes (circled) can be identified.

flighty and require quick confident capture and effective handling. Equipment that might be required during the examination should be prepared in advance. Scales and weighing containers should be ready for the bird to be placed into. Any materials required to collect diagnostic samples should be within reach (e.g. swabs for micro-biology specimens, appropriate transport media, equip-ment for blood sampling), as should any drugs that may form part of the initial treatment.

Head

Many species have fleshy protuberances on the head. These can vary in appearance between breeds and sexes (Figures 8.6 to 8.8). On occasion they can be mistakenly interpreted as abnormalities. Examination should involve observation of the head to check that it is bilaterally sym-metrical and that the plumage is normal; oculonasal dis-charge can sometimes be seen dried on the feathers. The skull should be gently palpated for any asymmetry that may be disguised by the plumage. Similarly, the mandible should be palpated and its range of movement assessed.

Eyes

Magnification is advised for the ophthalmic examination to ensure that the eye and eyelids can be fully evaluated.

The handler should ensure that the eyelids are com-pletely open before the head is restrained. Any wounds, swellings or areas of abnormal pigmentation should be noted. The outer surface of the eyelids should be dry; any discharge or area of wet feathers is abnormal. The margin of the eyelid should be symmetrical and fit smoothly against the curvature of the eye. When the eyes are closed, the upper and lower eyelids should meet symmet-rically and completely protect the eye. The lower eyelid (palpebra inferior) is larger, more mobile and covers approximately two-thirds of the cornea. The upper eyelid (palpebra superior) is smaller and only protects the top third of the cornea in the normal bird.

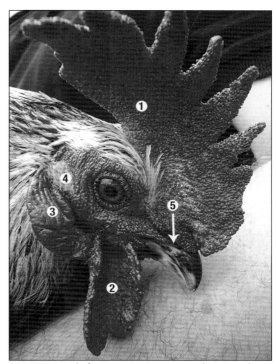

8.6 Head of a mature rooster. 1 = comb; 2 = wattles; 3 = ear lobe; 4 = ear coverts; 5 = naris.

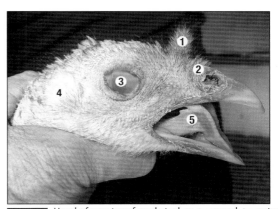

8.7 Head of a mature female turkey. 1 = snood; 2 = external naris with chronic rhinolith causing erosion of the tissues around the external nares; 3 = eye with nictitating membrane fully covering the cornea; 4 = ear coverts; 5 = tongue.

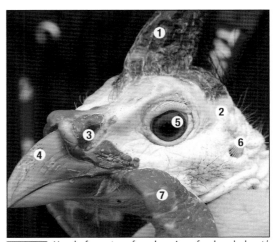

8.8 Head of a mature female guinea fowl. 1 = helmet/casque; 2 = headcap skin; 3 = nostril; 4 = beak; 5 = eye; 6 = ear; 7 = wattle.

The eyes should be compared and any asymmetry noted. Mild exophthalmos may be difficult to detect without a normal eye for comparison. The infraorbital sinus is a large paranasal sinus between the nasal and maxillary bone and extends around the eye. Distension of the infraorbital sinus is a common clinical sign of many upper respiratory tract diseases (Figure 8.9; see also Chapter 15).

The transparent nictitating membrane is an important structure which both lubricates and protects the eye. It should not be constantly visible in its normal state. This structure can completely cover the eye and has the important function of keeping the cornea moistened. It can be seen moving rapidly across the cornea. Handling the eye during the examination often results in the third eyelid coming across to protect the cornea, allowing its evaluation but restricting the view of the cornea (see Figure 8.7).

The conjunctival tissues are not normally visible. Parting the eyelids allows inspection of the conjunctiva. It should be moist, smooth and pink, unless the underlying tissues are pigmented. There should be no exudates present. Any pigment spots should be noted.

The cornea should be clear and moist with a smooth curved surface. Any visible vascularization, oedema (generalized or focal) or irregularities of the surface are abnormal. Fluorescein staining can be used to help detect and evaluate deficits of the corneal epithelium (Figure 8.10).

The iris should be circular (not ellipsoid), forming a sharp margin with the pupil. There is a wide variety of normal differences in the colour of the iris amongst species and breeds, as well as between the sexes. For example, with Pilgrim geese, fully grown ganders have blue eyes (Figure 8.11) whilst the females have brown eyes.

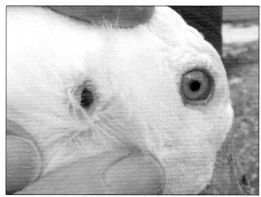

8.11 Head of a healthy mature Pilgrim gander with characteristic blue eyes (sexual dimorphism). The aural canal is located ventrocaudal to the eye and normally hidden by ear coverts.

Any discharge (crusts or mucus) in the eye or periocular area should be considered abnormal. The nasolacrimal duct has two puncta that drain fluid from the conjunctival area of the eye. Both puncta are located close to the medial canthus. In the chicken, the dorsal punctum has the largest opening. Fluorescein staining can be used to check the patency of the nasolacrimal duct. Patency can be affected by any disease process that causes periocular swelling.

See Chapter 14 for further information on the ophthalmological examination.

Ears

The aural canal is situated ventrocaudal to the lateral canthus of the eye. In some species it may be hidden by ear coverts (see Figures 8.11 and 8.12), whilst in others, mainly chickens and guinea fowl, there may be fleshy white, red or blue earlobes present. The external ear canals should be checked for excess cerumen, inflammation, swelling and developmental abnormalities such as a narrowed external ear canal.

Beak

The beak (also known as the rhamphotheca) is extensively modified between species as an anatomical adaptation for different feeding strategies. The beak is composed of keratin and covers the rostral parts of the mandible and maxilla. It should be symmetrical and the upper and lower beaks should come together with the lower beak just fitting inside

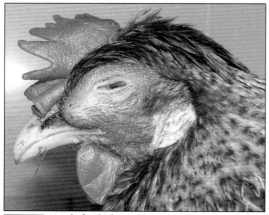

8.9 Head of a chicken with severe distention of the infraorbital sinus, causing distortion of the tissues around the eye.

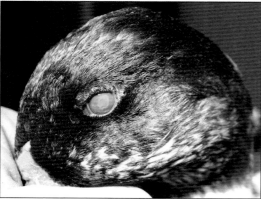

8.10 Duck with a corneal lesion. Fluorescein staining reveals a central ulcerative lesion in the corneal epithelium.

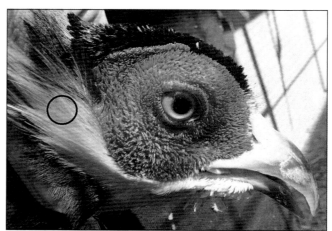

8.12 Large white feathers cover the opening to the aural canal (circled) in this blue-eared pheasant. Note the bare scarlet red facial skin surrounding the eye.

the upper beak. Keratin grows continuously to replace the part lost by normal wear. The edges of both the upper and lower beaks should be sharp. The beak should be checked for cracks and rigidity. Conditions causing demineralization of bone can result in a flexible beak.

Compared with the highly keratinized and continuously growing beaks of Galliformes (chickens, turkeys, guinea fowl and pheasants; see Figures 8.6, 8.7, 8.8 and 8.12), Anseriformes (ducks and geese) have softer more pliable beaks, making them more prone to traumatic injury. In ducks and geese there are horny lamellae along the edges of both the upper and lower beaks (Figure 8.13). These lamellae contain numerous sensitive nerve endings. Any injury to this area will be especially painful and, consequently, birds may be presented as anorectic due to a reluctance or inability to eat. In ducks and geese, the beak is covered by specialized skin and has a terminal/rostral 'nail' (Figure 8.14). Occasionally, wear or growth is not symmetrical, resulting in an overgrowth of the beak, which may need to be corrected. This is a common problem in Galliform birds.

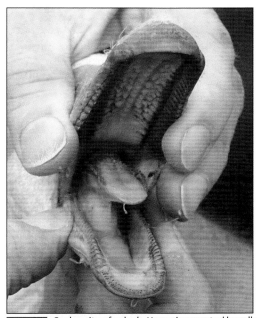

8.13 Oral cavity of a duck. Horny innervated lamellae can be seen along the edges of the upper and lower beaks. Note the horny papillae along the edge of the tongue that interdigitate with the lamellae, which aids in sieving food particles from water.

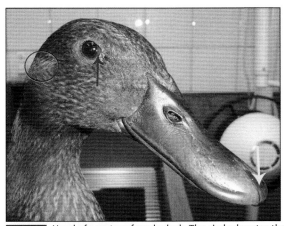

8.14 Head of a mature female duck. The circle denotes the ear coverts, whilst the red arrow indicates the visible nictitating membrane in the medial canthus. The terminal/rostral 'nail' is denoted by the yellow arrow.

Debeaking is the term used to describe partial removal of the beak. In most cases, it involves the removal of one-third or less of the upper beak, although sometimes the lower beak is also partially removed. Debeaked chickens and turkeys are most commonly encountered. Occasionally, ducks and pheasants are debeaked in order to prevent pecking injuries (see Chapter 19). Debeaking is illegal in some regions of the world (see Chapter 26 for the legal situation in the UK).

Nares

The nares of Galliformes are situated at the base of the beak, whereas the nares of Anseriformes are further forward. They should be symmetrical, round to oval, and free from any discharge. In some breeds of chicken, the comb and wattles may hide or even block the nasal openings. In many of the Anseriformes, there is an incomplete nasal septum and it is possible to look through one nasal opening and out the other (Figure 8.15).

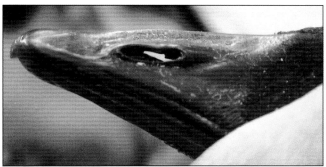

8.15 Head of a goose showing the nares. An incomplete nasal septum makes it possible to look through one nasal opening and out the other.

Comb and wattles

The comb and wattles of Galliformes vary in size and shape. They are usually red, although they may be bluish black, as seen in the Silkie breed. Both sexes have a comb and wattles. Chicks hatch without a comb or wattles; these develop as the chick matures. In turkeys, the comb is more commonly called a snood. In males, the snood hangs down over the beak and is semi-erectile, whereas in females the snood is smaller and does not change in size (see Figure 8.7). The snood changes colour if the bird becomes stressed, as well as during courtship. Under some management systems the snood is removed in 1-day-old turkeys to help prevent injury from pecking and fighting. Guinea fowl have a horn instead of a comb, which is sometimes referred to as the casque or 'helmet'. It is a bony structure that originates from the frontal bone and is covered in thin pigmented skin (see Figure 8.8).

Non-pigmented combs and wattles can provide some information on the circulatory system. Inadequate perfusion or anaemia will cause the comb and wattles to appear paler. When the blood is poorly oxygenated, they appear a bluish colour (cyanotic). Capillary refill time can be assessed by placing digital pressure on the comb or wattle and then measuring the time it takes for the colour to return. This should be <1 second; if the refill time is >1 second, this is taken as an indication of reduced peripheral circulation.

Swelling of the comb and wattles can be general or localized. Areas of localized swelling may be investigated further by analysis of a fine-needle aspirate. Abscesses caused by a variety of bacteria may be seen. Fowl cholera can result in swollen wattles and abscess formation (see Chapter 15). Avian influenza can also result in a swollen comb and wattles. Multiple focal nodular lesions are seen with the cutaneous form of fowlpox (see Chapter 13). Small wounds and localized areas of swelling or erythema are often due to bullying (see Chapter 19).

The development of secondary sexual characteristics (e.g. comb, wattles and caruncles) is under hormonal influence. Although a sex change is not possible, secondary sexual characteristics can change if there is an increase or decrease in male or female hormones as a result of underlying disease.

Oral cavity

Most birds will resist opening of the beak, but it is important not to be deterred as examination may reveal parasitic infestation or provide clues to infection or nutritional deficits. The mouth may be kept open by placing a thumb in the commissure. The colour of the mucosa should be evaluated and any odours present should be noted. The mucosa should be moist with no mucus accumulation. The oral cavity should be checked for any abnormal swellings, pigmentation or ulceration. White to yellow plaques in the oral cavity may be seen with diseases such as trichomoniasis and the diphtheritic form of fowlpox (see Chapter 16).

Tongue: The shape of the tongue varies widely between species; it is adapted to fit within the beak and for the diet of the species. It should be a uniform pink colour (unless pigmented) and bilaterally symmetrical. In both Galliformes and Anseriformes there is a transverse row of papillae at the base of the tongue called the lingual papillae (see Figure 8.13). Anseriformes have a well developed torus linguae, the function of which is to control the direction of movement of food within the oral cavity.

The tongue of Galliformes is non-protrusible and the anterior third is completely lacking in musculature. Due to the tongue being non-protrusible, paralysis is not often diagnosed, but even when it is identified, in most cases the bird still manages to transport food into the oesophagus. However, any major deviation in the upper or lower beak causes problems in manipulating food as birds rely on a closed beak to move the bolus. Retraction of the tongue pulls the food backwards into the oral cavity, using the backward facing lingual papillae to hook the food.

Wounds on the tongue heal more slowly in birds than in mammals due to the keratinized epithelium. Foreign bodies are sometimes found wrapped around the tongue; if they cause tongue tip necrosis, the bird usually manages well if the tongue is amputated rostral to the lingual papillae.

The area under the tongue should also be examined. A tongue depressor or a blunt probe can be used to expose this area. There should be no food accumulating in this area. Any asymmetrical swellings should be investigated. A finger can be gently pushed into the inter-ramal space (between the rami of the mandible) to 'tent up' the tissues and make examination easier.

Glottis: The glottis is situated just caudal to the base of the tongue. In Galliformes, the glottis should be easily visualized with the beak held open and the neck extended. In ducks and geese, it may be necessary to depress the tongue to visualize the glottis. There is no epiglottis in birds. Just caudal to the glottis are rows of backward pointing papillae. The surrounding tissues should be examined for any swelling, redness or discharge. Attention

should be paid to the rhythmical opening and closing of the glottis. If it is persistently open, this may be an indication of respiratory disease. It should be noted, however, that a very stressed bird can often have a persistently open glottis. No gurgles or crackles should be heard on either inspiration or expiration. Open-mouth breathing, if observed prior to handling, should be considered abnormal, although it may be due to stress on occasion. It is sometimes possible to visualize the parasitic nematode *Syngamus trachea*, also known as gapeworm, in the trachea through the glottis. This parasite is most commonly found in chickens, turkeys and guinea fowl.

Palate: The palate of the chicken contains several transverse rows of papillae. Numerous small openings should also be visible; these are the openings of the salivary glands. In ducks and geese the papillae are arranged in longitudinal rows. The horny lamellae are seen around the margins of the beak, and the two openings to the maxillary salivary glands can be identified in the rostral part of the palate. There is a slit-like opening in the palate into the nasal cavity. This is called the choana (Figure 8.16).

Choana: In ducks and geese, the choana is surrounded by backward pointing papillae. In Galliformes, the papillae are arranged in transverse rows. There should be no visible discharge coming from the choana. If any tissues can be visualized through the choana they should be moist and a normal pink colour. The infundibular cleft is just caudal to the choana, but is difficult to visualize. This is the opening to the pharyngotympanic tube (auditory tube). If a middle ear infection is present, this cleft may appear red and swollen. Endoscopy is usually required to examine this area (see Chapter 12).

Neck

Male turkeys have few or no feathers on the neck and the skin has a red or bluish iridescence, depending on the breed. As the turkey matures, the skin in this region becomes covered in fleshy nodular growths called caruncles (Figure 8.17). These are erectile structures that change

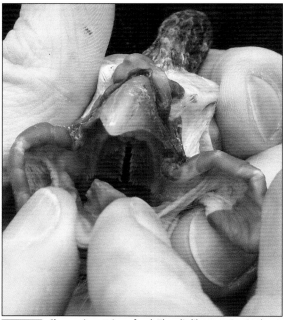

8.16 Choana in a guinea fowl. The slit-like opening in the palate communicates with the nasal cavity.

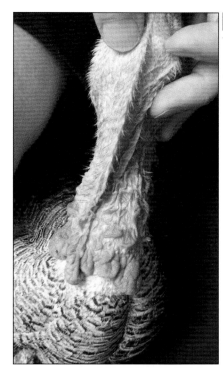

8.17 Caruncles on the neck of a female turkey. These are relatively small compared with those seen in mature male birds.

colour from red to blue when the bird is aroused. Their function is believed to be revealing the physical and reproductive status of the individual bird to potential mates and competitors, and they may also have a thermoregulatory function. Caruncles are also seen in some species of ornamental ducks. Another unique feature in turkeys is the beard. This is a tuft of modified feathers growing from the ventral midline of the chest of male and, occasionally, female birds (Figure 8.18). The beard is not moulted like the other feathers but grows continuously and its length is limited by wear on the ground whilst feeding.

The head and neck is mostly featherless in guinea fowl. The bare skin varies in colour from blue to bluish white. These birds have a sparse ridge of black filoplumes on the hind neck. As the name suggests, the Naked Neck breed of chicken also has a featherless neck. This breed needs protection from very cold weather.

All poultry have a sigmoid flexure of the cervical vertebrae, which in emaciated or very weak birds can protrude quite prominently. Occasionally, birds can be erroneously presented to the veterinary surgeon because the owner is concerned that the sigmoid flexure of the spine is an abnormality. Often these birds have lost weight or have an empty crop due to inappetence. The structures of the neck, blood vessels and trachea are very mobile. The trachea can be mobilized and held between a fold of skin and transilluminated (if non-pigmented) to detect tracheal foreign bodies (e.g. the gapeworm *Syngamus trachea*).

Crop

The crop is a diverticulum of the oesophagus where food can be stored temporarily, although it is mainly an area where food is softened prior to entry into the stomach. It is situated at the base of the sigmoid flexure and differs in size depending on the species, time of day and diet fed. Galliformes have a very well developed crop, which is situated on the right-hand side. Ducks and geese have a significantly smaller crop, which is not considered to be a true crop.

Palpation of the crop is a very important part of the examination. A normal crop should have a doughy consistency on palpation. An empty crop indicates that the bird is not eating. In the morning, before food is offered, the crop should be empty, indicating normal gut motility. If the crop appears to be full on palpation, this indicates crop stasis. In these cases, there may be a disease process within the crop or affecting gut motility in general (see Chapter 16). If a bird with crop stasis becomes dehydrated, fluid may be absorbed from the crop, causing the contents to dehydrate and feel more solid on palpation.

With the mouth kept open, the crop should be compressed gently; any abnormally foul or sour smell should be noted. Care must be taken not to cause regurgitation of the fluid, as this may be aspirated in weak birds. If a yeast-like smell is present this may be an indication of *Candida albicans* proliferation. This is often called sour crop and should be recorded as a clinical sign. It usually occurs secondary to prolonged crop emptying times (see Chapter 16). Any foul smell may indicate the presence of opportunistic pathogens. However, it should be borne in mind that this may not be the final diagnosis itself but merely a clinical sign of an underlying condition.

Occasionally birds are seen that have very distended crops but otherwise appear normal. Once other causes are ruled out, this is called 'pendulous crop'. This is seen most commonly in turkeys, but can also occur in chickens (Figure 8.19). The cause is unknown, but it is believed to be a combination of environmental and dietary factors together with a genetic predisposition. If recognized within

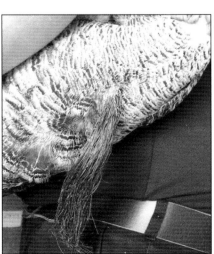

8.18 Turkey beard. This tuft of modified feathers is situated in the ventral midline of the chest in male and, occasionally, female birds.

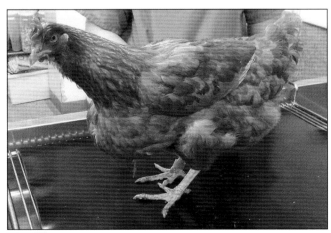

8.19 Distended crop in a chicken.

the first few days it is often reversible; however, if it persists for more than a week it is unlikely to be reversed due to damage of the supporting tissues.

Feathers and skin

The plumage is important for thermoregulation, waterproofing and flight, and has a role in communication with conspecifics. The condition of the plumage can be a reflection of general health. Any areas of feather loss or damage should be recorded. Check whether any feathers are broken off, leaving a portion of the shaft in the skin, or completely missing. Where feathers are missing, pin feathers (also known as blood feathers) should be seen to be emerging. The damaged feathers, along with apparently normal feathers bordering the affected area, should be examined for any abnormalities that may help reveal the cause. Fret marks (sometimes called stress lines) can be seen on feathers if there has been a nutritional crisis during their development. These marks appear as breaks in the feather colour as a result of interruption of growth and malformation of the feather barbs. The skin in the affected area should be examined for any associated changes. The type of feathers affected should be recorded and samples collected for microscopic examination.

It is important that the clinician does not confuse normal patterns of featherless tracts or moulting patterns (Figure 8.20) with pathology. The timescale of any plumage changes should be recorded, along with whether or not the changes are progressive. The owners should be asked whether they have noticed an increase in the number of feathers within the enclosure. (For further information on moulting in different species, the reader is referred to Chapter 3.) Chickens, ducks and turkeys can develop a seasonal brood patch. The brood patch is an area ventrally that is less densely feathered and the skin is highly vascularized for the transfer of body heat to the incubating eggs.

A thorough examination includes separation of the feathers to visualize the skin. The skin is almost transparent and in well nourished birds, especially ducks and geese, deposits of yellowish adipose tissue may be seen in the subcutis. However, it is usually difficult to examine the skin in Anseriformes due to their thick plumage. Any external parasites found should be identified and treated if necessary (see Chapter 13).

Located at the dorsal aspect of the base of the tail is the uropygeal gland (also known as the preen or oil gland; see Chapter 2) and it is usually larger in water birds. The ducts of the gland open into a papilla, which often has a little tuft of feathers called the uropygeal wick. These small feathers are usually oily in the healthy bird. This bilobed gland should be carefully palpated and it should be symmetrical with no obvious inflammation of the surrounding tissue.

Pectoral limb

The wings should be examined at rest, comparing each side. They should be held tightly against the body. A drooping wing may indicate a neurological problem but is more commonly caused by an abnormality in the bones, joints, ligaments or muscles (see Chapter 24).

Each wing should be palpated separately, starting at the pectoral girdle, to detect any asymmetry (Figure 8.21). The scapula extends caudally from the shoulder and is a long narrow bone parallel to the spine that extends approximately to the cranial border of the ilium. The paired clavicles join ventrally to form the furcula (see Chapter 2). The coracoid bones are the strongest of the pectoral girdle and are palpated laterally from the sternum to the shoulder joint. Oregon muscle disease can be diagnosed as swelling of the supracoracoideus muscle in chickens and turkeys (see Chapter 18). The range of movement of the shoulder joint should be assessed to determine whether it is normal.

The humerus should then be carefully palpated. This bone is pneumatized and air becomes palpable under the skin when it is allowed to escape (e.g. due to fracture). The range of movement of the elbow joint should be evaluated to determine whether it is normal. The radius and ulna are about equal in length. When the wings are folded these bones lie parallel to the humerus. In chickens, the ulna is more curved than in ducks and geese.

The distal radius and ulna articulate with the carpal bones, which in turn articulate with the carpometacarpal bones. If the bird has been pinioned, one wing will have been amputated at the level of the proximal carpometacarpal bone. Legally, pinioning can only be performed in the UK by a veterinary surgeon, and it should be noted that it is illegal to pinion farmed birds (see Chapter 26). Other regions of the world may have similar restrictions. The alula (the first digit) articulates with the proximal major carpometacarpal bone. At this point the wing should be completely extended and the remaining bones and joints carefully palpated to check for normal range of motion, as well as crepitus, deviation or instability. The thinly feathered underside of the wing should be checked for skin lesions, external parasites and any other abnormalities.

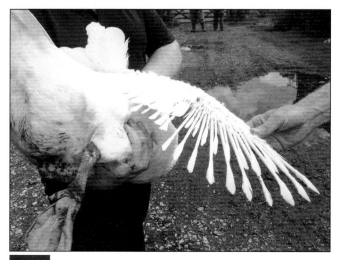

8.20 Emerging primary flight feathers in a moulting Pilgrim goose.

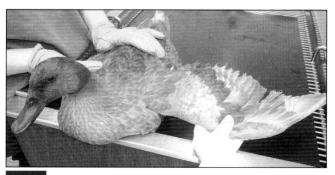

8.21 Examination of the extended wing of a female duck.

Pelvic limb

The legs should first be examined by observing the normal posture of the bird and noting whether the bodyweight is shared equally between both limbs. When the bird is restrained, the legs should be extended and compared for symmetry. Each leg should then be carefully palpated separately, starting at the hip joint. Each joint should be extended and flexed to detect any increase or decrease in range of movement and to identify any abnormal laxity. Areas of increased heat should be noted. If palpation of a limb generates a reaction that could be interpreted as a pain response, then the opposite leg should be palpated and the response compared.

The featherless areas of the limbs should be carefully inspected for damage to the scales; any changes in terms of appearance or feel should be noted. The scales on the feet should be smooth, straight and closely adhered to one another. Upturned scales may be the result of a scaly leg mite infestation, *Knemidocoptes*. Older birds usually have hyperkeratosis of the featherless areas on the legs and feet. The feet should feel evenly warm to the touch. The planter aspect of the feet should also be free from scratches, swelling, scabs or ulcerations. Areas of podo-dermatitis are more commonly seen in turkeys, ducks and geese (see Chapters 13 and 23). If a ring is present, it should be checked to ensure that it is not too tight.

Male turkeys, pheasants and some breeds of chickens (and on occasion older female birds) possess spurs which are used for fighting and self-defence (see Figure 8.5). They are mainly keratin covering a bony core and can be used as a dangerous weapon. The domesticated species of guinea fowl do not develop spurs. The reader is referred to Chapter 6 for information on safe handling techniques and to Chapter 23 for details on removal of spurs.

Vent

The vent is a slit-like opening from the cloaca. The dorsal and ventral lips of the vent are normally held inverted into the cloaca (Figure 8.22), but when a large faecal mass or an egg is being passed, the lips evert and the vent assumes a circular shape. In older hens the muscle tone around the vent may be poor, leaving the lips of the vent slightly parted. However, this is rarely a problem for the bird.

There should be no discharge from the vent and the surrounding area should be clean and free from faecal con-tamination. The presence of feathers or skin contaminated with faeces around the vent (pasted vent) may indicate intestinal disease or be a sign of weakness and warrants investigation. There should be no tissues protruding from the vent. Prolapse of the oviduct can be seen in females, and prolapse of the colon, cloaca or intestinal intussuscep-tion can be seen in both sexes (Figure 8.23). In male Anseriformes, prolapse of the phallus can also be seen (see Chapter 23). An abnormal discharge may be seen leaking from the vent, which is often referred to as 'vent gleet'. The underlying cause needs to be investigated in order to obtain a diagnosis. Differential diagnoses include any disease or abnormality leading to cloacal inflammation and/or infection. Partial cloacal prolapse and vent picking are other possible causes.

Cloaca

The cloaca should be examined by introducing a lubri-cated gloved finger through the vent and performing digital palpation. Space-occupying lesions causing asymmetry can be appreciated. Concretions of urates may be found

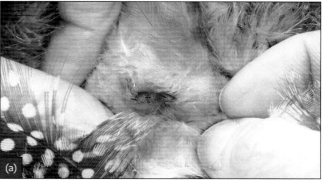
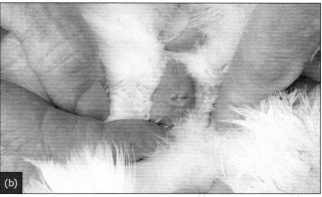

8.22 Normal appearance of the vent in (a) a guinea fowl and (b) a goose. The area around the vent is clean, the tissues appear pink and healthy, and the lips of the vent are held closely together and inverted into the cloaca.

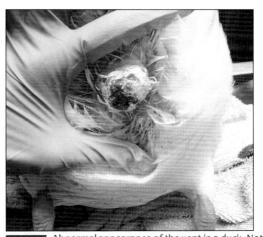

8.23 Abnormal appearance of the vent in a duck. Note the tissue protruding from the vent and the faecal soiling. A full examination should be performed in order to identify the prolapsed tissue as cloacal, intestinal, oviduct or phallus.

and eggs can sometimes be palpated. Abnormal struc-tures in the coelomic cavity can often be more readily appreciated with the aid of cloacal palpation (see below).

Phallus

Drakes and ganders possess a protrusible phallus, which when engorged projects cranially and ventrally from the vent. It is a spiral structure that can sometimes prolapse through the vent (see Chapter 23). It is normally palpable as a swelling on the ventral floor of the proctodeum (the most caudal compartment of the cloaca). The phallus can be exposed by applying pressure on either side of the vent to evert the cloacal folds (Figure 8.24). In some males, especially immature birds, it can be difficult to expose the

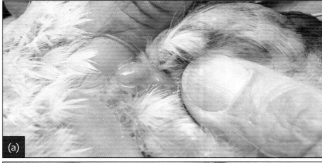

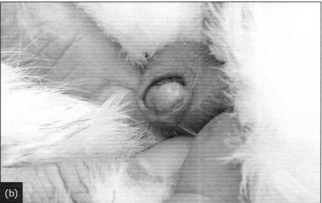

8.24 Partially exposed phallus of a mature (a) drake and (b) gander. Gentle pressure on either side of the vent causes the phallus to protrude, aiding examination and sexing.

phallus. The mucosa and mucocutaneous junction of the cloaca can be examined by gently everting with moistened cotton bud tips. In female waterfowl, a genital eminence is present, which should not be mistaken for a pathological change.

Coelomic space

In Galliformes, the ventral apterium (featherless area) runs down the midline, allowing the thin skin and underlying muscles or adipose tissue to be visualized. Use of an alcohol swab will enhance the examination by damping back the feathers and removing deposits on the skin. This area is not possible to examine in ducks and geese due to the thick covering of feathers. Distension of the coelomic space may be due to the accumulation of fluid within the coelomic cavity, organomegaly or the presence of space-occupying lesions. Cytology of aspirates, ultrasonography and radiography, as well as biochemistry and haematology screening provide information that may lead to a diagnosis. Poor muscle tone can mimic the appearance of distention, especially when the bird is standing; however, on palpation the coelomic cavity feels empty.

Palpation

Palpation is an important part of the clinical examination to assess body condition (see above). Palpation also reveals asymmetry of the musculature and the presence of any abnormal swelling. Digital palpation of the coelomic space via the cloaca may reveal hepatomegaly or posterior displacement of the ventriculus. With the bird in a standing position, the ventriculus should be palpable on the left-hand side. It can easily be mistaken for a mass or an egg; however, if normal, its contractions can be felt. The oviduct is also located on the left-hand side and its size depends on the reproductive status of the bird. Sexually active males can develop very large testes; however, they are situated too far forward to be palpable. The testes may be misdiagnosed as abnormal on radiography and ultrasonography because of their large size. If the coelomic cavity is filled with fluid, abdominocentesis will make the bird more comfortable, provide a diagnostic sample and subsequently allow more successful palpation.

Auscultation

Although birds often show outward signs of respiratory disease, it is important to auscultate the trachea, lungs, and thoracic and abdominal air sacs. A paediatric stethoscope is the best instrument for use in birds. The stethoscope should be placed just ventral to the notarium, and then moved caudally on either side to allow evaluation of the lungs as well as the thoracic and abdominal air sacs. Increased expiratory sounds are often associated with pathology of the lower respiratory tract, whereas increased inspiratory sounds are often associated with pathology of the upper respiratory tract.

Droppings

A specimen of droppings should be assessed as part of the routine examination. Ideally, owners should be asked to bring in a fresh sample on a carefully folded piece of paper. In birds, urine and faeces are excreted together. Urine is a combination of the white material in the droppings and the clear fluid sometimes seen around the faeces. The volume of fluid present in the droppings depends on the species and the diet. When polyuria is present there will be an increase in the amount of clear fluid around the faeces. Increased levels of stress (e.g. associated with capture and transportation) or diets with a high water content also result in more liquid droppings.

In Galliformes, two types of faeces are passed. The first type is the normal faeces, which are diet-dependent, various shades of greyish-green colour and passed in conjunction with white urates. The second type is the caecal faeces. These are only passed a few times a day and come from the caecal pouches. They are more homogeneous in consistency, appear soft and sticky, and are more odorous than normal faeces. Occasionally, they have a frothy appearance and can vary in colour from mustard to dark brown. The faeces passed by waterfowl are generally more variable in colour and consistency, and are considerably more liquid than those passed by Galliformes.

The presence of blood, mucus or any pseudomembranous material is abnormal. Blood passed with the faeces indicates pathology of the caudal part of the gastrointestinal tract. It may also originate from the reproductive tract, cloaca or there may be a haematuria. The presence of black tarry faeces is an indication of bleeding from the small intestine or more proximal areas of the gastrointestinal tract. For more information on abnormal faeces, the reader is referred to Chapter 16.

Emergency treatment

Initial evaluation

Initial triage begins with the receptionist (see above). When the bird is presented at the veterinary practice, the initial visual assessment should be brief and aimed towards evaluating whether the patient is stable enough for a full clinical examination. The following parameters should be evaluated to determine whether the bird is a medical or traumatic emergency:

- Respiration rate and effort; open-mouth breathing; discharge from the external nares
- Ocular discharge; periocular swelling; abnormal appearance of the eyes or eyelids
- Colour (combs and wattles of chickens and turkeys, the wattles around the eyes of male pheasants; those birds without fleshy structures of the head need to have their oral mucous membranes, conjunctival tissues and vent evaluated during the clinical examination)
- Level of consciousness
- Behaviour
- Neuromuscular abnormalities (weakness or paralysis of the neck muscles; lameness; drooping wing; abnormalities of posture; dysphonia).

It is necessary to start immediate stabilization of any bird showing the following clinical signs:

- Hypothermia
- Dyspnoea
- Bleeding and hypovolaemic shock
- Collapse
- Severe obvious pain (fractures and other traumatic injuries; prolapse; distended coelomic space or crop; egg binding) (see Chapter 22 for information on analgesia).

As birds often mask disease until they are severely ill, minimal handling should always be prioritized as increasing the level of stress in a sick bird may have a fatal outcome. It is wise to prepare the owner for the risks involved with handling a debilitated bird, especially if it is not used to human contact (e.g. pheasants and guinea fowl). It is not uncommon for a bird to collapse during examination. In these cases, the bird requires stabilization before a complete examination can be undertaken.

Fractures should be viewed as an emergency; however, radiography can be postponed until the patient is stabilized and has received appropriate analgesia. Relevant diagnostic samples should be collected and initial treatment provided along with supportive care. Repair of the fracture should wait until the bird is stable.

Admitting the bird

If a debilitated bird is admitted to the practice, it should be accommodated under ideal conditions as it may decline very rapidly. The patient should be placed in an intensive care cage or other appropriate enclosure (see Chapter 6). In order to minimize stress the environment should be:

- Warm
- Dimly lit
- Quiet
- Away from the sight and sound of predatory animals
- Free from unnecessary cage furniture that the animal may harm itself on (e.g. perches, toys, bowls).

Once emergency treatment has been provided, a thorough history should be collected from the owner.

Stabilization

Hypothermia

Hypothermia should be diagnosed and rapidly corrected. The bird should never feel cold to the touch, although the distal limbs may be several degrees colder than the core body temperature. A wet or fluffed up bird should raise the suspicion of hypothermia. The bird should be placed in a warm hospital environment, with the temperature set at approximately 25–36°C, depending on the species and the degree of hypothermia. The temperature of the bird should be measured every 15–20 minutes. The aim should be to have the patient normothermic within 2 hours. It is important not to allow the temperature to rise above the normal body temperature as this can also be harmful to the bird. Normothermic poultry should be hospitalized with an environmental temperature of <25°C.

Dyspnoea

Open-mouth breathing, changes in the mucous membrane colour, respiratory noises, and full body movement during inspiration or expiration may indicate that the patient is hypoxic and should immediately be provided with oxygen-enriched air. If available, the bird should be placed in an oxygen cage or anaesthetic induction chamber, as many birds find a facemask stressful. If the dyspnoea is being caused by a tracheal obstruction, an emergency procedure to place an air sac tube will be required (see Chapter 22). If the bird is dyspnoeic and open-mouth breathing, nebulization with hypertonic saline may help by osmotically drawing fluid into the airway, rehydrating the lining of the airways and resulting in improved mucociliary clearance.

Fluid therapy

The main objective of fluid therapy is to correct fluid deficits and provide for daily maintenance requirements. Fluids are required for dehydrated birds and for the stabilization of hypovolaemic shock and electrolyte imbalance. Fluids should be warmed to body temperature prior to administration. A bird in the early stages of shock often presents with hypothermia, hypotension, prolonged capillary refill time (>1 second) and tachycardia. The fluid deficit is estimated using the following equation:

Estimated dehydration (%) x Bodyweight (g)
= Fluid deficit (ml)

Routes of administration

Fluids may be administered via enteral, intravenous or intraosseous routes (see Chapter 9). Subcutaneous fluid administration is not ideal due to the very small subcuticular space. Fluid administration via the intracoelomic route is contraindicated in birds due to the presence of air sacs. Fluids can be given by continuous infusion, but are more commonly delivered in boluses due to the difficulty in protecting the infusion line.

Enteral administration: Enteral rehydration is sufficient for stabilized birds with mild dehydration and to meet maintenance requirements. The major disadvantage of this route of administration is the risk of aspiration. Preferably, a curved stainless steel feeding tube should be used as it is easier to direct. However, a soft rubber tube or a giving set tube can be adapted for this use. Ideally, the tube should already be attached to a preloaded syringe. Whilst holding the bird in an upright position, the beak must be opened and supported in order to pass the tube to the right of the glottis and into the crop. The crop should be palpated to ensure correct placement before the fluid is delivered.

Intravenous administration: Intravenous fluid administration is indicated in birds with significant blood loss (loss >25–30% of total blood volume). The primary advantage of this route of administration is the replacement of large fluid volumes within a short period of time. If the bird is collapsed, it may be beneficial to place an intravenous jugular catheter; usually no feathers need to be plucked due to the apterium over the puncture site. See Chapter 9 for information on the placement of intravenous catheters.

Intraosseous administration: Intraosseous administration may be preferred in small birds or in those presenting with extreme debilitation and veins too collapsed to permit venepuncture. Fluids may be administered in any bone with a bone marrow cavity. Preferred sites are the distal ulna and proximal tibiotarsus (see Chapter 9 for information on the placement of intraosseous catheters). Pneumatic bones such as the humerus and femur are unsuitable. Both colloids and crystalloids can be given via this route. The response seen is equivalent to that observed with fluids administered via the intravenous route.

Types of fluid

Crystalloids: Crystalloids are the fluids of choice to reverse dehydration and to provide maintenance fluids during the recovery phase. The most commonly used crystalloid solutions are isotonic glucose saline, Hartmann's solution and lactated Ringer's solution. The advantage of lactated Ringer's solution and Hartmann's solution is that as the lactate is metabolized in the liver, bicarbonate is produced, which helps correct the acidosis seen in most avian emergencies. Crystalloids are administered slowly at a dose of 3 ml/kg intravenously or intraosseously.

When administered intravenously or intraosseously, crystalloids expand the intravascular space in the short-term before being rapidly distributed to all body fluid compartments. Hypovolaemic patients that are not dehydrated benefit from an initial bolus of hypertonic saline combined with a colloid for a more medium-term expansion of intravascular volume. The 7.5% saline solution can be given at a dose of 3 ml/kg over 10 minutes combined with 3 ml/kg of a colloid.

Colloids: Colloids are considered intravascular volume expanders. They are essential in the treatment of hypovolaemic shock as the large molecular weight particles do not readily pass through the walls of the vasculature and therefore have the potential to replace deficient plasma proteins. The combination of colloids and crystalloids in the treatment of hypovolaemic shock therapy reduces the crystalloid fluid requirement by 40–60%. There are three types of colloids available:

- Synthetic colloids
- Oxygen-carrying colloids
- Natural colloids (for blood transfusion).

Synthetic colloids: The major advantages of using synthetic colloids compared with the alternatives are availability, cost and low risk. The major disadvantage is that they do not transport oxygen to the tissues. Synthetic colloids expand the intravascular volume by approximately 1.4 times the volume infused. They are best administered with isotonic crystalloids to reduce interstitial volume depletion. This is especially important in dehydrated birds.

Oxygen-carrying colloids: Haemoglobin-based oxygen-carrying colloids, although expensive, have the advantage of being readily available for emergency cases as they can be stored at room temperature and have a 3-year shelf-life. With both a colloid effect and being a potent oxygen carrier, this type of fluid is up to 10 times more effective than whole blood when administered during resuscitation of animals in hypovolaemic shock. Low volumes can be administered and boluses of 5 ml/kg over a few minutes have been given without side effects. There have been no clinical trials to establish safe dose rates in backyard poultry; however, Oxyglobin has been administered to psittacine birds in hypovolaemic shock at doses up to 30 ml/kg divided over 24 hours. Oxygen-carrying colloids are superior to whole blood because they contain no antigens; therefore cross-matching is not required and there is no possibility of transfusion reactions. Generally, when the packed cell volume (PCV) falls below 20% in acute conditions or below 12% in chronic disease processes, a colloid with oxygen-carrying ability should be chosen.

Blood transfusion (natural colloids): The benefits of blood transfusions are currently unclear and not well documented in poultry. Blood is a complete and physiological volume expander, although it does not promote blood flow as well as some acellular fluids (e.g. hetastarch) and therefore is not ideal for acute blood loss of large volumes. Blood transfusions appear to be most clinically beneficial to birds suffering from chronic anaemia with a PCV below 20%. The goal of blood transfusion is to stabilize the patient whilst diagnostic tests are performed to determine the cause of the anaemia, bearing in mind that a transfusion may alter (and therefore complicate) interpretation of subsequent haematological investigations.

Ideally, healthy homologous (same species) donors should be used, but if unavailable then a transfusion from a heterologous (different species) bird can be used, especially in a patient with significant ongoing bleeding. However, it should be noted that Oxyglobin is a superior choice to a heterologous match. Information regarding blood groups in avian species is limited, but chickens have been shown to have at least 28 different blood group antigens. A volume of 1% of the donor bird's weight in blood can safely be collected. It should be used fresh and ideally a cross-match should be performed before the transfusion. Acid citrate dextrose at a dose of 0.15 ml per millilitre of blood is the most commonly use anticoagulant. Agglutination and haemolysis should be checked for before any repeat transfusions by mixing donor serum with recipient red blood cells on one slide and donor red cells with recipient serum on another. Blood should be at or close to body temperature when it is administered. Whole blood can be administered intravenously or intraosseously by slow bolus or by infusion with a syringe pump at a dose of 10–20 ml/kg into the catheter.

Nutritional support

Enteral nutritional support should be provided as soon as the hypovolaemia has been corrected and is indicated in birds that have a functional gastrointestinal tract, are not severely dyspnoeic and are conscious enough to avoid crop reflux.

Aims of nutritional support

The aims of nutritional support are:

- To provide an adequate nutritional intake
- To prevent the negative effects of malnutrition

- To preserve gastrointestinal tract structure and function in critical illness
- To achieve better outcomes when treating a range of conditions.

Indications for enteral nutrition

The indications for enteral nutrition include:

- Impaired ingestion
- Inability to consume adequate nutrition orally
- Impaired digestion, absorption or metabolism
- Severe wasting or depressed growth.

Anorexic patients must be provided with nutritional support as part of the treatment plan. There should be a daily reassessment of the patient's nutritional requirements and changes made as needed.

Complications of nutritional support

The complications encountered when providing nutritional support include:

- Inadequate nutritional intake
- Iatrogenic damage
- Aspiration pneumonia
- Metabolic complications (e.g. refeeding syndrome)
- Gastrointestinal dysfunction.

Severely dehydrated birds must be rehydrated with normal blood pressure restored prior to initializing nutritional support. Delivering food to the gastrointestinal tract of a bird which is not adequately perfused may lead to mucosal damage and loss of barrier function.

Feeding recommendations

The recommendations for feeding include:

- Small volumes should be fed frequently
- Estimated energy requirements should not be exceeded
- Manufacturer recommendations should be followed regarding the quantity to be fed and the dilution factors
- If the animal is very weak, there will be a risk of aspiration pneumonia. Thus, only very small volumes should be fed
- After prolonged anorexia, small volumes (approximately one-third of requirements) should be fed initially and gradually built up to the estimated requirements over 4–5 days
- Requirements should be reassessed daily for the first 7 days
- Appetite stimulants should not be relied upon as they do not result in an adequate nutritional intake.

When to stop nutritional support

It is a common misconception that whilst nutritional support is ongoing the animal will not eat voluntarily. As the underlying condition is corrected, the bird's appetite will return and they will show interest in food and begin eating.

- Feeding should not be reduced or suspended solely to check whether the bird's appetite has returned.
- Reducing or stopping nutritional support is based on assessment of recovery from the underlying condition.

- Ideally, birds should be weaned off nutritional support following discharge from hospital whilst recovering in their own environment.

Types of enteral nutrition

There are several types of enteral nutrition:

1. Simple nutritional mixes (e.g. Critical Care Formula). These are suitable for very short-term nutritional support. They are not a complete nutritional diet but are useful in an acute crisis situation.
2. Elemental diets (e.g. Emeraid® Nutritional Care System – three different formulations are available, which can be mixed together in different proportions to achieve the correct nutritional balance for the species being treated). These are critical care diets that provide liquid nutrients in an easily assimilated form so that the gastrointestinal tract does not have to work to digest food and has time to heal. After the clinical status of the bird improves, most animals are ready to move on to recovery diets. Elemental diets can be fed for an extended period of time in cases of maldigestion and malabsorption.
3. Complete foods in a powder or liquid formulation that can be delivered via a tube (e.g. Oxbow Care System or appropriate commercial diet ground down into a powder – as for the Emeraid® Nutritional Care System, a variety of formulations are available which can be mixed together to achieve the correct nutritional balance for the species being treated). These are sometimes called recovery diets and require a functional gastrointestinal tract.

Enteral nutritional support can be delivered via a crop feeding tube. Both metal and flexible plastic or rubber crop feeding tubes are available. The flexible tubes are safer as there is a reduced risk of perforating the oesophagus. It should be noted that crop feeding carries an increased risk of aspiration pneumonia in weak or dyspnoeic birds. It may also be difficult in uncooperative birds, especially pheasants and guinea fowl.

The collapsed bird

A collapsed bird often requires stabilization prior to investigation of the potential causes.

1. Perform a brief physical examination with minimal handling to reduce stress.
2. Place the bird in a warm (25–36°C depending on the species), quiet, dimly lit room away from the sight and sound of any potential predators.
3. If the bird is dyspnoeic, provide oxygen enrichment; even just increasing the oxygen level to 40% will have a significant effect.
4. Provide water and food within reach of the bird; however, be aware of the risks of injury and drowning if the bird is unable to make controlled movements.
5. Collect blood or other samples for diagnostic testing (with the assistance of trained staff to keep the bird's stress levels to a minimum).
6. If the bird is judged stable enough, provide an initial enteral bolus of glucose saline at a dose of 10 ml/kg bodyweight.
7. Establish a complete history for the bird.
8. When stable, perform a full clinical examination.

References and further reading

Altman RB, Clubb SL, Dorrestein GM and Quesenberry K (1997) *Avian Medicine and Surgery*. WB Saunders, Philadelphia

Bowles H, Lichtenberger M and Lennox A (2007) Emergency and critical care of pet birds. *Veterinary Clinics of North America: Exotic Animal Practice* **10**, 345–394

Carey JR and Judge DS (2000) *Longevity Records: Life Spans of Mammals, Birds, Amphibians, Reptiles and Fish*. Odense University Press, Odense

Carpenter J (2013) *Avian and Exotic Formulary, 4th edn*. Elsevier Saunders, Missouri

Greenacre CB and Morishita TY (2014) *Backyard Poultry Medicine and Surgery: A Guide for Veterinary Practitioners*. Wiley-Blackwell, Oxford

Harrison GJ and Lightfoot TL (2006) *Clinical Avian Medicine*. Spix, Florida

King AS and McLelland J (1975) *Outlines of Avian Anatomy*. Bailliere Tindall, London

Lichtenberger M (2007) Shock and cardiopulmonary-cerebral resuscitation in small mammals and birds. *Veterinary Clinics of North America: Exotic Animal Practice* **10**, 275–291

Lichtenberger ML (2004) Principles of shock and fluid therapy in special species. In: *Seminars in Avian and Exotic Pet Medicine*, ed. AM Fudge, pp. 142–153. WB Saunders, Missouri

Nickel R, Schummer A and Seiferle E (1977) *Anatomy of the Domestic Birds*. Verlag, Hamburg

Pattison M, McMullin P, Bradbury JM and Alexander D (2008) *Poultry Diseases, 6th edn*. Saunders Elsevier, Philadelphia

Quesenberry KE and Hillyer EV (1994) Supportive care and emergency therapy. In: *Avian Medicine: Principles and Application*, ed. BW Ritchie, GJ Harrison and LR Harrison, pp. 382–416. Wingers, Lake Worth

Raftery A (2005) The initial presentation: triage and critical care. In: *BSAVA Manual of Psittacine Birds, 2nd edn*, ed. N Harcourt-Brown and J Chitty, pp. 35–49. BSAVA Publications, Gloucester

Randall C (1991) *Diseases and Disorders of the Domestic Fowl and Turkey, 2nd edn*. Mosby, London

Tully TN, Dorrestein GM and Jones AJ (2009) *Handbook of Avian Medicine, 2nd edn*. Saunders Elsevier, Edinburgh

Useful website

AnAge: The Animal Ageing and Longevity Database
www.genomics.senescence.info/species/

Chapter 9

Clinical techniques

Neil Forbes

This chapter describes routes of administration for medicines, methods for sexing poultry and euthanasia techniques. Other clinical techniques are described in appropriate chapters: blood and faecal sampling in Chapter 10; sampling feathers and skin in Chapter 13; and tissue biopsy in Chapters 12 and 23.

Administration of medication

Appropriate therapeutics, precautions, dosages, routes and frequency of administration are discussed in Appendix 2.

Oral administration

In food

Depending on the number of birds to be treated, therapeutic products may be compounded in food, which is ideal if practical and available (see Chapter 26 for legal aspects of prescribing protocol for compounding in food).

If small numbers are involved, palatable preparations may be mixed with food for consumption by a small group of birds. Medications (appropriate to the total weight of the group of birds) may be mixed with an appropriate volume of wet food (e.g. soaked bread or mash layers) and provided in food troughs with sufficient space to avoid excessive competition. If wet mash or soaked bread is inappropriate for the species to be treated, a suitable volume of corn can be mixed with sufficient vegetable oil to coat the corn, and a powdered medication mixed well with this, prior to feeding.

'Self-administration' of medication in this manner is based on the concept that heavier birds will eat more and consume more medication. Such an approach is only justifiable where there is a wide therapeutic/toxicity safety margin.

In drinking water

Medication provided in drinking water may be appropriate when a whole group of birds needs to be treated. However, it should only be used where:

- There is a wide therapeutic/toxicity safety margin
- The therapeutic agent is stable in water for a suitable period
- The agent does not interact with the water container

- The agent is not distasteful to the point of reducing fluid intake
- Patients are not consuming significant water in their food
- The medicated water is the only source of drinking water available.

Where an automated drinking water system is in use, it is necessary to fill and medicate the header tank and turn off the water supply to the tank until the medicated water has been consumed. Medication provided should be appropriate to the total weight of the group of birds being treated.

> **PRACTICAL TIP**
>
> The weight of a sample of patients can be recorded, averaged and multiplied by the group number to calculate the total group weight

Direct administration

Direct oral administration is preferred when dealing with individual patients or small groups.

> **PRACTICAL TIP**
>
> It is advisable for the clinician to demonstrate methods of administration, in order to optimize client compliance

Restraint: Restraint for oral administration is often best achieved by one person, with the patient wrapped in a towel and with the bird's feet on the ground in an upright position. A second person then restrains the bird's head in their left hand, opening the beak with the thumb and index finger of the right hand. Once the mouth is open, the index finger or thumb of the left hand is placed in the cheek of the bird, between the jaws, to act as a gag.

Liquid medication: If the volume of medication is small (e.g. 0.5 ml to a 1 kg bird), it is acceptable to administer the medication by syringe into the mouth. If the volume is greater, it is best administered by gavage tube, so that it is deposited into the crop to obviate risks of its entering the trachea. A gavage tube can be as simple as a section of giving set tubing attached to a syringe, or a commercially sourced metal gavage tube can be used.

1. With the bird suitably restrained, the gavage tube is introduced into the bird's mouth from the bird's left hand side, angled across the pharynx (Figure 9.1).
2. The tube is passed down the right-hand side of the oesophagus, behind the glottis (which is readily seen in the mid-caudal tongue), using gravity alone. The tube should not be forced as this may cause damage to the oesophagus.
3. The tube is passed at least 3 cm below the glottis and the contents expressed into the crop.

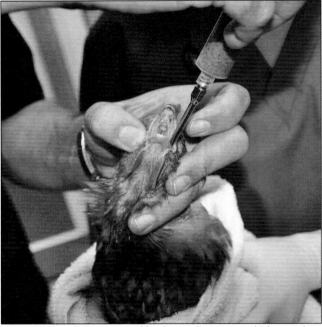

9.1 The administration of food or medication to a chicken can be achieved using a gavage tube.

Tablets: For direct administration, it is preferable to use a formulation with a diameter larger than that of the opening of the glottis and choana, so that inadvertent intratracheal administration by the owner is rendered impossible.

Depending on the size of the bird's mouth and the administrator's index finger, the tablet may be placed on top of an upturned index finger (Figure 9.2), passed into the open mouth and pressed against the dorsal aspect of the mouth. The finger is then passed caudally into the

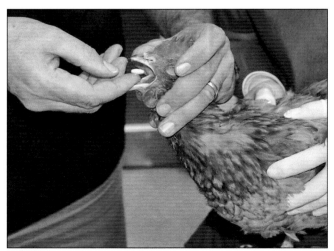

9.2 Administering a tablet to a chicken.

pharynx, which will naturally pronate so the tablet will pass safely down the oesophagus. Alternatively, a standard cat/dog 'pill popper' may be used to ensure that the tablet is placed in the pharynx, caudal to the glottis.

Ducks, geese and swans: It is important not to open the mouth by applying significant pressure to the tips of the beak, as beak fractures can occur. Rather, the index finger is slid up to the commissure and applied as a gag at this point. Giving tablets is generally easy using the method described above, even to small ducks. If it is not possible, a gavage tube or 'pill popper' should be used.

Injection
Restraint

It is preferable if the bird is restrained by an assistant. It may be held in a standing position on a table (see Figure 9.2) whilst the administrator holds the head with one hand and administers medication with the other. Alternatively, the bird may be held in an upright position with both its feet restrained in one hand, whilst the other hand is used to abduct a wing or restrain the head (Figure 9.3).

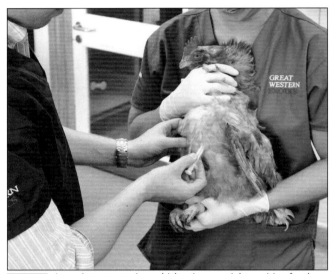

9.3 An assistant restrains a chicken in an upright position for the administration of an intramuscular injection.

Subcutaneous injection

- Small volumes of medications may be administered over the pectoral muscles (Figure 9.4).
- Larger volumes, as for subcutaneous fluid therapy, may be administered between the shoulder blades (preferable) or, if great care is taken, into the inguinal web (Figure 9.5) between the sternum and the medial thigh.

Intramuscular injection

An initial intramuscular injection may be advisable to expedite achievement of the minimum inhibitory concentration, especially if there is delayed crop emptying. Repeated intramuscular injections are generally avoided due to: the need for aseptic procedure; pain and damage to the breast muscle; and the availability of easier, less invasive routes. If repeated injections are required, these should be given intravenously if possible. Where this is impossible, sequential intramuscular injections should be given in different positions (Figure 9.6).

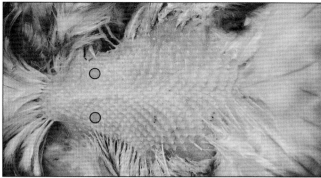

9.4 Subcutaneous injection sites (circled) over the pectoral muscles of a chicken.

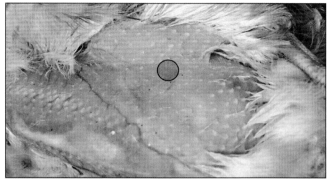

9.5 Subcutaneous injection site (circled) in the inguinal web of a chicken.

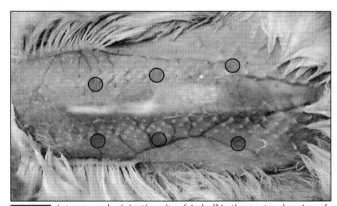

9.6 Intramuscular injection sites (circled) in the pectoral region of a chicken. If repeated injections are required, the sites should be rotated.

WARNING

Particular care is required when giving intramuscular injections to young birds, as they typically have little muscle mass and a soft sternum, so a hypodermic needle can be readily and inadvertently passed through the sternum and into the thoracic cavity

Intravenous injection and infusion

The intravenous route is the route of choice for fluid therapy and for repeated or frequent injections. The predominant access points are:

- Superficial ulnar (superficial basilic) vein (Figure 9.7a). Tape is applied to both sides of the catheter to act as an anchor whilst the catheter is sewn against the wing (Figure 9.7b)

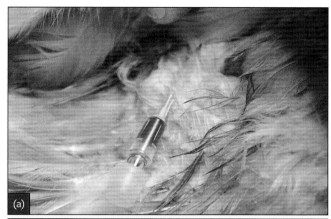

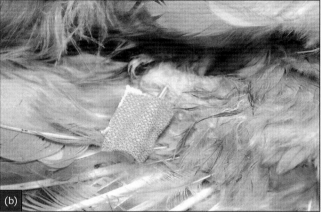

9.7 (a) A catheter placed in the superficial ulnar vein of a chicken. (b) Tape has been placed around the hub of the catheter to aid suturing into place.

- Medial tarsal vein (Figure 9.8). This is particularly useful in waterfowl, as long as the site can be kept clean. A 22–26 G plastic catheter with a metal stylet (e.g. Jelco, Sureflow) is used and is simply taped in place against the leg.

Intravenous catheters should be managed and maintained in an aseptic manner. Whilst in mammals they may be replaced every 48 hours, this may not be prudent in avian patients due to the limitation of possible access points if prolonged administration is anticipated.

The right (or left) jugular vein may be used for one-off injections, but this is not an easy location in which to maintain an intravenous catheter for repeated use. Almost all birds have a featherless tract (apterium) down either side of the neck; once this is located and the feathers either side are wetted with disinfectant or surgical spirit, the jugular vein is easily raised and accessed (Figure 9.9).

Intraperitoneal injection

Whilst the intraperitoneal route is invaluable in mammals, due to the complexities and risks associated with the anatomical position of the abdominal air sacs (situated bilaterally just medial to the abdominal wall), intraperitoneal injection in birds is not recommended.

Intraosseous injection

This is a very efficient route of access to the vascular system, although the intravenous route is typically less invasive and carries lower inherent risks in most cases.

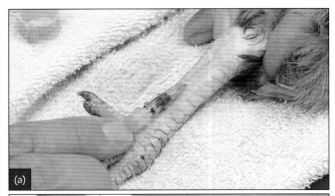

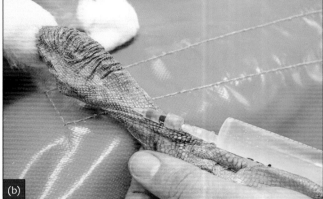

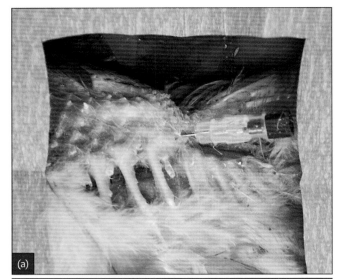

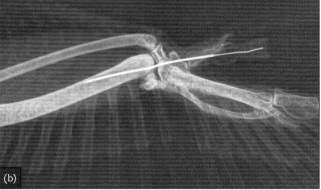

9.8 An intravenous catheter being placed into the medial tarsal vein of (a) a chicken and (b) a swan. (Saline solution with added electrolytes is being injected.)

9.10 (a) An intraosseous catheter placed in the distal ulna of a chicken. (b) The radiograph confirms the correct placement.

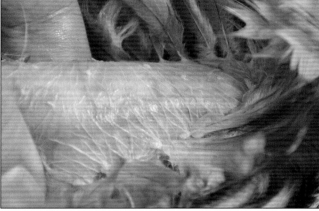

9.9 The right jugular vein can be seen running down the apterium in this chicken.

The intraosseous route is typically only required in a patient with severe dehydration or circulatory collapse, such that the veins are inaccessible, or in very young or small birds.

Intraosseous access is via the distal ulna or proximal tibiotarsus:

- For the ulna – the distal ulna is approached and the ulnar carpal bone is pushed ventrally to access the articular surface (Figure 9.10)
- For the tibiotarsus – the stifle is flexed to allow access to the articular surface of the proximal tibiotarsus from the lateral aspect (Figure 9.11).

The procedure is carried out under general anaesthesia, as it will involve hypodermic needle penetration through bone, with associated pain. A spinal needle (typically 20–22 G of suitable length) is used. The site is prepared in

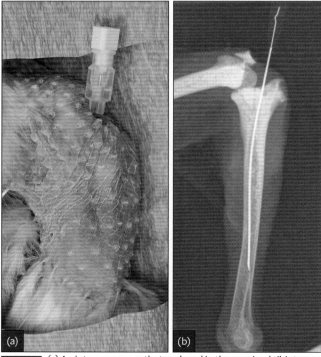

9.11 (a) An intraosseous catheter placed in the proximal tibiotarsus of a chicken. (b) The radiograph confirms the correct placement.

an aseptic manner. The needle is rotated and pressure applied to advance through the articular surface and into the medullary cavity. The intraosseous catheter must be capped off and maintained in an aseptic manner, but can be left in place for repeated use over a 48-hour period.

WARNING

Pneumatized avian bones (e.g. the femur and humerus) must be avoided for intraosseous injection, so as to avoid drowning

---

Nutritional support

Nutritional support is essential for anorexic or catabolic patients. A range of suitable foods are available (e.g. Emeraid® Omnivore diet). The diets should be mixed and fed as per the manufacturer's instructions (e.g. for the Emeraid® Omnivore diet, this is generally administered at a rate of 3% bodyweight and repeated three times daily). The administration technique is similar to that for oral fluids (see Figure 9.1). Clinicians should always demonstrate how to orally administer fluids and food to owners of those patients that require supplementation.

Sexing poultry

Although backyard poultry are frequently kept as pets, there are often other important motivating factors for keeping these birds, such as breeding and egg production. It is essential to know the sex of the birds in order to achieve such aims. In addition, successful management techniques require the correct ratio of males to females, which in some cases will be a 100% bias towards females.

Most poultry species show conspicuous sexual dimorphism as adults. However, dimorphism in juvenile poultry is typically subtle, or not apparent externally, providing a challenge to those trying to sex young birds. An additional challenge is that many poultry species have a large degree of breed-related polymorphism, which may limit secondary sexual characteristics to certain breeds or may act to obscure sexually dimorphic features. It is important to remember that certain poultry types represent a group of species rather than a single species (e.g. ducks). Figure 9.12 summarizes physical characteristics that can be observed to aid sexing.

Sex-linked colouring and feathering

In birds, males are the homogametic sex (two copies of the same sex chromosome) and females are the heterogametic sex (two different sex chromosomes). Avian sex chromosomes are denoted by Z and W, to distinguish them from the XX/XY system used in mammals. Hence, males are ZZ and females are ZW.

If an allele for plumage colour is located on the Z chromosome, the first generation offspring of the crosses between certain breeds of chicken will exhibit sex-linked plumage. These inheritance patterns are exploited by breeders to provide a non-invasive and relatively reliable way of sexing chicks.

Feature	Males	Females	Age seen (typical)
Chickens (Figure 9.13)			
Plumage	Often brighter and more exuberant (tail has sickle feathers) than females. Some cockerels have an inherited 'hen feathering' trait	Often less brightly coloured and less exuberant than males	From 6 months (i.e. maturity)
Feather shape	Tips of the neck feathers are usually pointed	Tips of the neck feathers are usually rounded	From 10 weeks
Body shape	Typically more slender appearance than females	Typically more squat and rounded appearance than males	From maturity
Comb and wattles	Usually larger and comb more erect	Usually less developed and comb may be less erect than males	Combs on males are typically larger by 4 weeks of age
Spurs	Always	Occasionally (especially when older) (Figure 9.14)	Males commence spur development at 4–6 weeks
Behaviour	Mounting behaviour. May be aggressive towards people	Will crouch for mating. Less likely to be aggressive towards people than males	From 4–6 months
Crowing	Common, especially at dawn	Rare	From around 6 months (may be earlier)
Ducks – mallard (Figure 9.15)			
Plumage	Often brighter than females	Often duller than males	From 6–12 months
Many species of duck have eclipse (winter) and breeding (spring and summer) plumage, which is much brighter in males			
Central tail feather(s)	Curved (the 'drake feather')	Straight	From 20–24 weeks
Body size	Usually larger than females	Usually smaller than males	From young and particularly at maturity
Phallus	Present (see Chapter 8)	Absent	Possibly from day 1, but much easier to identify from 3 weeks of age
Behaviour	More aggressive than females. Mounting behaviour and forced copulation	Less aggressive than males. Laying	Sexual maturity (9–12 months)
Voice	Soft rasp	Loud/clear quack	From 6–10 weeks

9.12 Physical and behavioural characteristics varying between male and female poultry that can aid sexing. (continues) ▶

Feature	Males	Females	Age seen (typical)
Ducks – Muscovy (Figure 9.16)			
Body size	Usually larger and stockier than females	Usually smaller and more slender than males	From young and particularly at maturity
Caruncles	Develop sooner and are more prominent than in females	Develop later. More variable in extent and typically less prominent	From 6 months
Feet and legs	Tend to be larger/wider than that of females	Tend to be smaller/thinner than in males	From young and particularly at maturity
Phallus	Present	Absent	Possibly from day 1, but much easier to identify from 3 weeks of age
Behaviour	More aggressive towards other birds than females. Mounting behaviour and forced copulation	Less aggressive than males. Laying	From sexual maturity
Voice	Hoarse, raspy, hissing	Trill	From 12 weeks
Turkeys (Figure 9.17)			
Body size	Usually larger than females	Usually smaller and more slender than males	From 8 weeks
Face colour	Darker red or blue (later)	More pink	From 8 weeks
Snood	Longer in males	Shorter in females	From 3–4 months
Caruncles	More developed than in females	Less developed than in males	
Beard of whiskers	Usually present protruding from the chest	Rarely present	
Neck feathers	Do not cover the head	Extend to the top of the head	
Legs	Longer with wider shank in males	Shorter with narrower shank in females	From 8 weeks
Spurs	Present	Usually absent, may be present in older birds	Start appearing from 10 weeks
Tail fan	Often displayed ('strutting')	Rarely displayed	From 9 months
Voice	Gobble	No gobble. Soft clucks and yelps	From around 6 months
Geese			
Plumage	May differ in a few breeds		
Body size	Usually larger than females	Usually smaller than males	From young and particularly at maturity
Eye colour (purebred Pilgrim geese)	Blue	Brown	From maturity
Knobs	If knobbed breed, usually larger in males	If knobbed breed, usually smaller in females	From 3 months
Phallus	Present (see Figure 9.20)	Absent	From day 1 in most species but much easier to identify from 3 weeks of age
Voice	More likely to be shrill and high pitched	More likely to be lower, deeper and harsher noise	From 3 months
Guinea fowl			
Helmet	Slightly larger in males	Slightly smaller in females	Adult
Wattles	Larger and thicker in males	Smaller and thinner in females	Between 12 and 15 weeks
Vent	Large heart- or butterfly-shaped ventral cloacal protuberance	Smaller, flatter, book-shaped protuberance	Possibly from 10 weeks
Voice	Always one syllable cry	Two-tone cry ('buck wheat–buck wheat' or 'come back–come back') unless excited, then one syllable	From 2 months
Pheasants (significant variation between species) (Figure 9.18)			
Plumage	Usually brightly coloured, long tails. Characteristic bright breast colouration commences at 6–8 weeks. From 4 weeks bars on wings are diagonal	Usually less brightly coloured, short tails. From 4 weeks bars on the tail are perpendicular to the shaft (rachis)	From first moult at 6–9 months
Body size	Usually larger than females	Usually smaller than males	Adult
Head shape (may be useful in certain species)	More square in males	More sloping in females	Young chick
Wattle shape and size (may be useful in certain species)	More extensive, especially dorsally	Less extensive	Young chick
Spurs	Present	Absent or only spur bumps	Development commences from 6 weeks

9.12 (continued) Physical and behavioural characteristics varying between male and female poultry that can aid sexing. (continues) ▶

Feature	Males	Females	Age seen (typical)
Peafowl (Indian) (Figure 9.19)			
Plumage	Iridescent blue-green or green. In the first year male birds have black and white bard on the wings, shoulders and back	Dull green, brown and grey. In the first year female birds have clear brown dusky feathers on the wings, shoulder and back	First blue feathers come through on the neck of the male bird at 6 months
Crest	Present	Present	
Neck and legs	Tend to be longer in males	Tend to be shorter in females	From a few months old
Train (tail)	Highly elongated with 'eyes'	Absent	2–3 years old
Behaviour	Will display tail feathers for mating or as a warning	Will display tail feathers as a warning	Sexual behaviours are demonstrated from 3 years of age

9.12 (continued) Physical and behavioural characteristics varying between male and female poultry that can aid sexing.

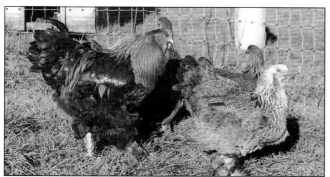

9.13 The male partridge form of the Cochin breed of chicken (left) has a marked difference in colour and pattern to that of the female (right and background). In some other colour forms and breeds of chicken, cockerels and hens may show little or no difference in colouration.
(Courtesy of R Poland with thanks to M Boarder)

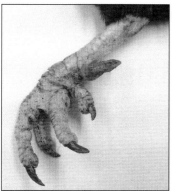

9.14 Spur development on the medial aspect of the right leg of a 5-year-old Welsummer hen. The spur on the left leg had not developed beyond a small knub.

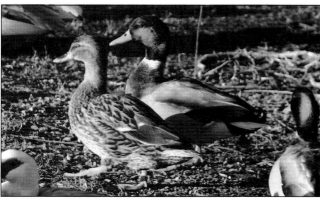

9.15 Male (right) and female (left) mallard ducks show marked dimorphism in terms of feather colour and pattern.
(Courtesy of R Poland)

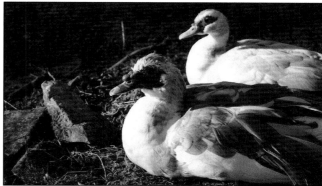

9.16 The male Muscovy duck (left) typically has more developed caruncles and more red colouring on the side of the head than the female (right).
(Courtesy of R Poland with thanks to M Boarder)

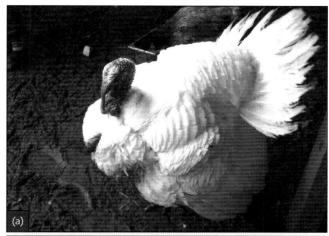

(a)

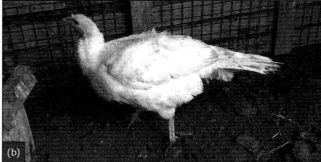

(b)

9.17 (a) The male turkey usually has a beard, which is generally absent in (b) the female. The male also has a more developed snood, and the neck feathers do not cover as far up the neck as they do in the female.
(Courtesy of L Vale)

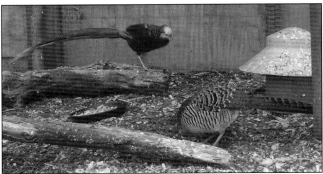

9.18 The male (left) and female (right) golden pheasant are a good example of sexual dimorphism with the male demonstrating a brightly coloured plumage in comparison with the female.

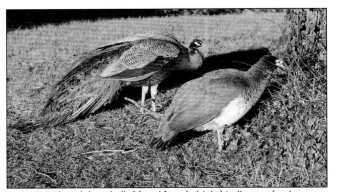

9.19 The adult male (left) and female (right) Indian peafowl are easily distinguishable from one another based on the brightly coloured plumage and long train of the peacock compared with the duller coloured plumage and short tail of the peahen.
(Courtesy of R Poland)

The red sex link in chickens

When hens with a silver factor are crossed with red cockerels, male offspring hatch out white (silver) whilst female offspring hatch out buff or red. Potential crosses include:

- White Plymouth Rock female X red New Hampshire male > Gold Comet
- Silver Laced Wynandotte female X red New Hampshire male > Cinnamon Queen
- Rhode Island White female X Rhode Island Red male
- Delaware female X Rhode Island Red male.

The particular genes involved depend on the cross, but in red sex-linked birds, the plumage colour is determined by two alleles: the silver (S) and gold (s) alleles carried on the Z chromosome. As S is dominant to s, the male must be homozygous recessive to show the red colour. In the crosses detailed above, male offspring receive one copy of the Z chromosome from the dam (carrying the dominant S allele), so will always be silver; female offspring will never be silver because their single copy of the Z chromosome comes from the homozygous recessive (ss) sire. Since the male offspring are heterozygous (Ss), they cannot be used for further red sex-linked crosses.

The black sex link in chickens

Black sex linkage may be observed when a barred hen is crossed with a non-barred cockerel, resulting in solid black female offspring and non-solid coloured male offspring. Since the barred allele is dominant, a non-barred

male must be homozygous for the recessive non-barred allele. The sex link also relies on the offspring carrying the autosomal 'extended black gene', so at least one of the parents must be homozygous for that gene. Most breeds can be used for the sire, as long as he is not barred or carrying a dominant white gene. Commercially, Barred Plymouth Rock females are typically used.

Delayed feathering in chickens

Certain breeds of chicken, such as the Barred Plymouth Rock, have a genetically determined delay in feather production during the early stages of growth. This delay is determined by a gene at the K locus on the Z chromosome. There are four alleles at this locus, ranging from extremely slow feathering to fast normal feathering. These alleles exhibit a dominance hierarchy, with the slow feathering allele being the most dominant, and the fast normal feathering allele being the least dominant. By crossing a homozygous fast normal feathering male with a delayed feathering female, the resulting male offspring will have slower feather growth than the female offspring. This can be seen in 1-day-old chicks, but is most obvious in 10-day-old chicks, and can be assessed by comparing the length of the primary remiges and the coverlets. In fast normal feathering birds, the primary remiges will be longer than the coverlets, whilst in slow feathering birds they may be the same length or shorter.

Other species

Sex-linked colouring is used to sex some breeds of turkeys and geese. Sex-linked delayed feathering is also used in some breeds of turkey to aid sexing, and the down of 1-day-old goslings can be used to sex certain breeds of geese.

Vent sexing

This is a skilled technique and is highly dependent on the experience of the technician. It is reported to carry a small risk of iatrogenic damage to the chick, especially when performed by inexperienced people. It is usually performed when the chick is 1-day-old but may be performed in older birds.

Chickens

The procedure for vent sexing chickens is as follows:

1. Faeces are expelled from the cloaca by gently pressing on either side of the abdomen in a cranial to caudal motion.
2. The chick is supported on its back in the palm of the hand with its head pointing towards the operator's elbow and vent pointing upwards. It should be supported by the middle and ring fingers across the breast.
3. The vent is everted using the index finger of the hand in which the chick is being held. The index finger is placed adjacent to the dorsal rim of the vent and the thumb of the other hand is placed adjacent to the ventral rim or side of the vent. Moving the index finger and thumb in a circular motion then applying pressure will help to achieve eversion.
4. Males are identified by the presence of a small prominence on the ventral wall of the cloaca, which is the rudimentary non-protrusible phallus. Some female chickens will also have a prominence at the entrance of

the oviduct into the cloaca, which may be hard to differentiate from that of the male. In females the prominence is likely to be smaller and to be reducible under digital compression, whereas in males the phallus is likely to be larger and remain firm when pressed.

Other species

A similar technique is used to that in chickens, but the phallus of ducks and geese is a more developed structure (Figure 9.20). In older ducks and geese, the phallus can be quite large and it may be difficult to evert the vent.

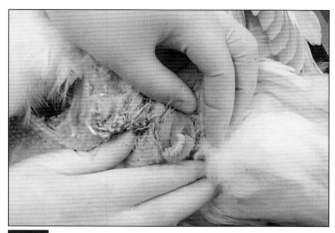

9.20 The phallus of an adult gander.

Laparoscopy

Laparoscopy can be used to visualize the gonads of birds, including poultry. It is relatively invasive and requires general anaesthesia, so tends to be reserved for use in birds of high genetic value and where non-invasive techniques are not sufficiently reliable.

Molecular techniques

Polymerase chain reaction (PCR) analysis of samples, typically blood or feathers, is widely available from commercial laboratories and relies on amplification of DNA sequences located on the W chromosome.

Euthanasia

Euthanasia of poultry raises several issues beyond those of euthanasia of other species usually encountered by small animal practitioners. Poultry may need to be euthanased in order to ensure their welfare, but they may also be killed for meat production or if they are not suitable for their intended purpose. Although a veterinary surgeon is unlikely to be involved other than for welfare purposes, it is essential that they are able to advise their clients on all aspects of humane killing. Regardless of the reason for killing, or the technique employed, it is the moral and legal responsibility of the person carrying out the procedure to eliminate any avoidable excitement, pain or suffering. The following section discusses the techniques used for euthanasia, and readers are directed to the Humane Slaughter Association (www.hsa.org.uk) for further information on the killing of poultry for other purposes. Some legal aspects of the slaughter of poultry are discussed in Chapter 26.

Many veterinary surgeons prefer to euthanase poultry birds in a clinical setting using chemical techniques; however, the food-producing origins of poultry mean that a number of mechanical techniques for the killing of poultry are available. There are circumstances where mechanical techniques may be preferable, since they may in fact cause less stress due to the speed of delivery.

Chemical euthanasia

Chemical euthanasia relies upon the administration of pentobarbital through the intravenous route. Prior to administration, chemical restraint may be employed to minimize stress and aid handling. This can be achieved by inducing gaseous anaesthesia (e.g. with isoflurane or sevoflurane) or by injectable sedation (e.g. diazepam, midazolam, ketamine ± medetomidine).

Pentobarbital is highly irritating to all tissues and so should only be administered via the intravenous route (e.g. superficial ulnar or medial tarsal veins; see above). In addition, the occipital sinus provides a very effective site for the administration of pentobarbital. This is achieved with the bird restrained in a normal physiological position. The clinician (if right-handed) restrains the bird's head in a flexed position with their left hand. The index finger of the right hand is used to locate a depression between the occiput and atlas. The hypodermic needle is placed in the midline at this point and advanced 2–3 mm (depending on bird size) before commencing barbiturate injection. Once the bird loses consciousness, the needle may be advanced into the brainstem for further barbiturate administration. This technique typically avoids the leg and wing flapping associated with many avian euthanasia techniques.

Mechanical euthanasia
Cervical dislocation

When performed by trained individuals, this technique appears to be humane. If performed near to the head, dislocation of the cervical vertebral column from the skull damages the lower brain region, with separation of the brain from the brainstem and carotid arteries, causing rapid unconsciousness. This is best accomplished using a stretching motion rather than by crushing the vertebrae. Applying a rotating movement to the neck can dislocate small birds' necks. No prior sedation or anaesthesia is employed, but proper training is vital in order to perform the technique without compromising animal welfare.

Adult poultry should be held by the shanks of both legs with one hand, and the head grasped immediately behind the skull with the other hand. The neck is then extended, twisted (pushing the knuckles into the back of the neck) and dislocated using a sharp downward and backward thrust. It is vital that the pull is firm, decisive and efficient. After neck dislocation, the operator should feel the neck for an obvious separation of the cervical vertebrae. To ensure death, the bird's throat should be cut after cervical dislocation.

The necks of larger or heavily muscled birds such as broiler breeders, turkeys, geese and waterfowl are extremely difficult to dislocate. It is therefore recommended that other methods, such as captive bolt or gas euthanasia, be used for birds >3 kg. If this is not possible, neck dislocation may be appropriate in some circumstances.

See the American Veterinary Medical Association (AVMA) guidelines on euthanasia (https://www.avma.org/KB/Policies/Documents/euthanasia.pdf) for more information.

PRACTICAL TIP

With neck dislocation, wing flapping and other body movements may persist for several minutes after cervical dislocation, although if the vertebrae have been properly dislocated these are reflex reactions. Restraining the bird's wings prior to performing the dislocation can prevent involuntary flapping

Other mechanical techniques

Other mechanical techniques, such as decapitation and percussive and electrical stunning, are used but discussion of these procedures is beyond the scope of this manual. As with all techniques, it is essential that the operator is fully trained and experienced in performing these procedures.

Euthanasia of hatchlings

Commercially, high concentrations of carbon dioxide are used for humane euthanasia of hatchlings. The placing of conscious chicks in a freezer is not recognized as a humane or permitted method of euthanasia. Any efficient and instant method of rendering the chick unconscious, such as crushing the cranium, is acceptable, although in a veterinary context, sedation or anaesthesia should always precede such techniques.

Disposal of dead birds

It is important that clinicians advise clients about the correct way in which to dispose of poultry carcases; see Chapter 26 for further information.

Acknowledgements

The section in this chapter on sexing poultry was written by Guy Poland.

Useful website

Welfare of animals at the Time of Killing
https://www.gov.uk/government/collections/welfare-of-animals-at-the-time-of-killing

Chapter 10

Clinical pathology

Helene Pendl and Karin Kreyenbühl

External *versus* in-house laboratory diagnostics

General considerations

Avian patients, in general, require a rapid and precise laboratory diagnostic work-up as clinical findings often do not correlate with the severity of the disease. Medical management of backyard poultry is a balancing act between individual care for pets and flock medicine ensuring safety for public health. Clinical pathology needs to achieve both objectives by providing a good mixture of diagnostic tests. Laboratory tests are performed to diagnose or exclude a certain disease, document the progress of a disease, for a prognosis or to set-up a database for specific questions.

In-house laboratories: prospects and limitations

In-house laboratory procedures should focus on rapid, simple and cost-effective techniques. Haematology, cytology, parasitology and selected parameters of clinical chemistry provide a good overview of the disease process and should give an idea for initial therapy and selection of further procedures. Efficacy and success of an in-house laboratory is dependent on the equipment available, sample preparation and expertise of the examiner. This is particularly true for diagnostic microscopy as applied in parasitology, cytology and haematology. Reliable in-house assessment of cytological specimens and blood films requires intensive education in the first place and then regular training to maintain expertise. Therefore, diagnostic success will only be achieved with review of a sufficient number of cases per day. Textbooks and practical courses provide a first entry into the field. Experience is best gained by second evaluation by a specialist. Thus, in the first instance, samples should be evaluated in-house and by an external laboratory; these samples will then serve as a reference collection for training and comparison. With increasing experience, only the more complicated cases need to be sent out for a second opinion. This approach allows for practice-specific training and quality control, both in terms of species, cases and sample preparation. Investment in a good quality microscope will simplify and speed up evaluation. It should be equipped with a minimum of four objectives: 4x, 10x, 40x and 100x, resulting in a total magnification of X40, X100, X400 and X1000, respectively. Dark field or phase contrast is helpful for the detection of flagellates and motile bacteria.

External laboratories

Further diagnostic work-up (such as histopathological and microbiological evaluation) is best performed by external laboratories with specialist knowledge in avian medicine. Besides commercial laboratories, academic institutions and public health services will provide appropriate services. In cases of a suspected epidemic or risk to public safety, a flock medical approach is required for rapid aetiological diagnosis. In these instances, access to polymerase chain reaction (PCR) and serological diagnostics from facilities specializing in poultry medicine is essential to generate results in a timely manner.

Reference values

Proper interpretation of numerical parameters in clinical pathology requires comparison to physiological reference values. Factors such as age, gender, hormonal status and environmental conditions have been proven to influence results under physiological conditions. Different techniques and definitions of reference groups in the literature additionally contribute to the high variability of given reference values. Thus, published data cited in Figures 10.19, 10.34 and 10.35 are intended as rough guidelines to begin with and should be replaced by practice-specific reference intervals as soon as possible. Ideally, this is achieved by generating flock-specific or even individual bird profiles by regular health checks.

Optimization of work and costs

The samples collected during a disease investigation should cover all possible differential diagnoses, even if they are not all used in the end. Recommendations for sample collection are summarized in Figure 10.1. Establishment of standard operating procedures (SOPs), such as the evaluation protocol for avian blood films (see Figure 10.6) and the checklist for avian post-mortem samples (Figure 10.2; see also Chapter 25) may be time-consuming in the first instance but are helpful to rationalize work flows in terms of staff education, time and cost-effectiveness. Consistent labelling of samples and computer-assisted archiving of results will allow rapid access to previous data, which is particularly useful for retrospective studies and the evaluation of serial samples. An example of a label used in practice is given in Figure 10.24 with the identification number in the first line (Z = cytology; yy/mm/dd = date; ss = case number), the scientific name of the species in the second line, the type of stain in the third line and the organ, sample number and additional remarks in the last line.

Site	Sample
Skin	• Swab (wet or dry) for cytology and microbiology • Scrape or acetate tape imprint for cytology and parasitology • Fine-needle aspiration of ulcers and/or underlying tissue for cytology
Feathers	• Full feather: direct microscopy to examine for anatomical aberrations and parasites • Calamus/pulp/follicle: biopsy sample for histology and virology; squash/acetate tape imprint for cytology; swab for microbiology
Eyes, nares, oropharynx, trachea, cloaca	• Swab (wet or dry) for cytology, microbiology, parasitology and polymerase chain reaction (PCR) • Solid masses: see below • Nares/trachea/cloaca: flushes into EDTA (ethylenediaminetetraacetic acid) for direct wet-mount or sediment smears for cytology, swabs for microbiology and PCR
Blood	• Whole blood sample: haematology (EDTA sample for cell counts; native sample for blood film); microbiology (swab) • Plasma/serum sample: heparin; serology; clinical chemistry
Fluid (cystic structures, abscesses, synovial fluid, ascites)	• Fluid: fine-needle aspirate into EDTA, native or sediment smear for cytology; swab for microbiology and PCR • Cystic wall/solid contents: fine-needle aspirate or squash preparation for cytology
Solid masses	• External/superficial: fine-needle aspirate, scrape or actate tape imprint for cytology • Ulcerated/exudative: additional swab for cytology and microbiology • Internal: ultrasound-guided (ideally) fine-needle aspiration
Faeces	• Voided samples or cloacal swabs: direct wet mount flotation for parasitology; Gram-stain and culture for microbiology; Wright-Giemsa stain for cytology
Post-mortem examination (see Figure 10.2)	• Acetate tape imprints, scrapes and aspirates for cytology from lesions together with squash preparations from the five large parenchymata (heart, lung, kidney, spleen, liver) • Full tissue blocks: preserved in formalin at room temperature for histology; frozen for virology • Swabs for microbiology and PCR • Smears (e.g. from gastrointestinal tract for parasitology)

10.1 Recommendations for sample collection in routine diagnostic procedures.

Checklist for avian post-mortem samples

Name/ID: .... Date: ....

History: ....

....

Histology (H)/virology (V)/cytology (C)

Gastrointestinal

	H	V	C
Liver	☐	☐	☐
Pancreas	☐	☐	☐
Proventriculus	☐	☐	☐
Ventriculus	☐	☐	☐
Small intestine	☐	☐	☐
Large intestine	☐	☐	☐
Cloaca	☐	☐	☐
	☐	☐	☐

Cardiorespiratory

	H	V	C
Heart	☐	☐	☐
Vessels	☐	☐	☐
Trachea	☐	☐	☐
Lung	☐	☐	☐
Airsac	☐	☐	☐
	☐	☐	☐
	☐	☐	☐
	☐	☐	☐

Haematopoietic

	H	V	C
Peripheral blood	☐	☐	☐
Spleen	☐	☐	☐
Bone marrow	☐	☐	☐
Bursa of Fabricius	☐	☐	☐
Thymus	☐	☐	☐
	☐	☐	☐
	☐	☐	☐

Urogenital

	H	V	C
Kidney	☐	☐	☐
Ovary	☐	☐	☐
Oviduct	☐	☐	☐
Testis	☐	☐	☐
	☐	☐	☐
	☐	☐	☐
	☐	☐	☐

Endocrine skin

	H	V	C
Thyroid	☐	☐	☐
Parathyroid	☐	☐	☐
Ultimobranchial	☐	☐	☐
Adrenal	☐	☐	☐
Skin	☐	☐	☐
Feather	☐	☐	☐
	☐	☐	☐

Neuromuscular

	H	V	C
Cerebrum	☐	☐	☐
Cerebellum	☐	☐	☐
Spinal C*	☐	☐	☐
Peripheral neuro	☐	☐	☐
Bone	☐	☐	☐
Sc muscle	☐	☐	☐
	☐	☐	☐

* Sampling of vertebral column in chicks: Please transect at the lumbosacral area to include Glycogen body (*Corpus gelatinosum*). Organs written in **bold** letters should be included in every histopath collection to assure an optimal histopathologic evaluation of the case. Organs written in **bold** and ***italic*** letters are of special interest in chicks. Histology: tissue in 6–8% formalin of high quality, buffered to ph 7.2 (standard buffers required, no calcium carbonate), Virology: frozen tissue; Cytology: slide preparations of imprints, fine-needle aspirates, swabs, scrapings.

Microbiology (M)/parasitology (P)

Organ/tissue	M	P	Remarks
....	☐	☐	....
....	☐	☐	....

10.2 Checklist for sample collection during a post-mortem examination.

Haematology

Collection of blood samples

A healthy bird will tolerate a total blood loss of approximately 1% of its bodyweight without adverse side effects (i.e. a sample of 5 ml can be obtained from a 500 g bird). To be on the safe side, even in the case of severely debilitated patients or unexpected haemorrhage during sampling, the volume should be reduced to 0.5–0.7%. A volume of 0.2 ml is sufficient for a routine blood cell count. Clinical chemistry requires 0.5–3 ml depending on the packed cell volume (PCV) of the individual bird and the number of parameters to be measured. Common sites for venepuncture include the jugular vein, the basilic vein and the caudal tibial vein. The jugular vein is difficult to visualize in ducks and geese as anseriforms lack the feather-free area (apterium) over the vessel that is present in gallinaceous birds. To minimize suction power and avoid collapse of the thin-walled vessels, blood samples are most effectively collected using a combination of a small lumen syringe (1–3 ml) and a short length, large lumen needle (22–25 G). Bending the needle at a 25–30-degree angle from the hub prior to venepuncture will facilitate smooth entry into the vein.

Handling and processing blood samples

To maintain an optimal mixing ratio of blood sample to anticoagulant, containers should always be filled up to the mark. In cases of small sample volumes, miniature blood collection tubes designed for human paediatric use can be used. Heparin is the anticoagulant of choice, as heparinized full blood or plasma samples can be used for cell counts, PCR diagnostics, toxicity and plasma chemistry. Samples collected into ethylenediaminetetraacetic acid (EDTA) are not appropriate for plasma enzyme assays as metal ions necessary for maximum activity will be chelated.

Both haematological and biochemical measurements are ideally obtained from fresh blood samples. In the case of plasma chemistry, plasma and cells should be separated immediately after collection to prevent leakage of intracellular enzymes into the plasma and consumption of nutrients by blood cells. Storage and shipment times need to be kept to a minimum under cooled conditions, otherwise cell degeneration, haemolysis and bacterial growth (due to the non-sterile nature of avian blood) will interfere with many parameters.

Blood films are ideally produced without anticoagulant from the last drop from the hub of the needle. Anticoagulants, although necessary for transport and storage of samples, have an adverse effect on haematological results. Heparin alters cell morphology in blood films, but is still preferable to EDTA, which is known to cause artificial *in vitro* haemolysis in certain bird species, including exotic gallinaceous species such as curassows and guans. This may also be the case for more common backyard poultry species.

Packed cell volume and haematocrit

Determination

PCV is defined as the relative portion of the cell-containing column to the full column of a centrifuged haematocrit tube. The haematocrit (HCT), in contrast, only relates the red cell column to the full column (Figure 10.3). The difference is usually of little practical significance, but may be important in cases of massive leucocytic responses with increased buffy coat. Methodically, the determination of

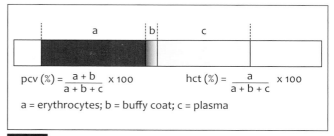

$$\text{pcv } (\%) = \frac{a + b}{a + b + c} \times 100 \qquad \text{hct } (\%) = \frac{a}{a + b + c} \times 100$$

a = erythrocytes; b = buffy coat; c = plasma

10.3 Columnar portions of a centrifuged haematocrit tube.

the PCV and HCT is the same for mammals and birds. The use of a microhaematocrit centrifuge is advantageous for small sample sizes. The timespan for maximum cell compression is device-dependent and should be adjusted according to the individual machine. This is simply performed by running the centrifuge with a filled microhaematocrit tube at appropriate speed and determining the time of maximum cell compression with repeated measurements. This should also be checked on machines with preset modes.

Changes in the cellular column

Due to the presence of up to 10% immature erythrocytes even in healthy adult birds, a smooth transition can be seen between the red cell column and the buffy coat. Physiologically, chicks have lower total HCT values and higher proportions of immature cells, which move towards adult values as they reach sexual maturity. Quantitative changes in the HCT are of either cellular (absolute) or plasmatic (relative) origin and can be differentiated by measuring the total protein content. A decrease in HCT value reflects anaemia and a rise points towards polycythaemia. A buffy coat >1.5% indicates leucocytosis or thrombocytosis; values >10% are strongly suggestive of leukaemic neoplasia. Qualitative changes can be observed in the transition area between the two cell columns. An abrupt change from red to white indicates a right shift; a broadened light red transition area indicates a left shift of erythrocytes. In severe cases, the latter can result in a pinkish buffy coat with a complete mixture of immature erythrocytes, leucocytes and thrombocytes rendering a clear measurement of the HCT impossible.

Changes in the plasma column

The clear blood plasma column in the centrifuged haematocrit tube can take on different colours in birds, mainly influenced by lipochromes (carotenoids) ingested with the diet. Red and yellow tinges are most frequently seen, the latter being particularly common in granivorous species. The intensity of the plasma colour varies with the volume of carotenoid intake. Some plasma colour changes indicate alterations in the metabolic state. A milky-white appearance is typical for lipaemia. This can be seen postprandially or may be caused by a malfunction in lipid metabolism. If present in a female bird, the list of differential diagnoses should include hyperoestrogenism due to a physiological reproductive state or pathological alterations of the reproductive tract. The latter is usually accompanied by a depressive anaemia. Haemolysis leads to a clear red plasma colour and can be artificial or pathological in origin. In contrast to samples with carotenoid-related reddening of the plasma column, haemolytic samples display an additional loss of the column layers, resulting in an overall blurred appearance of the haematocrit tube.

Blood films

Preparation

Blood films are ideally produced without anticoagulant from the last drop from the hub of the needle. The method of choice for blood film preparation is the wedge smear technique (Figure 10.4). Using a bevel-edged slide for streaking the sample minimizes the number of ruptured cells in the blood film. The drop of blood should be completely distributed on the slide, resulting in a film with a thinning vane at the end. Only these samples will contain a monolayer of cells located approximately between the second and last third of the film, which is crucial for a proper examination.

Staining

The best staining results are achieved with air-dried blood films. Alcohol fixation will affect staining properties of the granules in heterophils and basophils. Changes range from slight aberrations to optically empty, colourless structures. A Wright-Giemsa staining protocol, outlined in Figure 10.5, has been demonstrated to be of superior value for avian blood films. Quick stain kits may cause a severe loss of granular structures in heterophils, jeopardizing the diagnosis of subtle pathological changes

Colourant
• 3 g Wright powder[a]
• 0.3 g Giemsa powder[b]
• 5 ml glycerine
• 1000 ml absolute methanol (acetone-free)[c]
• Filter and store in a dark vial
• Stable for several weeks

Staining protocol
Using air-dried blood films:
1. Flood blood film with colourant for 3 minutes.
2. Add an equal volume of buffer with a pH of 6.8[d].
3. Mix gently by blowing with a pipette or straw until a metallic green sheen appears on the surface.
4. Allow to stand for 6 minutes.
5. Rinse and flood the blood film with buffer for 1 minute.
6. Wash copiously with buffer.
7. Wipe the back of the blood film to remove any excess stain.
8. Prop in a rack until dry or use a hairdryer.
9. Mount with mounting medium[e] and coverslip.

10.5 A Wright-Giemsa staining protocol for avian blood films. Examples: [a] Merck® No 1.09278.0025; [b] Merck® No 1.09203.0025; [c] Merck® No 1.06009.1000; [d] Merck® No 1.11374.0100; [e] Entellan® Neu, Merck® No 1.07961.0100. (Samour, personal communication)

in cell morphology. This is most commonly caused by a drop of alcohol concentration due to evaporation, as commercially available quick staining kits are often stored in containers without screw tops. Good closure of the jar lids and regular renewal of dyes is important for any staining protocol to receive consistent results. Basophils exhibit signs of disintegration in the majority of cases, even with Wright-Giemsa staining, and sometimes disappear completely in quick stained samples. The optical quality of the stained blood film is increased when mounted with a coverslip and a mounting medium. For non-permanent purposes mounting with a drop of immersion oil and a coverslip will give equal results. This is particularly advantageous for evaluation with the 40x objective.

Evaluation

Technical quality: To avoid counting errors, an assessment of the technical quality of the blood film and cell morph-ology is recommended before performing numerical counts. The protocol outlined in Figure 10.6 meets these demands as its design follows a strict order (i.e. from upper left to lower right of the form). Examination begins with a search for aggregates of thrombocytes. In cases where aggregates are present, an estimate of the total number of thrombocytes is not possible. For evaluation of technical quality, a semi-quantitative scale from 1 (not acceptable) to 5 (excellent) is useful. Any observed artefacts due to sampling, processing, transport, storage, fixation and staining must be considered.

Cytomorphology – general considerations: In comparison to mammals, avian blood cells show unique morphological characteristics. Mature erythrocytes and thrombocytes contain a nucleus; the neutrophil corresponding heterophils display visible granules. Due to these differences, several cell types in avian blood films are difficult to characterize correctly. This is particularly the case for the three types of granulocyte (Figures 10.7 and 10.8), and for small lymphocytes, thrombocytes (Figure 10.9) and erythrocytes.

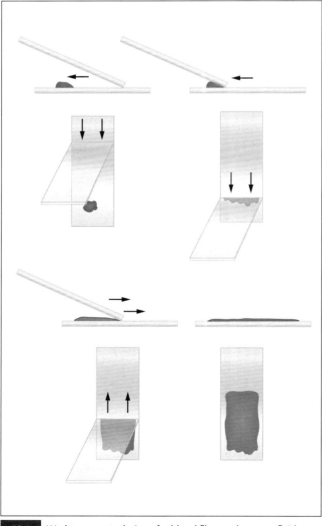

10.4 Wedge smear technique for blood films and opaque fluids.

ID:................................ **Name:**.................................... **Date:**.............................

Morphology			Counts							

Morphology

10x Objective: thrombocyte aggregates?

Yes ☐   No ☐

Technical quality
1 *(Not acceptable)* ☐   2 *(Problematic)* ☐   3 *(Acceptable)* ☐
4 *(Good)* ☐   5 *(Excellent)* ☐

Erythrocytes
HCT = PI^b =
1 *(Homogenous)* ☐   2 *(Slightly irregular)* ☐   3 *(Moderately irregular)* ☐
4 *(Severly irregular)* ☐   5 *(Extremely irregular)* ☐

Thrombocytes
(Look for: vacuoles, irregular cell membrane, cytoplasmic blebs)

>50% reactive?
Yes ☐   No ☐

Heterophils
(Look for: degranulation, vacuoles, cytoplasmic basophilia, non-lobulated nucleus)

Toxic/immature
Yes ☐   No ☐

Mononuclear cells
(Look for: cytoplasmic blebs, cytoplasmic basophilia, visible Golgi apparatus vacuoles, magenta bodies)

>50% reactive?
Ly: Yes ☐ No ☐
Mo: Yes ☐ No ☐

Remarks/other findings

Diagnoses – summary *(Numerical and morphological)*

1. Erythrocytes

2. Thrombocytes

3. Leucocytes

4. Other

Counts

Estimation[a]		Differential count					
Thr	Leuko	H	L	M	E	B	NDB
1	1						
2	2						
3	3						
4	4						
5	5						
6	6						
7	7						
8	8						
9	9						
10	10						
11	11						
12	12						
13	13						
14	14						
15	15						
16	16						
17	17						
18	18						
19	19						
20	20						
Σ	Σ	Σ					
Σx875	Σx875	%					

Correction formula in case of HCT outside 35–55%

☐ x ☐ : 45 = ☐
Σx875   HCT   Corrected value

☐ x ☐ : 45 = ☐
Σx875   HCT   Corrected value

10.6 Standardized protocol for avian blood film evaluation. [a] Estimation according to Campbell and Ellis (2007): total number of counted cells in 20 oil immersion fields x 875 = total estimated count. [b] Polychromatic index according to Dein (1983). B = basophils; E = eosinophils; H = heterophils; HCT = haematocrit; L = lymphocytes; Leuko = leucocytes; M = monocytes; NDB = non-definable blood cells; Thr = thrombocytes.

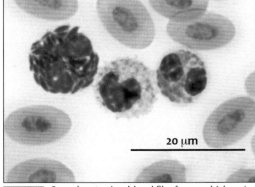

10.7 Granulocytes in a blood film from a chicken. Left to right: heterophil, basophil and eosinophil. The polychromatic index (PI) of the erythrocytes is 1.
(Wright-Giemsa stain)

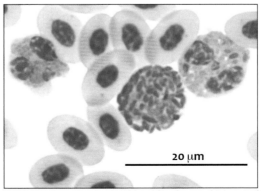

10.8 Granulocytes in a blood film from a chicken. Left to right: eosinophil, physiological heterophil and toxic heterophil. The polychromatic index (PI) of the erythrocytes is 1.
(Wright-Giemsa stain)

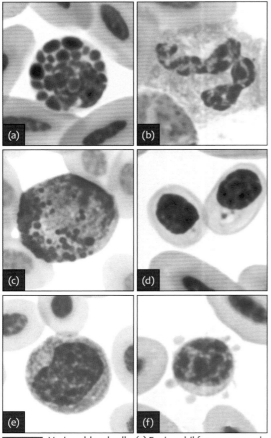

10.9 Various blood cells. (a) Eosinophil from a peacock. (b) Eosinophil from a goose. (c) Immature granulocyte from a chicken. (d) Thrombocytes from a peacock. (e) Reactive monocyte from a chicken. (f) Reactive lymphocyte from a turkey.
(Wright-Giemsa stain)

Cytomorphology of erythrocytes: Erythrocytes are seen as elliptic cells with an elliptical nucleus and a homogeneous eosinophilic cytoplasm. Mature cells with a pathologically low haemoglobin content are defined as hypochromic cells and typically have a faint perinuclear rim of weaker coloration (Figure 10.10). In contrast, the term polychromatic erythrocyte refers to immature cells with a physiologically low haemoglobin content and summarizes all immature developmental stages of the erythrocytic line. Due to the variable characteristics of the different maturation stages, polychromatic cells display a

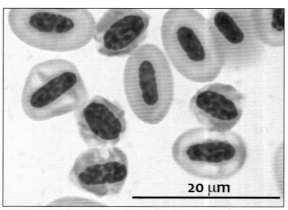

10.10 Erythrocytes in a blood film from a duck (species unknown). Note the left shift, hypochromasia and haemolysis. The polychromatic index (PI) of the erythrocytes is 3–4.
(Wright-Giemsa stain)

very heterogeneous morphology. In general, polychromatic erythrocytes have a less elliptic, paler and more basophilic appearance with a less condensed nucleus. The percentage of polychromatic erythrocytes in a blood film is determined by the polychromatic index (PI) (Figure 10.11). This semi-quantitative classification, using a scale from 1 to 5, allows an assessment of the degree of left shift in the red cell population and corresponds well with the examiner's subjective overall impression on first inspection (Dein, 1983).

Cytomorphology of leucocytes and thrombocytes:

Granulocytes: Criteria for the identification of granulocytes are summarized in Figure 10.12. The artefactual variability of heterophil and basophil morphology serves as a distinctive feature for the differentiation from eosinophils. The latter are resistant to artefactual alterations and show a species-specific appearance (see Figure 10.9). Morphological alterations mainly affect heterophilic granulocytes and are subsumed under the term toxic left shift. Toxic changes include cytoplasmic basophilia, loss of granulation (see Figure 10.8) and formation of vacuoles (see Figure 10.30). They are frequently accompanied by a left shift of the heterophilic line. Immature cells present with a basophilic cytoplasm and a variable segmentation of the nucleus. In addition to mature granules, immature round primary granules with basophilic coloration can also be found in the cytoplasm (see Figure 10.9). The more primary granules are present, the less differentiated the cell is. A toxic left shift always has to be considered as a sign of severe imbalance between cell production and demand. The immature cells lack the full spectrum of defence mechanisms present under physiological conditions. The immune reaction is likely to be inadequate or insufficient. The prognosis declines with increasing grade of toxicity/immaturity and declining total cell counts. Phagocytosis of heterophils by monocytes is rarely seen in blood films. It indicates an intravascular inflammatory reaction (e.g. toxaemia) or an autoimmune reaction.

Monocytes, lymphocytes and thrombocytes: Guidelines for the differentiation of monocytes, lymphocytes and thrombocytes are detailed in Figure 10.13. Signs of reactivity in thrombocytes consist of an irregular, undulated cell membrane with or without cytoplasmic vacuolation. Morphological changes in lymphocytes and monocytes include loss of the coarse chromatin structure, cytoplasmic basophilia, vacuolation and bleb formation (i.e. constriction of vesicles from the cell membrane) (see Figure 10.9). Blood films with altered cell morphology frequently pose difficulties in terms of differentiating reactive lymphocytes and thrombocytes from polychromatic erythrocytes. Guidelines for identification are given in Figure 10.14. Morphological alterations always indicate increased cell reactivity, with or without an increased number of immature cells in terms of a left shift.

Spirochaetes, Rickettsia *and haematozoa:* In the acute phase of spirochetosis, *Borrelia ansrina* (seen in chickens, turkeys, pheasants, geese and ducks) can be detected as long filament spiral structures in stained blood films viewed under X1000 magnification. They are highly motile in fresh native wet mounts viewed with dark field illumination or phase contrast. *Rickettsia* of the genus *Aegyptianella* (seen in chickens, turkeys and guinea fowl) appear as round, basophilic, more or less granular inclusions of variable size (0.3–4 µm) in the cytoplasm of affected erythrocytes.

Index	Estimated portion of polychromic cells in the total red blood cell counts (%)	Overall impression	Morphological criteria	Interpretation
1 (see Figures 10.7 and 10.8)	0	Homogeneous	Erythrocytes homogeneous in form and structure; absent or few polychromatic cells	Physiological to suspicion of a right shift; depression of erythropoiesis
2	<10	Slightly irregular	Some polychromatic cells	Physiological
3	10–20	Moderately irregular	Polychromatic cells regularly seen	Slight regenerative left shift; erythropoiesis slightly increased
4 (see Figure 10.10)	20–50	Clearly irregular	Considerable number of polychromatic cells; slight poikilocytosis	Regenerative to degenerative left shift; erythropoiesis increased
5	>50	Severely irregular	Large number of polychromatic cells; considerable poikilocytosis	Severe degenerative left shift; erythropoiesis severely increased

10.11 Polychromatic index (PI).
(Modified according to Dein, 1983)

Criteria	Heterophil	Eosinophil	Basophil
Key feature	Similar for all species; low in contrast; susceptible to artefacts	Species-specific variability; rich in contrast; little susceptibility to artefacts	Technique-dependent variability; tendency for disintegration; very susceptible to artefacts
Cytoplasm	Colourless; eosinophilic tinge in cases of granular disintegration	Colourless to basophilic	Colourless, basophilic or eosinophilic
Granulation	Elliptic; eosinophilic; occasionally brick red tinge; signs of degranulation or isolated stain of central bodies (round red granules in colourless rod)	Round (rods in *Anseriformes*); eosinophilic; clearly visible; no central bodies	Basophilic to reddish white due to tendency for disintegration; rarely densely packed with small dark violet granules
Nucleus	Lobulated; less clearly structured	Lobulated; intensive colouration; clearly structured	Non-lobulated; roundish; poorly structured

10.12 Differentiation of heterophils, eosinophils and basophils.
(Modified according to Lucas and Jamroz, 1961 and Campbell and Ellis, 2007)

Criteria	Monocyte	Lymphocyte	Thrombocyte
Key feature	Large, delicately structured cell with clearly visible contents	Medium to large cell with coarse structures and clearly visible contents	Small to medium pyknotic cell with poorly defined structures
Size	Medium to large	Small with almost no plasma to large with abundant plasma	Small to medium; occasionally in cases of aggregation only the nuclei are visible
Form	Round; irregular when in contact with adjacent cells		Round to oval; polymorphic in aggregations
Cytoplasm	Blue-grey; foamy; occasionally orange-red tinge close to the nucleus; vacuoles; formation of cytoplasmic blebs (sign of activation)	Homogeneous; basophilic; occasionally vacuoles; formation of cytoplasmic blebs (sign of activation)	Colourless to slightly grey; fine reticular structure; undulated membrane (sign of activation)
Granulation	Dust-like azurophilic granules close to the nucleus	Occasionally azurophilic granules or magenta bodies	Reddish to violet pole bodies close to the nucleus
Nuclear position	Rather eccentric	Rather central	No preference
Nucleocytoplasmic ratio	Moderate to high	Low to moderate	Low to moderate
Nuclear form	Rather irregular; occasionally kidney-shaped with more or less deep, smooth indentation	Roundish; occasionally sharp indentation due to artificial folding	Round to oval; polymorphic in aggregations
Nuclear structure	Small chromatin clumps integrated into nuclear reticulum; light appearance	Coarse chromatin clumps within the nuclear reticulum; very dense in small lymphocytes	Dense to pyknotic; dark appearance

10.13 Differentiation of monocytes, lymphocytes and thrombocytes.
(Modified according to Lucas and Jamroz, 1961 and Campbell and Ellis, 2007)

Criteria	Reactive lymphocyte[a]	Reactive thrombocyte[b]	Polychromatic erythrocyte[c]
Key feature	Well structured, rather clear cell; does not fit into the erythrocytic line of the blood film	Less structured, rather dark cell; morphology variable; does not fit into the erythrocytic line of the blood film	Well structured, rather dark cell; rich in contrast; fits into the erythrocytic line of the blood film
Form	Round	Variable; irregular cell margins	Round to elliptic
Cytoplasm	Basophilic; occasionally Golgi apparatus visible as clear area close to the nucleus; vacuoles; cytoplasmic bleb formation	Colourless to basophilic grey; vacuoles; undulated membrane; cytoplasmic bleb formation	Depending on stage of maturation clearly basophilic or polychromatic grey
Granulation	Azurophilic granules or magenta bodies	Pole bodies close to the nucleus, occasionally disintegrating	Absent
Nucleus	Violet basophilic colour; coarse chromatin clumps; finely structured or homogeneous	Black basophilic; round to elliptic; polymorphic; frequently pyknotic	Black basophilic; increasing pyknosis; structure rich in contrast

10.14 Differentiation of reactive lymphocytes, thrombocytes and polychromatic erythrocytes. [a] Morphology of a lymphocyte in stage of activation. [b] Morphology of a thrombocyte in stage of activation. [c] Morphology of an immature, juvenile erythrocyte.
(Modified according to Lucas and Jamroz, 1961 and Campbell and Ellis, 2007)

Spirochaetosis and aegyptianellosis are more frequently encountered in free range poultry flocks. Their occurrence is strictly associated with the presence of the tick, *Argas persicus*. *A. persicus* is found worldwide in tropical and subtropical countries.

Developmental stages of haemoparasites are commonly found in blood films of non-domestic bird species and are mostly considered incidental findings with low or unknown pathogenicity. Clinical disease has been reported in all orders of backyard poultry for the genera *Haemoproteus*, *Plasmodium* and *Leucocytozoon*. Flying arthropods act as vectors for the whole group. Higher prevalence has to be expected in open housing systems than in closed facilities. Recent findings suggest that *Haemoproteus* spp. adapted to European songbirds as their natural host may cause fatal outbreaks of malaria in captive collections of psittacine birds from South America and Australasia (Olias *et al.*, 2010). Similar scenarios are conceivable for exotic backyard poultry species.

Haemoproteid gametocytes are visible as fine granular structures in the cytoplasm of erythrocytes (*Haemoproteus*, *Plasmodium* and *Leucocytozoon*) and leucocytes (*Leucocytozoon*). At an advanced stage of development, gametocytes of *Plasmodium* spp. and *Leucocytozoon* spp. displace the nucleus of the host cell laterally. In contrast, *Haemoproteus* gametocytes surround the host nucleus resulting in a more or less pronounced horseshoe form of the parasite (Figure 10.15). The intensively stained and large macrogametocytes of *Leucocytozoon* distort the host cell and often appear as elongated structures with one or two tails at the poles. Roundish tailless forms may also occur and can be misinterpreted as a granulocyte with peculiar morphology.

Differential count: For the differential count, at least 100 leucocytes have to be defined as heterophils (H), lymphocytes (L), monocytes (M), eosinophils (E), basophils (B) or non-definable blood cells (NDBs) (see Figure 10.6). The latter category includes all white blood cells which cannot be further differentiated due to their immature appearance. Using the wedge smear technique, monocytes and heterophils tend to concentrate at the longitudinal borders of the smear, whereas small lymphocytes stay in the centre. Viewing the blood film perpendicular to the smear direction (see Figure 10.4) counteracts related errors in the differential count. Differentiation of large lymphocytes from monocytes in routine stains is often not possible even for the experienced examiner. Consequently, uncertainty in differential counts needs to be taken into consideration when interpreting results.

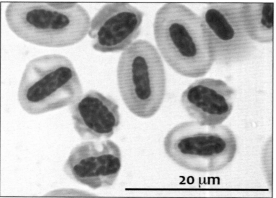

20 μm

10.15 Great tit (*Parus major*) with a concurrent infestation with *Haemoproteus* (left gametocyte) and *Plasmodium* (right gametocyte).
(Wright-Giemsa stain)

Total blood cell counts

As erythrocytes and thrombocytes in birds remain nucleated throughout maturity, their similarity to lymphocytes hampers automated counting. Recent experimental studies on flow cytometry based blood cell counting in chickens and turkeys return promising results (Seliger *et al.*, 2012; Lindenwald *et al.*, 2019). Distinction, however, becomes more challenging in samples from diseased individuals with altered cell morphology. Therefore, time-consuming and labour-intensive manual methods currently still represent the gold standard for haematology in birds. Formulas for these methods are summarized in Figure 10.16.

For a direct count of erythrocytes, thrombocytes and leucocytes, the blood sample is diluted 1:200 with Natt and Herrick's solution (Figure 10.17) using a red blood cell diluting pipette. The dilution is placed in one half of a counting chamber (haemocytometer) with improved Neubauer ruling. The filled haemocytometer is stored in a humidity chamber (covered Petri dish with a wet piece of cotton swab) for at least 10 minutes to allow full sedimentation of all cells into one focussing plane.

- Total red blood cell count (TRBC) – all red blood cells in the corner and central squares of the large central square are counted following the L rule (Figure 10.18). Cells that touch the centre line of the triple rules on the left and bottom of the square are counted. Cells that touch the centre line of the triple rules on the right and top are not counted.

Chamber methods

Direct method using Natt and Herrick's solution:
- Total red blood cell count (cells/μl) = count in 5 small squares x 10,000
- Total white blood cell count (cells/μl) = (count in 9 large squares + 10%) x 200

Semi-direct method using the Avian Leukopet™
- Total white blood cell count (cells/μl) = Avian Leukopet™ count x 1778/(heterophils (%) + eosinophils (%))

Estimations from blood films

Method by Campbell and Ellis (2007) using oil immersion magnification:
- Total white blood cell count (cells/μlest) = number of leucocytes in 20 fields x 875

Corrected if packed cell volume (PCV) is outside the range of 35–55%
- Total white blood cell countcorr = total white blood cell count (cells/μlest) x observed PCV/45%

Method by Lane (1987) using X40 magnification
- Total white blood cell count (cells/μlest) = number of leucocytes in 20 fields x 100

Report of number with range of error

Total white blood cell count (cells/μlest)	Range of error
<25.000	± 2000
25.000–40.000	± 4000
40.000–65.000	± 5000
65.000–140.000	± 10,000
>140.000	± 20,000

Example:
- Total white blood cell count (cells/μlest) = 40.000
- Range of error = ± 5000
- Reference interval = 35.000–45.000 (cells/μl)

10.16 Formulae for different methods of total blood cell counts. (Formulae for total white blood cell counts also apply for thrombocyte counts.)

- NaCl = 3.88 g
- Na$_2$SO4 = 2.50 g
- Na$_2$HPO$_4$ x 12(H$_2$O) = 2.91 g
- KH$_2$PO$_4$ = 0.25 g
- Formalin (37%) = 7.50 ml
- Methyl violet 2B = 0.10 g
- Distilled water = ad 1000 ml

Leave for 12h at room temperature, then filter and store

10.17 Natt and Herrick's solution.

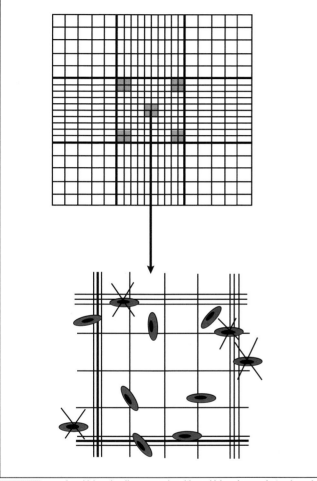

10.18 Total red blood cell count. The diluted blood sample is placed in one half of a haemocytometer counting chamber with improved Neubauer ruling. The red blood cells present in the corner and central squares of the large central square are counted following the L rule (see text).

- Total white blood cell count (TWBC) – the leucocytes in all nine large squares of one half of the haemocytometer counting chamber are counted and then 10% is added to the count. The same method is applicable to the total thrombocyte count (TTC). Success with this method requires training in cell differentiation. However, sometimes leucocytes and thrombocytes are hard to distinguish, even for experienced examiners. To diminish miscounts in these cases, a combined count of all non-red blood cells is undertaken. A true total white blood cell/thrombocyte count is achieved by performing a differential count, including thrombocytes, on a stained blood film and recalculating the total numbers of each portion by multiplying the percentage by the total number obtained from the chamber count.

Semi-direct counts

A semi-direct leucocyte count is performed using 1% phloxine B solution (Avian Leukopet™). The phloxine dye stains exclusively eosinophils and heterophils, which are seen as round, refractile, orange-red dots in the counting chamber. After filling a haemocytometer with a 1:200 dilution, all orange-red cells in both halves of the counting chamber (i.e. all cells in the 18 large squares) are counted. Relative heterophil and eosinophil numbers are determined with a differential count performed on a stained blood film. The TWBC is calculated using the formula in Figure 10.16. This method has an increased risk for a greater margin of error in cases of low granulocyte numbers.

Estimated counts

Estimated counts from the blood film save time and costs, but require a technically perfect blood film with a monolayer devoid of cluster cells. The number of all leucocytes in twenty 40x objective fields (Lane, 1987) or twenty oil immersion fields (Campbell and Ellis, 2007) are counted and multiplied by an estimation factor, as outlined in Figure 10.16. Reporting results with a range of error, as outlined in the method described by Lane (1987), takes into consideration that precision will decrease with increasing cell numbers. Eyepiece graticules with square grids may enhance precision but will not have a positive effect on accuracy. Compared with haemocytometer methods, estimations reveal higher and wider reference intervals (Wiskott, 2002). Published reference intervals for estimation methods do not exist, and counts depend on the specific magnification properties of the microscope. Thus, the establishment of practice- or laboratory-specific reference intervals is of particular importance for estimated counts.

Haemogram
General considerations

A blood panel represents the actual status of circulating cells in the peripheral bloodstream. Many influencing factors cause conspicuous variations, which result in haematological analysis being a very sensitive diagnostic tool with low specificity. With the exception of the detection of haemoparasites and leukaemic neoplasia, aetiological diagnoses in haematology are rare. However, the general health status of the patient can be assessed. Serial blood samples yield important information regarding the progress of the disease, the prognosis and the efficacy of treatment.

Aspects to consider when interpreting a haematological result include:

- Comparison to reference ranges (Figure 10.19)
- Physiological and technical causes
- The severity or frequency of changes
- The tendency of development
- The function of the cells affected
- Correlation to other results.

The immune system is subject to permanent changes. Transition from physiological to pathological is gradual. Physiological results do not rule out a disease but document a missing haematological reaction. Depending on the stage of the disease, infections with *Aspergillus* spp., for example, may be associated with all types of results from highly reactive in the active stage with accessible antigen, to completely physiological in the quiescent stage with antigen compartmented in granulomas.

Species	PCV (%)	TRBC (x 10^{12}/l)	Hb (g/l)	TWBC (x 10^9/l)	Het. (x 10^9/l)	Lym. (x 10^9/l)	Mon. (x 10^9/l)	Eso. (x 10^9/l)	Bas. (x 10^9/l)
Galliformes									
Domestic fowl[ab]	23–55	1.3–4.5	70–186	9–32	1.4–16.0	2.6–26.9	0.1–2.2	0–1	0–2.6
Domestic turkey[a]	30–45	1.7–3.7	88–134	16–25.5	4.6–13.3	5.6–12.2	0.5–2.6	0–1.3	0.2–2.3
Pheasant[ac]	28–42	1.2–3.5	80–112	18–39	2.1–11.7	11.3–24.9	0.2–2.7	0–0.3	0–0.9
Guinea fowl[d]	35–43	2.1–3.0	108–158	12–32.7	1.2–7.7	7.7–31.3	0.1–0.4	0.2–0.8	0.1–0.4
Peafowl[e]	33–44	1.9–2.8	120–172	4.8–18.3	1.3–9.1	1.6–9.4	0–0.1	0–0.5	0–0.4
Anseriformes									
Duck (not specified)[f]	35–50	2.5–3.7	111–140	14–24	7.4–16.6	3.7–12	0–0.5	0–0.2	0–0.2
Mallard[b]	34–52	1.6–3.6	98–164	23.4–24.8	6.5–15.4	12.2–16.6	0.5–0.9	0–0.1	0.5–0.9
Wood duck[c]	42–49	2.6–3.1	137–162	17.9–29.3	5.7–11.0	11.5–15.1	0.4–1.7	0–0.5	0.2–0.6
Canada goose[ac]	38–58	1.6–2.7	127–191	13.0–21.8	3.0–9.2	6.0–13.7	0.1–1.3	0–0.4	0.3–1.5
White-fronted goose[g]	41–45	2.7–3.1	132–163						

10.19 Haematology reference intervals in selected galliform and anseriform species. It should be noted that these are guidelines for initial orientation; replacement with practice-specific ranges is recommended. Bas. = basophils; Eso. = eosinophils; Hb = haemoglobin; Het. = heterophils; Lym. = lymphocytes; Mon. = monocytes; PCV = packed cell volume; TRBC = total red blood count; TWBC = total white blood count.
([a]Carpenter and Marion, 2012; [b]Wakenell and Campbell et al., 2011; [c]Ritchie et al., 1994; [d]Nalubamba et al., 2010; [e]Samour et al., 2010; [f]Fudge, 2000; [g]Samour, 2000)

Interpretation of the erythrogram

To diagnose the type of aberration, it is usually sufficient to evaluate haematocrit changes with regard to cytomorphology in the blood film. Haematological diagnoses and possible aetiologies for the most common findings are summarized in Figure 10.20. In selected cases, haemoglobin content, total red blood cell count and the calculation of red cell indices are necessary to reach a conclusion.

Interpretation of the leucogram and thrombogram

Guidelines for the interpretation of the leucogram and thrombogram are given in Figure 10.21. In principle, the assessment follows three key statements:

- Always interpret absolute numbers
- Use cytomorphology as the differentiating key
- Always form a haematological diagnosis based on cell function first.

Always interpret absolute numbers: Cell counts need to be read in absolute numbers. For example, a relative differential count of 80% heterophils and 20% lymphocytes with an absolute leucocyte count of 60,000 cells/µl indicates heterophilia; whereas a cell count of 10,000 cells/µl indicates an absolute lymphopenia. The first instance points towards a heavy reaction of the innate immune system, as would be expected with acute or subacute inflammation. The second case indicates a depression of lymphocytes and can be the result of handling stress (transport or treatment) or immunosuppression caused by a pathogen.

Finding	Haematological diagnosis		Possible causes (examples)

HCT increased Dehydration ruled out PI = 2–3	Increased erythropoiesis	Polycythaemia	• Absolute primary: *Polycythaemia vera* rare
			• Absolute secondary due to tissue hypoxia:
			  • Adaptation to high altitudes
			  • Defective oxygen binding in erythrocytes
			  • Chronic respiratory or cardiovascular disease (pneumonia, cardiomyopathy, atherosclerosis, ascites, rachitis deformations of the ribs, expansive abdominal processes)

HCT decreased Overhydration ruled out PI = 2–5 depending on phase and degree		Haemorrhagic anaemia	• Trauma (injuries, bloodsucking parasites) • Coagulopathies (factor deficiencies, hepatopathies, toxins, infections, septicaemia) • Ulcers, neoplasia (secondary tissue haemorrhage, coagulopathies)
HCT decreased PI = 4–5		Haemolytic anaemia	• Congenital defects • (Auto)immune reactions (haemoparasites, septicaemia, toxaemia, intoxications) • Neoplasia, burns
HCT decreased Overhydration ruled out PI = 1–2 Occasionally hypochromasia	Decreased erythropoiesis	Depressive anaemia	• Iron/haemoglobin deficiency (malnutrition, chronic emaciating conditions, lead and zinc intoxication) • Deficiency in erythropoietic factors (hepatopathies, nephropathies, hypothyroidism, hyperoestrogenism, deficiency in vitamin B12 or folic acid) • Bone marrow damage (infections, toxins, drugs, neoplasia)

10.20 Interpretation of the erythrogram using haematocrit values and cytomorphology. HCT = haematocrit; PI = polychromatic index.
(Modified according to Lucas and Jamroz, 1961; Fudge, 2000; Campbell and Ellis, 2007; Davison et al., 2008)

Cell type	Increased number (examples)	Decreased number (examples)
Heterophil	• Innate immune reaction • Non-specific phagocytosis of microorganisms (infection), cell debris (trauma, tissue breakdown, foreign material) • Microbicidal activity • Wound healing, tissue repair • With toxic left shift: depletion of mature cell pools, excessive demand, guarded prognosis (septicaemia, toxaemia, massive tissue necrosis)	• Physiological morphology: artefactual (separation of cellular components in the storage tube) • Toxic left shift: damage or exhaustion of granulopoiesis, grave prognosis (overwhelming septicaemia, fenbendazole intoxication) • Bone marrow depression (pancytopenia)
Eosinophil	• Significance not fully understood • Sign for delayed rather than immediate hypersensitivity reactions • Poor correlation to parasitic disease • Reported with severe tissue trauma • Skin disease (feather plucking, self-mutilation, flying accidents, carnivore attacks, drug injections, post-surgical recovery) • Respiratory disease (smoke inhalation) • Infectious disease (mycoplasmosis, West Nile virus, mycobacteriosis, streptococcosis, staphylococcosis, listeriosis, erysipelas)	• Bone marrow depression (pancytopenia)
Basophil	• Significance not fully understood • Life-threatening stress situations (hyperthermia, water deprivation) • Reported with severe tissue trauma, especially skin and respiratory disease (see Eosinophil)	• Bone marrow depression (pancytopenia)
Lymphocyte	• Acquired immune reaction • Humoral (production of immunoglobulins and cell mediators) and cell-mediated immune response • Marked lymphocytosis with signs of reactivity: lymphoid neoplasia or leukemoid inflammatory reaction with pronounced antigenic challenge	• Increased migration to extravasal compartments in primary stages of infection • True suppression of lymphocyte proliferation • Stress, corticosteroid therapy • Immunoevasive strategies of microorganisms (chronic viral infections, *Aspergillus* spp., *Mycobacterium* spp., Gram-negative septicaemia) • Drugs and toxins (tetracyclines, tylosin, gentamicin, mycotoxins, lead) • Neoplasia • Bone marrow depression (pancytopenia)
Monocyte	• Innate and acquired immune reaction • Phagocytosis (see Heterophil) • Granuloma and giant cell formation (microbial infection, wound healing, tissue repair) • Antigen-specific interaction (immunoglobulin (Ig)M, IgY) • Antigen presentation for lymphocytes	• Amonocytosis in combination with toxic heteropenia, thrombocytopenia, anaemia suggestive of myelophthisis, prognosis guarded • Bone marrow depression (pancytopenia)
Thrombocyte	• Response to haemorrhage (thrombus formation, haemostasis) • Rebound effect after thrombocytopenia • Innate immune reaction • Non-specific phagocytosis (see Heterophil) • Wound healing, tissue repair	• Artefact (aggregation in blood sample) • Excessive demand (coagulopathies, massive haemorrhage) • Decreased thrombopoiesis: bone marrow depression (toxins, septicaemia, pancytopenia)

10.21 Guidelines for the interpretation of the leucogram and thrombogram.
(Modified according to Lucas and Jamroz, 1961; Maxwell, 1993; Fudge, 2000; Campbell and Ellis, 2007; Davison et al., 2008)

Use cytomorphology as the differentiating key: Compared with numerical parameters changes in cell morphology are less affected by physiological, environmental and artefactual variation. Often the presence of cells with morphological abnormalities is a more reliable index of inflammation than cell counts. Assessment of cellular morphology allows for further specification of numerical findings. A normocytosis of 15,000 cells/µl with a normal differential count and physiological cytomorphology does not provide evidence for a clinically relevant immune reaction. In contrast, identical numerical results with a toxic left shift of heterophils and reactivity of mononuclear cells indicates a massive immune reaction with the possibility of damage or exhaustion of granulopoiesis with an overall poor prognosis.

Always form a haematological diagnosis based on cell function first: Haematological diagnosis based on cell function needs to be separated from the aetiological differential diagnoses to prevent the diagnostic plan from becoming too narrow. For example, heterophils act as rather non-specific phagocytes of the avian immune system. Thus, heterophilia first and foremost indicates an increased demand for phagocytosis. Aetiologically, this may be correlated to a bacterial infection, but can also be seen in cases of increased phagocytosis of cell debris such as wound healing or loss of tissue due to toxic, metabolic, neoplastic and infectious causes other than bacteria.

Cytology

Cytology is a rapid, low-stress, low-risk and low-cost diagnostic tool, ideal for daily routine in practice. Sample collection can be performed using minimally invasive techniques without sedation. Simple processing allows for rapid results and repeated collections within the same appointment. A collection of mounted slides is helpful for future reference. If evaluation is outsourced, a check for adequacy and artefacts on a stained second sample is helpful before shipment of the unstained slide.

Cytology *versus* histopathology

Cytology in combination with diagnostic imaging, during surgery or post-mortem examination, increases the amount of information gathered and in case of diagnosis saves time and costs for histopathology. The diagnostic value of cytology has increased considerably over the last decade and it is now considered complementary rather than subordinate to histopathology. Cytomorphological deviations are better depicted in cytological samples than in histological sections, due to extended spreading of the cells and decreased thickness of the sample. This makes cytology superior to histopathology in the detection of intracellular pathogens and lesions, and the assessment of poorly differentiated round cell tumours, where diagnosis is mainly based on cytomorphological features. On the contrary, the small sample size and limited number of cells in cytological specimens has the potential risk to evaluate a non-representative sample. This is particularly the case with solid masses of well differentiated connective tissue. Histopathology is the method of choice in cases where evaluation of tissue architecture is necessary for correct assessment. Examples include differentiation of granulomatous inflammation from fibrosarcoma or rating the degree of infiltrative behaviour as a criterion for tumour grading

Sample collection, preparation and staining

The choice of collection method depends on the character and accessibility of the tissue in question. Tissue that spontaneously sheds individual cells, such as blood, fluid or epithelia, will require less aggressive methods than connective tissue, which naturally does not exfoliate cells. Fine-needle aspiration (FNA), impression smears, scrapings, swabs and squash preparations are the most commonly used techniques to obtain cytological samples. Cytological specimens need to be prepared and air-dried immediately after collection. Any delay will result in cell degeneration or microbial overgrowth. Routine overview stains are the same as used for haematology. Useful complementary stains include Gram stain for the differentiation of bacteria (Figure 10.22), acid-fast stain for mycobacteria and *Cryptosporidium*, modified Giménez stain for *Chlamydophila*, and new methylene blue stain for mast cells, intracellular parasites, fungal hyphae, lipid droplets and fibrin (Campbell and Ellis, 2007).

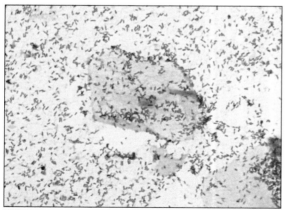

10.22 Bacterial overgrowth with ≥90% Gram-negative bacteria from a pharyngeal swab taken from a fancy breed hen.
(Gram stain; Courtesy of Dr Peter Wencel)

Fine-needle aspiration

Fluids: Fine-needle aspirates of fluids need to be processed in different ways depending on their physical properties. Opaque fluids are spread on to a slide using the blood film method (see Figure 10.4). For translucent fluids of low cellularity, the line smear concentration technique is used to ensure sufficient cell concentration at the end of the smear. In cases of very hypocellular samples, centrifugation at low speed and preparation of solely the sediment may be required.

Solid masses: FNA of solid masses is performed with or without negative pressure during cell collection. The latter is of benefit in highly vascularized tissue. Retrieval of the cells from the lesion is always performed without the use of a vacuum to avoid aspiration of the material from the needle lumen into the syringe. The sample is then expelled on to a slide and spread by gently squashing with a pressure to ensure sufficient cell separation with minimal cell destruction (see Figures 10.23 and 10.27). A multi-directional aspiration within the lesion will enhance the probability of a representative sample. For the same reason ultrasound-guided aspiration is recommended for investigating internal masses.

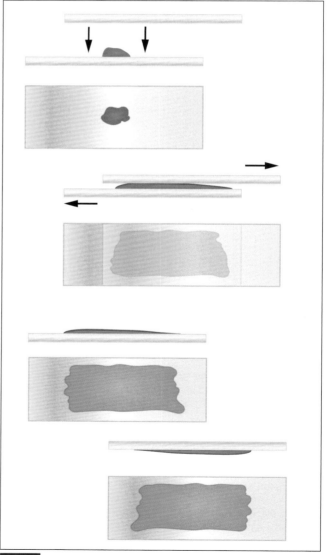

10.23 Squash preparation technique.

Impression smears, scrapings, swabs and squash preparations

Impression smears from biopsy or post-mortem specimens are best produced if excess blood on the freshly cut surface is first removed by blotting with lint-free paper. Otherwise high numbers of haemic cells may overlay diagnostic features (Figures 10.24 to 10.26). Scrapings performed with a scalpel blade perpendicular to the surface of the tissue or squash preparations of small full tissue samples will result in highly cellular preparations with higher diagnostic reliability than impression smears. This is of special advantage for the detection of intracellular structures such as viral, chlamydial, or mycoplasmal inclusion bodies and protozoans. Additionally, scrapings will remove sufficient material from firm, non-exfoliative tissue such as solid masses of connective tissue (Figure 10.27). In cases of dry superficial lesions, prolonged scraping until blood or serum appears will help adhere the material to the slide. The material is retrieved using a moistened swab and then rolled (not smeared) on the slide to avoid cell damage. Moistening the swab with a drop of blood plasma or serum from the bird will also enhance adhesion of the material on to the slide.

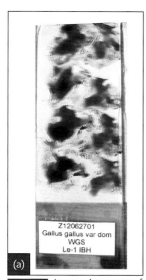 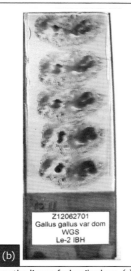

(a) (b)

10.24 Impression smears from the liver of a broiler hen. (a) Without removal of excess blood. (b) After removal of excess blood. IBH = inclusion body hepatitis; Le = liver. (Wright-Giemsa stain)

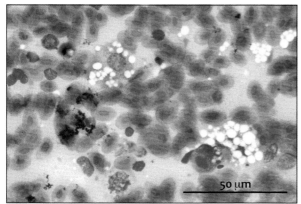

10.25 Photomicrograph of the slide in Figure 10.24a. Excess blood hampers the detection of the intranuclear inclusion body right above the size bar.

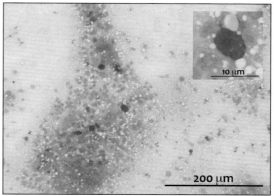

10.26 Photomicrograph of the slide in Figure 10.24b. Clear view of several prominent intranuclear polymorphic basophilic inclusion bodies suggestive of *Adenovirus* spp. (confirmed by histology).

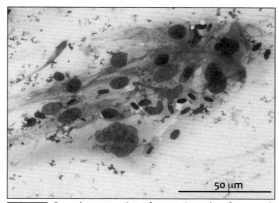

10.27 Squash preparation of a scraping taken from a subcutaneous mass in a fancy breed hen. Cytology revealed the mass to be a sarcoma. Note the aggregate of mesenchymal cells and the cell at the bottom of the slide showing nuclear signs of malignancy. (Wright-Giemsa stain)

Evaluation

Assessment of cytological specimens should follow a systematic approach, similar to the standardized evaluation of blood films. Cytological samples are first scanned at low power for their overall quality and sufficient number of representative flecks. Subsequently, all suitable 'spots' are evaluated under higher magnification. The examination should begin with an assessment of the slide cellularity and the determination of tissue types present, including their proportion within the slide (see Figure 10.27). Characteristics of epithelial, mesenchymal and round cells are summarized in Figures 10.28, 10.29 and 10.30. Occasionally, aetiological agents such as microorganisms (see Figures 10.22, 10.26 and 10.31), parasites or non-vital structures such as cholesterol or urate structures are detected.

The sample should then be evaluated for signs of increased cell reactivity and signs of malignancy. Cytomorphological criteria for increased cell reactivity or immaturity are the same as outlined for haemic cells (see above). Inflammation can be caused by infectious (parasites, microorganisms), non-infectious (traumatic, chemical, thermal) and neoplastic processes. Classification of inflammatory reactions into purulent, granulomatous, eosinophilic and lymphoplasmacellular allows for conclusions to be reached regarding the pathogenesis (Figure 10.32). However, it should be remembered that in birds macrophages and lymphocytes invade lesions within hours. Thus, a mixed cell (pleocellular) inflammatory reaction is most commonly seen, indicating a fully active immune response (see Figure 10.30).

Cell type	Slide cellularity	Appearance on the slide	Cytomorphology
Epithelial (see Figure 10.29)	Moderate to high	Predominantly clusters; acinar or tubular arrangements possible; increased number of individual cells in malignancy	Tissue dependent: small to large (squamous cells are very large); round, cuboidal, columnar, microvilli, cilia possible; distinct cell margins in individually placed cells
Mesenchymal (see Figure 10.27)	Low to moderate (possibly high in malignant neoplasia)	Aggregates and single cells; cells often uniformly directed; eosinophilic back-ground matrix in osteoid/chondroid tissue	Spindle-shaped with one or two tails (fibrous); roundish (osseous, chondrous); indistinct; fading cell margins
Round (see Figure 10.30)	High	Even distribution	Small to medium sized; different types (see Haematology); distinct cell margins

10.28 Determination of the tissue cell type in cytological samples. (Modified according to Mischke, 2005; Cowell et al., 2008)

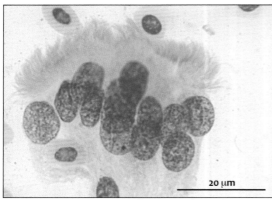

10.29 Impression smear of lung tissue from a laying hen showing physiological respiratory epithelium. (Wright-Giemsa stain)

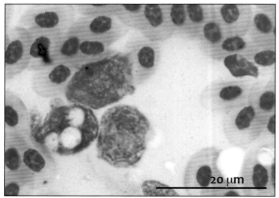

10.30 Impression smear of lung tissue from a laying hen showing pleocellular inflammation with signs of reactivity and toxicity. (Wright-Giemsa stain)

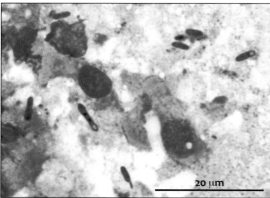

10.31 Mid-gut swab from a 24-week-old laying hen showing spore-bearing cigar-shaped bacteria, suggestive of *Clostridium*. (Wright-Giemsa stain)

When considering the grading of a neoplasm, it has to be emphasized that general cytological criteria such as hypercellularity, anisocytosis, macrocytosis and pleomorphism also occur as sequelae of irritation and inflammation. Malignancy should be suspected in cases where nuclear criteria are observed simultaneously (Figure 10.33). Regular detection of three or more criteria of malignancy within the same cell is strongly suggestive of a malignant process. Anisocytosis is seen in the mesenchymal aggregate in Figure 10.27. Cytoplasmic tails and the tendency to oval nuclei suggest a fibrous rather than an osseous or chondrous origin. The cell at the bottom of Figure 10.27 shows three signs of nuclear malignancy (polynucleosis, aniso-nucleosis and poikilonucleosis), indicative of a sarcoma.

Type of inflammation	Cytology	Interpretation
Purulent	≥80% heterophils	• Acute phase reaction • Increased phagocytic (cell debris, microorganisms) or microbicidal activity • Microbiological culture recommended if signs of heterophilic toxicity; bacterial and fungal pathogens more likely than viral
Pleocellular	Mixed populations of heterophils, macrophages and lymphocytes	• Most common type in birds • Fully active immune response • Always search for intracellular microbial or parasitic structures
Granulo-matous	≥50% macrophages; giant cells and epithelial cells possible; heterophils and lymphocytes variable	• Response to necrotic tissue rather than an infectious pathogen • Does not necessarily suggest chronicity • Secondary wound healing, granuloma or scar formation • Encapsulation of persistent pathogens: fungi (aspergillosis), mycobacteria, foreign body reactions (xanthomatosis), protozoans (frounce)
Eosinophilic	≥10% eosinophils	• Hypersensitivity reaction of rather delayed than immediate type (see also Figure 10.21)
Lympho-plasmacellular	≥50% lymphocytes and plasma cells	• Secondary rather than humoral reaction • Chronic infections without prominent tissue necrosis • Viral pathogens more likely than bacterial and fungal • Immune-mediated disease

10.32 Types of inflammation in birds and their interpretation. (Modified according to Mischke, 2005; Campbell and Ellis, 2007; Cowell et al., 2008)

Term	Description
Nucleus	
Increased nucleocytosomal ratio (N:C)	In non-lymphoid tissue an N:C ratio ≥1:2 is suggestive
Macrokaryosis and anisokaryosis	Large (>20 μm) in ≥3 erythrocytes is strongly suggestive
Polynucleosis	More than one nucleus per cell **Please note:** physiological in osteoclasts, inflammatory multinucleated giant cells. Binucleation in hepatocytes suggestive of irritation/attempts of repair; uneven numbers strongly suggestive
Increased mitotic figures	Strongly suggestive if lack of symmetrical alignment of chromosomes and 'ropey cord-like' chromatin patterns
Nuclear moulding	Closely packed and deformed nuclei within one or two neighbouring cells
Nucleolus	
Macronucleosis	Strongly suggestive if ≥5 μm (4–5 μm is the average length of an erythrocytes nucleus)
Polynucleolosis and anisonucleosis	>2 per nucleus and different sizes
Poikilonucleosis	Abnormal shape (angular shape is strongly suggestive)

10.33 Nuclear criteria of malignancy.
(Modified according to Mischke, 2005; Cowell et al., 2008)

Biochemistry and electrolytes

Comprehensive published serum biochemical profiles in poultry species are scarce. The reference values given in Figures 10.34 and 10.35 are intended as rough guidelines for first orientation prior to the generation of practice-specific ranges. The guidelines for interpretation detailed in Figure 10.36 are recommendations for bird species in general.

Species	ALP (IU/l)	Amylase (IU/l)	AST (IU/l)	CK (IU/l)	LDH (IU/l)	Na (mmol/l)	K (mmol/l)
Galliformes							
Domestic fowl [abc]	10–106		(174.8)		(636)	131–171	3–7.3
Domestic turkey [a]						149–155	6–6.4
Pheasant [ad]	742–1878		247–432		588–1698		
Guinea fowl [e]						149–157	
Peafowl [f]	140–457	1364–2555	49–198	906–2784	98–437		
Anseriformes							
Duck (not specified) [g]			12–73	165–378	120–246		
Mallard [hi]	21–67	2000–3450	11–21		67–282	145–155	4.6–7.6
Wood duck [a]	160–780		45–123	110–480	30–205	141–149	3.9–4.7
Canada goose [ah]	29–115	25–754	58–92		221–381	138–146	2.8–4.0
White-fronted goose [e]	34–122	253–656	80–126		192–324	141–151	2.7–3.9

10.34 Serum chemistry reference intervals for selected galliform and anseriform species – enzymes and electrolytes. ALP = alkaline phosphatase; AST = aspartate aminotransferase; CK = creatine kinase; K = potassium; LDH = lactate dehydrogenase; Na = sodium.
(Modified according to [a]Carpenter and Marion, 2012; [b]Simaraks et al., 2004; [c]Lumeij, 1997; [d]Nazifi et al., 2011; [e]Samour, 2000; [f]Samour et al., 2010; [g]Fudge, 2000; [h]Ritchie et al., 1994; [i]Olayemi et al., 2002)

Species	Bile acids (μmol/l)	Ca (mmol/l)	Chol. (mmol/l)	TP (g/l)	Albumin (g/l)	Globulin (g/l)	Glucose (mmol/l)	P (mmol/l)	Uric acid (mmol/l)
Galliformes									
Domestic fowl [a]		3.3–5.9	2.2–5.5	33–55	13–28	15–41	12.6–16.7	2.0–2.6	149–482
Domestic turkey [a]		2.9–9.7	2.1–3.3	49–76	30–59	17–19	15.3–23.6	1.7–2.3	202–309
Pheasant [ab]		2.1–3.1	2.8–4.0	36–50	26–27	19–21	10.6–15.1	1.92–3.23	333–357
Guinea fowl [c]				35–44					172–303
Peafowl [d]	25–88	2.9–3.9	2.7–5.2				18.0–27.3	1.26–4.1	48–345
Anseriformes									
Duck (not specified) [e]	22–82	2.2–3.2	2.69–6.31	35–55	17–22	35–60	7.0–17.7		119–701
Mallard [f]		1.9–2.8		31–47	11–19		7.5–13.8	0.61–1.3	161–434
Wood duck [a]	22–60	1.9–2.6		21–33	15–21	6–12	12.8–14.9	0.6–1.3	149–767
Canada goose [af]		2.4–2.7	3.7–5.1	41–55	19–23	22–34	10.5–13.4	0.6–1.2	357–631
White-fronted goose [b]		2.4–2.7	3.1–3.8	40–48	15–20	24–30	10.7–15.5	0.8–1.4	583–702

10.35 Serum chemistry reference intervals for selected galliform and anseriform species – nutrients and metabolites. Ca = calcium; Chol. = cholesterol; P = phosphorus; TP = total protein.
(Modified according to [a]Carpenter and Marion, 2012; [b]Nazifi et al., 2011; [c]Samour, 2000; [d]Samour et al., 2010; [e]Fudge, 2000; [f]Ritchie et al., 1994)

Parameter	Increased	Decreased
Enzymes		
Alkaline phosphatase	Increased bone metabolism (growth, fracture healing, egg laying, hyperparathyroidism); enteritis	Dietary zinc deficiency
Amylase	Acute pancreatitis; pancreatic necrosis; enteritis	Not considered to be of clinical significance
Aspartate aminotransferase	Advanced cell damage (necrosis) in liver and muscle	Severe loss of liver tissue
Creatine kinase	Haemolysis; increased turnover of muscle tissue (training, myopathies due to stress, malnutrition, neurological disorders, toxins, trauma)	Bacterial contamination of sample
Lactate dehydrogenase	Haemolysis; liver, heart or muscle damage	Severe loss of liver tissue
Electrolytes		
Sodium	Dehydration; salt poisoning; nutritional	Renal disease; overhydration
Potassium	Haemolysis; nutritional; severe tissue damage; acidosis; dehydration	EDTA contamination; diuretic therapy; alkalosis; overhydration; dietary deficiency
Nutrients and metabolites		
Bile acids	Lipaemia; haemolysis; loss of liver function	Liver cirrhosis; microhepatia
Calcium	Lipaemia; hyperproteinaemia; bacterial contamination; conditions with increased bone turnover (preovulatory state, hyperoestrogenism, hypervitaminosis D3, osteolytic neoplasia, primary hyperparathyroidism, pseudohyperparathyroidism)	EDTA contamination; bacterial contamination; young bird; metabolic and nutritional disorders; lead poisoning; hypoproteinaemia; glucocorticoid administration
Cholesterol	Increased fat metabolism (postprandial, high-fat diet, female reproductive activity, hepatic lipidosis, hypothyroidism, starvation); bile duct obstruction	Not considered to be of clinical significance
Total protein	Lipaemia; preovulatory state; inflammation; dehydration; chronic infection	Catabolic state (chronic disease, malabsorption, malnutrition, starvation); renal disease; blood loss
Albumin	Haemoconcentration due to dehydration	Inflammation; catabolic state (chronic disease, malabsorption, malnutrition, starvation)
Globulin	Inflammation; gamma globulinopathy; lymphoproliferative or myeloproliferative disease	Clinically relevant only for gamma globulins: immunosuppression affecting development of B lymphocytes
Glucose	Postprandial; acute stress; diabetes; female reproductive activity; corticosteroids	Unseparated blood; bacterial contamination; hepatic dysfunction; septicaemia; neoplasia; catabolic status (chronic disease, malabsorption, malnutrition, starvation)
Phosphorus	Lipaemia; haemolysis; postprandial; nutritional secondary hyperparathyroidism; hypoparathyroidism; egg laying	EDTA; hypovitaminosis D; malabsorption; chronic glucocorticoid therapy
Uric acid	Lipaemia; increased protein catabolism (starvation, chronic disease, tissue damage); decreased elimination (renal disease)	Overhydration; juvenile bird; decreased production (end-stage liver disease)

10.36 Guidelines for the interpretation of serum chemistry profiles in avian patients.
(Data from Carpenter and Marion, 2012; modified according to Lumeij, 1997; Fudge, 2000)

The following key points are valid for many bird species:

- Having ruled out a postprandial increase, an elevated level of bile acids is a reliable indicator of impaired liver function
- Simultaneously increased levels of creatine kinase (CK), aspartate aminotransferase (AST) and lactate dehydrogenase (LDH) always point towards muscle tissue damage, whereas elevations of AST and LDH without CK involvement most likely indicate hepatic disease
- Elevated AST (a mitochondrial enzyme) levels are always a sign of severe cell damage (e.g. necrosis).

Parasitology

Common parasitological examinations undertaken in poultry medicine include skin scrapings and acetate tape impressions for ectoparasites and faecal examinations for endoparasites. Tracheal flushes, as well as transillumination of the trachea using a torch, will detect parasites in the respiratory tract such as gapeworms (*Syngamus* spp. and *Cyathostomum*), mites and *Cryptosporidium*. Direct cotton tip wet smears are useful to detect flagellates.

Scrapings, swabs and acetate tape impressions

Arthropods

Skin mites such as *Knemidocoptes* and *Epidermoptes* spp. are diagnosed by microscopic evaluation of dermal crusts and deep skin scrapings at low magnification. A deep skin scraping is best achieved by squeezing an affected skin area between the thumb and forefinger of one hand and scraping the skin surface bluntly with a scalpel blade in the other until the first petechiae occur. Boiling or overnight storage of the material in 10% potassium hydroxide (KOH) prior to examination will enhance the visibility of the parasites. Acetate tape impressions are useful to identify ectoparasites found on birds or the surfaces of their housing, such as mites and lice. The tape is gently pressed on the skin or surface with suspected ectoparasites and then attached on to a glass slide for microscopic examination at low magnification (Figures 10.37 to 10.39).

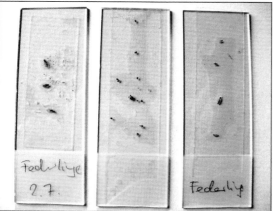

10.37 Acetate tape impressions of lice (left and right) and mites (centre) from a chicken.

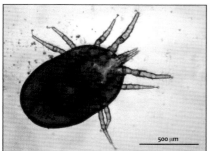

10.38 Acetate tape impression from a chicken showing the red chicken mite (*Dermanyssus gallinae*). The morphologically similar northern fowl mite (*Ornithonyssus sylviarum*) has more pointed caudal ends of the dorsal and anal plates and readily visible chelicerae.

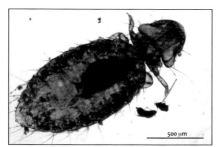

10.39 Acetate tape impression from a chicken showing the instar of the chicken head louse (*Cuclutogaster heterographa*).

Flagellates

Motile protozoans are best viewed in fresh, direct wet smears from the crop or oral cavity (*Trichomonas* spp.), of the caecal contents (*Histomonas* spp.) or of the duodenal contents (*Hexamita* spp.). To maintain motility a warm environment during microscopy is helpful and can be achieved by using a drop of warm water or saline for dilution or by using a small heat-producing lightbulb. Phase contrast or special stains are necessary to visualize subcellular structures.

- *Trichomonas* spp. are pear-shaped (5–9 μm in length and 2–9 μm in width) with four flagella protruding from the anterior pole of the body and an undulating membrane on one side.
- *Hexamita* spp. are comparatively long (6–12 μm) and thin (2–5 μm) organisms with eight prominent flagella originating symmetrically from different parts of the body. Their rapid body movements are characterized by sudden twitches.

- *Histomonas meleagridis* is difficult to distinguish from macrophages in its round non-amoeboid tissue form (3–16 μm) and shows high pleomorphic variability with occasionally one single flagellum in its intraluminal stage in the caecum.

Faecal examination

Parasitological evaluation of faecal samples will reveal parasites of the intestinal, respiratory and, occasionally, vascular systems (*Ornithobilharzia* spp. in anseriforms). Structures to search for include entire parasites (nematodes, cestodes, protozoans, arthropods), their parts (proglottids of tapeworms) and their developmental stages (eggs, larvae, oocysts). Experience is required to distinguish between true parasites and pseudoparasitic structures such as artefacts (air bubbles), plant and fungal material (cells, pollen, hyphae, spores), tissue and transient parasites from prey, and accidentally ingested living organisms (eggs and larvae from free-living nematodes).

Sample collection

Faecal samples are best collected immediately after voiding and should be examined as soon as possible following collection. Samples that cannot be processed immediately need to be wrapped safely to avoid dehydration and stored in a refrigerator. If the time between collection and evaluation is likely to exceed 24 hours, dilution of the sample with 10% formol after collection is recommended to prevent embryonation. The minimum amount of faeces necessary for examination is 5 g. Deposition of paper under the roosts decreases environmental contamination. Sampling at different times of day is recommended, as shedding intensity follows a circadian rhythm in many parasites.

Macroscopic evaluation

Macroscopic evaluation sometimes reveals a presumptive diagnosis. Tapeworms and their proglottids are easily detected in fresh faecal samples as moving, segmented structures. Larger nematodes may be preliminary classified according to size, form and colour ('red worms' for *Syngamus*). Concentration of macroscopically visible parasites is achieved by filtering the sample through a thin meshed sieve. Residues are then washed into a petri dish and allowed to sediment for 10 minutes. Small and thin nematodes are easily detected by examining the petri dish against a dark background.

Direct mounts

Direct microscopic evaluation is performed using a drop of tap water or physiological saline solution placed in the centre of a glass slide and gently mixed with a small amount of faeces. The mixture is then covered with a coverslip and should have a homogeneous translucent texture. Examination should begin under low magnification with an almost closed aperture. The slide should be scanned systematically so that all areas of the sample are assessed. Preparation with diluted iodine solution stains the eggshells of *Ornithobilharzia* and protozoal cysts. Addition of a dilute (1%) methylene blue solution will further enhance the visibility of parasitic eggs, as plant material and dust turns blue whilst ova stay yellow-brown. The direct method is a quick and simple technique, which reveals the presence of small worms, larvae, eggs and oocysts. However, it may be less reliable in cases of heavy contamination with pseudoparasitic structures or give rise to false-negative results with low-grade infestations. Detection of different life stages of one or more parasite species in a direct mount always indicates a moderate to high infestation. When seen in conjunction with clinical signs (e.g. diarrhoea, ruffled feathers), treatment is indicated.

Flotation

In cases where macroscopic evaluation and direct mounts have returned negative results, flotation is recommended. Worm eggs will float on the surface of solutions that have a higher specific gravity than themselves. Depending on the specific gravity (SG) of the flotation solution, nematode eggs (SG >1.15) or eggs from trematodes and cestodes (SG >1.35) will float. However, it should be recognized that the higher the SG of the solution, the more pseudoparasitic structures will also float, requiring intermediate steps of washing and filtration. Deformation of eggs and other structures occurs with flotation techniques and worsens with increasing time and SG of the solution.

Flotation solutions: Concentrated solutions with stable specific gravities are commercially available. Cost-effective homemade solutions can be prepared from water and salt or sugar. An excessive amount of dry salt or sugar is mixed with water. Boiling, frequent stirring and allowing the solution to stand for several days will result in a saturated supernatant above the sediment of undissolved material. The solution is best stored in a glass jar fitted with a tap. Regular checks for density with a densimeter are recommended. Saline solutions are superior to sugar-based ones in terms of cost and stability. For daily practice, a combination of saturated saline (NaCl; SG = 1.2 at 20°C) for nematodes and most cestodes, and zinc chloride (ZnCl₂; SG = 1.50 at 20°C) for trematodes and some cestodes has proven to be useful.

Preparation and evaluation: For preparation, a narrow-necked glass test tube or commercially available plastic vial with integrated sieve (Figure 10.40) is filled half full with 5 g of faeces and concentration solution, mixed until the faecal components have dissolved, and then filled until surface tension is visible on the very top. The mixture is allowed to stand for 10–15 minutes and then covered with a coverslip for 1 minute. The coverslip is lifted in a perpendicular manner and placed directly on to a glass slide. Alternatively, the egg-containing surface of the fluid can be transferred to the glass slide with a fine-wire loop as used in bacteriology. Evaluation begins by systematic scanning of the slide at low magnification with an almost closed aperture. The degree of infestation is determined semi-quantitatively from + (low;

one parasite per sample) to +++ (high; more than 10 parasites per sample). For a more precise assessment of the parasitic burden, the use of counting chamber based methods such as the McMaster or the FLOTAC technique will allow for the quantification of the parasitic load as number of eggs per gram faeces (EPG) or number of eggs per day (EPD) in 24hr samples. Both techniques, however, require additional equipment and are usually carried out in commercial laboratory settings.

Coccidia

Coccidial oocysts are small, translucent, round to oval structures approximately 15–30 μm in diameter, depending on the species (Figure 10.41). They can be distinguished from air bubbles by their refractile nature at different depths of focus. For a species-specific diagnosis a combination of oocyst size, the location in the gut and appearance of the lesion is necessary. Although detectable in living birds, coccidial infestations are best diagnosed at necropsy by swabbing or squashing several areas of the gastrointestinal tract. *Eimeria truncata*, the causative agent of renal coccidiosis in geese, is only found in the kidneys and the cloaca close to the opening of the ureters.

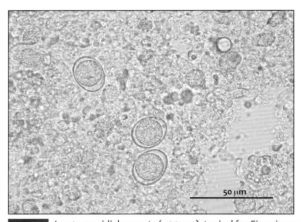

10.41 Large coccidial oocysts (~ 30 μm), typical for *Eimeria maxima*, from a mid-gut swab in a 24-week-old laying hen (same case as in Figure 10.31).

Cryptosporidium

Cryptosporidium spp. are easily distinguished from coccidians by their small size (2–6 μm) and their more or less firm location on the apical border of internal surface epithelia. Enteric or respiratory epithelium is most commonly affected. Vigorous swabbing of the cloaca, choana or trachea with a moist cotton tip will detach *Cryptosporidium* infected cells from the surface. In Wright-Giemsa stained samples, the detection of granular basophilic roundish meronts and gametocytes *budding* from the apical surface of epithelial cells is diagnostic. Mature oocysts, however, remain colourless, and are therefore difficult to distinguish from fat droplets and starch granules. In contrast to yeast cells (for which they are easily confused), intact mature *Cryptosporidium* oocysts stain bright pink in acid-fast stains.

Helminths

Helminth eggs are classified by their size, form, poles, contents and specific adnexes. An identification key for the differentiation of common worm eggs in faecal samples is given in Figure 10.42. Figure 10.43 provides an

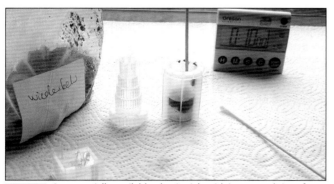

10.40 Commercially available plastic vials with integrated sieve for faecal flotation.

Features						Species
With polar filaments (long thread-like appendages)						Notocotylus Catatropis
Without polar filaments	With polar plugs (cork-like structures)					Capillaria (Aonchotheca, Baruscapillaria, Eucoleus)
	Without polar plugs	With embryo	<40 μm with larvae			Echinuria
			>40 μm with spine			Ornithobilharzia
			With transparent poles			Tetrameres
			Hexacanth embryo			Hymenolepis[a] Raillietina[a] Davainea[a]
		Without embryo	With polar opercula (flat caps)	Clearly visible opercula (ellipsoid)		Syngamus
				Operculum hard to visualize (ovoid)		Cyathostoma (Syngamus bronchialis)
			Without operculum – unsegmented, granular contents	<75 μm, ± parallel side walls		Heterakis
				>75 μm, ± barrel-shaped side walls		Ascaridia
			Without operculum – segmented contents	<75 μm, parallel side walls		Trichostrongylus
				>85 μm, barrel-shaped side walls		Amidostomum

10.42 Key to the most common worm eggs of backyard poultry. [a] Cestodes are determined more accurately by examining the whole worm or the proglottids.
(Reproduced from Thienpont et al., 2003 with permission from the publisher)

Location	Chickens, turkeys, guinea fowl	Ducks, geese, swans	Pheasants, peafowl
Nematodes			
Oral cavity, oesophagus, crop	Capillaria sp.	Capillaria sp. Echinura uncinata Amidostomum anseris	Capillaria sp.
Proventriculus	Tropisurus sp. Tetrameres sp. Dispharynx sp.	Tetrameres sp.	Tropisurus sp. Dispharynx sp.
Gizzard	Acuaria sp.	Echinura uncinata Amidostomum anseris	Acuaria sp.
Small intestine	Capillaria sp. Ascaridia sp.	Capillaria sp. Ascaridia sp.	Capillaria sp. Ascaridia sp.
Caecum	Heterakis sp. Trichostrongylus tenuis Capillaria sp.	Heterakis sp. Trichostrongylus tenuis Capillaria sp.	Heterakis sp. Trichostrongylus tenuis Capillaria sp.
Trachea	Syngamus trachea	Syngamus trachea Syngamus bronchialis	Syngamus trachea
Brain[a]	Bailascaris procyonis		Bailascaris procyonis
Eye[a]	Oxyspirura mansoni		Oxyspirura mansoni
Cestodes			
Intestine	Davainaea sp. Railletina sp. Hymenolepis sp. Choanotaenia sp.	Hymenolepis sp. Ligula sp.	Railletina sp. Hymenolepis sp. Choanotaenia sp.
Trematodes			
Intestine	Echinostoma sp. Echinoparyphium sp.	Echinostoma sp. Echinoparyphium sp.	
Rectum	Notocotylus sp. Catatropis sp.	Notocotylus sp. Catatropis sp.	Notocotylus sp.
Cloaca/oviduct	Prosthogonimus sp.	Prosthogonimus sp.	Prosthogonimus sp.
Vascular system		Ornithobilharzia sp.	

10.43 Anatomical location of common worms in backyard poultry.
(Reproduced from Thienpont et al., 2003 with permission from the publisher; [a] Modified according to Arends et al., 2003)

overview of the anatomical location of common worms. All cestode eggs (onchospheres) contain a hexacanth embryo (Figure 10.44); species identification is carried out on complete worms or gravid proglottids. Capillaria eggs are typically lemon-shaped with asymmetrical sides and prominent pole plugs (Figure 10.45). Eggs of Heterakis spp. can be differentiated from Ascaridia spp. by their smaller size and strictly parallel sides (Figure 10.46).

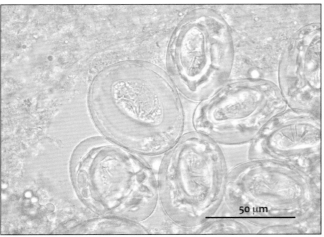

10.44 Direct faecal mount from a fancy breed hen showing cestode onchospheres with hexacanth embryos within a proglottid.

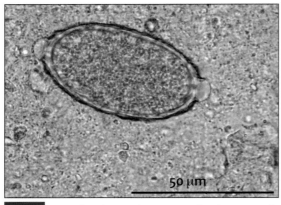

10.45 Direct faecal mount from a goose showing an egg of *Capillaria* sp.

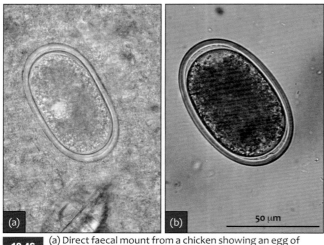

10.46 (a) Direct faecal mount from a chicken showing an egg of *Heterakis* spp. (b) Faecal flotation from a chicken showing an egg of *Ascaridia* spp.

References and further reading

Arends JJ, McDougald LR, Norton RA et al. (2003) Section IV – Parasitic diseases. In: Diseases of Poultry, 11th edn, ed. YM Saif et al., pp. 905–1023. Iowa State Press, Ames, Iowa

Campbell TW and Ellis CK (2007) Avian and Exotic Animal Hematology and Cytology. Blackwell Publishing Professional, Ames, Iowa

Campbell TW, Smith SA and Zimmermann KL (2011) Hematology of waterfowl and raptors. In: Schalm's Veterinary Hematology, 6th edn, ed. DJ Weiss and KJ Wardrop, p. 979. Wiley Blackwell, Hoboken, New Jersey

Carpenter JW and Marion CJ (2012) Exotic Animal Formulary, 4th edn, pp. 347–349 and 368–372. Elsevier Saunders, St Louis, Missouri

Cowell RL, Tyler RD, Meinkoth JH et al. (2008) Diagnostic Cytology and Hematology of the Dog and the Cat, 3rd edn. Mosby Elsevier, St. Louis, Missouri

Davison F, Kaspers B and Schat KA (2008) Avian Immunology. Academic Press Elsevier, London

Dein FJ (1983) Avian hematology: erythrocytes and anemia. Proceedings of the Annual Meeting of the Association of Avian Veterinarians, pp. 10–23

Fudge AM (2000) Laboratory reference ranges for selected avian, mammalian and reptilian species. In: Laboratory Medicine: Avian and Exotic Pets, 1st edn, ed. AM Fudge, pp. 375–400. WB Saunders, Philadelphia

Hawkey CM and Dennett TB (1989) A Colour Atlas of Comparative Veterinary Hematology. Wolfe Medical Publications Ltd, London

Howlett JC (2000) Clinical and diagnostic procedures. In: Avian Medicine, 1st edn, ed. JH Samour, pp 28–42. Mosby Harcourt Publishers Limited, London

Lane RA (1987) Avian Hematology: Basic Cell Identification and WBC Count Determination. Proceedings of the 1st International Conference on Zoological and Avian Medicine, Oahu, Hawaii, pp. 290–297

Lindenwald R, Pendl H, Scholtes H, Schuberth HJ and Rautenschlein S (2019) Flow-cytometric analysis of circulating leukocyte populations in turkeys: Establishment of a whole blood analysis approach and investigations on possible influencing factors. Veterinary Immunology and Immunopathology 210, 46–54

Lucas AM and Jamroz C (1961) Atlas of Avian Hematology. US Department of Agriculture, Washington

Lumeij JT (1997) Avian clinical biochemistry. In: Clinical Biochemistry of Domestic Animals, 5th edn, ed. JJ Kaneko et al., pp. 857–879. Academic Press, San Diego, California

Maxwell MH (1993) Avian blood leucocyte responses to stress. World's Poultry Science Journal 49, 34–43

Mischke R (2005) Zytologisches Praktikum für die Veterinärmedizin (Cytological practical training for veterinary medicine). Schlütersche Verlagsgesellschaft, Hannover, Germany

Nalubamba KS, Mudenda MB and Masuku M (2010) Indices of health: clinical hematology and body weights of free-range Guinea fowl (Numida meleagris) from the southern province of Zambia. International Journal of Poultry Science 9, 1083–1086

Nazifi S, Mosleh N, Ranjbar VR et al. (2012) Reference values of serum biochemical parameters in adult male and female ring-necked pheasants (Phasianus colchicus). Comparative Clinical Pathology 21, 981–984

Olayemi FO, Oyewale JO and Omolewa OF (2002) Plasma chemistry values in the young and adult Nigerian duck (Anas Platyrhynchos). Israel Journal of Veterinary Medicine 57, 4

Olias P, Wegelin M, Zenker W et al. (2010) Avian malaria deaths in parrots, Europe. Emerging Infectious Diseases 17, 950–952

Pendl H and Wencel P (2017) Avian Diagnostic Microscopy–Basic and Advanced Course. 3rd International Conference on Avian Herpetological and Exotic Mammal Medicine (ICARE); March 25th–29th 2017; Venice; pp. 242–260

Ritchie BW, Harrison GJ and Harrison LR (1994) Appendix I: Hematology and biochemistry. In: Avian Medicine: Principles and Application, pp. 1340–1346. Wingers Publishing Inc., Lake Worth, Florida

Samour JH (2000) Appendix II: Hematology reference values and Appendix III: Blood chemistry reference values. In: Avian Medicine, pp. 335–337 and pp. 362–365. Mosby Harcourt Publishers Limited, London

Seliger C, Schaerer B, Kohn M et al. (2012) A rapid high-precision flow cytometry based technique for total white blood cell counting in chickens. Veterinary Immunology and Immunopathology 145, 86–99

Simaraks S, Chinrasri O and Aengwanich S (2004) Hematological, electrolyte and serum biochemical values of the Thai indigenous chickens (Gallus domesticus) in northeastern Thailand. Songklanakarin Journal of Science and Technology 26, 425–430

Thienpont D, Rochette F and Vanparijs OFJ (2003) Diagnosing Helminthiasis by Coprological Examinations. Janssen Research Foundation, Beerse, Belgium

Wakenell PS (2011) Hematology of chickens and turkeys. In: Schalm's Veterinary Hematology, 6th edn, ed. DJ Weiss and KJ Wardrop, pp. 965–966. Wiley Blackwell, Hoboken, New Jersey

Wiskott M (2002) Vergleich verschiedener Methoden zur Leucozytenzählung bei Vögeln. Doctoral thesis, Diss med vet Wien

Chapter 11

Imaging techniques

Maria-Elisabeth Krautwald-Junghanns and Johanna Storm

In recent years, imaging techniques have become increasingly important as diagnostic tools in pet, zoo and wild bird medicine. Most scientific publications on imaging techniques in poultry, however, are experimental studies dealing with birds commercially produced for human consumption. Such studies emphasize aspects of commercial interest, such as the ultrasonographic examination of the female genital apparatus in laying hens or analysis of the composition of pectoral muscles via magnetic resonance imaging (MRI) and computed tomography (CT) in poultry raised for human consumption. Other studies relate to welfare aspects, such as the measurement of bone density using CT and/or MRI, particularly in relation to the development of osteoporosis. Newer applications of non-invasive imaging techniques in poultry are based on these past scientific studies, as well as experience in the field of companion bird medicine, and allow diagnosis not only of changes in the skeletal system (such as fractures or rickets) but also of infectious diseases.

Most owners of poultry lack the close relationship with their pet bird that owners of parrots or raptors often exhibit. As birds tend not to show specific clinical signs, disease may only be noticed when the process is in a fairly advanced stage. Consequently, the patient will often be critically ill at clinical presentation. This creates the need for the practitioner to perform a rapid health assessment to determine the underlying disease aetiology and initiate an adequate treatment protocol. As the number of available diagnostic methodologies for bird species is still somewhat limited, conventional radiography and ultrasonography, together with specific laboratory tests, allow a rapid diagnosis in the live bird.

The relatively small size and the fact that birds have pneumatized bones and internal air sacs that act as a negative contrast medium mean that far more revealing and instantly diagnostic images can be obtained compared with mammalian medicine. Most poultry breeds have a far greater body mass than the common species of companion birds, which provides for a greater variety of detail on radiography. It is also easier to examine poultry ultrasonographically because the larger body mass offers an improved range of coupling options. In general, ultrasonography is an easily performed, non-invasive and fast diagnostic procedure in backyard poultry. Ultrasonography often provides the practitioner with important supplementary information about diseases subsequent to an unclear radiographic result, especially with conditions relating to the genital tract, liver or kidneys.

Radiography

Films and exposure factors

A comprehensive discussion regarding the technical parameters of radiography is outwith the scope of this chapter. However, one of the greatest problems in avian radiography is loss of sharpness due to movement and high respiratory rates. Thus, short exposure times are needed (0.015–0.05 seconds or less). This requires the use of modern high-frequency or digital radiography equipment. The fact that the resolution of digital systems is lower than that of common film–screen combinations used in avian medicine is not of great importance in most backyard poultry compared with small pet birds as they are usually of higher body mass.

Exposure factors (kilovolts (kV) and milliamperes (mAs)) are dependent on the thickness and density of the object, type of apparatus, focus–film distance, film and screen types and processing of the film. For birds up to 2 kg in bodyweight, the kV values should not be higher than 45–55 kV in order to reduce scatter and therefore obtain images of high contrast with many shades of grey. The distance between the film and focus should be approximately 1 m. Reducing this distance will lower the required exposure, but picture quality may be affected by magnification and poor definition of parts of the object more distant from the film. Thus, for the most part high-definition film–screen combinations are used (rare-earth screens). Mammography films may be used, especially for the skeletal system; however, they also require higher exposure times. The use of grids is not necessary in most birds due to their small size.

For digital radiography, the reader should refer to the operating instructions and recommendations of the manufacturer of the equipment. It is important to note that the ability to perform post-processing image enhancement (including zooming, sharpening and contrast manipulation) using direct radiography and computed radiography systems does not provide a substitute for good radiographic technique, in particular the use of correct exposure settings. In fact, the overuse of such processing techniques can introduce artefacts that may lead to incorrect diagnosis.

Restraint

Although mainly performed under general anaesthesia in the UK due to health and safety legislation, radiography may be carried out without anaesthesia in birds <2 kg in bodyweight, with the conscious bird restrained on a custom-made radiotranslucent fixation plate (Figure 11.1). The head is fixed with a clamp positioned over the bird's neck, the feet are fixed with straps and the wings are restrained with tapes or weights. Sedation or general anaesthesia may be necessary in excitable birds, but is not usually required for routine radiography in animals accustomed to human contact.

Manual restraint of the conscious patient for radiographic examination may be preferred for very sick birds, those that may be likely to suffer from shock and larger animals weighing >2 kg. With this method, the hands of the person restraining the bird should never be placed within the primary X-ray beam, and should be protected from scatter radiation by the use of lead gloves (Figure 11.2). It can sometimes be difficult to hold smaller patients adequately whilst wearing lead gloves, and in those instances when the bird simply has to be restrained with bare hands to position it correctly, an assistant must always cover the positioner's hands with lead gloves or other type of lead protection. Thin, radiation-protective, lead-free gloves are commercially available and can be worn to restrain smaller

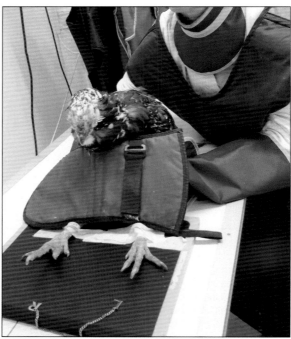

11.2 Patient positioning for a ventrodorsal view of the feet of an Orloff chicken using manual restraint. Note: it is important to keep the hands of the person restraining the bird outside the primary X-ray beam, even when wearing lead gloves. Other personal protective equipment such as a lead apron and thyroid gland protective collar should also be worn.

patients; these gloves are not much thicker than disposable latex operating gloves, and feel very similar. They allow proper restraint of the smallest patients, which with the thicker lead gloves is near impossible. Human cardiologists, who need to protect their hands from secondary scatter radiation whilst visually controlling the correct placement of stents and catheters in hearts and other vessels using fluoroscopy, routinely wear these gloves. It should be borne in mind, however, that these gloves only provide protection from scatter radiation, so additional protection is required if the hands of the positioner are to be placed within the primary X-ray beam. It is safe practice to also wear a lead apron and, where possible, a thyroid gland protective lead neck collar.

In instances where radiography is being used either specifically to exclude one single suspected condition (e.g. the presence of a calcified egg in a dyspnoeic bird with suspected dystocia or ingested toxic particles, particularly in waterfowl), or when it is essential to obtain a quick survey radiograph, then it can prove far safer and perfectly sufficient to simply place the debilitated bird in a physiological 'sitting position' directly on to the plate. For a dorsoventral (DV) view, the bird can either sit unrestrained directly on top of the plate if very weak and immobile, or sit/stand quietly and devoid of stressors within a radiolucent or dark cardboard box placed on top of the radiographic plate. The orthogonal view can then be obtained using a horizontal beam centred on to a plate positioned upright lateral to the patient. A procedure such as this can be performed quickly and safely without the application of major restraint, sedation or general anaesthesia. Even if the resulting radiographic image could hardly be regarded as a 'proper' all-round diagnostic image, such a provisional radiographic assessment will allow the practitioner to initiate the proper essential and immediate treatment protocol, and may make the difference between death or survival of a critically ill patient.

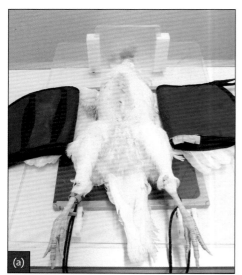

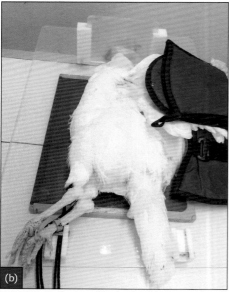

11.1 Patient positioning for (a) a ventrodorsal and (b) a lateral view of a chicken using a radiotranslucent fixation plate. Note: the bird is conscious during the procedure. For the lateral view, to avoid tilting of the body, radiotranslucent material such as a towel can be placed between the wings.

A 'proper' diagnostic radiograph can always be performed at a later stage on a stabilized patient that is more likely to survive extended restraint or a general anaesthetic.

In some bird species presented as clinical cases, it is often simpler and faster to anaesthetize the individual for radiography. Whilst chickens, ducks, geese and peacocks tend not to be too difficult to handle, some backyard poultry, such as guinea fowl, pheasants and especially francolins (*Francolinus* species), tend to be very nervous. Pheasants may display extremely excitable behaviour and it is not uncommon for gentle and straightforward capture, handling and restraint for radiographic examination to cause considerable feather loss. Anaesthesia tends to result in more feathers remaining on the bird and less landing on the table or on the consulting room floor. Anaesthetized patients are positioned using radiolucent adhesive tape placed over the feet, wings and neck and stuck to the cassette itself or to a radiotranslucent sheet placed over it. Low residue, easy to peel surgical tape can be safely stuck to avian plumage as well as to the most delicate of avian skins (Figure 11.3). The adhesive tape helps to restrain the unconscious bird with the tautness required to take a precise diagnostic image without adhering to the patient's feathers too closely. The radiographer can then carefully remove the tape from the skin and plumage following the examination without causing any feather loss or injuries to the bird's skin. When positioning chickens and other round-bodied birds in dorsal recumbency, tilting from the ideal position can be prevented by simply placing towels or other radiotranslucent positioning tools next to the bird to prop it up firmly.

Radiographic views

As radiography simplifies a complex three-dimensional (3D) body into a two-dimensional (2D) picture, it is of particular importance to obtain at least two views before attempting to assess a condition or reach a diagnosis. Relying only on one view can easily lead to the wrong conclusion and an avoidable misdiagnosis (Figure 11.4). In general, a ventrodorsal (VD) and lateral view should be obtained. Care should be taken to ensure that the patient is positioned correctly prior to exposure, as an accurate diagnosis cannot be reached without precise positioning.

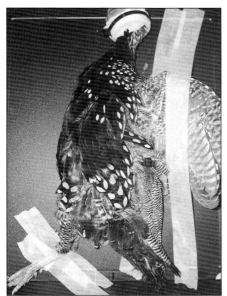

11.3 Patient positioning for a lateral view of a Pakistani partridge. General anaesthesia has been provided with isoflurane gas and the feet and wings have been fixed into position with adhesive tape.

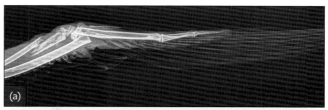
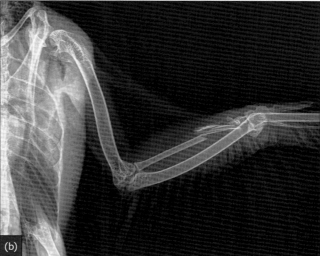

11.4 (a) Caudocranial view of the wing of a duck showing a distal fracture of the radius and ulna. (b) Mediolateral view of the wing of a duck with a distal fracture of the radius. In contrast to (a) a fracture of the ulna may be easily overlooked on this view.

Ventrodorsal view

Patient positioning for a VD view needs to be meticulously judged by eye and by palpation to ensure that the sternum overlies the vertebral column. In order to avoid superimposition, the legs should be stretched as far caudally as possible so as not to overlie any abdominal structures. The wings should be stretched outwards away from the body (see Figure 11.1a), which helps to stabilize the position. If correct positioning is not achieved, then the two sides of the body cannot be compared accurately, which is especially important in the VD view. Apparent distortion of various structures and body cavities may be seen, which has no clinical significance, and the air sacs on one side may look smaller than those on the other side of the body. The shadow of the liver and the position of the gizzard may become distorted, risking misdiagnosis. The typically symmetrical hourglass shape formed by the heart and liver shadows that are seen on radiographs of psittacine birds, is only rarely seen in the chicken, due to the large amount of ingesta normally present in the intestines. Under normal circumstances, variations in the symmetry and relative position of organs, the pectoral and pelvic girdles, hip and femur, the heart and liver shadows, as well as the axillary diverticula/caudal air sacs can be assessed on a VD view (Figures 11.5 and 11.6). However, when there is an egg present (Figure 11.7), the space the egg occupies and the consequent displacement of surrounding organs will obscure most detail in the abdomen.

Lateral view

For the lateral view, the bird should be placed in right lateral recumbency. Care must be exercised when placing avian patients in this position if they are already suffering

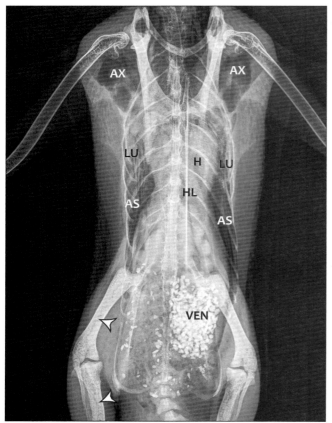

11.5 Ventrodorsal view of a female Indian Runner duck. The medullary bone in the femur and tibiotarsus (note the increased radiodensity) is denoted by the arrowheads. AS = caudal air sac region; AX = axillary air sacs; H = heart; HL = the 'waist' of the hourglass shape caused by the heart and liver shadows; LU = lung region; VEN = ventriculus.

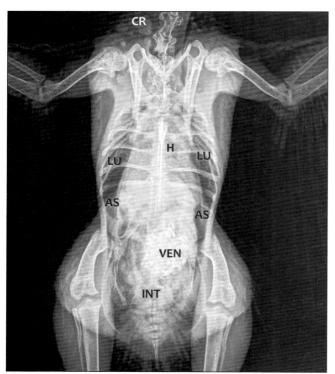

11.6 Ventrodorsal view of a Japanese Bantam. Note that there is no hourglass shape created by the heart and liver shadows and that the bones of the legs are relatively short (compared with Figure 11.15). AS = caudal air sac region; CR = crop; H = heart; INT = intestines; LU = lung region; VEN = ventriculus.

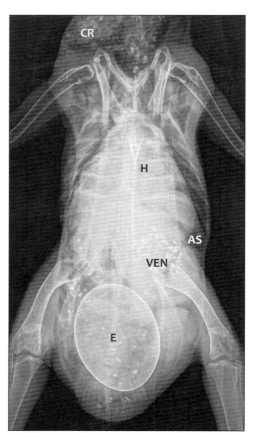

11.7 Ventrodorsal view of a chicken prior to laying an egg. Due to the space-occupying process (developed egg), the inner organs such as the heart, lungs, air sacs and liver cannot be properly assessed. AS = caudal air sacs; CR = crop; E = egg; H =heart; VEN = ventriculus.

any signs of respiratory depression, as it is likely to compound the dyspnoea even further. In the true lateral position, the two hip joints and two shoulder joints should be superimposed (see Figure 11.1b). Both wings are held dorsally above the body using tape or weights. To prevent the body from being drawn into an oblique position, a radiotranslucent pad should be placed between the wings. The legs need to be stretched caudally as far as possible to avoid superimposition (Figure 11.8). On this view it is possible to visualize the spine, heart and major blood vessels, the lung structure and the main bronchus, part of the caudal air sacs, the gastrointestinal tract and, in part, the gonads (Figures 11.9 and 11.10). The kidneys and spleen often cannot be seen due to the presence of ingesta in the intestines. As with the VD view, the presence of an egg will obscure most detail in the abdomen (Figure 11.11).

Mediolateral view

When obtaining a mediolateral view of the wings (with the patient placed in either lateral or ventral recumbency), care should be taken to ensure that not only are both wings in a flat position and as close to the radiographic film as possible, but also that they are extended symmetrically and to the same degree (Figure 11.12). For a mediolateral view of the hindlimbs, the bird should be placed in lateral recumbency with the extremity to be examined as close to the cassette as possible. Each limb should be examined in turn.

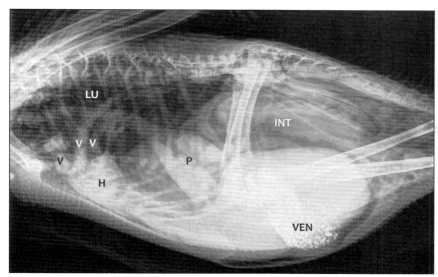

11.8 Lateral view of a goose. Due to the poor positioning (the legs have not been pulled caudally as far as possible), there is superimposition in the caudal body cavity and the organs cannot be properly assessed. H = heart; INT = intestines; LU = lung region; P = proventriculus; V = large heart vessels; VEN = ventriculus.

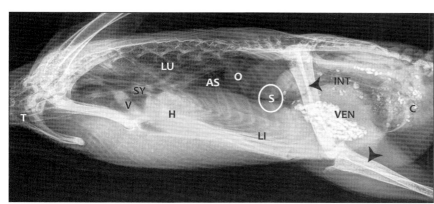

11.9 Lateral view of a female Indian Runner duck. The medullary bone in the femur and tibiotarsus (note the increased radiodensity) is denoted by the arrowheads. AS = caudal air sac region; C = cloaca; H = heart; INT = intestines; LI = liver region; LU = lung region; O = region of the ovary; S = spleen; SY = typically elongated syrinx; T = trachea; V = large heart vessel; VEN = ventriculus.

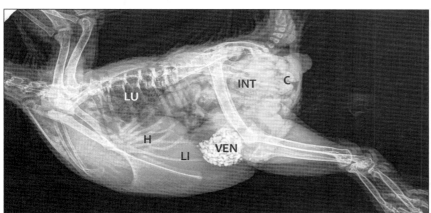

11.10 Lateral view of a Japanese Bantam. Note that due to the normally ingesta-filled and distended intestines, the caudal air sacs are not usually visible in Galliformes. In addition, the bones of the hindlimbs are relatively short (compared with Figure 11.15) and the pygostyle points dorsally. C = cloaca; H = heart; INT = intestines; LI = liver region; LU = lung region; VEN = ventriculus.

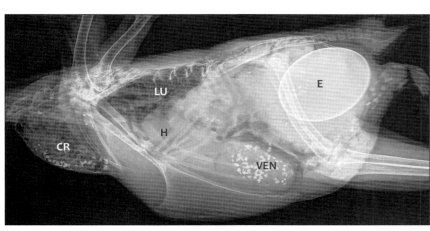

11.11 Lateral view of a chicken prior to laying an egg. Due to the space-occupying process (developed egg), the inner organs such as the heart, lung, air sacs and liver cannot be properly assessed. CR = crop; E = egg; H = heart; LU = lung region; VEN = ventriculus.

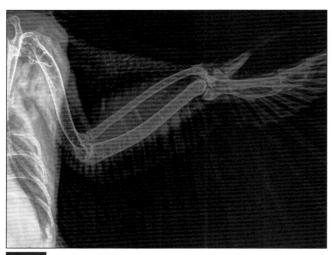

11.12 Mediolateral view of the wing of a Game Bantam.

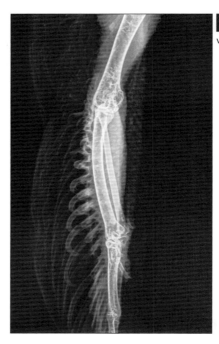

11.14 Caudocranial view of the wing of a Game Bantam.

Caudocranial view

For a caudocranial view of the wings, the patient has to be positioned with its head down and legs elevated with the dorsal wing edge touching the table/cassette. The wing is then extended laterally as far as possible and placed on to the cassette, so that its cranial border lies parallel to the edge of the cassette (Figures 11.13 and 11.14). An endo-tracheal tube should be placed to prevent the potential regurgitation and inhalation of ingesta, as in this particular position previous starvation of the patient can prove an insufficient precaution to avoid unwanted material from entering the trachea.

Dorsoplantar view

For a dorsoplantar view of the hindlimbs, the bird should be positioned in dorsal recumbency (as described for the VD view). When obtaining radiographs of the legs and feet (see Figures 11.15 and 11.20), it is important to achieve positional symmetry of both legs to allow any significant differences between the left and right limbs to be ident-ified. If the toes need to be imaged, they should be indiv-idually positioned as close as possible to the cassette using adhesive tape (see Figure 11.2).

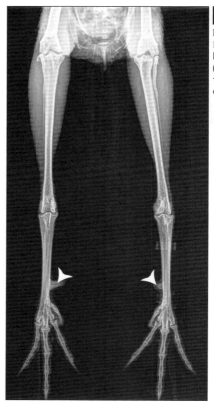

11.15 Ventrodorsal view of the legs of a Bantam cockerel. Note the typically long legs of this breed (compared with Figure 11.6). The arrowheads denote the spurs.

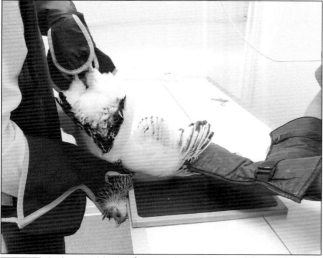

11.13 Patient positioning for a caudocranial view of the wing of a chicken.

Cranial views

To assess diseases involving the head of a bird, exact positioning is a prerequisite. Motion artefacts can only be avoided by heavy sedation or general anaesthesia. It is important to position the head of the bird very meticu-lously in dorsal, ventral and lateral recumbency to obtain views (see Figure 11.16). Further images can be obtained at 30- and 75-degree angles.

Normal anatomical variations

The radiographic anatomy of a healthy bird may display certain natural variations within the same species, depending on the bird's age, sex, reproductive status and environment. There are also many breed- and species-specific variations that need to be recognized. Some examples of anatomical variation in poultry include:

- The development of a crest in the Polish chicken and Crested duck (Figure 11.16)
- The development of a tracheal loop or coil or the bulla tympaniformis in some waterfowl (Figure 11.17)
- Polydactyly in the Faverolle (Figure 11.18)
- A shortened tibiotarsal bone in Japanese Bantam (see Figure 11.6) and Chabo chickens
- The typical metatarsal spur of males in many poultry species (see Figures 11.15 and 11.18).

Contrast studies

Contrast medium is infrequently used in backyard poultry, but when it is used, barium sulphate is the contrast agent of choice. It is used to outline the gastrointestinal tract (Figure 11.19). Indications for contrast radiography include:

- Diseases of the gastrointestinal tract with retarded or accelerated passage of ingesta
- Suspected abnormal contents of the gastrointestinal tract
- Diseases with alteration of the gastrointestinal tract walls
- Instances when it is necessary to outline the gastrointestinal tract against neighbouring organs.

The bird should have a more or less empty gastrointestinal tract in order to judge transit time. Anaesthesia should

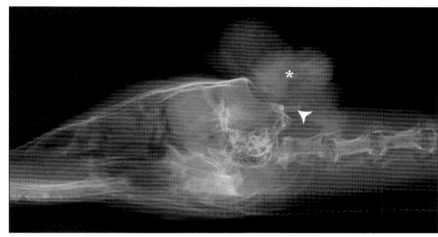

11.16 Lateral view of the skull of a Crested duck. The arrowhead denotes the bony protuberantia of the crest. * = crest.

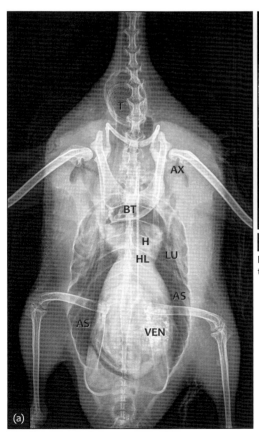

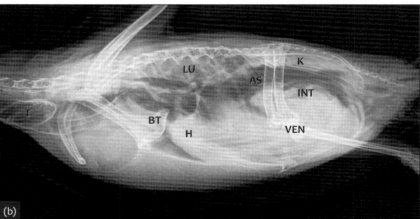

11.17 (a) Ventrodorsal and (b) lateral view of a goldeneye. AS = caudal air sac region; AX = axillary air sacs; BT = bulla tympaniformis; H = heart; HL = the 'waist' of the hourglass shape caused by the heart and liver shadows; INT = intestines; K = region of the kidneys; LU = lung region; T = physiological widening of the trachea; VEN = ventriculus.

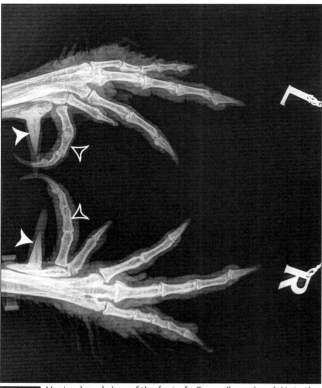

not be used for these studies as this may cause almost complete cessation of gastrointestinal motility. When perforations of the gastrointestinal tract are suspected, non-absorbable barium contrast media should be avoided. Organic non-ionic iodine contrast media may be administered in these cases. However, it should be noted that the gastric transit time of iodine contrast media is far quicker (about twice as fast) than that of barium contrast media.

A survey radiograph should always be obtained prior to the administration of any contrast medium. The barium sulphate suspension can then be instilled into the crop via an oesophageal tube made from any suitable diameter plastic or rubber tubing fitted to the Luer tip of a hypodermic syringe. A specialized rigid metal catheter (i.e. gavage crop tube) for use in birds, with a ball-shaped, smooth distal end, can be utilized in patients likely to bite a softer tube. Rigid tubes should be well lubricated. The quantity of barium in the suspension should be adjusted depending upon the patient's condition and the exhibited signs. Weaker suspensions help differentiate the gastrointestinal tract from its neighbouring organs, whilst a more concentrated suspension is better suited for identifying diagnostic changes within the gastrointestinal tract itself.

The usual dose is 20 ml/kg of a 25–45% suspension. After administration, the bird should be held upright for a few minutes in order to avoid regurgitation of the suspension. The time taken for the suspension to reach the various parts of the alimentary canal depends on the drugs used for premedication and anaesthesia, as well as any pathological conditions that may be present. On average, and in a

11.18 Ventrodorsal view of the feet of a Faverolle cockerel. Note the polydactyly (open arrowheads) and spur (solid arrowheads).

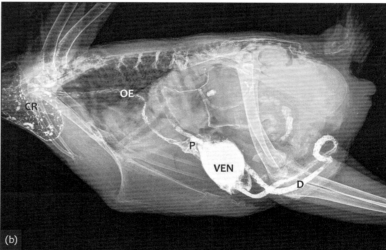

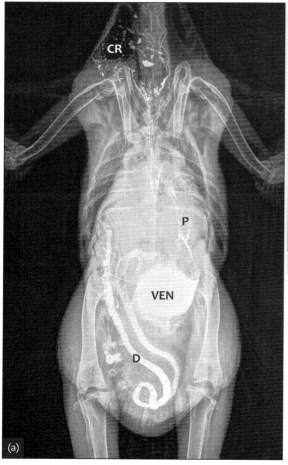

11.19 (a) Ventrodorsal and (b) lateral view of a chicken 50 minutes after the ingestion of barium sulphate contrast medium. CR = crop; D = duodenal loop; OE = oesophagus; P = proventriculus; VEN = ventriculus.

healthy bird that has been fasted, barium will reach the proventriculus and gizzard within 5–10 minutes and the small intestine within 30–60 minutes. It should reach the cloaca after 3–4 hours at the latest in granivorous (seed eating) species.

Barium sulphate suspension or one of the iodine contrast agents such as iohexol or iopamidol (10 mg/kg of a 250 mg iodine/ml solution) can also be used retrograde to outline the cloaca and rectum of avian patients.

Special care needs to be exercised to avoid the possible regurgitation and aspiration of barium and other compounds by the patient whilst performing radiographic contrast studies. For this reason, it is recommended that the patient is fasted prior to the administration of the contrast medium. The crop of the bird should always be checked for food contents by gentle palpation. A bird that has been presented at the veterinary clinic well fed and with a crop full of grain should at least be allowed sufficient time to turn over the crop contents, whilst having food and water withheld, before attempting the administration of any contrast medium.

Patient positioning for the radiographic study needs to be undertaken with care. If there is still sufficient liquid barium in the crop when the bird is restrained and positioned for a VD view, then the liquid can potentially flow into the mouth of the bird and be inhaled. Positioning for a lateral view, where the bird's wings are folded backwards above its head before it is placed in lateral recumbency, can be particularly difficult as the conscious bird may regurgitate the barium contrast medium whilst trying to avoid the handler's restraint.

There is also a small but considerable risk of causing ileus through the administration of a hygroscopic contrast suspension, especially when administered to an already dehydrated patient. Due to the desiccating properties of contrast media, it is imperative that the patient receive an adequate volume of fluid prior to the procedure. Administering 20 ml/kg of a saline solution subcutaneously should prove sufficient.

Urography

Urographic investigations have very limited diagnostic value in the bird, due to the lack of clear differentiation between the medulla and cortex in the kidneys and the fact that they lack both a bladder and urethra. Urography may help to differentiate the kidneys from surrounding tissue, which cannot be achieved with normal survey radiography or ultrasonography (e.g. ovarian cysts and tumours of the gonads). In addition, urography can also be used to determine whether the ureters are functional (i.e. to look for the presence of uroliths). Patients found to be dehydrated should receive sufficient rehydration prior to attempting urography. The contrast agent, an organic iodine compound with an iodine content of 300–400 mg iodine/ml, should be warmed to body temperature prior to being administered slowly intravenously, via the ulnar vein, to the sedated bird at a dose of 2 ml/kg bodyweight. Only highly concentrated compounds that are specifically indicated for urography should be used, otherwise the resultant inadequate contrast of the anatomical structures being visualized will render the study non-diagnostic.

Sinography

For visualization of the nasal passages and sinuses, soluble contrast agents (e.g. non-ionic iodine compounds) can be administered directly into the region of the head under investigation. However, it should be noted that superimposition of the infraorbital sinus can make the interpretation of sinographic radiographs difficult. Delineation of the sinus can be achieved by injecting 0.1–1 ml (depending on the size of the bird) of a 200–250 mg iodine/ml solution directly into the paranasal sinus. The contrast agent should be immediately flushed with sterile saline solution following completion of the investigation, in order to minimize any possible local tissue irritation, oedema or periorbital swelling. It should also be noted that in the majority of cases where contrast studies would be indicated (e.g. disease processes associated with rhinitis and/or sinusitis, or where there is suspicion of an intranasal tumour of head trauma), CT would yield a far more diagnostic picture.

Angiography

Angiography can be particularly helpful in clinical cases where echocardiography cannot be performed. It is also helpful for depicting aneurysms. Angiocardiography is not considered a substitute for echocardiography, but it can have additional diagnostic value. In aquatic birds, where no coupling sites are available and it is not possible to extract feathers due to animal welfare reasons, it offers a good alternative. Angiocardiography should always be performed under general anaesthesia. The iodine-based contrast agent (e.g. iopamidol: 370 mg iodine/ml solution) at a dose of 2–4 mg/kg should be slowly injected through an intravenous catheter that has been placed either in the jugular or basilic vein. A series of lateral and/or VD radiographs should then be obtained as quickly as possible. Due to the rapid heartbeat, it is difficult to assess cardiac contractility in birds, but ventricular hypertrophy and dilatation, aneurysms and stenosis of blood vessels and heart valves can, in principle, be diagnosed with angiography.

Musculoskeletal system

Radiography is essential in the field of avian orthopaedic surgery and immensely helpful in assessing the degree of distortion and prognosis in bone disease.

When reviewing radiographic images of the skeleton for the diagnosis of orthopaedic problems, attention should also be paid to the surrounding musculature. A reduction in size of one of the pectoralis muscles due to atrophy can often be seen on a radiograph, although it may not be so obvious on palpation. It may also be possible to detect slight contraction and swelling of the muscle mass following rupture of the tendon. Signs of muscle injury are visible as a subtle increase in density when compared with the contralateral side. Some idea of how recent an injury to the skeleton is can be gauged by the condition of the neighbouring muscles. With very recent injuries, there is a noticeable increase in the size and density of the radiographic shadow. This usually decreases considerably, almost returning to normal, during the course of the next few days, providing the fracture is not compound and there is not superimposed infection.

Pathological alterations of the long bones most commonly occur in the legs (Figures 11.20 and 11.21) rather than in the wings (Figure 11.22) in backyard poultry. Fractures of the vertebral column usually involve the last thoracic vertebra cranial to the synsacrum; pelvic fractures hardly occur. Fractures of the long bones can be identified easily on radiographs (see Figure 11.4). Apart from diagnosing the type, extent, age (a fresh fracture has sharp edges, whereas older fractures have rounded edges) and displacement of a specific fracture, radiography allows the

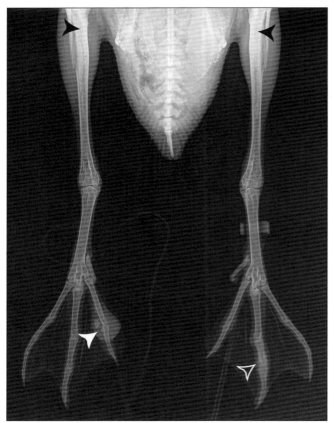

11.20 Ventrodorsal view of the legs of a female Indian Runner duck. This image clearly shows soft tissue swelling and reorganization in the right medial toe (white arrowhead), arthritis in the left toe (open arrowhead) and medullary bone in both proximal tibiotarsi (black arrowheads). Note also that due to the erect leg posture in this particular duck breed, the intra-articular space in the hock joint is extremely narrow.

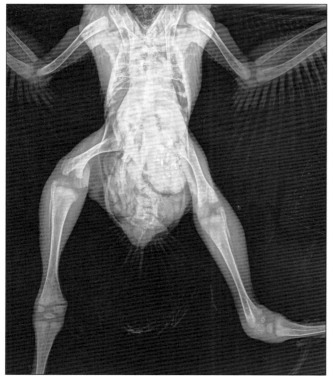

11.21 Ventrodorsal view of a young turkey with tibiotarsal rotation. Note the wide joint space, which is physiological in young birds.

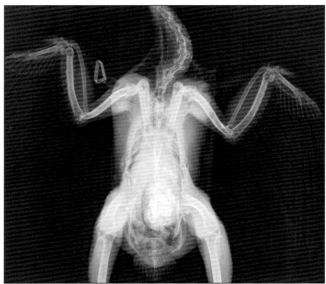

11.22 Ventrodorsal view of a red junglefowl with severe osteomyelitis in both ulnar bones and mild disease in both radial bones. This could be a sign of salmonellosis.

important process of fracture healing to be followed in the patient. In birds, physiological endosteal callus is hardly visible radiographically. When osteomyelitis is present in a long bone, new bone tends to be formed by the cortex and endosteum, rather than by the periosteum as is the case in mammals. Osteomyelitis is recognized radiographically from approximately 10–14 days after onset.

Metabolic bone disease can be a common finding in fast-growing fledglings that have been inadequately fed, where it is recognized as rickets. It occurs where fledglings have not received the required balanced alimentary calcium:phosphorus ratio (see Chapters 18 and 20). This results in a folding distortion of the thin and weak cortex of the long bones (see Figure 11.21). Gross distortion and pathological fractures occur first in the legs (as these are the first parts that have to carry the increasing weight of a rapidly growing body), then in the vertebral column (kyphosis), sternum and wings, which often results in the bird becoming permanently crippled. On occasion, one member of a clutch of chicks may develop the condition whilst its siblings seem perfectly normal. It is notable that this condition does not only occur in captivity but also in wild birds, especially in individuals belonging to the heron family.

Other conditions that can be recognized radiographically include:

- Osteoporosis (where the radiographic picture is similar to that of rickets)
- Neoplasia (Figure 11.23)
- Arthritis (see Figure 11.20).

Neoplasia tends to be predominantly osteolytic in birds. Arthritis in joints can be seen in birds with *Salmonella* infection (often in conjunction with hepatomegaly). Radiography of most of the limb joints in the bird is easy to perform, with the exception of the hip joint where the shape of the ileum makes outlining of the joint difficult.

In mycobacteriosis there is often localized osteolysis (Figure 11.24) together with surrounding sclerosis accompanied by focal densities in the long bones. These skeletal signs are often seen in conjunction with hepatomegaly and splenomegaly.

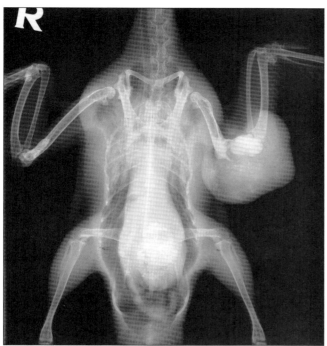

11.23 Ventrodorsal view of a male Mandarin duck showing chondrosarcoma of the periosteum in both wings.

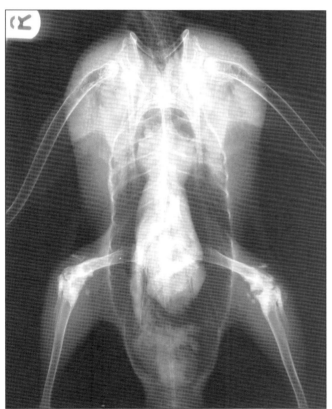

11.24 Ventrodorsal view of lesser whitefronted goose showing severe osteolysis in both knee joints due to tuberculosis.

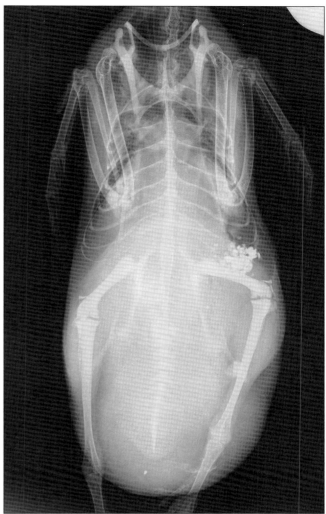

11.25 Ventrodorsal view of a female Indian Runner duck. Medullary bone is visible in the long bones of the legs and the shoulder girdle. It is not possible to differentiate the internal organs, with the exception of the displaced ventriculus, due to the presence of ascites (see also Figure 11.41).

subsequently become calcified. The bones appear much denser on radiographs. Formation of medullary bone may suggest the presence of a genital tract disease with a concurrent raised oestrogen level, e.g. in those cases of egg binding with laminated eggs, ovarian cysts or tumours (see Chapter 17).

Soft tissues

Since a radiograph constitutes a 2D shadow of a 3D body, it is absolutely essential to obtain both VD and lateral views. The VD view is especially valuable when assessing the symmetry of 'paired' organs (e.g. the lungs or air sacs) as it allows unilateral changes to be identified. The lateral view, on the other hand, offers better differentiation and verification of the shape and size of individual organs.

Respiratory tract

There are a few interspecies peculiarities of the respiratory tract of which the avian radiologist should be aware. In some species the trachea is elongated or has a tracheal loop (e.g. swans) (see Figures 11.9 and 11.17). There is also interspecific, and sometimes intraspecific, variation in the

A normal physiological condition, which is often found incidentally during radiography, is the formation of so-called medullary bone (see Figures 11.20, 11.22 and 11.25) in hens that have a high oestrogen level prior to egg laying (representing temporary calcium storage for the eggshell). It is recognized when assessing the medullary cavities of the long bones, which are normally filled with air but have

anatomy of the air sacs and in the pneumatization of the bones. In the male of some species of ducks and geese, there is a normal balloon-like irregular distension of the syrinx (bulla tympaniformis), which increases in size with age (see Figure 11.17).

In good quality lateral radiographs, the two lungs can be identified by their slight honeycomb appearance (see Figures 11.8 to 11.10). Any increase in density or areas of loss of the normal reticular pattern should be noted as these may represent pathological changes (Figure 11.26). The region of the air sacs should be carefully examined; however, it may not be possible to differentiate these structures due to the food-filled distended gastrointestinal tract or the presence of an egg (see Figures 11.10, 11.11 and 11.19). Absence of a clear outline of the caudal air sacs may also be due to other space-occupying lesions, adhesions or gross air sacculitis. Less severe air sacculitis is recognized on the VD view as general haziness of part or all of the air sac spaces. On the lateral view, dense striations represent the end-on view of thickened air sacs. On the VD view, the left and right thoracic and abdominal air sacs should always be compared for signs of a localized increase in density due to infection. An overall homogeneous 'ground glass' increase in density of both the thoracic and abdominal cavities, accompanied by obvious distension of the caudal abdomen, is usually due to peritonitis or ascites (see Figure 11.25).

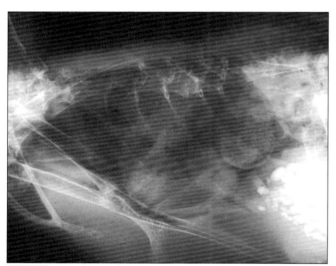

11.26 Lateral view of a peacock showing a lung granuloma due to mycobacteriosis.

The extrathoracic diverticula of the clavicular sacs can be seen in the pectoral muscle mass around the proximal end of the humerus (see Figure 11.5). There is considerable interspecific variation in these diverticula. Excessive distension of these air sacs indicates the presence of stenosis in the lower part of the respiratory tract.

Heart

One of the most obvious features visible on the VD view is the 'waist' between the shadow of the heart and that of the liver in graminivorous (grass eating) species. However, in most chickens this hourglass outline is less distinct or absent due to the food-filled distended gastrointestinal tract (see Figure 11.6) or the presence of an egg in the abdominal cavity (see Figure 11.7).

When examining the heart shadow, size, shape and radiodensity should be noted (Figure 11.27), as well as the

visibility of the great vessels (see Figure 11.8). However, radiographic signs are non-specific and may only give a general indication of cardiac disease. A diagnosis has to be supported by other techniques, such as echocardiography. An enlarged heart shadow (see Figure 11.25) may indicate any heart disease such as hydropericardium (sometimes seen with systemic infection and accompanied by liver insufficiency) or granulomatous lesions (often of mycobacterial origin). Increased radiodensity of any of the great vessels of the heart, particularly in elderly individuals, suggests calcification and possibly arteriosclerosis.

Gastrointestinal tract

On radiographs of the gastrointestinal tract, the crop is visible above the thoracic inlet, often partly filled with food (see Figures 11.7, 11.11 and 11.19). Any increase in size of the left side of the hepatic shadow may be caused by an increase in size of the proventriculus. Enlargement of the gastrointestinal tract with gas-filled contents is best seen on the lateral view (Figure 11.28) and differentiated with barium sulphate contrast medium. Enlargement of the proventriculus with the organ occupying much of the thoracoabdominal cavity (best seen with barium contrast studies)

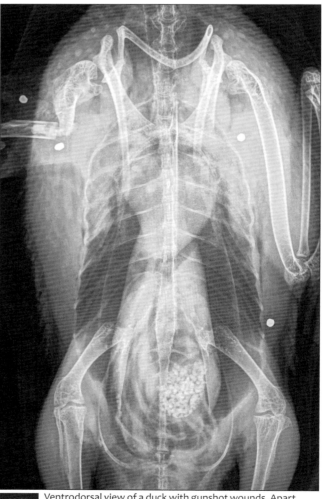

11.27 Ventrodorsal view of a duck with gunshot wounds. Apart from the radiodense shotgun pellets embedded within the soft tissues and the obvious humeral fracture, note that the heart apex and liver edges can be clearly differentiated. This is due to air sac rupture within this area and, as air is a negative contrast medium, the organs have become clearly outlined on the image. This is commonly seen following trauma.

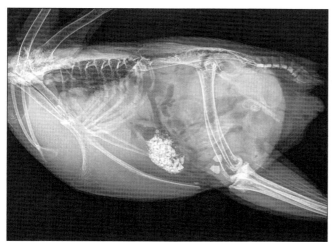

11.28 Lateral view of a pheasant showing enlarged and partially gas-filled intestinal loops as a result of a parasitic infection.

usually indicates motility disturbances of the gastrointestinal tract of infectious or non-infectious origin (e.g. foreign bodies, bezoars, parasite infestation). Proventricular dilatation disease, although well recognized in psittacine birds, has also been confirmed to affect many different species of wild waterfowl. Parasite infestation (e.g. with tapeworms or *Candida*) may also slow down gastric emptying and occasionally cause an enlarged proventricular shadow.

The ventriculus (or gizzard) is easily recognized on the VD view in graminivorous birds (see Figures 11.5 and 11.10) by the presence of retained grit, and it normally occupies a position just to the left of the midline and just below an imaginary line joining the two hips. If a bird has been given only soluble oyster shell grit or has been deprived of grit altogether, then the gizzard may not be identifiable by this method. Space-occupying lesions may be responsible for displacing the normal position of the gizzard shadow. In graminivorous birds, excessive grit may cause impaction or indicate malfunction of the gastrointestinal tract. Foreign bodies such as fish hooks, lead shot and nails are not uncommonly seen lodged in the oesophagus, proventriculus or gizzard of waterfowl (Figure 11.29). They may occasionally pass further along the alimentary canal.

Disease of the lower gastrointestinal tract may lead to increased density and greater visualization of the intestinal loops. This is sometimes accompanied by gas filling and distension (see Figure 11.28). These signs may be indicative of microbiological or parasitic infection. However, gas filling is normal in gamebirds and some waterfowl. Foreign

body obstruction of the intestine in birds is not usually accompanied by a build-up of gas, as is the case in mammals. There may, however, be enlargement and greater visualization of the intestine. Gastrointestinal disease is also indicated by the presence of grit and, when using barium contrast medium, undigested seed in the intestine.

Liver

The radiographic shadow of the liver is the caudal part of the hourglass silhouette (when seen) in graminivorous species (see Figure 11.17). Hepatomegaly (Figure 11.30) may alter the outline and also lead to displacement of the proventriculus, which is visible on a lateral view (best seen with barium sulphate contrast studies). Hepatomegaly may be seen most commonly in cases of infection (usually viral or bacterial). Ascites reduces the ability to differentiate the internal organs on radiographs (see Figure 11.25). It often occurs secondary to heart failure and/or various other hepatopathies of infectious and non-infectious aetiology. Ascites may also be seen accompanying egg peritonitis in older hens. Birds with ascites are often in severe respiratory distress, so good images of this condition are not easy to obtain. In cases of ascites, ultrasonography is the imaging modality of choice as the fluid provides an ideal contrast medium for this technique (see Figure 11.41). The liver margins can be seen exceptionally clearly in patients in which severe trauma has led to rupture of the surrounding air sacs (see Figure 11.27).

Spleen

The spleen is rarely seen in most poultry species on the lateral view. When visible it appears as a relatively small, round or oval shadow situated between the angle of the proventriculus and the gizzard (see Figure 11.9). Although the spleen may not always be recognizable in healthy birds, it is more easily seen when enlarged due to infection or neoplasia (Figure 11.31).

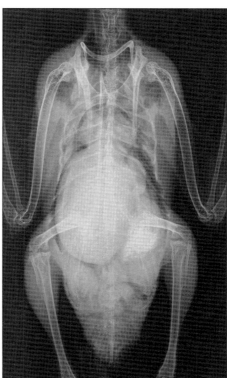

11.30 Ventrodorsal view of a painted shelduck showing massive liver enlargement due to neoplasia.

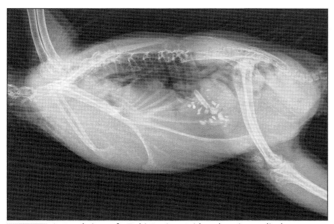

11.29 Lateral view of a Pakistani partridge showing radiodense foreign bodies within the ventriculus.

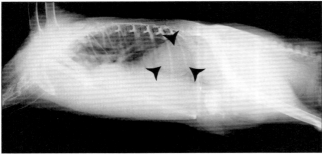

11.31 Lateral view of an Indian Runner duck showing an enlarged spleen (arrowheads).

Kidneys

The lateral view may provide information about the size and radiodensity of the kidneys, but these are not easily identifiable in poultry. Active gonads (see Figures 11.9 and 11.32) must not be confused with kidney enlargement. On the VD view, the gastrointestinal tract is superimposed on the kidneys; thus only severe renal abnormalities can be identified. Enlargement of the renal shadow is interpreted as a non-specific sign of many generalized infections, as well as non-infectious conditions such as kidney cysts and neoplasia (differentiation may be easily performed using ultrasonography in most cases). With severe dehydration, gout and vitamin A deficiency, there tends to be an increase in the density of the kidney shadow, but this is difficult to evaluate.

Reproductive tract

Gonadal imaging should be used to differentiate pathological enlargement from physiological activity (Figure 11.32), with the patient history and clinical findings providing the necessary indications. Gonadal neoplasia, especially in chickens, may occur due to Marek's disease or leucosis and causes massive enlargement of the organ, resulting in pressure on the air sacs and ventrocaudal displacement of the gastrointestinal tract (seen more clearly with barium sulphate contrast studies). Alterations in the size and shape of the gonads may also occur with cystic ovaries, and differentiation of these cases is best achieved using ultrasonography.

Ultrasonography may also be useful when a rudimentary left oviductal cyst or egg yolk peritonitis (Figure 11.33) is suspected, as these conditions cannot be diagnosed by radiography alone; only a diffuse shadowing of the soft tissues in the caudal abdomen can be seen radiographically. Ultrasound-guided coelomocentesis may also be performed in these cases. In addition, salpingitis cannot be diagnosed on radiography.

In birds with egg retention, the egg can often be palpated, provided it is calcified and not situated too deep within the coelomic cavity. In these cases, radiography is not only necessary to provide information about the form, size, number and position of any eggs (see Figures 11.7 and 11.11), but it can also be helpful when determining whether surgical or non-surgical removal should be attempted. Unfortunately, it is not possible to differentiate eggs lacking a calcified shell altogether, eggs with a very thin shell (Figure 11.34), laminated eggs and other soft tissue masses (e.g. tumours or cysts) within the thoraco-abdominal cavity on radiography. Ultrasonography is the method of choice for differentiation in these cases (see Figures 11.35 and 11.47). However, visualization of medullary bone on radiography (see Figures 11.5 and 11.9; see also Chapter 18) and

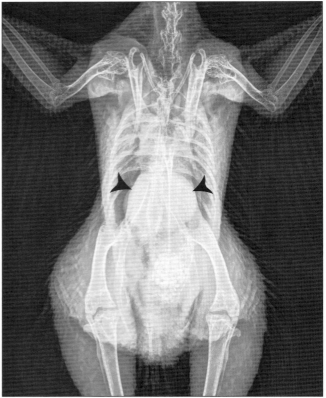

11.32 Ventrodorsal view of a Game Bantam showing active testes (arrowheads). These should not be confused with kidney tumours. Note the extremely well developed musculature of the hindlimbs.

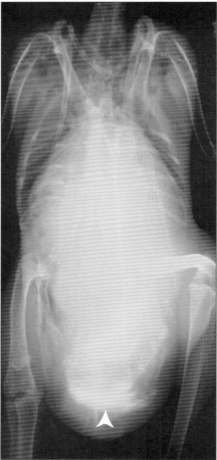

11.33 Ventrodorsal view of a female partridge with egg yolk peritonitis (compare with Figure 11.48). There is no differentiation of the internal organs and egg structures are visible in the caudal abdomen (arrowhead).

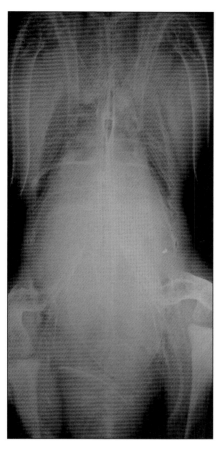

11.34 Ventrodorsal view of a chicken with soft-shelled eggs.

contrast studies of the gastrointestinal tract can be useful in reaching a diagnosis. Other changes that occur in conjunction with an increased oestrogen level, such as cystic changes of the ovaries and oviduct or gonadomas, cannot be conclusively ruled out by radiography alone. Thus, the identification of medullary bone is only helpful in radiographs with otherwise unclear findings.

Ultrasonography

Ultrasonography is often useful in complementing the images obtained by radiography (e.g. in cases of egg binding, ascites or suspected neoplasia). It can even be used as the sole imaging modality for a rapid diagnosis, instead of radiography. In contrast to radiography, ultrasonography provides information about the internal structural changes occurring within the soft tissue organs and their cross-sectional topography. However, it should be borne in mind that obtaining diagnostic ultrasonograms is more dependent on the technique used and the level of expertise of the examiner than radiography, and that interpretation of the images is more subjective. Serial ultrasound examinations can be used to follow the therapeutic progress of a specific treatment.

Ultrasonography is the most important imaging modality for examination of the cardiovascular and urogenital systems, as well as the liver. For some disease processes, such as pericardial effusion and ascites (see Figure 11.41), ultrasonography may be the only useful means of diagnosis in the live bird. When differentiating between hydropericardium and cardiomegaly it is invaluable, as well as when it comes to examining the liver parenchyma of a patient with hepatomegaly (see Figures 11.43 and 11.44),

where it can be used to differentiate between neoplastic and inflammatory changes and to guide liver biopsy. When investigating changes in the reproductive tract of female birds, ultrasonography can be of primary importance, particularly when assessing radiolucent masses such as laminated eggs (see Figure 11.47).

It should be noted that whereas in a healthy bird ultrasonographic visualization of the internal organs may be difficult due to a fully developed calcified egg or a full gastrointestinal tract, this is not the case in a diseased bird. Organ enlargement and the resulting air sac displacement, as well as fluid accumulation, improve image quality and diagnostic potential.

Equipment

The capital investment in equipment is initially high, but once acquired the running costs are minimal. For this reason, purchase solely for use in avian practice is highly unlikely, although a clinician may have access to the equipment if it is available in the practice for use in other species. In this case, purchase of a small probe suitable for bird cases should be considered.

A comprehensive discussion regarding the technical parameters of ultrasonography is outwith the scope of this chapter and the reader is referred to other texts for information (Krautwald-Junghanns *et al.*, 2011). Ultrasound examination in birds requires electronic transducers (probes) with small coupling surfaces (micro-convex or phased array transducers are preferable in smaller birds; linear transducers may be used in birds ≥500 g in bodyweight) and frequencies of between 5 MHz and 12 MHz. The size of the transducer is important, especially in smaller birds. The best results are obtained using transducers developed for human paediatric medicine or those developed for surgical or gynaecological use.

Coupling sites

Avian anatomy restricts the number of locations where the transducer can be brought into close contact with the skin. As close contact is essential to achieve optimal imaging quality, only two coupling sites are suitable in birds:

- Ventromedian site caudal to the sternum (Figure 11.35)
- Parasternal site caudal to the last rib (Figure 11.36).

Of these two approaches, the ventromedian is the most useful and the transducer is applied in the midline, directly caudal to the keel. The parasternal approach may be used in birds with sufficient space between the last rib and the pelvic bones. The transducer is applied on the right side of the bird because, if placed on the left side, the contents of the gizzard can disturb the penetration of the ultrasound waves. The leg of the bird is pulled either forwards or backwards and the transducer has to be pressed slightly to the body wall to compress the underlying air sacs.

Feathers in these areas need to be parted or plucked. Separating the feathers is sufficient in most cases. In hens, the featherless area behind the sternum (brood patch) can make plucking redundant if using the ventromedian coupling site. If examining aquatic birds, feather plucking should be kept to an absolute minimum, as excessive feather loss could lead to hypothermia and in extreme cases the patient may lose their ability to swim. Moreover, it is sometimes difficult to remove sufficient feathers at the ventromedian coupling site in ducks and geese.

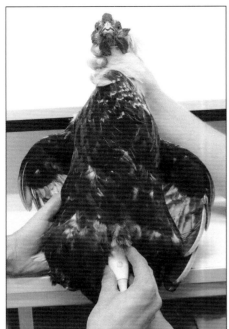

11.35 Patient positioning for an ultrasound examination of an Orloff chicken using the ventromedian coupling site. Once the feathers are parted and acoustic gel applied, the transducer is positioned caudal to the sternum.

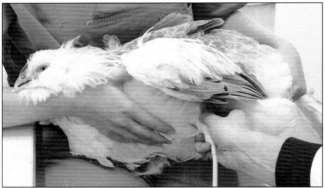

11.36 Patient positioning for an ultrasound examination of a Faverolle using the parasternal coupling site. Once the feathers are parted and acoustic gel applied, the transducer is positioned caudal to the last rib.

A commercially available water-soluble acoustic gel should be applied generously to the coupling site to ensure good contact between the transducer and the skin. These gels are well tolerated and can be removed easily from feathers and skin following the examination.

Patient preparation and positioning

Since the penetration of the ultrasound beam can be disturbed by contents in the gastrointestinal tract, birds should be fasted prior to examination. This is especially important when using the ventromedian coupling site. However, caution should be exercised in critically ill birds that have had a reduced appetite over a prolonged period of time, as in these cases fasting may neither be possible nor necessary.

For routine assessments, an assistant (or even the patient's owner) can hold the bird in either dorsal or lateral recumbency (see Figures 11.35 and 11.36) or in an upright position. In patients displaying clinical signs of heart disease or dyspnoea, lying in dorsal recumbency can cause circulatory problems and should therefore be avoided. It is generally advised to restrain the patient in as upright a position as possible for the examination.

Anaesthesia and sedation are commonly not necessary for routine ultrasonography.

Heart

Any pathological heart condition is an indication for a cardiac ultrasonographic examination (with the exception of waterfowl and any aquatic birds; see above). The great advantage of an ultrasonographic examination of the avian heart is visualization of the internal structures. This allows assessment of the anatomy and functional status quickly and efficiently. However, due to the anatomical peculiarities of the avian heart, the protocols or standardized views recommended for echocardiography in mammals cannot be applied to birds.

B-mode echocardiography (2D) is the established examination technique in birds. M-mode echocardiography, which is used to assess wall thickness and contractility in mammals, is not useful in birds since the avian heart can only be visualized in longitudinal and semi-transverse views. B-mode echocardiography can be used to subjectively assess structures and take precise measurements. Reference ranges have been reported for several avian species, but not yet, to the authors' knowledge, for backyard poultry.

The size of the ventricles, the thickness of the interventricular septum and the contractility of the ventricles, and the left and right atrioventricular valves are important parameters to evaluate the morphology and function of the heart (Figure 11.37). The most frequently identified pathological findings include hydropericardium and hypertrophy

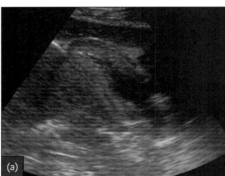

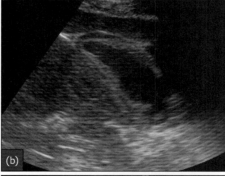

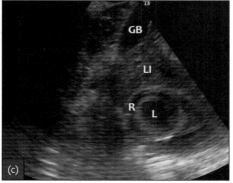

11.37 Echocardiograms of a Game Bantam. (a) Ventromedian view during systole. (b) Ventromedian view during diastole. (c) Parasternal short-axis view. GB = gallbladder; L = left ventricle; LI = liver; R = right ventricle.

or dilatation of the right ventricle, which are often caused by right-sided congestive heart failure. Doppler ultrasonography is used in avian patients to determine the rate of inflow as well as outflow of blood; this rate is plotted as a curve against time. Reference ranges have not yet been published for poultry species.

Gastrointestinal tract

The gastrointestinal tract (especially the intestinal loops) is visible during almost every examination (Figure 11.38), and therefore it is important to be familiar with its ultrasonographic appearance. Indications for ultrasonography are rare, as most information can be gained from radiography. Ultrasound examinations of the gastrointestinal tract in diseased birds are under-recorded, and so the value of ultrasonography for this purpose is still limited in comparison to radiography. Often a diagnosis is made coincidentally during examination.

The gastrointestinal tract should be as empty as possible prior to examination or, ideally, contain only fluid. Neither solid food particles nor gas can be penetrated by ultrasound waves due to absorption and reflection. Whilst imaging of the crop and oesophagus in the majority of avian patients is not possible due to the lack of coupling sites, the ventriculus is easily viewed from both the median (Figure 11.39) and lateral coupling sites, especially in grit-consuming graminivorous birds. Grit is often observed during routine examinations as hyperechoic particles with distant shadows. The particles of grit are surrounded by a hypoechoic region, which varies in size depending upon the amount of food ingested. The ventriculus produces an acoustic shadow because the grit totally reflects the ultrasound waves.

Gastric muscle is visible as a round or oval hypoechoic zone. Transducer frequencies >12 MHz allow assessment of the koilin layer in the gizzard. The cranially situated proventriculus can be imaged in smaller gramnivores only if it is enlarged. Identifying the ventriculus first and then angling the transducer can localize it. The proventriculus is usually round in cross-section, has a medium degree of echogenicity and hyperechoic contents in the form of food particles, some of which produce distal acoustic shadows.

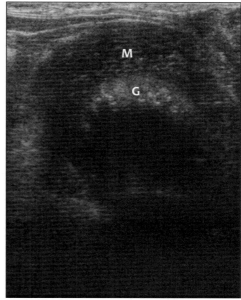

11.39 Ultrasonogram of a goose obtained using a ventromedian approach showing the ventriculus. G = grit; M = muscle.

The intestines can be identified by peristaltic activity during examination and the presence of ingesta within the lumen (see Figures 11.38 and 11.40). Both longitudinal and cross-sectional views of the intestinal loops may be observed at any one time. Layers within the intestinal walls can be recognized to a certain degree, and sometimes granulomatous lesions may be identified. Intestinal loops in birds weighing <1 kg can only be examined with transducers that offer a frequency of at least 10 MHz. With such transducers, both the luminal contents and intestinal wall layers can be visualized. In addition, intestinal peristalsis can be recognized and thus it is possible to differentiate the salpinx from the gastrointestinal tract. The duodenum is easily identifiable in cross-section by its U shape.

The cloaca can be examined from the ventrodorsal coupling site by tipping the transducer caudally. Depending on the consistency of the cloacal contents, it can show different levels of echogenicity. The wall of the cloaca can be visualized by flushing out all the faecal material with warm saline solution and then administering sufficient warm water to improve the diagnostic quality of the image. The cloaca has a narrow and hyperechoic oval form with a regular margin. In birds weighing >2 kg an intracloacal

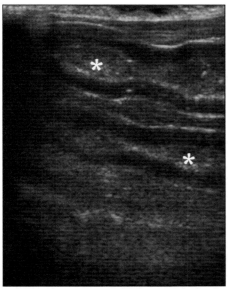

11.38 Ultrasonogram of a pheasant obtained using a ventromedian approach. The intestinal loops, which are filled with ingesta (*), are clearly visible.

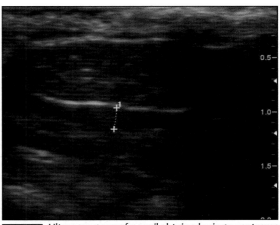

11.40 Ultrasonogram of a quail obtained using a ventromedian approach showing distended intestinal loops due to parasitic infection.

ultrasonographic examination can be achieved. With this coupling site, the normal kidney and the gonads can also be easily visualized. However, to date this coupling site has only been used for experimental purposes and with fully anaesthetized birds.

Contrast studies are also useful for examining the gastrointestinal tract. In these cases, water that has been warmed to the animal's body temperature and administered orally at a dose of 20 ml/kg is used as the contrast medium. The transit time of the liquid is extremely fast, and the water greatly improves the quality of the images.

Liver

Ultrasonography has resulted in a greater understanding of the internal structure of parenchymatous organs, including the liver. Important indications for an ultrasound examination include the differentiation of infectious from neoplastic processes in a patient in which radiography has revealed hepatomegaly as the main diagnosis. It is also invaluable in cases where ascites is suspected (Figure 11.41). It should be noted that ascitic fluid can be helpful in identifying the internal organs on ultrasonography.

Normal liver parenchyma appears as finely granulated with medium homogeneous echogenicity on ultrasonography (Figure 11.42). Imaging of the liver can be difficult if the surrounding organs show severe dilatation or if the gastrointestinal tract is filled with ingesta. For investigation of the liver, the transducer should be placed on the midline, caudal to the xiphoid, and aimed in a craniodorsal direction (see Figure 11.35). Liver tissue is spotted with small to medium-sized anechoic areas which, depending on the plane, appear round, oval or long with a hyperechoic wall and can be clearly differentiated from the parenchyma. These areas represent the liver vessels (Figure 11.42); it should be noted that differentiation of the portal vein and hepatic veins is not possible in birds. The edges of the liver appear sharp. Measurements cannot usually be obtained as the liver can only be evaluated in sections. The gallbladder can be partially identified, depending on its state of fullness, as an oval or rounded body of anechoic contents (see Figure 11.37). Changes in the gallbladder are rare.

Abnormalities of the liver parenchyma that can be identified on ultrasonography include:

- Inflammation (Figure 11.43)
- Neoplasia (Figure 11.44)
- Calcification
- Granulomas
- Cystic and fatty degeneration.

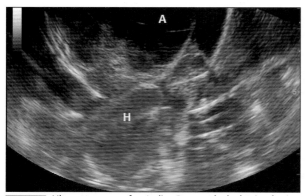

11.41 Ultrasonogram of an Indian Runner duck obtained using a ventromedian approach showing ascites due to liver congestion. A = ascites; H = heart.

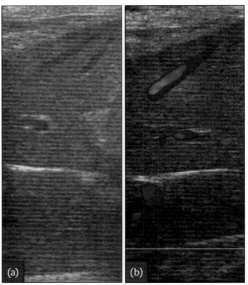

11.42 (a) Ultrasonogram of a chicken obtained using a ventromedian approach showing the liver parenchyma and large hepatic vessels. (b) Doppler ultrasonogram of a chicken obtained using a ventromedian approach showing the blood flow in the hepatic vessels.

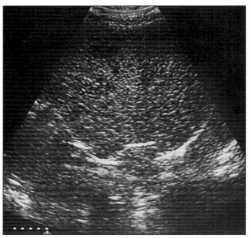

11.43 Ultrasonogram of a goose obtained using a ventromedian approach showing increased homogeneous echogenicity of the liver parenchyma. The diagnosis was confirmed as hepatitis due to *Salmonella* infection.

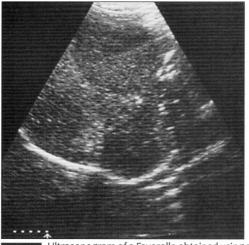

11.44 Ultrasonogram of a Faverolle obtained using a ventromedian approach showing the irregular structure and heterogeneous echogenicity of the liver parenchyma. The diagnosis was confirmed as liver neoplasia due to leucosis.

The presence of dilated vessels (e.g. as seen with liver congestion) is also a frequent abnormal finding on ultrasonography. Whilst it is not possible to predict the histological nature of a lesion from its ultrasonographic appearance alone, an ultrasound-guided biopsy sample may be taken from defined regions of the liver parenchyma using the same procedure as in mammals. Ultrasound-guided fine-needle biopsy samples can be taken safely and without associated complications in most avian patients.

Kidneys

Routine ultrasonographic examination of normal kidneys is not possible due to their position within the sacrum and the surrounding abdominal air sacs. However, in cases of kidney enlargement, the size and parenchyma can be assessed easily not only in large birds but also in smaller patients. Differentiation of renal inflammation, neoplasia and cysts is possible. Uric acid deposits and calcification cause reflections (increased echogenicity) and the renal tissue appears less homogeneous. However, the identification of renal gout by ultrasonography alone is difficult and other techniques (radiography, endoscopy, blood chemistry, biopsy) should be used to confirm the diagnosis.

Reproductive tract

Demonstration of the gonads is only possible in sexually active birds. The ultrasonographic appearance of active ovaries is characterized by the presence of follicles of different sizes, representing various stages of development (Figure 11.45). The retention of follicles after cessation of egg-laying activity can be easily diagnosed by a series of ultrasonographic examinations. The active oviduct can be distinguished due to the presence of eggs (Figure 11.46) and lack of contractility, in comparison with the intestine. When a fully calcified egg is positioned just prior to be laid, it can make an ultrasound examination impossible, as the ultrasound waves are unable to penetrate the egg and instead are reflected by the eggshell. Thus, an ultrasound examination is only indicated in cases of dystocia when a clear diagnosis cannot be reached by radiography alone.

The differentiation of structures such as cysts and neoplasms is possible with ultrasonography. Salpingitis, soft-shelled and laminated eggs (Figure 11.47) are also routinely recognized during an ultrasonographic examination. Advanced inflammatory processes of the oviduct can be recognized as an increased thickness of the oviduct wall.

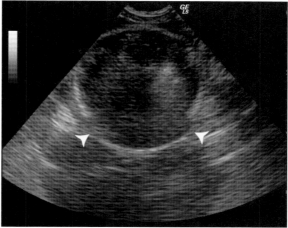

11.46 Ultrasonogram of a chicken obtained using a ventromedian approach showing an intact calcified egg. Note that due to artefacts, the eggshell may be misinterpreted as being broken (arrowheads).

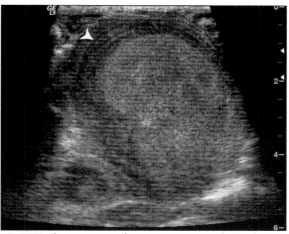

11.47 Ultrasonogram of a Japanese Bantam obtained using a ventromedian approach showing a laminated egg. Note the typical onion-like structure (arrowhead).

Egg yolk peritonitis is a common problem in laying hens. In these cases, the abdomen would appear as heterogeneous on ultrasonography, with the changes proportional to the severity of the case, with partially visible laminated eggs, fibrinous exudate and fluid (Figure 11.48).

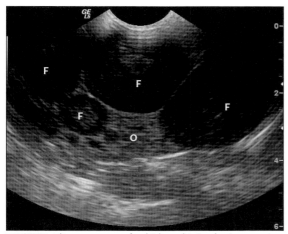

11.45 Ultrasonogram of a chicken obtained using a ventromedian approach showing an active ovary (O). F = follicle.

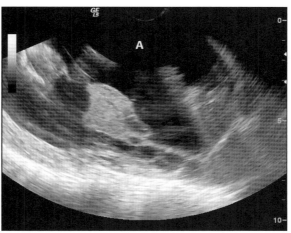

11.48 Ultrasonogram of an Indian Runner duck obtained using a ventromedian approach showing egg peritonitis. A = ascites.

Computed tomography and magnetic resonance imaging

As mentioned previously, the use of CT and MRI has been described mainly in relation to experimental studies in poultry. These studies tend to focus primarily on aspects of commercial interest (e.g. composition of the pectoral muscle in broilers) or animal welfare (e.g. measurement of bone density in laying hens related specifically to the development of osteoporosis). The advantage of CT and MRI is that the body is viewed in 3D; thus there is no superimposition of organ structures in the final images and individual scanning planes can be viewed without any distortion. Due to the relatively small body size of birds, they can be placed across the gantry opening (Figure 11.49) for sagittal images or longitudinal to the machine for transverse images. Those patients weighing up to 1 kg can be examined in fairly thin slices. The disadvantages of both modalities are the extremely high capital investment and the high operating costs.

CT is a radiographic method of producing cross-sectional images of a body. (Note that the higher radiation dose required to complete a CT scan, compared with a conventional radiographic examination, is not of significance in birds because of their much smaller size and the fact that they are relatively insensitive to X-rays.) Modern CT scanners only require 1–2 minutes to evaluate an avian patient (which constitutes a major advantage over MRI). CT is therefore a rapid method for examining the skeleton, particularly the spine (e.g. spinal fractures) and skull, as well as the soft tissues, especially the lungs. CT images can also be used to obtain radiodensity measurements (Figure 11.50), which are many times more accurate than those possible through the subjective differentiation of grey shades on radiographs by the human eye, and these can be extremely useful for patients with central nervous system (CNS) signs, respiratory disease or tissue swellings with no clear cause. CT enables imaging of abnormalities affecting the lungs and pulmonary vessels, as well as measurement of entire lung field density, thereby providing a precise clinical picture of early respiratory disease. In addition, CT provides an effective way of monitoring the

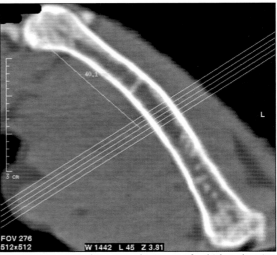

11.50 Computed tomographic image of a chicken showing how to obtain bone density measurements of the tibiotarsus.

effect of therapy. Urography, sinography and angiocardiography using iodinated contrast media are also possible.

MRI creates 3D images of the patient using an external magnetic field. The choice of coils has an important impact on the image quality. Usually superficial coils are used for birds. MRI is most useful for the visualization of different structures of the CNS, abnormalities in the soft tissues (Figure 11.51) and tumours, and provides images with exceptionally good soft tissue contrast. There is no exposure to radiation and no artefacts are caused by bones, as seen with CT. With neither method should any magnetic objects, such as foreign bodies or microchips, be in or near the bird's body as they may cause artefacts or injury to the patient.

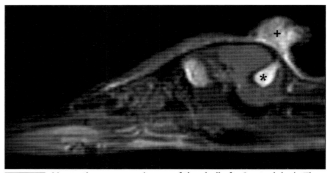

11.51 Magnetic resonance image of the skull of a Crested duck. The crest (+) and the lipoma (∗) within the cerebellum are easily identifiable.

Patient preparation and positioning

Usually, no special preparation of the avian patient is required. However, it would be wise to examine a patient that has been fasted, so food and water should be withheld for a short period prior to the CT/MRI scan. As the examination is time is very short with CT, a general anaesthetic is not always required. Discretion has to be exercised when deciding whether general anaesthesia or sedation is needed, and factors such as the bird's state of health and excitability as well as the goal of the study should be taken into consideration. It can often be sufficient to restrain the patient using a radiotranslucent fixation plate (see Figure 11.49) used for conventional radiography. If used, then the

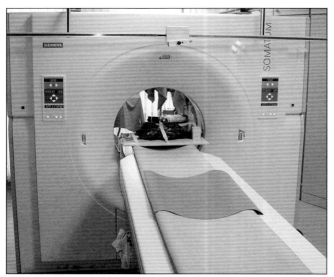

11.49 Patient positioning for computed tomography using a restraint plate. As the examination only takes a few minutes and the equipment is not noisy (in contrast to magnetic resonance imaging), it is possible to perform the assessment without sedation in most birds.

fixation plate should not contain any metal screws or other components that could produce artefacts. To minimize movement artefacts, it may be necessary to either sedate the bird or quieten it down by loose placement of a light-weight dark cloth over its eyes. Birds under general anaesthesia can be positioned with the use of a radiotranslucent fixation plate. MRI requires general anaesthesia in every case because of the associated noise (which is quite considerable and can alarm avian patients), low operating temperature and the relatively long examination time. In very sick patients this may be a considerable risk, so the faster examination time associated with CT may make it a superior technique for the examination of birds.

Dorsal recumbency is preferred for CT/MRI and care must be taken to obtain positional symmetry, which is essential for correct interpretation of the images. Depending on the aim of the study, or in cases where the patient is displaying signs of cardiovascular insufficiency or severe dyspnoea, a more tilted position (with the head positioned higher than the feet) is indicated. Ventral recumbency is also possible as long as care is taken to avoid mechanical interference with the patient's ability to breathe. For the examination, the bird is placed either across the gantry mouth for sagittal scanning or longitudinal to the machine for transverse scanning. The advantage of obtaining sagittal images is that the whole length of the body can be examined and a better degree of orientation of the anatomical structures can be provided. Compared with transverse scanning, sagittal scanning allows for fewer sections to complete the examination.

References and further reading

Bartels T, Krautwald-Junghanns ME, Portmann S *et al.* (2000) The use of conventional radiography and computer-assisted tomography as instruments for demonstration of gross pathological lesions in the cranium and cerebrum in the crested breed of the domestic duck (*Anas platyrhynchos* f.dom.). *Avian Pathology* **29**, 101–108

Krautwald-Junghanns ME, Pees M, Reese S and Tully T (2011) *Diagnostic Imaging of Exotic Pets*. Schluetersche Verlagsanstalt, Hannover

Melnychuk VL, Cooper MW, Kirby JD, Rorie RW and Anthony NB (2002) Use of ultrasonography to characterize ovarian status in chicken. *Poultry Science* **81**, 892–895

Mitchell AD, Rosebrough RW, Taicher GZ and Kovner I (2011) *In vivo* measurement of body composition of chickens using quantitative magnetic resonance. *Poultry Science* **90**, 1712–1719

Oviedo-Rondon EO, Parker J and Clemente-Hernandez S (2007) Application of real-time ultrasound technology to estimate *in vivo* breast muscle weight of broiler chickens. *British Poultry Science* **48**, 154–161

Chapter 12

Endoscopy, biopsy and endosurgery

Michael Lierz

Endoscopy is the term used to describe direct visualization of an internal cavity, including the organs, using an endoscope. It includes laparoscopy, choanoscopy, otoscopy, rhinoscopy, tracheobronchoscopy, gastroscopy and cloacoscopy. In addition, endoscopy can also be used to guide minimally invasive surgical procedures (including tissue sampling), which are becoming increasingly important in practice. As endoscopy allows direct visualization and evaluation of the internal organs (size, shape, colour, surface, early alterations), it is superior to radiography as a diagnostic tool for specific abnormalities. However, endoscopy should not be considered as a replacement for radiography, which provides an overview of the whole body. Radiography also provides valuable information about the potential risks associated with an endoscopic procedure (e.g. the presence of ascitic fluid). Thus, endoscopy should be used as an additional diagnostic tool based on radiographic findings.

As endoscopy is an invasive technique, patients need to be anaesthetized prior to the procedure (see Chapter 22). However, compared with other invasive techniques, endoscopy is relatively simple and easy to perform. The main challenge is the interpretation of the images obtained, which requires a high level of practice and experience. As well as being of use in individual birds, endoscopy is also valuable for diagnosing conditions affecting a flock, and offers an alternative to sacrificial necropsy. Many flock diseases cause typical organ abnormalities, which can be easily visualized via endoscopy. In comparison with diagnostic necropsy, where the owner usually only allows euthanasia of a very limited number of birds, a large number of birds can undergo endoscopic examination over a short period of time, providing an excellent overview of flock health.

Equipment

The air sac system in birds provides a unique opportunity to employ endoscopy as a diagnostic tool without the need for insufflation (with the exception of gastroscopy and cloacoscopy). Thus, the technical requirements of the equipment are generally low. When buying a complete endoscopy set-up, the author recommends purchasing the equipment from the same manufacturer to ensure all parts are compatible.

Basic equipment

The following basic equipment is required to perform endoscopy in birds:

- Endoscope (with working channel for instruments)
- Light source (xenon or halogen light) and light cable
- Biopsy and grasping forceps
- Small curved forceps
- Scalpel blade or a small pair of scissors
- Haemostatic agents and vascular clips
- Resorbable suture material (1–1.5 metric (5/0–4/0 USP); see Chapter 23 for a review of suture material selection).

Endoscope selection

Rigid endoscopes are required for the majority of cases in backyard poultry. However, in some of the larger pheasant species, flexible endoscopes may be advantageous for gastroscopy (i.e. to examine the crop, proventriculus and ventriculus). There are two main types of rigid endoscope:

- Endoscopes with several single lenses – these are cheaper but the image quality is lower (especially contrast)
- Endoscopes with rod lenses (Hopkins endoscopes) – these are more expensive but the image quality is better.

It is important that clinicians compare a range of different endoscopes (in terms of border sharpness, depth of focus) in order to select an instrument best suited to their requirements.

Diameter and length

Endoscopes are available in a variety of sizes (Figure 12.1).

- 1.9 mm diameter – smallest scope available with acceptable image quality.
- 2.7 mm diameter – best compromise between image quality and diameter for small patients such as quail.
- 4 mm diameter – excellent image quality, especially for record documentation. This is the best choice for most poultry species.
- Length is variable but should not be <13 cm; 19 cm is standard and recommended.

Viewing angle

Endoscopes are available with a choice of two viewing angles (Figure 12.2).

- 0-degree viewing angle – straight forward view, superior for record documentation; similar view achieved if the endoscope is turned on its optical axes.
- 30-degree viewing angle – forward oblique telescope; allows visualization of a larger area by rotating the endoscope on its optical axes.

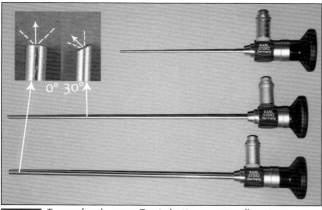

12.1 Types of endoscope. Top to bottom: 1.9 mm diameter scope, 2.7 mm diameter scope and 4 mm diameter scope. The different viewing angles available (0 degrees and 30 degrees) are shown in the top left-hand corner of the figure.

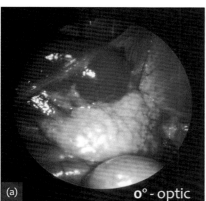
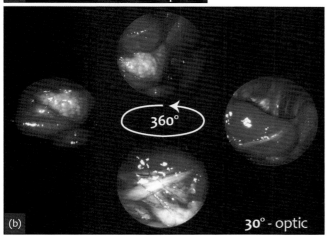

12.2 (a) View through a 4 mm, 0-degree endoscope, which allows only a straight forward view. (b) View through a 2.7 mm, 30-degree endoscope. The 30-degree angle allows a panoramic view by turning the scope around its optical axes.

Working channel

The diameter of the working channel varies according to the size of the endoscope. The working channel protects the scope from damage and allows the introduction of instruments, as well as air and/or water, for endoscopic procedures. Basic endoscopic instruments include:

- Flexible biopsy forceps (1.8 mm diameter) with ellipsoid cups (grasp deeper into tissue) or round cups
- Flexible grasping forceps for granuloma and foreign body removal.

Additional equipment

The following additional equipment may also be useful for endoscopy in poultry:

- Flexible aspiration needle with cover (22 G) for puncturing of cysts or direct administration of medication (Figure 12.3)
- Equipment for endoscope-guided surgery (including diode laser and high frequency electrosurgery unit)
- Equipment trolley
- Camera and monitor for use during diagnostic and surgical procedures (also advantageous for record documentation)
- Method for capturing and storing images or videos (essential for forensic cases and useful to show owners when discussing the patient and/or procedure)
- Mobile endoscopy unit, including light source, camera, monitor and digital storage system, which can be useful for flock visits.

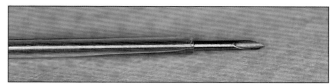

12.3 A flexible 22 G needle in a plastic sleeve can be used for the endoscopic administration of medication and the collection of aspirate biopsy samples.

Equipment care

- Bending and torsion of the endoscope should be avoided.
- Endoscopic instruments should always be used within a working channel.
- The manufacturer's recommendations for cleaning and disinfecting the endoscope should be followed. Gross debris (e.g. blood, tissue) should be removed from the endoscope prior to disinfection and sterilization.
  - Gas sterilization – uncommon.
  - Heat sterilization – not recommended as it may reduce the functional lifespan of the scope (e.g. may loosen the optical lenses).
  - Disinfectant bath – the manufacturer's recommendations for the concentration of disinfectant and the contact time should be followed. The contact time should not be extended as this can cause precipitations to form on the lens (resulting in a 'milky' image) and may decrease the flexibility of instruments such as forceps and scissors.
- The endoscope and instruments should be rinsed with sterile water following disinfection to avoid causing irritation when used in the next patient.
- The equipment should be dried using sterile towels or alcohol.

Patient preparation and contraindications

Fasting prior to endoscopic procedures is important in backyard poultry for a number of reasons, including:

- Endoscopy is performed under general anaesthesia
- To ensure that no food remains in the crop or gastrointestinal tract. The presence of food prevents a

good view of the abdomen as other organs, in particular the air sac, are compromised by an extended intestinal tract. Gastroscopy is nearly impossible with a filled crop.

Food should be withheld for at least 6–8 hours and water withdrawn 2 hours before the procedure. Further preoperative considerations are discussed in Chapter 22. If tissue biopsy is planned, supplementary vitamin K administration should be considered.

Obesity is common in backyard poultry and can reduce the view within the body cavity (Figure 12.4). This in turn increases the risk of organ damage by the scope or other endoscopic instruments. In addition, removing growing feathers from moulting birds may lead to haemorrhaging, which may also obscure the view.

The most important contraindication for abdominal endoscopy is ascites. This occurs regularly in poultry patients as a result of inflammation of the oviduct, oviductal cysts, liver disease or egg yolk peritonitis. During endoscopy, a connection is established between the air sacs and the abdominal cavity, leading to the drainage of fluid into the air sacs and consequently the lung. This can lead to drowning of the bird.

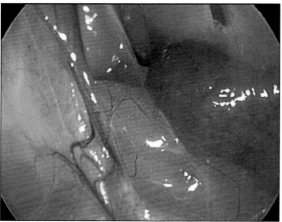

12.4 Excessive fat deposits are commonly seen in poultry and can obscure the view of other internal organs.

Tracheobronchoscopy

Tracheobronchoscopy is a common procedure in backyard poultry. Respiratory diseases are frequently seen in these birds and tracheobronchoscopy can be used to differentiate between conditions. The bird should be anaesthetized and placed in an upright position with the neck extended. The tongue should be pulled cranially and the endoscope passed through the glottis (Figure 12.5). The scope should then be advanced gently down the trachea to the level of the syrinx, where the trachea bifurcates into the two main bronchi. The diameter of the endoscope should be a maximum of two-thirds the diameter of the trachea, allowing the bird to breathe during the procedure. It is usually possible to complete the examination between the time the administration of anaesthesia is ceased and when the patient begins to recover. In cases where an extended evaluation or surgical procedure is required, air sac perfusion anaesthesia should be provided (see Chapter 22).

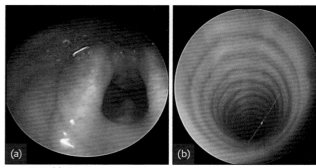

12.5 (a) The opening of the trachea is located at the base of the tongue. (b) The tracheal rings in birds are closed and the mucosa appears slightly red.

Insufflation

The expansion of hollow organs is necessary for endoscopy. This is achieved using air or water insufflation.

Water insufflation is performed via the working channel of the endoscope using two taps: one tap is required for water inlet and the other tap is required for water outlet. A third tap for biopsy or grasping forceps is also recommended (Figure 12.6). The water inlet tap is attached to an infusion bottle via a tube. The infusion bottle should be elevated above the level of the bird. A second tube is attached to the water outlet tap, ending in a collecting bin. Using the inlet and outlet taps, the volume of water entering the digestive system can be regulated and the organ expanded as required for examination. It is essential that the water is pre-warmed to avoid inducing hypothermia in the patient.

Air insufflation also requires the use of a working channel and three taps, and follows the same principles as water insufflation. Air insufflation is achieved via pressure using either a pressure bottle or pump. Medical pumps or aquarium air pumps are suitable for this purpose.

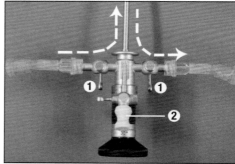

12.6 For gastroscopy and cloacoscopy, a working channel is required for water insufflation to allow examination of the hollow organs. 1 = inlet (left) and outlet (right) water taps; 2 = working channel for endoscopic instruments. The arrows indicate the direction of water flow.

The use of air insufflation is usually quicker and associated with less risk than water insufflation. Thus, air insufflation can be useful for short procedures such as the removal of a foreign body. However, the washing effect of water is sometimes an advantage as it removes mucus and faeces, and some anatomical structures (e.g. papillae) are only visible using water insufflation. The disadvantage of water insufflation is that, during gastroscopy, water may rinse backwards into the oral cavity and be aspirated

Gastroscopy

Gastroscopy allows evaluation of the oesophagus, crop, proventriculus and, in larger birds, the ventriculus. Foreign bodies are commonly ingested by backyard poultry (particularly chickens) and gastroscopy is indicated for the removal of these objects, as well as for diagnostic purposes. Gastroscopy can be performed using a flexible endoscope. In larger birds, a long gastroscope might be an advantage, but it is also possible to introduce a rigid endoscope through an ingluviotomy incision. It is vital that food is withheld for a period of 6–8 hours prior to the procedure to ensure that the gastrointestinal tract is empty. Placement of an endotracheal tube is recommended. The bird should be anaesthetized and placed in ventral recumbency with the head lower than the body. The endoscope should be inserted into the oesophagus and advanced under visual control (Figure 12.7). Only gentle pressure should be applied to avoid oesophageal perforation. As gastroscopy is performed using a working channel for air or water insufflation, mucosal biopsy samples can be easily obtained and are of great diagnostic value. Foreign bodies are removed using grasping forceps or sling cages.

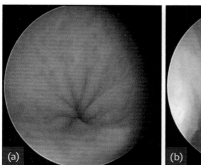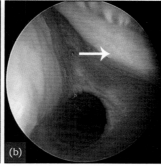

12.7 (a) When entering the oesophagus, the mucosal folds are clearly visible. Insufflation with air or water increases the pressure within the oesophagus, causing it to expand. (b) The mucosal fold (arrowed) can be used to locate the entrance to the crop.

Cloacoscopy

Indications for cloacoscopy in backyard poultry include investigation of trauma caused by cannibalism, evaluation of the origin of bleeding in cases of cloacal haemorrhage (cloaca, intestine, ureter, uterus) and examination of the oviduct or rectum. The bird should be anaesthetized and placed in dorsal recumbency. Insufflation is required for cloacoscopy (see above). The endoscope should be inserted into the cloaca (Figure 12.8) and the rectum. If

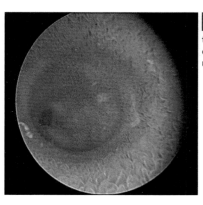

12.8 Endoscopic view upon entering the cloaca. Papillae are clearly visible when water is used for insufflation.

possible, the urethral and oviduct openings are evaluated. In sexually active female birds, the uterus can be entered and examined. Reproductive disorders involving the uterus are common (especially in chickens) and endoscopy is a valuable tool for assessment. Faeces and urine are always present and need to be removed for a more detailed examination. A band of urates may be seen originating from the ostium of the ureter when water is used for insufflation of the cloaca.

Laparoscopy

Laparoscopy in backyard poultry is performed to evaluate all internal organs. The approach to the body cavity depends on the diagnostic goal of the procedure. In most cases, a left-sided approach is used, as female birds only have a left ovary. However, a right-sided approach may be appropriate if radiography indicates alterations in this area. It is highly recommended that all organs within the body cavity are assessed as unsuspected lesions are regularly present.

The bird should be anaesthetized and placed in right lateral recumbency with the left wing extended dorsocranially. The left leg may also be pulled either cranially or caudally (preferred) (Figure 12.9a). A few feathers are plucked at the incision site to allow disinfection and surgical preparation of the skin. To locate the incision site, a triangle is drawn using the last rib as the cranial border and the iliotibialis muscle as the caudal border (Figure 12.9b). The incision is made in the middle of this triangle, starting 0.5 cm ventral to the acetabulum.

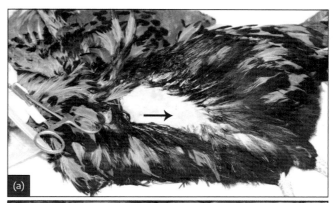

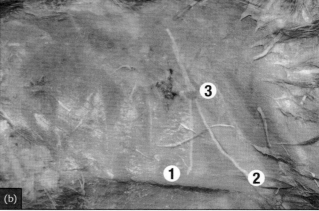

12.9 Patient positioning for laparoscopy. (a) The chicken has been placed in lateral recumbency with the wing pulled dorsally and the legs pulled caudally. The arrow indicates the incision site. (b) The incision site (3) is located using a triangle drawn from behind the last rib (1) to the cranial border of the iliotibialis muscle (2).

The iliobiaialis muscle, which can obscure the approach to the body cavity, should be pushed caudally using forceps or a trocar (Figure 12.10) so that the fascia can be visualized. The abdominal wall and underlying air sac are penetrated by increasing the pressure on the body wall using the forceps or trocar, which should be oriented ventrocranially. Dorsal orientation must be avoided as the kidney can be easily lacerated, causing severe bleeding. Penetration is marked by a 'popping' sound. Depending on the orientation of the forceps or trocar, the abdominal or cranial thoracic air sac is entered (Figure 12.11). The importance of using a blunt instrument for this procedure cannot be overemphasized. It is difficult to control the exact level of penetration during this procedure and serious damage with accompanying haemorrhage can occur if a sharp trocar or other pointed instrument is used.

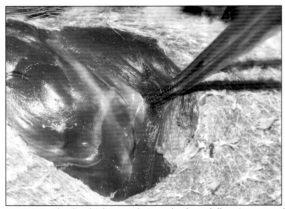

12.10 The iliotibialis muscle is pushed caudally using curved forceps to allow visualization of the body wall. (The skin has been removed for better demonstration.)

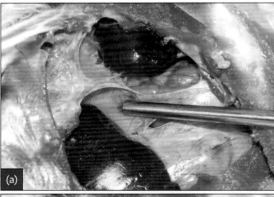

(a)

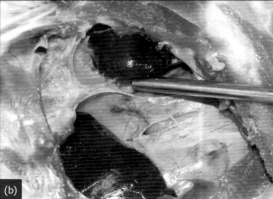

(b)

12.11 Depending on the orientation of the forceps or trocar when penetrating the body wall, either (a) the caudal thoracic air sac or (b) the abdominal air sac will be entered.

The endoscope is then inserted via the trocar or between the legs of the forceps into the body cavity. It is held at its tip by the thumb and forefinger with the ball of the thumb resting on the bird or table (Figure 12.12). This allows permanent contact with the bird and prevents uncontrolled deeper insertion in the case of bird movement. The internal organs can then be evaluated (Figure 12.13). In small birds or species such as bantams, the

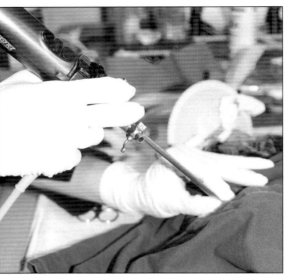

12.12 Correct handling technique for the endoscope: the hand of the clinician should be in contact with the bird at all times.

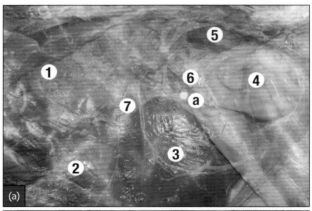

(a)

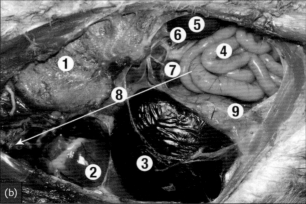

(b)

12.13 (a) Gross anatomy of the bird from a left lateral view. a (yellow circle) = entrance for the endoscope; 1 = lung; 2 = heart; 3 = liver; 4 = intestine; 5 = kidney; 6 = spleen; 7 = proventriculus. (b) Gross anatomy of the body cavity. The arrow demonstrates the direction of the endoscope for full exploration of the body cavity. 1 = lung; 2 = heart; 3 = liver; 4 = intestine; 5 = kidney; 6 = gonads and adrenal gland; 7 = spleen; 8 = proventriculus; 9 = ventriculus.

gonads may be visualized without further advancement of the endoscope. In larger species or those with opaque air sacs, the abdominal air sac may need to be punctured in order to obtain a clear view of the adrenal gland, gonads and cranial division of the kidney (Figure 12.14a). Necessary punctures of air sacs do not harm the bird as the holes close quickly. Cranial to the kidney, the caudal aspect of the lung is visible. Ventral to the kidney, the ureter and uterus or ductus deferens are visible. Further ventrally, intestinal loops may be seen. Cranioventral to the kidney, the proventriculus, ventriculus, liver and, in some cases, the spleen may be visible (Figure 12.14b).

Upon entering the caudal thoracic air sac, the liver, proventriculus and the ostium to the lung can be visualized (Figure 12.14c). Depending on the size of the bird, the ostium allows retrograde evaluation of the lung, including the smaller bronchi (Figure 12.15). Advancing the endoscope further cranially, the cranial thoracic air sac is reached and further parts of the lung and liver, as well as the heart, are visible. With experience, the clinician can slowly guide the endoscope further cranially towards the heart base, where the main blood vessels and brachial plexus can be evaluated. Advancing the scope over the heart base, the trachea and thyroid glands can be identified (see Figure 12.20). Following laparoscopy, skin closure can be performed by placing one or two single knots or by using tissue glue (see Chapter 23).

Sex determination

Most backyard poultry species are sexually dimorphic. The sex of the bird can usually be determined within the first few weeks of life (by 8–10 weeks old) and, in some breeds, on the day of hatching. However, in cases where the sex of the bird is not obvious visually, endoscopic sexing can be helpful. Compared with DNA analysis, where only sex determination is possible, endoscopy allows evaluation of the internal organs, as well as assessment of gonad activity and functionality (physiological breeding performance).

Female birds

In female birds, the gonads are visible ventrally at the cranial pole of the kidney. A suspensory ligament is seen crossing the cranial pole of the kidney towards the dorsal body wall (Figure 12.16) and is the main anatomical feature used to determine sex. This ligament should be carefully assessed because if it is damaged or absent, the breeding performance of the bird is questionable. Removal of the

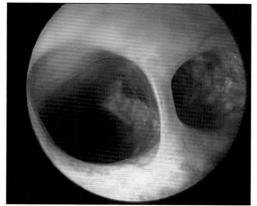

12.15 The connection between the caudal thoracic air sac and lung allows a retrograde internal exploration of the lung and evaluation of the honeycomb structure. This type of view is not possible via tracheobronchoscopy.

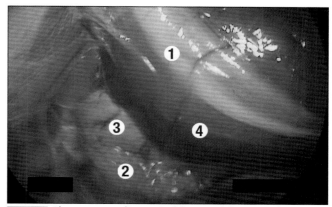

12.16 The suspensory ligament of the ovary is important in determining sex in poultry. 1 = suspensory ligament; 2 = ovary; 3 = adrenal gland; 4 = kidney.

suspensory ligament has been used as a technique for sterilization. In poultry only the left ovary is present. It may be flat with a cobblestone appearance in birds with inactive ovaries, or appear as a 'cluster of grapes' when there is follicular development. Inflammation of the follicles may be present, which can reduce the reproductive performance of the bird. The uterus is seen in close contact with the ureter, and evaluation of its size can provide an indication about previous breeding and/or laying activities.

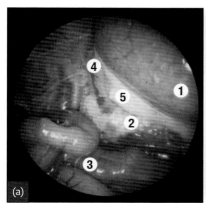 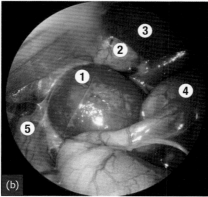 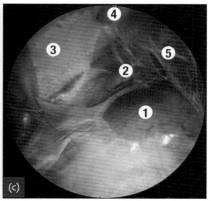

12.14 (a) Endoscopic view upon entering the abdominal air sac. 1 = kidney; 2 = ovary; 3 = intestine; 4 = adrenal gland; 5= uterus/ureter. (b) Endoscopic view upon entering the abdominal air sac with the scope positioned at a slightly more downwards angle than in (a). 1 = spleen; 2 = adrenal gland; 3 = kidney; 4 = intestine; 5 = proventriculus. (c) Endoscopic view upon entering the caudal thoracic air sac. 1 = liver; 2 = proventriculus; 3 = lung; 4 = retrograde entrance into the lung; 5 = hole in the air sac (made by surgeon to access the abdominal air sac).

Male birds

In male birds, the gonads are visible ventrally at the cranial pole of the kidney. The ductus deferens is seen in close contact with the ureter and the paired white testicles are usually oval-shaped with 2–3 vessels crossing the surface (Figure 12.17). Male birds do not have a suspensory ligament. In birds with transparent air sacs, both testicles may be visualized from a left lateral approach. Testicular biopsy is a very valuable tool for the investigation of infertility in breeding birds.

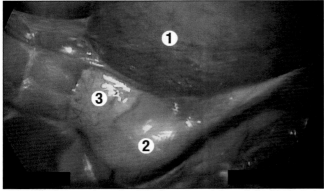

12.17 The gonads can be difficult to assess in juvenile birds. The lack of a suspensory ligament in this case indicates a male bird. 1 = kidney; 2 = testicle; 3 = adrenal gland.

Evaluation of internal organs

Figure 12.18 summarizes the normal endoscopic appearance of the internal organs of birds, as well as detailing the common abnormalities encountered and the possible causes for these alterations.

PRACTICAL TIP
Yellow to white foci seen in the surface of the kidney are often uric acid crystals and may be indicative of renal gout. These foci may also occur in cases of exsiccosis, as uric acid is actively excreted. After the administration of fluid to correct any dehydration, the kidney is re-examined. In cases of gout, the foci are still present

The caudal coelom is divided into three compartments by the post-hepatic septum (see Chapter 2). This septum is the principal peritoneal fat depot, making laparoscopy more difficult than the same procedure in psittacines or raptors. In addition, it is very common to have a significant ascites secondary to yolk coelomitis in females (see Chapter 17). Any coelomic fluid accumulation will increase the risk of laparoscopy.

Structure	Normal appearance	Abnormalities	Common causes
Tracheobronchoscopy			
Trachea	Mucosa is light red/pink and shiny; visibly closed tracheal rings; no exudate (see Figure 12.5b)	Swollen red mucosa; hidden tracheal rings (Figure 12.19)	Tracheitis (viral, bacterial, fungal, parasitic); infectious bronchitis; infectious laryngotracheitis
		Exudates	Viral, bacterial or parasitic infection; infectious laryngotracheitis if exudate is haemorrhagic
		Granulomas (especially at the syrinx); foreign bodies	Fungal or bacterial infection; foreign bodies
		Strictures; tumours	
		Nematode worms	*Syngamus trachea*
Gastroscopy			
Oesophagus, crop and proventriculus	Surface varies with species; usually the oesophagus is smooth and the crop has furrows (see Figure 12.7); mucosa is homogeneous and light red/pink	Plaques; haemorrhage; focal dark red areas	Trauma; ulceration; irritation due to the presence of foreign bodies; infection
		Yellow coating	Trichomoniasis; wet pox; *Candida*; hypovitaminosis A
		Yellow–white spots	Trichomoniasis; *Capillaria*
Cloacoscopy			
Cloaca	Divided into three parts; the mucosa is light red/pink (see Figure 12.8)	Reddened mucosa	Irritation; inflammation; infection
		Cauliflower appearance; traumatized	Neoplasia; cannibalism
Laparoscopy			
Trachea, bronchi and thyroid glands	The trachea and bronchi appear as white tubes with complete tracheal rings; thyroid glands are lens-shaped, light red and attached to the trachea near the syrinx (Figure 12.20)	Glassy colour of thyroid glands	Hypothyroidism (biopsy is required for confirmation)
Air sacs	Clear and transparent with just a few vessels and, on occasion, fatty infiltrates (Figure 12.21a). Pathognomonic images are rare; areas of alteration should be biopsied. In laying chickens, regular opaque appearance due to fat inclusion is present. Peritoneum usually thicker compared with other birds	Increased vascularity; thickening of air sac wall	Mild inflammation; early infection; environmental (smoke, spray)
		Granulomas (Figure 12.21b); yellow coating; foreign material (e.g. pus, egg yolk material in layers) (Figure 12.22)	Aspergillosis; foreign bodies; bacterial infection (*Ornithobacterium rhinotracheale* (ORT), pasteurellosis). Opaque air sacs could also be due to mycoplasmosis

12.18 Normal endoscopic appearance of the internal organs of birds, common abnormalities and the possible reasons for these alterations. (continues)

▶

Structure	Normal appearance	Abnormalities	Common causes
Laparoscopy continued			
Lung	Pink–reddish colour, prominent structure. Bronchi can be entered through the caudal thoracic air sac (see Figures 12.14c and 12.15)	Blur of structures; colour changes (yellow); occasionally the presence of foreign material	Pneumonia; gout; ORT; pasteurellosis
		Haemorrhage	Trauma
		Focal black spots	Anthracosis (birds living in cities, passive smoking)
Heart and pericardium	Pericardium is transparent. Fat at the heart base and tip. Main heart vessels are seen as thick white tubes. Located next to the heart is the brachial plexus (fine yellow–white cross stripe net shape)	Milky pericardium	Pericarditis; pericardial effusion (drain with a 22 G flexible needle; see Figure 12.3); gout
		Missing heart fat	Starvation; chronic disease; guarded prognosis
		White to yellow coating	Pericarditis; bacterial infection (ORT, pasteurellosis)
Proventriculus	Elongated (usually) white organ, dorsal to the liver, with a smooth surface (Figure 12.23)	Focal haemorrhage; enlargement	Ulceration; foreign bodies; impacted with food or straw
Ventriculus	Not visible in all routine examinations. Massive muscular structure	Focal haemorrhage	Ulceration; foreign bodies; nematodes (geese)
Intestine	Tube-like structure. Smooth surface with many vessels. Colour depends on ingesta (usually grey)	White foci; foreign material (pus)	Endoparasites; bacterial granulomas (*Escherichia coli*); peritonitis; egg yolk peritonitis
Kidney and sacral plexus	Three parts: brown–red–orange, star-shaped structure on surface; adrenal gland and gonad at cranial pole; ventrally attached ureter and uterus (deferent duct) (see Figures 12.17 and 12.24). Kidney biopsy is often rewarding. With a 30-degree endoscope, the sacral plexus is detectable dorsal to the kidney	Star-shaped structure not visible (kidney swelling)	General disease or kidney problem (biopsy indicated); infectious bronchitis
		Yellow to white foci on surface	Uric acid; gout; dehydration
		Yellow colour	Obesity
		Pale colour	Anaemia
		Single yellow–white spots	Abscesses; neoplasia; cysts
		Nerve swelling	Marek's disease
Adrenal gland	Slightly cranial to the gonads, usually yellow and small. May vary in size, colour and shape. Might be confused with or obscured by gonads (see Figure 12.16)	Increase in size and/or vascularization	Stress; associated with disease
Pancreas	Found within the duodenal loop (Figure 12.25). White–yellow colour with a homogeneous structure	Colour changes; glassy appearance; uneven surface (biopsy indicated); petechial haemorrhage	Pancreatitis; neoplasia; influenza virus infection
Liver	Uniform brown–red colour with a sharp border (Figure 12.26). It is the central organ of metabolism. Biopsy is very rewarding, even without visible abnormalities (e.g. indicated by relevant blood values)	Round stump liver border	General disease; infection; fatty liver
		Uniform yellow colour	Fatty liver
		Swollen; yellow–grey colour; mealy appearance	Amyloidosis
		Focal red areas (Figure 12.27)	Haemorrhage (trauma); siderosis
		Multiple white foci (Figure 12.28)	Necrosis (hollow); herpesvirus; salmonellosis; histomoniasis; tuberculosis; abscesses; other bacterial infection; neoplasia
		Coating of the liver capsule	Often seen in conjunction with air sac coatings (bacterial, fungal, parasitic infections)
		Neoplasia	Tumours related to Marek's disease; leucosis
Spleen	Reddish-purple-brown colour, sometimes speckled (see Figure 12.14b)	Increased size (Figure 12.29)	Immune response (disease, check for *Chlamydia*); haemorrhagic enteritis in turkeys
		Yellow colour	Obesity; fatty spleen
		White foci	Necrosis (e.g. herpesvirus); granulomas (tuberculosis)
		Neoplasia	Tumours related to Marek's disease; leucosis
		Marbled appearance	Pericarditis; bacterial infection (ORT, pasteurellosis); adenovirus

12.18 (continued) Normal endoscopic appearance of the internal organs of birds, common abnormalities and the possible reasons for these alterations.

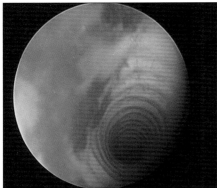

12.19 Reddening of the tracheal mucosa is a clear sign of irritation or inflammation. The presence of blood in the trachea, as in this case, indicates severe disease such as infectious laryngotracheitis. The clinician should also be aware that iatrogenic damage to the trachea (mucosal irritation and haemorrhage) can occur with inappropriate handling of the endoscope.

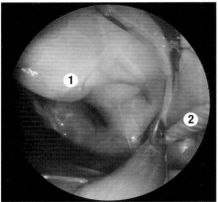

12.20 Endoscopic view of the thyroid glands and trachea after bypassing the heart. 1 = thyroid glands; 2 = trachea.

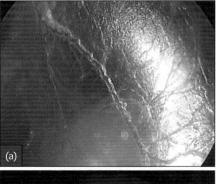

(a)

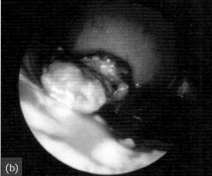

(b)

12.21 (a) The air sac of a healthy bird is like a window. The internal organs behind the air sac can be seen and only a few vessels are present. (b) Granuloma detached from the wall within the caudal thoracic air sac.

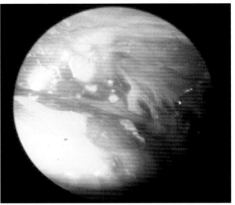

12.22 The presence of foreign material is a clear sign of infection and can be easily sampled for cytology and microbiology during endoscopy. In chickens, this foreign material can also be egg yolk, resulting in aseptic egg yolk peritonitis.

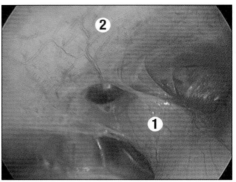

12.23 The proventriculus (1) is a compact organ above the liver and below the lung (2).

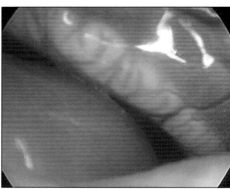

12.24 Endoscopic view of the deferent duct of a sexually active cock. The festoon appearance makes identification easy.

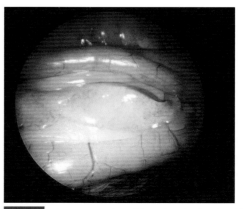

12.25 The pancreas is visible within the duodenal loop.

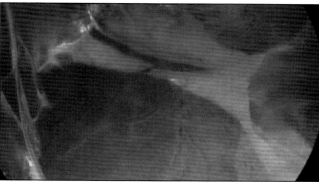

12.26 Endoscopic view of the liver. Note the homogeneous brown-red colour and sharp border.

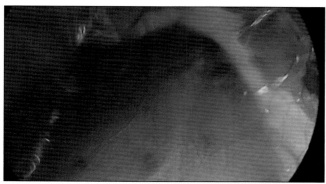

12.27 Colour change in the liver is always a pathological alteration. In this case, haemosiderosis is present. Note that haemorrhage may have a similar appearance.

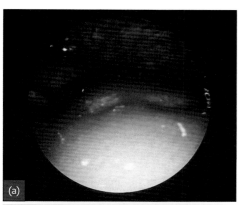

(a)

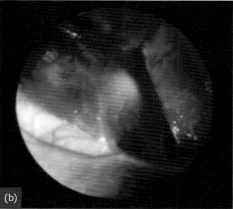

(b)

12.28 Multiple white foci within the liver typically represent (a) areas of necrosis or (b) granulomas/tubercles. Granulomas and tubercles are usually visible above the surface of the liver, whereas areas of necrosis appear below the surface. Differential diagnoses include *Escherichia coli*, *Salmonella*, tuberculosis, herpesvirus and histomoniasis.

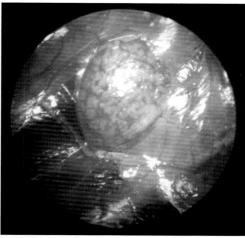

12.29 A swollen spleen is regularly seen with systemic infections. Colour changes or areas of necrosis (as seen in this case) are occasionally visible. Splenic biopsy may be of value if the infectious agent cannot be detected by other means. Differential diagnoses include herpesvirus or adenovirus.

Complications during and after endoscopy

Usually, complications during or after endoscopy are rare, apart from anaesthetic emergency events (see Chapter 22). Organ damage, in particular of the kidney, by the endoscope or instruments, and the resulting haemorrhage, are the main complications. In cases of severe gastritis or inflammation of the uterus, perforation of these organs may occur. Haemorrhage should be controlled by electro-coagulation, diode laser (endoscopically guided) or sterile sticks of cotton wool. The bird should be placed at a 45-degree angle with the head lifted so that the blood stays in the caudal air sacs and does not drain into the lungs. Complications following endoscopy can occur in the form of emphysema, due to inadequate closure of the entry point. Emphysema, if it occurs, should be punctured regularly (or drained) until the defect closes.

In cases of insufficient cleaning or sterilization of the endoscopic equipment, internal granulomatous infection or disease transmission might occur. Thus, birds from different sources should not be scoped in close succession, unless adequate sterilization time of the equipment between patients can be guaranteed.

Endoscope-guided biopsy

Indications

Organ biopsy is an invaluable tool for the diagnosis of any alterations or clinical disease. In general, the decision to perform a biopsy is made far too late. During any routine endoscopic examination, a biopsy should be performed (Lierz *et al.*, 1998). Many infectious diseases have similar clinical signs, especially in poultry, and demonstration of the pathogen is vital. Pathogens can be most easily identified in biopsy samples with further laboratory investigation. Endoscope-guided biopsy allows sampling of organs under direct visualization and therefore is superior to other biopsy techniques. Samples can be collected from altered areas, and complications (e.g. haemorrhage) are immediately visible.

- Polyuria, polydipsia or altered blood values indicates a kidney biopsy.
- Elevated blood levels of bile acids indicates a liver biopsy.
- The presence of milky air sacs indicates an air sac biopsy.
- An unclear lung structure indicates a lung biopsy.

Equipment

In general, biopsy of the lung, liver, kidney, spleen, gonads, proventriculus, ventriculus, thyroid gland and mucosal membranes of the oesophagus, crop and cloaca is possible using biopsy forceps within a working channel. Aspiration biopsy is possible using a long flexible needle with a Teflon™ cover (see Figure 12.3).

Technique

When investigating a general alteration of the liver, the biopsy sample should be taken from the border where there are fewer vessels. The insertion point for the endoscope is the preferred area for an air sac biopsy. In cases of focal abnormalities, these areas should be sampled. Where blood values need to be evaluated, the blood sample should be drawn prior to endoscopy, as the procedure in conjunction with organ biopsy can lead to alterations in certain blood values (Lierz *et al.*, 1998).

Endosurgery

Endoscope-guided surgery in birds is a relatively new field that has only recently been described (Lierz, 2004; Hernandez-Divers, 2005; Lierz, 2005). With experience, it will develop further and allow procedures to be performed that were not previously possible.

Basic endoscope-guided surgery is a single-entry technique (e.g. for biopsy). A single instrument is directed through a working channel into the visual field of the endoscope. This means that the instrument cannot be used independently from the endoscope. By adding an additional instrument channel (cannula with trocar) next to the insertion point for the endoscope, double-entry techniques can be performed. This allows the surgeon to work with two different instruments. By adding a second cannula with trocar as a working channel and placing the endoscope between both trocars, triple-entry techniques can be performed. This allows the surgeon to work with two different instruments independently from the endoscope. After insertion of the cannula (usually stainless steel, graphite or plastic), the trocar is removed and the instrument inserted into the visual field of the endoscope. Technique selection aims to balance good surgical access for the procedure being performed with minimal tissue damage.

An important point to consider during endoscopic surgery is haemostasis; tools to maintain it are therefore vital. Electrocautery or lasers are typically used for this purpose. Instruments for endoscope-guided surgery can usually be connected to electrosurgical units, whereas lasers are operated independently. Necessary equipment includes dissection forceps, scissors and grasping forceps; these should be monopolar so that they can be connected to the radiosurgery unit. In addition, bipolar forceps and a monopolar sling are essential. Experienced surgeons may extend their equipment to include palpation probes, needle holders and knot tiers. Before undertaking endoscope-guided surgery, specific training is highly recommended; practice first on euthanased birds.

Surgical procedures

Many endoscope-guided procedures are possible, including the removal or vaporization (via laser) of tracheal or air sac granulomas (Figure 12.30) and papillomas. Endoscopically guided diode lasers are commonly used with success to vaporize granulomas in emergency situations, in order to restore respiratory function. In addition, tumour resection as well as sterilization and castration of birds can be performed endoscopically (Lierz, 2005). The latter technique is regularly requested by backyard poultry owners to prevent cocks from fighting or crowing; however, the legality of castration procedures varies between countries (e.g. in the UK it is prohibited in farmed birds and may only be carried out as part of a conservation breeding programme).

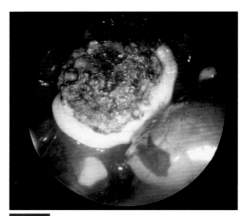

12.30 Large *Aspergillus* granuloma during laser ablation.

Patient preparation and port placement

Patient preparation for endosurgery is similar to that for a routine endoscopic examination (see above). The surgical field for double- or triple-entry techniques is wider and feathers have to be plucked cranially and caudally to the insertion site for the endoscope. The standard gonadal approach (e.g. for sterilization, castration and cysts) is from the left side for female birds or from either side for male birds. For double-entry techniques, the additional working channel is placed cranioventral to the endoscope, between the last two ribs (Figure 12.31). In triple-entry techniques, the second working channel is placed ventrocaudal to the endoscope (Figure 12.32a), leaving the scope centrally placed between both working channels. An alternative approach is to pull the leg cranially and enter the body cavity ventral to the flexor cruris medialis muscle, caudal to the last rib (Lierz *et al.*, 2008). However, in most backyard species, pulling the leg caudally is advantageous.

In any multiple-entry technique, the instrument ports and the endoscope should be placed as far apart as possible to ensure the correct triangulation of the endoscope and instruments within the bird (Figure 12.32bc). Thus, triple-entry techniques are only possible in birds weighing >400 g (which is the case in many backyard

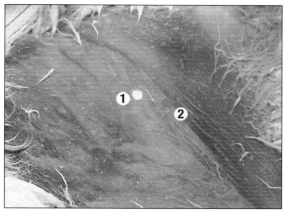

12.31 Double-entry technique for minimally invasive surgery in birds. The insertions points for the endoscope (2) and additional working channel for instruments (1) are shown.

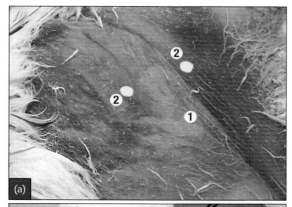

(a)

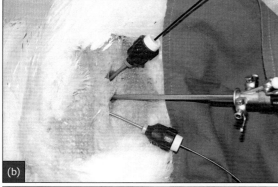

(b)

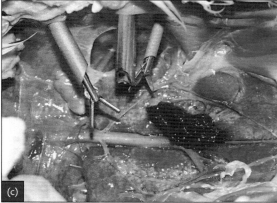

(c)

12.32 Triple-entry technique for minimally invasive surgery in birds. (a) The insertion points for the endoscope (1) and two additional working channels for instruments (2) are shown. (b) Correct placement of the endoscope and cannulas for triple-entry techniques in a chicken. (c) Correct triangulation of the endoscope (middle) and instruments is vital for successful surgery.

poultry species). However, for most indications, single- or double-entry techniques are sufficient. In particular, with the use of a diode laser directed through the working channel of the endoscope, granulomas, gonads and tumours can be vaporized using only a single-entry technique. In single- and double-entry techniques, the endoscopist controls both the endoscope and the instrument; in triple-entry techniques, the endoscopist controls both instruments whilst the endoscope either rests on a sandbag or is handled by an assistant. The radiosurgery or diode laser unit is activated by a foot pedal.

Sterilization and ovariectomy of female birds

Sterilization of female birds is seldom requested for backyard poultry species. It should also be noted that in chickens, sterilization does not prevent ovulation (as it does in some other bird species) (Pye *et al.*, 2001) and thus poses a risk to the individual bird. However, ovariectomy is sometimes performed to prevent reproductive disorders, which are common in chickens. In adult birds, the ovary is a very fragile organ and endoscopic removal represents a high risk of lethal haemorrhage. In juvenile birds, removal of the ovary is best achieved using a diode laser to vaporize all hormone-producing tissue (Figure 12.33). However, as the ovary grows quickly in chickens, this procedure has to be performed before the bird is 8 weeks old. In ornamental species (e.g. pheasants), the birds can be older.

In cases where sterilization is requested, an endoscopic procedure should be performed only in juvenile birds. In adult birds, conventional surgery rather than endosurgery is recommended. A single-entry technique can be used. A pair of grasping forceps is introduced through the working channel of the endoscope. The infundibulum is grasped and the oviduct can be removed from the underlying tissue by gently pulling. Using this technique it is possible to remove nearly the entire oviduct whilst avoiding excessive haemorrhage. Development of these female birds is un-eventful (including development of the ovary) and the birds are hormonally active. This technique is recommended rather than obliteration of the oviduct by electrosurgery, as in poultry the oviduct may fill with albumin (egg white) during hormonal activity.

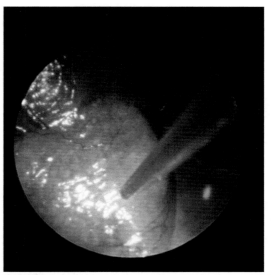

12.33 A diode laser can be used to vaporize the ovary in juvenile birds.

Sterilization of male birds

Sterilization of male birds is usually requested for some ornamental pheasant species. Sterilized cocks of the same or different species are used to stimulate females to lay eggs. These eggs are then artificially inseminated using semen from birds of the same species or certain genetically valuable males. Sterilization can be performed in either juvenile or adult birds. For the less experienced surgeon, it is much easier to perform sterilization in the sexually active bird, as the deferent duct is more easily located compared with in the juvenile bird. In juvenile birds, the deferent duct can be removed by pulling it out through the working channel of the endoscope using a pair of grasping forceps. Using this method in Japanese quail, it was demonstrated that the testicles developed uneventfully and that testosterone blood levels increased with sexual maturity, in a similar way to unsterilized males. In addition, the sexual behaviour of the sterilized males was unaltered (Jones and Redig, 2003). The same procedure can be performed in adult birds; however, the deferent duct is usually too large to be pulled out through the working channel, but it can be removed with the endoscope. This requires re-entry of the bird several times (if using a single-entry technique) or a double-entry technique. Alternatively, the deferent duct may be obliterated by electrosurgery. In some adult birds of large breeds or species (e.g. turkeys), endoscopic sterilization is easier using a double- or triple-entry technique. Using grasping forceps, the testicle is elevated from the underlying tissue, raising the deferent duct as well. Using a second working channel, a pair of scissors can be introduced to cut the deferent duct (Figure 12.34). At least 1 cm of the deferent duct needs to be removed in order to avoid reunion of the cut ends and a re-establishment of functionality.

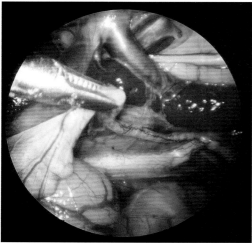

12.34 Sterilization of an adult male bird. The deferent duct is elevated and cut using a pair of scissors. This procedure must be performed in two locations in order to remove at least 1 cm of the duct to prevent reunion.

Castration of male birds

Castration of male birds is frequently requested, particularly in chickens. For owners who raise chicks, disposal of surplus male birds is often not an option. However, as they start crowing and fighting, problems occur which may be overcome with castration. Male birds should be castrated as early as possible, as the risk of lethal haemorrhage increases dramatically with age. In juvenile birds, the optimal age for castration is up to 6 weeks old. In juvenile birds, the testicle can be grasped and removed using a radiosurgical sling, which obliterates the vessels as it is closed. Vaporization using a diode laser is advantageous in very young birds where the testicle is often closely attached to the adrenal gland and kidney vessel (Figure 12.35).

For castration of adult birds, a double- or preferably triple-entry technique is used. The testicle is elevated from the kidney using grasping forceps. The mesorchium is cut using monopolar coagulation scissors. The main vessels supplying the testicle should be obliterated using monopolar or bipolar grasping forceps. Owners need to be informed that in sexually active birds (note that chickens are sexually active year-round), the risk of lethal haemorrhage is considerably higher and conventional surgery can be advantageous in these cases.

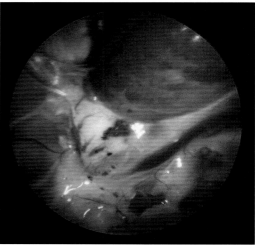

12.35 Cranial pole of the kidney of a male bird 3 months following castration using a diode laser. Note the absence of testicular tissue.

Further applications

Castration and sterilization are excellent procedures to learn the techniques of endoscopic surgery. They also represent the routine application of these techniques as every procedure is very similar. Other applications, such as tumour or granuloma resection, are always different according to the location of the lesion and the severity of the disease. Thus, practitioners should attempt to hone their skills during routine procedures before proceeding to less predictable surgery.

Removal or vaporization of granulomas is a frequent indication for endosurgery, in particular if lesions (single or multiple) cause problems by blocking the airway. In the case of generalized disease, endosurgery alone will not solve the problem; treatment of the underlying cause is always necessary. Using a diode laser via the working channel of the endoscope, granulomas, papillomas and tumours can be completely vaporized or removed from the underlying tissue and extracted using grasping forceps. Larger lesions can be cut into pieces and removed individually. Alternatively, an electrocautery probe can be inserted into the working channel of the endoscope to detach the lesion from the underlying tissue. In principle, both techniques are comparable, minimizing the risk of haemorrhage. In experienced hands, a diode laser can offer more precision.

Risks

The main risk associated with endoscopic surgery is uncontrolled haemorrhage. The risk of bleeding is greater than during diagnostic endoscopic procedures. Thus, all measures must be taken to avoid large vessels. When using coagulation or vaporization techniques, care must be taken to avoid damaging the underlying tissues. The power used during these procedures should, therefore, be kept to a minimum and only increased if necessary. For example, laser vaporization of small lesions should start at 0.5 Watts and be increased slowly to 1 Watt. In rare cases, higher power is necessary but should never exceed 2 Watts.

The risk of cutting or removing the wrong tissue, such as the ureter instead of the oviduct or deferent duct, is always present. It is essential, therefore, that the surgeon has a detailed knowledge of the relevant anatomy, and experience should be gained with cadaver specimens or birds under general anaesthesia where euthanasia is planned (legal aspects must be considered in some countries). Training endosurgery should be followed by necropsy to confirm that the procedure carried out had the required result.

It should also be borne in mind that electrosurgery and lasers apply a high amount of power to a minimal point. As birds are usually anaesthetized with isoflurane inhalation in oxygen, the use of lasers might cause a fire within the body cavity when the oxygen concentration inside the bird is high (Lierz *et al.*, 2006). Thus, it is advisable not to use pure oxygen for anaesthesia in patients when use of a laser is planned; lowering the oxygen concentration by mixing it with pressurized air in the anaesthetic machine is highly advisable.

References and further reading

Baileys RE (1953) Surgery for sexing and observing gonad condition in birds. *Auk* **70**, 497–500

Birkhead TR and Pellatt JE (1989) Vasectomy in small passerine birds. *Veterinary Record* **125**, 646

Hernandez-Divers SJ (2005) Minimally invasive endoscopic surgery of birds. *Journal of Avian Medicine and Surgery* **19(2)**, 107–120

Hochleithner M (1997) Endoscopy. In: *Avian Medicine and Surgery*, ed. RB Altman, SL Clubb, GM Dorrestein and K Quesenberry, pp. 800–805. WB Saunders, Philadelphia

Jones R and Redig PT (2003) Endoscopy guided vasectomy in the immature Japanese Quail (*Coturnix coturnix japonica*). *Proceedings of the 7th Conference of the European Association of Avian Veterinarians and the 5th Scientific Meeting of the European College of Avian Medicine and Surgery*, Tenerife, Spain, pp. 117–123

Lierz M (2004) Endoskopie. In: *Leitsymptome bei Papageien und Sittichen*, ed. M Pees, pp. 185–194. Enke Verlag, Stuttgart

Lierz M (2006) Diagnostic value of endoscopy and biopsy. In: *Clinical Avian Medicine, Volume II*, ed. G Harrison and T Lightfoot, pp. 631–652. Spix Publishing Inc., Palm Beach, Florida

Lierz M (2008) Endoscopy, biopsy and endosurgery. In: *BSAVA Manual of Raptors, Pigeons and Passerine Birds*, ed. J Chitty and M Lierz, pp. 128–142. BSAVA Publications, Gloucester

Lierz M, Ewringmann A and Goebel T (1998) Blood chemistry values in wild raptors and their changes after liver biopsy. *Berl Muench Tierarztl Wochenschr* **111**, 295–301

Lierz M and Hafez HM (2004) Endoscopic guided surgery in birds – sterilisation and castration. *Proceedings of the XIV DVG Conference about Avian Diseases*, Munich, Germany, pp. 26–31

Lierz M and Hafez HM (2005) Endoscopy guided multiple entry surgery in birds. *Proceedings of the 8th Conference of the European Association of Avian Veterinarians and the 6th Scientific ECAMS Meeting*, Arles, France, pp. 184–189

Lierz P, Lierz M, Gustorff B and Felleiter P (2006) Management of intratracheal fire during laser surgery in veterinary medicine. *The Internet Journal of Veterinary Medicine* (http://ispub.com/IJVM/2/2/9312)

McDonald SE (1987) Endoscopic examination. In: *Companion Bird Medicine*, ed. EW Burr, pp. 166–174. Iowa State University Press, Ames

Pye GW, Bennett RA, Plunske R and Davidson J (2001) Endoscopic salpingohysterectomy of juvenile cockatiels (*Nymphicus hollandicus*). *Journal of Avian Medicine and Surgery* **15**, 90–94

Taylor M (1994) Endoscopic examination and biopsy techniques. In: *Avian Principles and Application*, ed. BW Ritchie *et al.*, pp. 327–354, Wingers Publishing Inc., Florida

Chapter 13

Disorders of the integument

John Chitty

Feather and skin diseases, especially parasitism, are common reasons for poultry owners to contact a veterinary surgeon (veterinarian). As well as being the easiest part of the bird to see, the visual appearance of birds (especially when showing) is a major part of their appeal. Feather and skin disorders are, therefore, often accorded an importance out of proportion with their clinical significance. Conversely, some feather and skin disorders may appear minor yet reflect serious internal disease.

Anatomy and physiology

The anatomy and physiology of birds is discussed in Chapter 2. In the main, the skin of poultry is similar to that of other bird species and is described in full by Lucas and Stettenheim (1972). However, there are some important points to note:

- Gallinaceous birds are quite 'loose-feathered' and feathers are easily lost if handled roughly. The loss of feathers also results in reduced waterproofing
- Waterfowl have very good feather waterproofing via a tight feather structure and extensive interlocking barbules. Under the outer layer of feathers, they have a layer of down feathers to provide thermal insulation. They lack obvious apterylae, which means that feathers need to be removed prior to venepuncture
- Poultry have more extensive intradermal and subdermal fat deposits than other birds. This often results in yellowing of the skin and can make visualization of the subcutaneous blood vessels more difficult
- Hormone-linked skin and feather changes (e.g. wattle development and long tail feathers in cockerels) may be seen from 6–8 weeks of age in male birds. Surgical or chemical castration will result in a reduction of these features
- Moulting may occur annually in some species (e.g. in chickens as they enter the non-laying period in the autumn) or twice a year in other birds (e.g. in waterfowl where males enter an eclipse moult out of season when their feathers are comparatively dull). Peacock tail feathers grow prior to the breeding season and are lost soon afterwards; this is presumed to be linked to fluctuating hormone levels.

History and clinical examination

With all species, it is important to consider the whole bird and not just the integument. Thus, a full history (Figure 13.1) and clinical examination are mandatory in all but the simplest of cases. Specific dermatological sampling techniques are summarized in Figure 13.2 and discussed further in Chapter 10 (see also Chitty, 2005). Further diagnostic investigations (e.g. haematology/biochemistry, radiography and endoscopy) are required in complex cases or where there may be an underlying systemic disease.

- Number of birds in the flock and the number affected
- Age range of the flock and the age range of birds affected
- Routine parasite control (internal and external)
- Housing
- State of lay/egg production
- Number of birds in the flock that are moulting
- Access to dust bath or water (waterfowl)
- Diet
- Initial lesions or areas of feather loss (and how these have changed)
- Response to treatment
- Other medical history

13.1 Important aspects of the clinical history.

Technique	Indication	Notes
Skin scrape	Crusts; hyperkeratotic lesions	Performed as for dogs and cats. Note that the cells tend to present in sheets or 'rafts'
Feather digest	Feather damage; changes in calamus	The feather is digested in warmed 10% potassium hydroxide for 6–12 hours and then centrifuged
Pulp cytology	Feather damage	Rectrices or remiges may be removed, the calamus incised and the contents scraped on to a slide for examination. With smaller body feathers, a drop of pulp may be extracted by squeezing (the first drop should be discarded as it will be contaminated with blood) or by needle aspiration
Skin acetate	Excessive scale; hyperkeratotic lesions; crusts; exudative lesions	Performed as for dogs and cats. Romanowsky-type stains are normally used for examination

13.2 Specific dermatological sampling techniques. (continues) ▶

Technique	Indication	Notes
Biopsy	Unusual lesions; cases that fail to respond to rational therapy or where other diagnostic tests indicate the need for biopsy	The biopsy sample should always include a feather follicle; however, a flight feather follicle should never be removed as this will result in permanent loss of the feather. The skin should not be aseptically prepared as this will result in removal of the surface cells. Bird skin contains a mesh of muscles linking feather follicles, so when a section of skin is removed the muscles contract, resulting in a tiny curled biopsy sample and a very large skin defect, especially if an excisional biopsy has been performed. Instead, a piece of transparent adhesive tape should be placed over the skin and a sample taken through the tape using a biopsy punch. Care should be taken to avoid damaging the underlying tissues. The sample (with the tape attached) should be placed in formol saline and submitted for histopathology

13.2 (continued) Specific dermatological sampling techniques.

Feather disorders

Feather loss or damage

A distinction must always be made between physiological feather loss (e.g. moulting) and pathological feather loss. Where the cause is physiological, one or more of the following features is usually present:

- The bird appears normal with no other pathological findings
- Absence (or very small numbers) of ectoparasites
- No observed aggression from other birds
- Feathers are lost intact and the base of the calamus is closed off
- Growing (replacement) feathers are present
- Other moulting birds are present in the group
- Spontaneous recovery.

When the moult is abnormal or asynchronous, the cause is likely to be pathological. Some birds (particularly ex-battery hens) may have pre-existing feather and feather follicle loss. In these cases, feathers do not always grow back and special attention must be paid to providing additional shelter from wet and/or cold conditions. Reasons for pathological feather loss include:

- Physical rubbing
- Plucking/pecking by other birds
- Trauma
- Malnutrition
- Abnormal moult
- Ectoparasite infestation
- Bacterial infection
- Fungal infection.

Physical causes of feather loss and damage

Physical causes of feather loss and/or damage should not be overlooked. Careful observation and obtaining a good history (Figure 13.3) are vital for confirming the diagnosis.

- How many birds are affected?
- Are all birds affected to the same extent?
- Has there been a recent addition to the existing flock?
- Is a cockerel present?
- Have any aggressive interactions between birds been noted? Is a potential aggressor identifiable?

13.3 Questions that form part of the clinical history when investigating whether feather loss or damage is caused by plucking or pecking by other birds.

The distribution of feather loss is a major indicator of the cause. For example, feather loss over the dorsal head and circumferentially around the neck indicates rubbing of the neck feathers as the bird pushes its head through a fence or narrow feeder to obtain food. Whereas feather loss over the dorsal head, neck and around the vent indicates plucking and/or pecking by other birds (Figure 13.4) (see Chapter 19). If feather loss due to plucking or pecking by other birds is suspected, appropriate changes to the management regimen should be implemented, and the feathers should regrow. Mating injuries can also result in feather loss or damage. In these cases, the use of a breeding saddle may be useful. If the clinical history is not conclusive, a clinical examination should be carried out to rule out clinical disease.

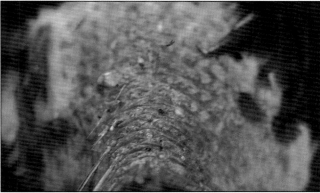

13.4 Behavioural feather plucking. Feathers have been lost from the dorsum over the tail. Note the reddening of the exposed skin. This does not appear to be inflammatory in origin and is not centred on the damaged feather follicles.
(© John Chitty)

Trauma

As poultry are loose-feathered, they will readily lose feathers if attacked. There may be a history of trauma, the presence of wounds, or a significant loss of feathers may be observed at the trauma site. Feathers tend to regrow spontaneously.

Malnutrition

Interruption in growth due to periods of malnutrition (as well as systemic disease or endoparasitism) may result in the formation of fret (stress) marks in the feathers. These visible lines often occur in the same place on a number of feathers if there is a systemic problem. Feathers are weakened at these marks and are easily broken. A full dietary evaluation may assist in determining the diagnosis, although the clinical signs are often obvious. The diet should be corrected and the growth of new feathers observed. It is important to remember that fret marks on existing feathers may not reflect the current clinical or dietary status of the bird. In the author's experience, essential amino acid supplementation may be useful.

Abnormal moult

An abnormal moult generally occurs when the husbandry or weather conditions are not consistent (i.e. they allow the moult to start but not to be completed). Typically, either the feathers are lost but not immediately replaced or the moult is continuous. Attention should be paid to:

- Diet – particularly protein and essential amino acid content. Vitamin levels (including vitamin A) are also of importance. If the feed is found to be balanced, then it is worth checking for feed spoilage and storage conditions, especially if owners have 'economized' by buying large bags of feed to last longer. The addition of a general vitamin and amino acid supplement can be of some assistance
- Light cycles – as birds normally moult in the autumn, it may be advantageous to reduce access to light to 6 hours daily. It should also be explained to the owner that this may reduce or stop egg laying. In the domestic situation, this may be achieved by using a light-proof house for roosting
- Stressors – including overcrowding, poor social structure and lack of enrichment (see also Chapter 19)
- Internal disease.

Some birds appear to have a 'normal' abnormal moult and may show signs of a protracted or asynchronous moult every year, even though no underlying factors appear to be present and the bird seems healthy. In other cases, the moult may vary in terms of rate and degree from year to year. In these instances, attention should be paid to providing adequate shelter from cold and wet conditions, and the bird should be carefully monitored throughout the moult.

Ectoparasite infestation

Lice: Chewing lice (*Menopon* genus in poultry and *Holomenopon* genus in waterfowl; Figure 13.5a) are commonly found on birds. In small numbers these are not generally considered to be pathogenic and control is not necessary as preening, dust bathing, swimming or diving, and wing flapping will control numbers in healthy birds. In unhealthy birds, numbers may become very heavy and feather damage may result (this is a potential cause of wet feather in waterfowl; see below). Large numbers of eggs may be laid on the feather bases around the vent, resulting in feather damage and further soiling and irritation around the vent (Figure 13.5bc). Louse infestations may be an indication of general health.

Mites: Feather mites are commonly seen and, like lice, are species- and site-specific. Mites are relatively non-pathogenic and feather damage will only occur with exceptionally heavy infestations when mites move off the feathers and on to the skin, causing irritation. Mite numbers are also an indicator of general health. Feather mites (Figure 13.6) can be distinguished from red mites (see below and Chapter 10) and northern mites (which are of much greater clinical importance) as they lack piercing mouthparts and have shorter legs designed for gripping feathers.

Treatment: There are many products marketed as suitable for treatment of ectoparasite infestations. However, few of these drugs have a veterinary authorization and their efficacy is variable. The prescribing cascade should be followed in all cases and appropriate egg-withholding periods adhered to (see Chapter 26). Specific product names are not given here as products vary between countries.

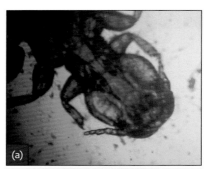
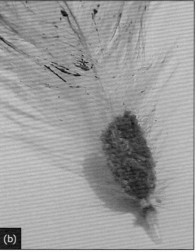
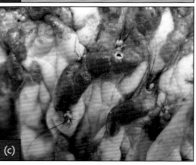
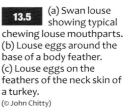

13.5 (a) Swan louse showing typical chewing louse mouthparts. (b) Louse eggs around the base of a body feather. (c) Louse eggs on the feathers of the neck skin of a turkey.
(© John Chitty)

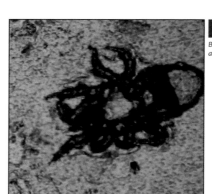

13.6 Feather mite.
(Reproduced from the *BSAVA Manual of Raptors, Pigeons and Passerine Birds*; © John Chitty)

- Most authorized ectoparasiticides are based on pyrethrum powder. This can be effective against feather mites, *Ornithonyssus* and lice. The application of powder can be difficult as the bird needs to be covered and powder must penetrate under and through plumage, which requires intensive handling. (The method of placing a bird in a sack and adding powder may be effective but is not recommended as it is likely to distress the bird and may cause powder to enter the eyes and respiratory system.)

- Herbal products are also available, which are popular with owners because they are 'natural', but do not appear to be particularly efficacious. They may have a role in prevention of problems, but not in therapy.
- Fipronil spray is very effective against feather mites and lice but is not authorized for use in food-producing species. However, it can be used in ornamental pheasants. Fipronil should be sprayed on to a cotton wool pad and applied to the back of the head, over and under each wing.

Bacterial infection

Bacterial disease is very rare, although feather loss may occur due to infection of the follicles (see below). Bacterial growth on feathers may occur in unhygienic situations and where there is soiling and contamination of the feathers. Cleaning and topical disinfection is recommended.

Fungal infection

Feather loss around the head and neck may be caused by favus infection (avian ringworm; see later).

Wet feather

Wet feather describes the breakdown of waterproofing mechanisms in waterfowl, resulting in an inability to repel water, a wet bedraggled appearance and increased risk of hypothermia. Waterproofing is mainly achieved by:

- Feather structure – the extensive interlocking barbules create a lattice with an airspace, such that an impervious air–water barrier is created
- Preening – regular preening helps maintain feature structure. It also helps to spread oils from the uropygial gland. Whilst these oils play no part in waterproofing, they do assist in preserving feather structure and flexibility. An absence of oil will result in 'premature ageing' of the feather
- Moulting – regular moulting and replacement of ageing feathers assist in overall plumage integrity.

Wet feather results from any process that interferes with these waterproofing mechanisms, including:

- Feather lice
- Contamination of feathers (e.g. oils, chemicals, surfactants, sooty mould, faeces, mud)
- Poor feather quality
- Loss of feathers over a large area, allowing water to enter 'under' other feathers
- Abnormal moult
- Uropygial gland disease, resulting in poor feather quality
- Reduced preening (e.g. following debilitating or system illness) or physical inability to preen (e.g. due to overcrowding). In a case seen by the author, the underlying cause appeared to be intestinal capillariasis in a group of thin ducks. Feather quality improved as the birds began to preen.

Treatment includes:

- Taking the animals off water. In some mild cases, this may only be for a short period of time; however, in most instances once feather integrity is lost, it will only be restored after the next moult
- Removing contaminants. Conventional washing-up liquid and gentle scrubbing usually suffices for removal of most contaminants
- Correcting any environmental problems
- Investigating and treating underlying diseases.

Skin disorders

Skin reddening

Skin reddening is common (Figure 13.7). The areas usually affected include contact areas, such as the crop, keel and ventrum, and around the vent, abdomen or dorsum where feathers have been lost. These lesions normally appear just as pigmented skin with no evidence of inflammation and they do not appear to be irritant to the bird or to cause other problems. In the author's opinion, these lesions represent a skin response to exposure or abrasion and are of little clinical significance. Instead, attention should be paid to the reasons for feather loss and skin exposure. Where skin reddening occurs on ventral contact areas, attention should be paid to possible causes of debility or systemic disease that result in the bird spending more time sitting. If the crop is affected and unduly pendulous, causes of crop impaction should be investigated.

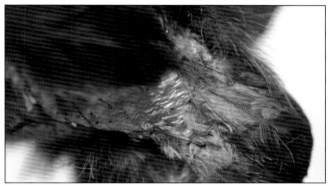

13.7 Skin reddening on the ventrum of a bird with a slightly pendulous abdomen.
(© John Chitty)

Irritation

Skin irritation may be seen in any region, but particularly featherless areas and especially the feet. In poultry, this may be seen as reddening of the feet and the history may suggest exposure to irritant substances, including plant toxins (e.g. giant hogweed). Waterfowl are more commonly affected and syndromes have been described where vesicles form over the foot webs, as well as on the beak and facial skin.

Photosensitization in Muscovy ducks

A particular syndrome of photosensitization has been described in Muscovy ducks, where vesicles form in the dorsal surface of the foot webs. The author has also seen similar clinical signs in swans as a result of bacterial embolic spread. Systemic antibiosis and the application of barrier creams, combined with keeping the bird away from water (and the use of sunblock cream where photosensitization is suspected) can be successful in treating the condition. If photosensitization is suspected, the diet of the bird should be evaluated for potential photosensitizing agents. Various plants and toxins may be implicated, both via external contact and by ingestion. A list of plants that are known to induce photosensitization can be found on the Twycross Zoo website (http://wildpro.twycrosszoo.org/S/00dis/Miscellaneous/Plant-Induced_Photosensitisation.htm)

Frostbite

Skin irritation needs to be distinguished from frostbite of the extremities. With frostbite, the lesions tend to be the full thickness of the web and are found on the very extremity of the digit and web. Whereas lesions caused by irritation or photosensitization are rarely the full thickness of the web and are located mid-web.

Mite infestation

Red mites

Red mites (*Dermanyssus*; Figure 13.8a) are one of the most common and significant ectoparasites of backyard poultry. These mites do not cause direct skin signs (other than extreme irritation), but because they are blood-sucking they do result in anaemia and debilitation, especially in young birds, where death may occur. Clinical signs include debility, lethargy and, occasionally, pale wattles (see Figure 13.14).

Red mites are photophobic and only emerge at night. Birds may show signs of irritation at night, as well as becoming restless and vocal. The lifecycle of the mite is spent primarily off the host, apart from when it feeds. There may be intervals of up to 6 months between feeds. The diagnosis is rarely confirmed by finding mites on the bird; instead, environmental checks must be performed. Typically, owners report finding mites on their skin (which can be very irritating) after entering the poultry house at night. If this has not been reported, a white sheet may be placed on the floor of the house at night and a light shone upon it. This will reveal numerous small dark mites moving rapidly away from the light. Mites can be collected on acetate strips and examination will reveal the typical piercing mouthparts (Figure 13.8b).

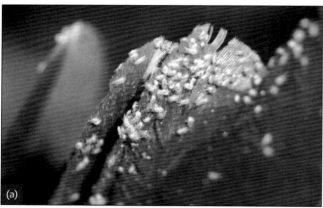

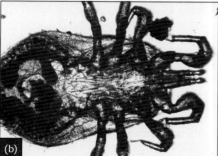

13.8 (a) Red mites (*Dermanyssus*) on the feathers of a cadaver. The post-mortem examination revealed a thin anaemic carcass, as well as vast numbers of mites. (b) The typical piercing mouthparts of the red mite.
(b, Reproduced from the *BSAVA Manual of Raptors, Pigeons and Passerine Birds*; © John Chitty)

Treatment: Bird-based treatment is capable of killing only a very small proportion of mites because much of their lifecycle is spent in the environment. The bird-based treatments described for feather mites (see above) may also be effective against red mites. Environmental control is of much greater importance and there are various options available:

- If light cycles can be controlled, intermittent short-cycle lighting regimes have been described as reducing mite numbers, presumably by reducing the amount of time available for these photophobic mites to feed
- The use of pyrethrum powders and permethrin sprays has been described. However, their penetration of housing materials is poor and thus these treatments are only effective in limiting mite numbers. Permethrin/pyriproxifen spray has a persistent action, so may be more effective overall
- Diatomaceous earth is frequently recommended as part of red mite control. It is often advised alongside disinfectants, although neither product appears to have a direct acaricidal action
- The careful use of blowtorches to penetrate into cracks and crevices has been described. However, this is a time-consuming and potentially dangerous process and is unlikely to clear an infestation
- The only guaranteed way to clear an infestation is to destroy the existing housing, especially if it is constructed of wood or brick. New housing constructed of plastic is recommended and all birds should be treated prior to being moved to the new accommodation.

Prevention: Prevention of red mite infestation is better than treatment; however, prevention is not easy. Birds may initially harbour only one or two mites, but this can rapidly amplify into a clinically significant problem. All new birds should be quarantined before being introduced to a flock; they should be treated for mites at both the beginning and end of this isolation period. The poultry house should also be checked regularly to ensure that red mite numbers are not building up. See also Chapter 7.

Northern mites

Northern mites (*Ornithonyssus*) are becoming more common. Similar to the red mite, this blood-sucking parasite does not cause skin lesions. However, unlike the red mite, this species spends its entire lifecycle on the bird, resulting in continuous irritation and a more rapid onset of anaemia and debilitation. The diagnosis is based on the clinical signs (similar to those seen with a red mite infestation, but with continuous restlessness and irritation) and on finding mites on the bird. Northern mites (Figure 13.9) should be

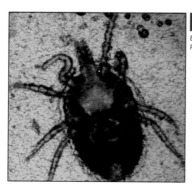

13.9 Northern mite.
(Reproduced from the *BSAVA Manual of Raptors, Pigeons and Passerine Birds*; © John Chitty)

differentiated from feather mites. It should be borne in mind that as Northern mites spend their entire lifecycle on the bird, infestation is much more easily treated and controlled as on-bird treatment is all that is required, e.g. ivermectin at 200 μg/kg administered percutaneously, orally or intramuscularly every 2 weeks for three occasions.

Epidermoptid mites

Epidermoptid mites are relatively common burrowing mites that cause feather loss and skin irritation, mainly of the face and neck ('depluming itch') (Figure 13.10). Secondary bacterial infections are sometimes seen. Severe manifestations may cause damage to the growing tissue of the beak. The diagnosis is confirmed by the clinical signs, and a skin scrape or biopsy. Treatment consists of ivermectin at a dose of 200 μg/kg administered percutaneously, orally or intramuscularly every 2 weeks for three occasions. All in-contact birds should be treated, even if they are not showing any clinical signs.

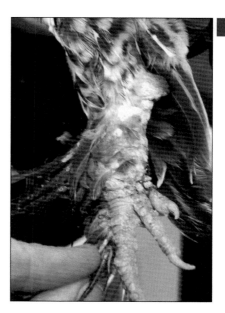

13.11 Scaly leg.
(© John Chitty)

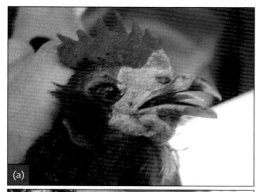

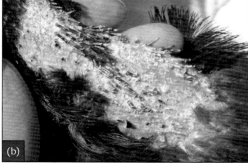

13.10 (a) Epidermoptid mite infestation. (b) Depluming itch on the neck of a peacock.
(© John Chitty)

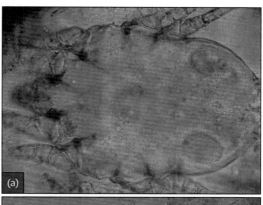

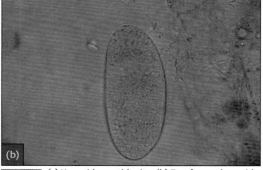

13.12 (a) Knemidocoptid mite. (b) Egg from a knemidocoptid mite identified on a skin scrape.
(© John Chitty)

Knemidocoptid mites

The knemidocoptid mite is probably the most common skin parasite of clinical importance. *Knemidocoptes pilae* is typically the cause of scaly leg in poultry. Scaly leg describes the formation of extensive crusts in the scaled skin of the feet and legs (Figure 13.11). There are varying degrees of irritation. Secondary bacterial infection and pododermatitis are common (see below). The species *Neocnemidocoptes gallinae* may cause a syndrome similar to that of depluming itch (see above). The diagnosis is confirmed by the clinical signs (if observed closely, winding burrows of the mites may be seen in the scale) and by a skin scrape (Figure 13.12).

Treatment for Knemidocoptid mites may be as for epidermoptid mites; however, topical therapy may also be of use. Traditionally, petroleum jelly or liquid paraffin were smeared over the legs of the birds to block burrows and

suffocate the mites. This is often sufficient in mild infestations and should be repeated weekly until the crusting has resolved. Alternatively, the author prefers to use a 1:50 mix of ivermectin and propylene glycol, which is coated on to the legs of birds twice a month. All in-contact birds must be treated. Owners should be instructed to wear rubber gloves whilst applying the medication and advised that this is not an authorized poultry treatment in most jurisdictions. Antibiosis may be required where there is a secondary infection. Many cases resolve completely, although not until after the next moult, and some scarring may remain. It is also important to note that birds may harbour these mites without any clinical signs and that the presence of clinical signs may represent immunosuppression or the presence of an underlying stressor.

Bacterial infection

Primary bacterial diseases are uncommon in backyard poultry. However, secondary infection of damaged skin is frequently seen and should be addressed and treated when suspected.

Breast blisters

Of the primary bacterial diseases encountered in practice, breast blisters in turkey stags and extremely large or obese chickens are the most common. Breast blisters represent chronic abrasion of this region in birds that are unable to keep their breast off the ground. A range of bacteria are associated with this condition, most likely representing opportunistic invasion. Treatment involves:

- Moving the bird to a clean dry environment
- Systemic antibiosis, ideally based on culture and sensitivity testing; however, the author often initiates treatment with co-amoxiclav whilst waiting for the results
- Cleaning and topical barrier creams for any damaged skin over the sternum
- A controlled weight loss programme.

In severe cases, bacterial infection may penetrate to the keel bone itself, resulting in osteomyelitis. This carries a poor prognosis and extensive surgery is likely to be required.

Dermatitis

Dermatitis involving *Staphylococcus* spp. penetrating the dermis and feather follicles has been described. Rarely, dermatitis is reported as a primary epidemic in birds (e.g. *Erysipelothrix rhusiopathiae* in broilers, turkeys and ducks). It is likely that poor environmental hygiene (e.g. contact with sheep, pigs and pig slurry in the case of erysipelosis) and underlying stressors (e.g. overcrowding) play a part in the aetiology of this condition. Vaccination against *Erysipelothrix* is available for turkeys in the UK and for chickens in some other countries.

Cellulitis and exudative dermatitis, caused by a range of bacteria, have been described in broilers. However, these conditions are extremely unusual in a backyard poultry flock, presumably due to lower stocking density, better hygiene and fewer stressors. Mycobacterial dermatitis has also been described, but is very rare. Nevertheless, it should be suspected in any case of granulomatous dermatitis and it is advisable to obtain biopsy samples in such cases owing to the zoonotic nature of the infection.

Abscesses

Bacterial abscesses are frequently seen with inspissated pus being identified in subcutaneous lesions following injury or skin penetration. They are commonly found between the toes or on the scaled part of the legs. Lumps of pus located in the subocular region may appear as subcutaneous abscesses but are actually located within the infraorbital sinus. Subcutaneous abscesses should be surgically excised and the abscess cavity flushed (chlorhexidine, povidone–iodine or 1:250 dilution F10 are also suitable) before the skin is closed. Where primary wound closure is not possible, secondary healing by granulation may be successful.

Fungal infection

Favus (also known as avian ringworm or white comb disease) is a very common finding in backyard poultry and is caused by *Trichophyton megnini*. Lesions appear as a white scale over the face and wattles (Figure 13.13a), spreading down the skin of the head and neck. Favus can also cause feather loss (Figure 13.13b), and a deep infection may result in damage to the eyelids and/or beak. The infection is spread to other birds by direct contact and/or fomites, but does not appear to be zoonotic. The diagnosis is confirmed by microscopic identification of the fungus in scrapes or biopsy samples taken from the affected areas. *T. megnini* does not seem to grow well on conventional ringworm media. Favus is treated using topical antifungal agents (e.g. iodine, F10) until the lesions resolve. In severe cases, topical miconazole spray may be used or systemic antifungal drugs, although it should be noted that none are authorized for use in food-producing animals. Very severe cases may require euthanasia.

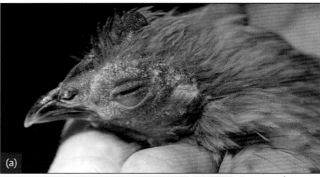

13.13 Favus on the (a) head and (b) neck of a hen. Note the scale and feather loss. (© John Chitty)

Viral infection

Poxvirus is an occasional finding in backyard poultry, particularly waterfowl. Lesions are seen in featherless areas (especially the face and foot webs) and consist of either raised plaques or pale yellow scabs. Transmission occurs either directly or via fly-borne spread. The diagnosis is confirmed by the presence of typical lesions and via biopsy. There is no treatment. However, lesions are usually self-limiting and there is little scarring unless there is a secondary infection. Topical antibiotics may be useful, especially if the lesions are located around the eyes. Care must be taken to prevent the spread of the virus to in-contact birds and strict barrier nursing is required. In severe cases with extensive lesions around the eyes, nares and mouth, supportive care may be required to help the bird to feed. Vaccination is possible but generally not indicated as the infection is not very common, nor is it particularly severe in most cases.

Papillomavirus has also been reported as a cause of raised plaques or nodules on the featherless skin of waterfowl.

Conditions of the wattle

Colour changes

Wattle colour and turgidity are excellent measures of internal health. A flaccid and/or discoloured wattle may be an indication of internal disease (Figure 13.14).

Appearance	Potential causes
Pale	Anaemia: evaluate and remove the underlying cause. The most common cause of anaemia is *Dermanyssus* infestation (see Chapter 21 for other causes of anaemia) Shock: evaluate and provide supportive treatment
Purple/blue	Cyanosis; severe respiratory disease
Black	Necrosis or dried blood: clean carefully, check for wounds and necrotic tissue. Note that this may be normal in some breeds (e.g. Silkies)
Yellow	Generally associated with extensive fat discoloration and/or pigmentation from high corn ration (Figure 13.15); jaundice (rare)
White spots	Poxvirus infection (Figure 13.16)
Crusting/ scaling	Favus; epidermoptid mites

13.14 Potential causes of changes in wattle colour and appearance.

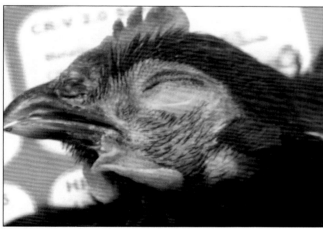

13.15 The yellow skin and wattle of this cadaver is not indicative of jaundice but of pigmentation from an exclusively corn diet. The cause of death was egg-related peritonitis.
(© John Chitty)

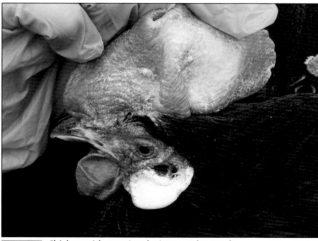

13.16 Chicken with poxvirus lesions on the comb.
(© John Chitty)

Damage

The wattle may be injured in fights or become necrotic following frostbite. Following trauma, the wattle may bleed extensively as it has a very rich blood supply. Haemostatic powders or potassium permanganate may be used to control haemorrhage. If the wattle has been extensively damaged, the wounds may be sutured closed (although it should be noted that they frequently break down due to inflammatory reactions) or amputated. Necrosis is initially managed using systemic antibiosis and topical barrier creams with the aim being to achieve a controlled slough of the necrotic regions. In severe cases, amputation of part or all of the wattle may be required.

Conditions of the beak

Beak disease

The beak is derived from skin and has a similar structure and growth pattern in poultry to that of other birds (see Chapter 2). Beak overgrowth is comparatively unusual in poultry compared with other bird species seen in practice. However, it does occur occasionally and is usually the result of either disease affecting the regions of the beak responsible for growth (e.g. mite infestation or favus) (Figure 13.17) or trauma to the beak such that the upper and lower jaws no longer align properly.

The beak tissue of poultry is comparatively soft compared with that of parrots and raptors, and very sensitive with many nerve endings. Thus, although it is easy to trim, it is also easy to traumatize the beak, and any trimming should be undertaken with care and with the aim of restoring the beak to its normal shape (or as close as possible). Clippers and files can be used; however, the author prefers to use a modeller's grinding tool. Beak trimming can normally be performed with the bird conscious.

Trauma

Beak trauma is common, especially in geese, where it is often seen following a fox attack. In these cases, typically areas of the beak are found to be missing. The regrowth of beak material is variable and can often result in large defects. However, birds with altered beaks seem to cope very well and reconstructive surgery and/or prostheses

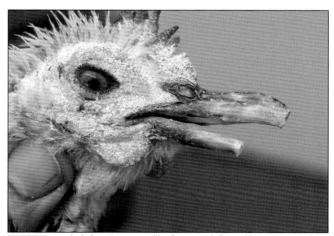

13.17 Beak deformity caused by favus with fungal invasion into the germinative areas of the beak.
(© John Chitty)

are rarely, if ever, required. The following supportive care is recommended:

- Antibiosis and analgesia immediately following the injury. The author generally administers co-amoxiclav and meloxicam
- Daily cleaning of the injury and the application of hydrophilic gel
- Assisted or tube feeding whilst the bird learns how to feed with an altered beak. Food should be provided as a mash (rather than as pellets) and 'greens' should be provided as large pieces to make prehension easier.

In the long term, regular trimming of the beak may be required as the upper and lower jaws may no longer align properly (Figure 13.18).

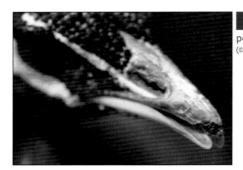

13.18 Misaligned beak of a peafowl.
(© John Chitty)

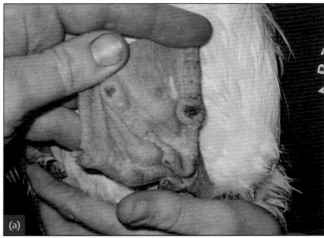

(a)

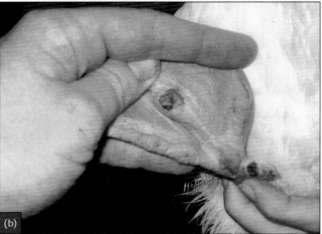

(b)

13.19 (a, b) Pododermatitis in a duck.
(© John Chitty)

Conditions of the feet

Pododermatitis

Pododermatitis is also known as 'bumblefoot' and is a common condition in poultry. To a certain extent, the condition in poultry can be considered similar to that encountered in raptors. However, the aetiology of pododermatitis in poultry appears to be simpler and the treatment success rate much higher. Unlike in raptors, where the majority of cases appear to result from the accumulation of endogenous bacteria and altered haemodynamics of the foot, pressure on the feet is the main cause of pododermatitis in poultry. Altered pressure on the weight-bearing surfaces of the foot results in skin lesions, which act as the point of entry for infection.

Pododermatitis is a two-footed problem. If lesions are present on only one foot, then the unaffected leg should be checked thoroughly (including radiography where necessary) to determine why there is altered weight-bearing and more pressure on the contralateral foot. The lesions seen with pododermatitis are similar to those found in raptors with granuloma and/or abscess formation. Waterfowl tend to form thick-walled granulomas over the joints of the digits, and it is not uncommon for the lesions to penetrate the joints (Figure 13.19). In other species of poultry, there tends to be extensive formation of caseous pus.

Common causes

The following are common causes of pododermatitis in poultry:

- Poor substrate – the use of inappropriate substrates appears to be the most important cause of pododermatitis. Abrasive solid surfaces commonly result in foot lesions. Concrete is probably the major

culprit, especially around artificial ponds where slipping and scraping as the birds enter the pond may exacerbate the problem. The use of wire flooring is commonly linked to foot lesions in chickens
- Hygiene – unhygienic conditions encourage bacterial colonization. Waterfowl may be more susceptible to pododermatitis in excessively dry conditions, as their feet may become bruised on dry ground and microcracks may form in the skin; whereas other species of poultry may be more susceptible to pododermatitis in excessively wet conditions
- Underlying skin conditions – underlying conditions affect weight-bearing as well as disrupt the integrity of the skin surface. Scaly leg (see above) is very commonly seen with pododermatitis
- Foot injuries – injuries affect weight-bearing in the contralateral limb and wounds may allow the entry of bacteria into the subcutaneous tissues
- Bodyweight – obese animals are particularly prone to pododermatitis and this makes treatment more difficult. Lesions in turkeys appear especially intractable
- Lack of movement – birds that do not move around very much are at an increased risk of pododermatitis. This lack of movement may reflect the underlying disease (e.g. osteoarthritis) or an environment without adequate stimulation (see Chapter 19). In waterfowl, failure to provide water deep enough for swimming also predisposes to pododermatitis.

Treatment

Systemic antibacterials are indicated in all cases with granuloma and/or abscess formation. Ideally, drug selection should be based on the results of culture and sensitivity testing. Swabs or biopsy specimens for culture should be obtained for the deeper parts of the lesion, as surface samples can be affected by environmental contaminants. Before the test results are received, it is appropriate to start presumptive therapy based on the most likely isolate. Some texts suggest that *Staphylococcus* spp. are almost exclusively involved; however, in reality, it appears that there is a wide range of potential bacterial pathogens that can cause pododermatitis, including *Escherichia coli*. In most cases, co-amoxiclav at a dose of 125–150 mg/kg orally q12h is a good way to initiate treatment, and can be amended based on laboratory results and clinical response. Analgesia is indicated in all cases. Non-steroidal anti-inflammatory drugs (NSAIDs; e.g. meloxicam) appear most useful. Analgesia will encourage movement and thereby improve haemodynamic flow in the feet. Topical treatments may also help to treat pododermatitis, including:

- Barrier creams (e.g. silver sulfadiazine or F10 ointment)
- Hydrophilic gels.

The choice of treatment depends on how open the lesions on the feet are and the likely level of infection and/or contamination. In many cases, depending on the class of the lesion (see Chapter 18), antimicrobial drugs, analgesia and topical creams or gels will be sufficient (over several weeks) to resolve the condition, as long as the underlying environmental factors are corrected:

- The substrate should be improved. Concrete and wire flooring should be avoided and deep litter (paper or hay and straw) provided. The substrate should not be too wet or dry, depending on the species of bird. Where ponds are lined with concrete, the use of rubber mats (either covering the whole pond or just where the birds spend the majority of their time, and where they enter and leave the water) can be helpful
- Environmental hygiene should be improved
- Any underlying diseases should be treated (e.g. provision of analgesia in cases of osteoarthritis or ivermectin for cases of scaly leg)
- Environmental and feeding enrichment should be provided to encourage movement. Waterfowl should be encouraged on to the water, so they spend as much time as possible swimming, thereby reducing weight-bearing on the feet
- The bodyweight of obese birds should be reduced in a controlled manner.

Where the above treatments are ineffective or the lesions are extensive, surgery may be indicated (see Chapter 23).

Conditions of the claws

The claws can be damaged and broken. Damaged or broken claws should be managed in poultry as for other bird species, with bleeding treated by cautery. If the haemorrhage cannot be controlled or there is extensive infection, surgical amputation of the toe may be required. Antibiosis and analgesia should be administered as indicated on an individual basis. Claw overgrowth is uncommon.

However, this may occur if there is insufficient wear or as a sequel to claw damage and/or infection. Claws of poultry can be clipped as for other bird species.

Neoplasia

A variety of tumours may affect the skin of poultry species. Subcutaneous tumours include haemangiopericytomas, lipomas and liposarcomas. These tumours should be diagnosed via biopsy and treated as in other species. Excision should be curative unless the tumour has metastasized. The decision to perform surgery should be based on the tumour type, the size of the tumour and the ability to close the skin defect. Avian leucosis virus is associated with some subcutaneous tumours (fibromas, fibrosarcomas, myxomas and myxosarcomas) and should be suspected when these tumour types are identified, especially when seen in more than one bird in the flock. Cutaneous tumours include:

- Squamous cell carcinoma – reasonably common and may be a sequel to chronic irritation and/or infection. Excision is relatively curative but in most cases the mass is too extensive to allow excision
- Feather folliculoma – this neoplasm is also referred to as a 'feather cyst' and is ideally treated by excision. (However, where cost is a problem, incision and evacuation of inspissated cyst material will alleviate discomfort, although this is not curative)
- Epithelioma
- Adenoma of the uropygial gland – if removed from waterfowl, careful attention should be paid postoperatively to feather waterproofing.

Wounds

Wounds are commonly seen in poultry and are often caused by a dog or fox attack, or by the spurs of a cockerel (see Chapter 19). Scalping of the head may occur following particularly aggressive pecking from other birds. If fresh, wounds may be cleaned and repaired in a conventional fashion (see Chapter 23). However, in most cases, wounds are contaminated and skin retraction and granulation may have already started. There may also be skin deficits. However, even very deep extensive wounds will heal well by secondary intention. In these cases, the bird should be anaesthetized and the wound thoroughly cleaned. Where possible, the skin should be closed in a conventional manner. Open areas may then be encouraged to granulate, either by regular cleaning and the application of hydrophilic gels or Manuka honey preparations, or by suturing pads over the defect. If using the latter method, the bird will require periodic anaesthesia to change the pad. Antibiotic cover (the author prefers co-amoxiclav) should be maintained until the granulation bed has formed.

References and further reading

Bailey T and Lloyd C (2008) Raptors: disorders of the feet. In: *BSAVA Manual of Raptors, Pigeons and Passerine Birds*, ed. J Chitty and M Lierz, pp. 176–189. BSAVA Publications, Gloucester

Chitty J (2005) Feather and skin disorders. In: *BSAVA Manual of Psittacine Birds, 2nd edn*, ed. N Harcourt-Brown and J Chitty, pp. 191–204. BSAVA Publications, Gloucester

Lucas AM and Stettenheim PR (1972) *Avian Anatomy: Integument Parts 1 & 2*. US Department of Agriculture, USA

Chapter 14

Ophthalmological and otic disorders

David L. Williams

Eyes

Very few diseases in poultry solely affect the eye, whereas many systemic diseases have ocular manifestations. Due to this, few comparative ophthalmologists have detailed knowledge of poultry ophthalmology, and extrapolation from what is known about the mammalian eye may not be appropriate given the considerable differences in anatomy and pathological responses to disease agents. The small size of the eye of commonly kept backyard poultry also complicates efforts to deal with ocular disease in these species.

However, the chick eye has been used extensively as a model for research in vision and some of this work can be used to gain an understanding of pathology that affects the eyes of poultry. Research into accommodation and the development of myopia has used the chick eye as a model (Lauber, 1991), whilst chick and quail eyes have been used extensively in understanding the normal development of the eye and problems in such defects as microphthalmia (Ehrlich *et al.*, 1989). The chicken cornea has been used in research on corneal ulcer healing (Ritchey *et al.*, 2011) and for refractive surgery, with the most recent studies investigating responses to laser-assisted keratomileusis (LASIK).

The vast majority of published work on eye diseases in poultry concerns birds in commercial flocks, rather than backyard poultry. However, there is a body of research concerned with poultry within the context of subsistence farming. In many regards, these studies have more in common with backyard poultry than commercial flocks, despite the substantial differences in climatic conditions that might apply, and as a result may prove particularly useful when treating poultry for ophthalmic conditions on an individual basis.

Normal anatomy

The avian eye (Figure 14.1) has a number of differences in anatomy from the mammalian eye, several of which have considerable consequences with regard to the diagnosis and treatment of ocular conditions in backyard poultry. Perhaps the most important difference is not in the globe itself but in the surrounding structures. The sinuses around the eye (Figure 14.2), particularly the infraorbital sinuses, impinge on the globe and pathology in these structures may have a significant impact on the eye. The glands of the orbit include the Harderian gland and lacrimal gland. These glands are important not only in production of ocular surface secretion, but also in immunological activity at the

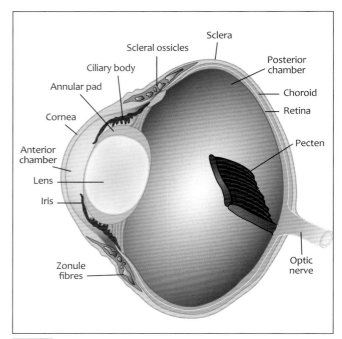

14.1 Cross-section of the avian eye.

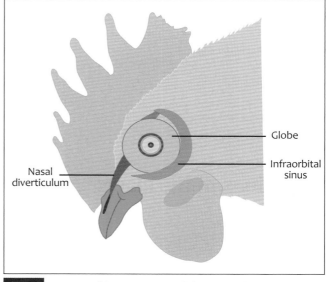

14.2 Location of the sinuses around the eye in a chicken.

ocular surface. In the eye itself, a ring of bony plates or ossicles supports the eye immediately behind the limbus. These ossicles and the role of the globe in maintaining the structure of the skull are of particular importance when considering enucleation or evisceration of the eye.

The conjunctiva has a similar appearance to that of mammals, but its population of immune cells plays an important role in systemic immunity (van Ginkel *et al.*, 2012). Conjunctival-associated lymphoid tissue is part of the more general mucosal-associated lymphoid tissue and has been particularly well characterized in bird species. Its presence allows successful vaccination using eye drop formulations of important pathogens such as Newcastle disease virus (Thekisoe *et al.*, 2004).

The globe in birds is an anterior–posteriorly flattened spheroid with a relatively wide cornea (see Figure 14.1) compared with the mammalian eye. There are also significant differences in the cornea, iris and posterior segment, which need to be taken into consideration when evaluating the structures of the avian eye. Like the human eye, but in contrast to most commonly encountered veterinary species, the avian cornea possesses a Bowman's layer. This is an acellular layer of immediately subepithelial stroma. It is difficult to know what influence this acellular layer has on corneal physiology, but the cornea of chickens and turkeys is remarkably thin. A study using ultrasonic pachymetry estimated the corneal thickness in adult White Leghorn chickens to be 0.25 mm (compared with 0.55 mm in the dog) (Montiani-Ferreira *et al.*, 2004), which may explain why backyard poultry appear to be relatively susceptible to penetrating injuries from trauma by compatriots or foreign bodies such as hay awns. Keratoglobus (an abnormal curvature of the central cornea) has been reported in commercial broilers, but is unlikely to be seen in backyard poultry (Landman *et al.*, 1998).

The avian iris comprises striated rather than smooth muscle and so is under conscious rather than autonomic nervous control (Yamashita and Sohal, 1986). This means that birds can communicate through voluntary rapid pupil dilatation and constriction, and may account for the bright coloration of the iris (Figure 14.3). The small size of the eyes in poultry species requires the lens to be spherical to give the shortest possible focal distance. The equator of the lens is firmly attached to the ciliary body to allow accommodation.

Of particular note is the marked difference between the posterior segments of the avian and mammalian eye. Birds have an avascular retina devoid of blood vessels. Instead, it is believed that the pecten provides oxygen and nutrients

to this highly metabolically active tissue. It is a pleated, comb-like structure that is vascular and pigmented like the choroid, the structure from which it arises. It is believed that small movements of the globe waft the pecten through the fluid posterior vitreous, allowing oxygen and nutrients to diffuse to the retinal periphery (Pettigrew *et al.*, 1990). The role of the pecten, however, is debated. In one study, chickens that underwent experimental ablation of the pecten did not show evidence of blindness, but did demonstrate an increase in vitreal pH, suggesting that the pecten has a role in pH regulation of the posterior segment (Brach, 1975).

Vision

Birds see in three primary colours, with ultraviolet cones in addition to the trichromatic photoreceptors (red, green and blue) encountered in humans. The colour vision of birds relies on both the absorptive properties of the visual photopigments and on the filtering effects of oil droplets residing in the cone cells. Being diurnal, chickens have a high rod:cone ratio. Unlike many other bird species, chickens do not appear to have an obvious macula for high visual resolution (Wood, 1917). They do, however, have a histologically apparent area centralis, which is a target site for efferent or centrifugal neurons from the midbrain and a retinal feature unique to birds. In his book, Wood illustrates the retinal detail of a vast range of birds, including the Brush turkey (Figure 14.4a), the Harlequin quail (Figure 14.4b), the Black-bellied duck (Figure 14.4c) and the quite beautiful retinal detail of the Blue snow goose (Figure 14.4d) but, surprisingly, not the chicken.

In avian species such as chickens where pecking for food close-up requires short-sighted vision but being aware of potential predators necessitates long-distance vision of the horizon, the eye is adapted to allow down gaze myopia but up gaze emmetropia. The refractive state of the eye is varied to match the viewing distances of different areas of the visual field (Shaeffel *et al.*, 1994).

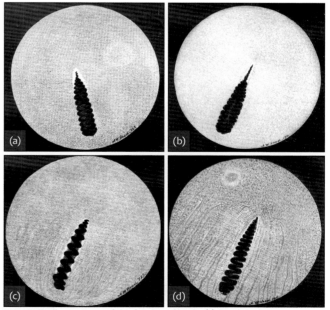

14.4 Illustrations of the fundus of birds. (a) Brush turkey. (b) Harlequin quail. (c) Black-bellied duck. (d) Blue snow goose. Note the variations in the form of the pecten in the four illustrations, and the area centralis or fovea in the Blue snow goose illustration.
(Reproduced from Wood (1917))

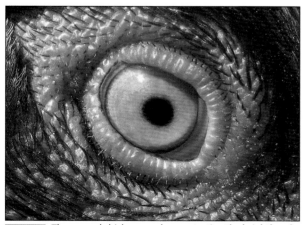

14.3 The normal chicken eye demonstrating the brightly coloured iris.

Estimates of the visual acuity of the chicken vary from between 1.9 and 2.2 cycles per degree (c/d) (DeMello *et al.*, 1992) to between 6.6 and 8 c/d (with a snellen equivalence of around 20/80). This is significantly better than that of rodents (1.5–2 c/d), comparable with those of cats or 5-month-old humans, and around a quarter to a fifth of that of adult humans. Gover *et al.* (2009) have shown that acuity is greater at higher light intensities. At the highest luminance level where cones provide visual function, acuity was measured at 6.5 c/d, reducing to 3.2 c/d at scotopic light intensities where rods account for vision.

Ophthalmological examination

Direct ophthalmoscopy is easily achieved in the consulting room or off-site.

1. Performing distant direct ophthalmoscopy with the ophthalmoscope held 20 cm away from the bird's head (Figure 14.5) and with the setting at 0 dioptres will reveal whether corneal or lens opacity is present.
2. Keeping the setting at 0 dioptres, closer assessment of the eye (approximately 5 cm from the head) will show the retina with a pink/orange reflex associated with the choroidal blood vessels, and the black or brown pleated pecten protruding from the posterior pole of the eye.
3. Move the setting on the ophthalmoscope to 10 dioptres and hold it at a distance of 10 cm from the surface of the eye. This will provide a magnified view of the lens and iris and show any cataracts in more detail.
4. Move the setting on the ophthalmoscope to 20 dioptres and hold it at a distance of 5 cm from the surface of the eye. This will provide a magnified view of the cornea and adnexa.

The small size of the eye in backyard poultry means that the slit lamp biomicroscope is a particularly valuable tool for examining the eyes of chickens, ducks and quail. This instrument provides a highly magnified view and the opportunity of forming an optical cross-section of the cornea and lens, but is not available in the majority of practices.

Ancillary tests in the examination of the eye in any species should include measurement of tear production with the Schirmer tear test and of intraocular pressure (IOP) by tonometry. One study on over 100 3-week-old chicks gives an IOP of 17.5 ± 0.1 mmHg using the Tonovet rebound tonometer (Figure 14.6) (Prashar *et al.*, 2007), but there are no published reports on the IOP in adult birds. A preliminary study performed by the author on 100 backyard hens

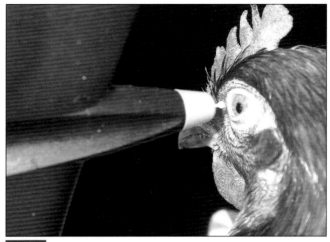

14.6 Use of the Tonovet rebound tonometer.

showed a considerably lower IOP with an average of 11.4 ± 1.2 mmHg; the study also demonstrated that the IOP reduced with age, being 12.7 ± 1 mmHg in birds 1.5 years old and 10.6 ± 0.9 mmHg in birds of 7 years of age, with a logarithmic function curve that might well allow for a much higher IOP in young chicks.

A substantial body of work exists on the production of immunoglobulins in tears by the Harderian gland (Baba *et al.*, 1990) and the value of vaccination for conditions such as Newcastle disease by eye drop on to the ocular surface (Thekisoe *et al.*, 2004). Despite this work, there are no published data on normal tear production as measured by the Schirmer tear test in any poultry species. In a preliminary study of backyard chickens by the author, a mean Schirmer tear test of 10.7 ± 1.7 mm/min was obtained using a modified Schirmer tear test strip (Figure 14.7). The major problem with using a standard Schirmer tear test strip is that in the small eyes of backyard poultry, the sizable curved end of the strip does not fit well into the lower conjunctival sac and causes considerable irritation. The study conducted by the author attempted to overcome this problem by reducing the width of the end of the strip and placing it under the upper eyelid (there is less movement in the upper lid than the lower lid) (Figure 14.8).

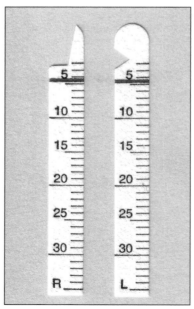

14.7 Modified Schirmer tear test strip (left) for use in backyard poultry. The normal tear test strip (right) is shown for comparison.

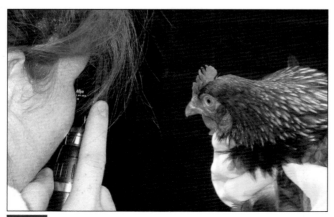

14.5 Examination of the eye using distant direct ophthalmoscopy.

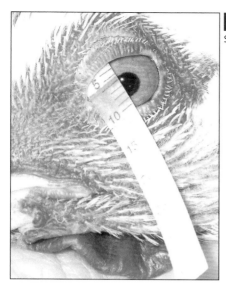

14.8 Use of the modified Schirmer tear test strip.

Clinical signs of disease

Adnexal disease

The majority of ocular diseases in non-commercial poultry involve the adnexal structures, from conjunctivitis to sinusitis, and recognizing the subtle signs of early disease in these periocular tissues can be very important for ensuring that the condition does not progress to the point where it becomes a significant health and welfare problem.

Sinusitis: As noted above, the cranial sinuses abut directly around the globe and thus inflammation of these structures (which is commonly seen in respiratory disease) has a profound influence on the eye. Mild upper respiratory disease causes nothing more than slight sinus enlargement (Figure 14.9a), which is evident as periorbital swelling, and particularly noted with regard to the diverticulum of the infraorbital sinus below the eye. With increasing severity, the inflammatory exudate closes the narrow entrance to the sinus and the inflammatory deposit becomes a 'fibricess' (Huchzermeyer and Cooper, 2000), with significant swelling of the sinuses either confined to the infraorbital sinus or extending around the eye (Figure 14.9bc). The heterophilic cell population forms a caseous mass rather than the liquid pus seen in mammals (Montali, 1988), requiring surgical resection rather than just a lancing incision, as might be sufficient in, for example, a cat.

As sinusitis is not only a direct local problem but also a sign of respiratory disease, it should not be ignored. A substantial number of different infectious organisms can

lead to sinusitis. Cytology, culture and sensitivity testing, as well as virus isolation and polymerase chain reaction (PCR) techniques should be employed to try and identify the microorganism responsible for the infection. Where it is not practical to determine the agent responsible through laboratory diagnosis, a presumptive diagnosis may be achievable based on the history and the bird can be treated accordingly. For example, where mycoplasmosis is suspected, authorized antibiotics such as tiamulin, tylosin or tilmicosin should be used. When a specific aetiology cannot be determined, the use of broad-spectrum antibiotics may be beneficial, particularly in the early stages of the disease. Once a caseous mass has formed in the sinus, drug penetration is very poor and successful treatment is difficult or impossible. Affected birds should be quarantined away from the rest of the flock, as many aetiological agents are highly contagious; however, this may be to no avail since agents such as *Mycoplasma* may be endemic in the flock and only causing problems in birds with an otherwise weakened immune system.

The infraorbital sinus can become so enlarged that its upward swelling closes the eyelids (see Figure 14.9b) and renders the animal blind on that side. In bilateral cases, which most are, this can lead to a total loss of vision. In these instances, birds have to be fed by hand and attempts to remove the inflammatory mass from the sinuses should be made. However, the masses are often so solid that curettage to promote dehiscence can be difficult. Even if curettage is possible, the large size of the inflammatory mass often pulls the periorbital tissues such that after removal the palpebral aperture is stretched sufficiently that it no longer apposes the anterior face of the globe.

Congenital abnormalities

Congenital abnormalities that might lead to death in the wild or euthanasia in a commercial setting, such as congenital microphthalmos, anophthalmos and cataract, may be tolerable in the context of pet poultry. Affected birds may need to be hand-reared and careful consideration must be given to the welfare needs of the individual, in particular the freedom to fulfil its natural behaviour. According to the Animal Welfare Act (2006) it is unlawful to keep an animal if one cannot fulfil its five freedoms, including freedom to avoid hunger and thirst, discomfort, pain, injury or disease, fear and distress, and freedom to fulfil its natural behaviours. Whether a blind chicken with severe microphthalmos or anophthalmos (Ehrlich *et al.*, 1989; Figure 14.10) can have what the Farm Animal Welfare Council considers 'a good life' or even 'a life worth living' (Green and Mellor, 2011) is unclear, although some pet poultry owners would argue that with care and attention

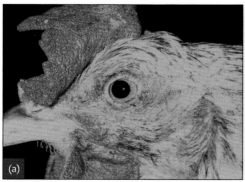
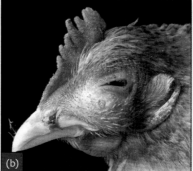
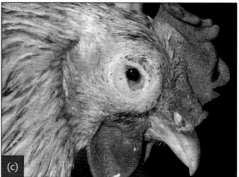

14.9 Sinus enlargement in disease states. (a) Slight infraorbital enlargement in mild respiratory disease. (b) More severe infraorbital sinus enlargement. (c) Sinus enlargement around the entire globe.

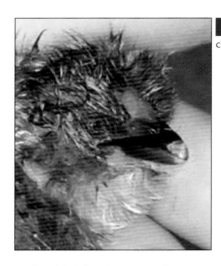

14.10 Anophthalmos in a 3-day-old chick.

such a bird that has never known any different can lead a fulfilled life. Legislation regarding animal welfare is discussed in Chapter 26.

Corneal ulceration

Erosion of the corneal epithelium or deeper involvement of the stroma can occur after external trauma or as a result of abrasion from swollen eyelids (Figure 14.11). In most cases profuse lacrimation is seen, which could be considered to be exactly what the ocular surface needs to maintain lubrication, as well as immunological support, given that immunoglobulin A is produced by lymphocytes in the Harderian gland. Topical antibiotics in a tear replacement base are ideal in such situations; as the bacterial populations in a backyard population are predominantly Gram-negative enterobacteria, an antibiotic such as gentamicin is recommended (rather than fusidic aid which is used in dogs and cats, as it is only active against Gram-positive cocci). In addition, the use of fusidic acid in poultry is not permitted under the prescribing cascade and it should be noted that the use of chloramphenicol is prohibited in poultry in the European Union. It should also be borne in mind that it is impossible to specify an appropriate withdrawal period for a medication such as a topical antibiotic without a relevant study, and unfortunately these are currently not available for such drugs.

In most cases, if perforation does occur, the fibrinoid aqueous resulting from such a trauma rapidly plugs the defect. In more severe cases, the iris can protrude through the perforation resulting in a staphyloma. In such cases,

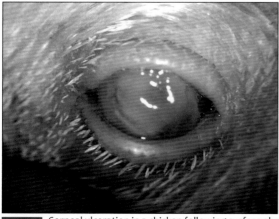

14.11 Corneal ulceration in a chicken following surface abrasion. (Courtesy of Dr N Biucimchi)

ocular evisceration (rather than enucleation) may be best option in order to relieve the pain resulting both from the trauma itself and the consequential long-term uveitis. The problem with enucleation is that as the globe occupies such a large proportion of the cranial volume, the removal of one eye leaves a large area of dead space and a potentially unbalanced bird. For this reason, evisceration (see below) is preferred.

Uveitis

Many, if not all, cases of corneal ulceration have a degree of uveitis, but intraocular inflammation can also occur when systemic bacterial infection leads to septicaemia. Pupil constriction and the presence of purulent material in the anterior chamber (hypopyon) are characteristic signs of severe uveitis. Earlier signs of uveitis include reddening of the iris (Figure 14.12) as a result of neovascularization; this condition used to be known as rubeosis iridis, but is now termed pre-iridal fibrovascular membrane. Often irritation associated with more severe inflammation can result in the eyelids being closed, and it can be difficult to differentiate this condition from severe conjunctivitis. Typically, there is less discharge between the closed eyelids in uveitis alone than in cases of conjunctivitis severe enough to cause blepharospasm.

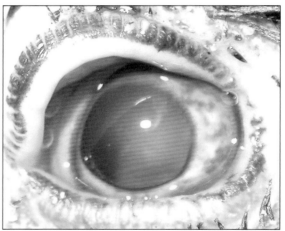

14.12 Reddening of the iris in early uveitis in a chicken with cataract (both conditions are probably associated with trauma).

Causes of disease
Infectious diseases

Infectious agents are a common cause of ocular disease in both commercial flocks and backyard birds. Mycoplasma and other bacterial species are most commonly implicated, but there are also several important viral agents that should be considered.

Viral infections:
Fowlpox: This condition, also known as avian pox, has different clinical characteristics in different species of bird. In chickens, it is characterized in the cutaneous form ('dry' form) by proliferative nodules on the unfeathered parts of the body, including the eyelid margins, whilst the fibrinoproliferative form ('wet' form) is characterized by necrotic lesions of the upper respiratory tract and gastrointestinal system.

The ocular lesions, if present at the lid margin, may involve nodules large enough to preclude vision (Figure 14.13). Such lesions are normally bacteriologically sterile,

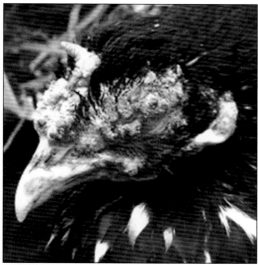

14.13 Cutaneous form of fowlpox in a chicken.
(Courtesy of V Roberts)

but secondary infections can result in hyperaemia and the accumulation of fibrinous exudate with increased lacrimation. Normally the globe itself is not affected, but trauma to the periocular area can occur if the lesions become pruritic, and in such cases damage to the eye itself may be seen. The diagnosis is normally made based on the characteristic appearance of the lesions and can be confirmed by cytological examination of impression smears obtained from the nodules. Biopsy is also diagnostic, but is perhaps best avoided since this can result in significant haemorrhage. Virus isolation is not generally required for diagnosis.

Marek's disease: This is a common lymphoproliferative condition caused by a herpesvirus with a tropism for neural tissue and lymphocytes. The proliferation of lymphocytes in the iris causes depigmentation, resulting in the condition being known by the colloquial terms 'grey eye' and 'pearly eye'. In the early stages of the disease, there may be a mixed lymphocyte and heterophil infiltrate around the peripheral capillaries of the iris, and iridal redness. More severe uveitis can involve hypopyon, hyphaema or synechiae with abnormally shaped pupils. Similar infiltrates can be seen in the choroid, ciliary body and pecten. Lens changes, including cataracts, may form with diffuse degeneration or coagulative necrosis, although the pathogenesis is unclear. Secondary glaucoma has been reported in cases where inflammatory cells have obliterated the iridocorneal angle drainage, although this is rare. Conjunctival swelling and thickening of the third eyelid can also occur. The ocular signs of Marek's disease may often be overlooked due to the obvious signs of paralysis, but they can be helpful in suggesting or supporting the diagnosis. Sheets of neoplastic lymphocytes may be found throughout the conjunctiva on histopathology, as well as the uvea and optic nerves. Whilst the diagnosis can usually be made on the clinical signs alone, confirmation can be achieved by isolation of the virus from the aqueous humour (Pandiri *et al.*, 2008).

Avian encephalomyelitis: As with Marek's disease, the ocular signs of avian encephalomyelitis are often missed due to the more prominent neurological presentation. The causative RNA virus causes epidemic tremors in young chickens, turkeys and pheasants, in most cases before the age of 5–6 weeks old (although it has been recorded in

birds up to 17 weeks old). Morbidity is usually reported to be 15% of the flock and mortality in affected birds is high. Corneal opacity and cataract formation are commonly seen in young chicks and turkey poults. These changes are caused by lymphoid proliferation and infiltration of the cornea, and lens epithelial proliferation. Iridal pallor with leucocoria (a cataractous lens that appears white through the pupil) is seen with changes involving lens epithelial necrosis with later proliferation of the anterior lens epithelium and formation of Morganian globules (deposits of protein from lens fibre degeneration). Cataracts in these patients can resemble a collapsed sac full of these globules within fluid from the degenerating lens cortex.

Avian influenza: Many viral diseases result in lacrimation, blepharitis and conjunctivitis (Figure 14.14); intraocular inflammation is sometimes also seen. Avian influenza is characterized by respiratory signs and high mortality, and the ocular signs noted include lacrimation, eyelid oedema, conjunctival petechiation and periocular oedema with a characteristic yellow tinge. Lymphoplasmacytic infiltration of the uvea and optic nerve with episcleral congestion is accompanied by a granulomatous blepharitis with vascular thrombosis in conjunctival blood vessels and vasculitis of vessels at the limbus. In addition to lymphoid proliferation and heterophil infiltration, these lid changes can occur as a result of periocular vasculitis and myonecrosis, often with concurrent bacterial infection. Given the severity of this disease and its potentially zoonotic and highly contagious nature, avian influenza is a notifiable disease and confirmation of the diagnosis is urgently required by serological tests or direct viral isolation from conjunctival swabs.

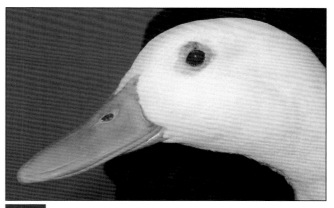

14.14 Conjunctivitis in a duck.

Newcastle disease: This is a highly contagious paramyxoviral condition that results in a drop in egg production and neurological signs; there is also a foamy ocular discharge, congestion, haemorrhage, oedema and necrosis of the conjunctiva and lids with velogenic strains; sometimes the eyelids are sealed shut and there is an associated opacity of the cornea and lens. Mesogenic strains result in respiratory signs rather than neurological ones, and thus the only ocular sign may be lacrimation, perhaps accompanied by foamy exudate in mild disease. Viral isolation from the aqueous humour is possible, but serology is more commonly used to confirm the diagnosis.

Infectious laryngotracheitis: This is an acute respiratory condition in chickens, pheasants and peafowl, and results in dyspnoea and serous ocular and nasal discharge, which may become purulent with secondary bacterial infection.

Conjunctival haemorrhage and hyperplastic conjunctival mucosa may also be seen. Histopathologically, the lesions are characterized by a heterophilic infiltrate and hyperplastic conjunctiva mucosa with syncytium formation in the epithelial cells, often including intranuclear inclusion bodies. Viral isolation is required to confirm the diagnosis.

Infectious bronchitis: This is a highly contagious coronavirus infection in turkeys and a co-pathogen in chickens. It causes a drop in egg production, as well as increased lacrimation and, on occasion, foamy discharge and periocular exudate. Concurrent infection with coliform bacteria leads to conjunctival hyperplasia and episcleritis, as part of a condition termed 'swollen head syndrome', with fibrino-heterophilic conjunctival inflammation. Serology and, on occasion, viral isolation provide a definitive diagnosis.

Duck enteritis: This is an acute contagious herpetic disease and is manifest in the eye by lacrimation, conjunctival congestion, photophobia and, in severe cases, the eyelids sealed shut. It occurs in ducks, geese and swans, in particular Muscovy ducks and Canadian geese. Corneal necrosis can be seen with ulceration of the corneal epithelium. This condition must be differentiated from an undetermined viral disease seen in goslings with a high mortality rate.

Notifiable diseases: Since avian viruses tend to be highly contagious, and both Newcastle disease and avian influenza are notifiable in the UK (other diseases may also be notifiable in other countries), determination of the causative agent responsible for the lacrimation, conjunctivitis and blepharitis is important. This may require histopathological investigation, virus isolation and culture of samples obtained from a euthanased affected individual. Veterinary surgeons (veterinarians) and keepers must ensure that they comply with local regulations with regard to the reporting of cases of birds possibly infected with notifiable diseases.

Bacterial infections: Bacterial infections of the periocular region and sinuses are far more prevalent than viral diseases. Details of the systemic pathology and diagnosis of these conditions can be found elsewhere in this manual; this chapter concentrates on the ocular signs and histopathology that lead to the differential diagnosis. Many bacterial agents can cause conjunctivitis.

- *Escherichia coli* causes systemic infection, with ocular lesions particularly seen in young birds, and manifests as a suppurative intraocular infection with corneal opacity and exudate in the anterior chamber, progressing to inflammation throughout the eye (panophthalmitis). *E. coli*-related disease is controlled through the use of antibiotics, including tylosin and amoxicillin. As noted above, coliform infection complicating viral diseases such as avian pneumovirus results in swollen head syndrome.
- *Salmonella* infection results in a dull appearance to the ocular surface, as well as a cloudy cornea and caseous exudate in the conjunctiva, which commonly leads to uveitis involving the iris, ciliary body and choroid, and subsequently panophthalmitis and complete blindness.
- Fowl cholera (caused by *Pasteurella multocida*) occurs predominantly in adult birds and is characterized by swollen and closed eyelids and periorbital swelling with discharge. Uveitis with synechiae and an anterior chamber exudate can occur, but is rarer. This often affects only one eye, but may be bilateral on occasion. Treatment for fowl cholera is described in Chapter 15.

- *Riemerella anatipestifer* is a bacterium closely related to the Pasteurellaceae and has been reported as causing infectious polyserositis in ducklings, with or without periocular swelling and uveitis (Leavitt and Ayroud, 1997).
- *Staphylococcus* spp. result in a fibrinosuppurative blepharitis and conjunctivitis in chickens, turkeys and quail. Systemic antibiosis following culture and sensitivity testing can resolve the lesions.
- *Bordetella* spp. cause upper respiratory infections in turkeys, with ocular and nasal discharge; dyspnoea and stunted growth are far more important signs than the ocular lesions. The treatment of *Bordetella* is described in Chapter 15.
- *Avibacterium paragallinarum* results in ocular and nasal discharge in chickens, along with subcutaneous oedema, swollen eyelids and a foamy discharge from the conjunctiva. For further information on treatment, see Chapter 15.
- *Chlamydophila psittaci* may cause blepharospasm, lacrimation and a serofibrinous or purulent discharge. This disease (known as ornithosis in non-psittacine birds) is characterized in turkeys by a unique swelling above the eye, resulting from severe inflammation of the supraorbital glands (also termed the nasal or salt glands), lying dorsomedial to the globe. For treatment protocols, the reader is referred to Chapter 15. *Chlamydophila psittaci* is highly zoonotic (causing psittacosis in humans) and appropriate measures must be taken to protect both owners and staff.
- Mycoplasmosis is predominantly a respiratory condition, but periorbital inflammation with swelling, lacrimation (often with a foamy appearance) and conjunctival vessel swelling may be seen. Keratoconjunctivitis has been reported with *Mycoplasma gallisepticum* in chickens (Nunoya et al., 1995). Often ocular lesions caused by *Mycoplasma* spp. are complicated by coliform infection, resulting in a caseous exudate. Mycoplasmosis is less common in backyard poultry than in commercial flocks, where overcrowding predisposes to transmission of infection. Ocular signs are commonly seen in pheasants and guinea fowl, where morbidity and mortality can be significantly higher than that seen in chickens and turkeys housed together (Bencina et al., 2003). The treatment and control of this condition is discussed further in Chapter 15.

Fungal infections: *Aspergillus fumigatus* and, less commonly, *A. flavus* can give rise to respiratory signs with a yellow caseous discharge from the eyes, resulting in swollen lids and cloudy corneal lesions. *Aspergillus*, a common cause of air sacculitis, can also result in infraorbital sinusitis. *A. fumigatus* has been reported to cause keratitis with subsequent intraocular invasion in a commercial facility. Whilst such infection may be seen in backyard poultry, progression to severe, sight-threatening disease is less likely with careful examination of individual animals; this is a good reason for careful flock examination.

Ocular lesions caused by candidiasis have been reported in ducks and, together with other fungal species, give rise to so-called avian ringworm, which affects the periocular skin, resulting in an appearance of 'fine flour sprinkled around the eye'. The diagnosis is confirmed by cytology and topical treatment with miconazole is effective. Readers are directed to Chapter 13 for further information.

Parasitic diseases: Toxoplasmosis results in a watery ocular discharge with swollen conjunctiva, as well as optic neuritis and blindness. Although seroconversion has been reported in the UK and Europe, the main disease seems to be identified in the Far East and South America, with a variety of bird species from turkeys to guinea fowl showing little in the way of clinical signs.

Cryptosporidiosis is a common condition in chickens and turkeys, but rarely gives rise to ocular signs in these species; however, in pheasants, ducks and peacocks, oculonasal discharge may be seen, along with corneal opacities in peacock chicks with severe chemosis. Further information can be found in Chapter 15.

Helminths of the order Oxyspirura and trematodes of the family Philophthalmidae can cause clinical signs ranging from mild conjunctivitis with a light *Oxyspirura mansoni* infestation to pronounced lacrimation and loss of body condition, as reported in severely affected ostriches in Florida; these signs can also be seen in other avian species, more commonly in warmer climes.

Cataracts

Lens opacities can arise due to infectious agents such as avian encephalomyelitis virus, Marek's disease virus, Newcastle disease virus and *E. coli* (see above). Cataracts may also occur due to nutritional deficiencies or have a hereditary basis, but most are likely to be age-related. It is for this reason that spontaneously occurring cataracts are rarely seen in relatively short-lived commercially reared birds.

A study of backyard hens by the author found the prevalence of cataracts to be low (<10% of hens aged 7–8 years old were affected by lens opacities). Many of the opacities identified in these birds may be associated with trauma (see Figure 14.12). Further research is needed in this area to confirm that cataracts are not a common problem in backyard poultry.

Retinal disease

Blindness caused by retinal disease is rare, although inherited defects have been reported (Curtis *et al.*, 1987). In birds that are blind as a result of retinal disease, an unusual syndrome of ocular enlargement occurs (Wilkinson *et al.*, 1991). This has been studied in detail in the hope that it will help understanding of globe enlargement in glaucoma.

Trauma

Injury from pecking or due to compatriots' spurs is relatively commonly seen in backyard poultry, especially with high stocking densities. Such injuries can result in corneal ulceration, opacity or even penetration.

Ankyloblepharon (where the eyelids fuse together, yielding a small palpebral aperture) can occur after lid injury (Figure 14.15) in any bird. Treatment is difficult as any surgical intervention appears to exacerbate the centripetal growth of the conjunctiva, further fusing together over the ocular surface.

Neoplasia

Neoplastic transformation is possible in any of the tissues of or around the avian globe, but such lesions are rarely reported. Dukes and Pettit (1983) documented ocular neoplasia in 21 chickens, 18 of which were lymphoproliferative lesions associated with Marek's disease. A third of the neoplasms involved orbital structures, predominantly the Harderian gland, whilst in five cases corneal infiltration was observed with or without corneal ulceration. In the

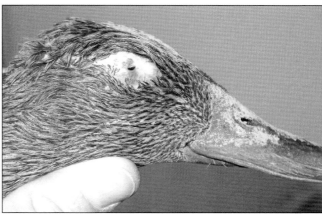

14.15 Ankyloblepharon as a result of lid regrowth following trauma in a duck.

majority of cases (14 birds), the iris was infiltrated and in seven cases cataract ensued. Retinal detachment or degeneration was only seen in three birds, and neoplastic infiltration of the optic nerve occurred in another three cases. Although uncommon, a diagnosis of spontaneous neoplasia (such as squamous cell carcinoma; Figure 14.16) should always be considered.

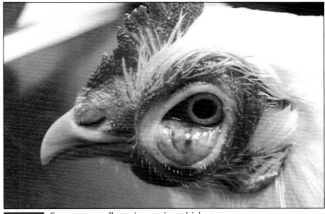

14.16 Squamous cell carcinoma in a chicken.
(Courtesy of V Roberts)

Ammonia toxicity

Occasionally seen with intensive poultry farming, conjunctivitis associated with high levels of ammonia can also be a problem in backyard poultry if sufficient care is not taken to clean out the house (Nimmermark *et al.*, 2003). Ammonia causes ocular irritation at concentrations >15 parts per million (Miles *et al.*, 2004; 2006). Measurement of ammonia levels may not be practical in a backyard setting, but any ammonia that can be smelled is indicative of excessive levels. Ocular lesions associated with ammonia toxicity are generally observed in young chickens with photophobia, lacrimation and conjunctival hyperaemia (Miles *et al.*, 2006). Birds generally sit with their eyes closed and lid swelling and oedema may be noted. A blue band in the inter-palpebral zone of the cornea is seen where epithelial devitalization and sloughing can occur. Remedying the environmental problem is essential on a flock basis but, for individual birds, lavage of the corneal surface and periorbital region reduces the irritation immediately.

Ocular surgery

Removal of the eye is, unfortunately, one of the main procedures performed by veterinary surgeons on poultry, whilst in other avian species surgery has ranged from cataract removal to corneal grafting. The avian eye takes up a considerable proportion of the cranial volume and is important in maintaining the structural integrity of the skull. This, together with the presence of scleral ossicles, which complicate the removal of the entire eye through the orbital face, renders evisceration a preferable option. The cornea is opened and a central disc of corneal tissue removed. The intraocular contents are removed with a curette or arrow swab and a pad of haemostatic felt is used to fill the globe. The lid margins are excised and the eyelids closed over the open face of the globe shell. This retains the volume component of the eye whilst alleviating the prolonged pain associated with uveitis or ocular surface disease. However, it should be noted that this technique is not appropriate where there is intraocular infection or neoplasia.

Ears

The chicken ear is widely used as a model for human auditory pathology, but is hardly noted at all in veterinary or poultry husbandry books. Its use as a model system is somewhat ironic, as the inner ear of birds differs from that of mammals, not only in its detailed anatomy, but also in its development and response to injury. Hair cells are essential for hearing and in mammals they are only produced during development. Thus, any damage to these cells, for example due to a loud noise, drug toxicity or infection, will result in permanent hearing loss. In birds and other non-mammalian vertebrates, however, the hair cells can be reformed from epithelial supporting cells.

Normal anatomy

The external ear canal of chickens and other poultry species is short, ending in a tympanic membrane that, like mammals, absorbs sound waves and transmits them to the inner ear fluids (Dooling *et al.*, 2000). Rather than the three ossicles of the mammalian ear, there are only two in birds: the columella and the stapes (Figure 14.17). A muscle attached to the tympanic membrane is activated when stimulated by tension from the membrane and attenuates the sound conducted to the labyrinth. Thus, in a rather different way to that of mammals, the avian middle ear acts as an impedance matching device that couples the energy of airborne sound waves to the movement of the fluid in the labyrinth (Saunders *et al.*, 2000).

As in all vertebrates, the auditory cavity of the avian ear has three chambers. The scala vestibuli and scala tympani contain perilymphatic fluid and lie on either side of the scala media, which contains endolymphatic fluid. The differences in sodium and potassium concentrations between the perilymph and endolymph maintain a voltage gradient (+15 mV), termed the endocochlear potential. The basilar papilla is the avian auditory receptor (compared with the organ of Corti in mammals), and in the domestic chicken it is an elongated curved structure approximately 3 mm in length. It consists of around 10,500 hair cells with associated supporting cells, nerve fibres, basement cells and the basilar membrane. The sensory band of the papilla is wide at the low-frequency end and narrows towards the high-frequency end.

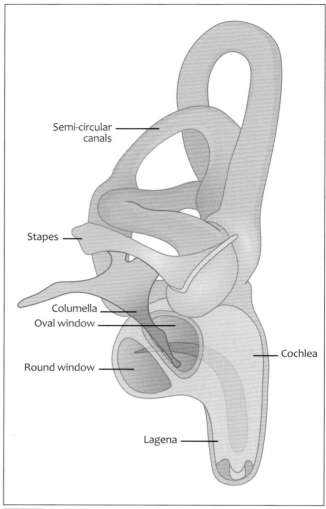

14.17 Anatomy of the ear of a chicken.

Labels: Semi-circular canals; Stapes; Columella; Oval window; Round window; Cochlea; Lagena

The noise levels in a commercial poultry house may be of sufficient intensity to cause hearing loss in birds (Smittkamp *et al.*, 2002). Cochlear degeneration has been shown to be much more severe in broilers than in layers, even at the same noise level, suggesting a genetic difference in susceptibility to cochlear damage (Durham *et al.*, 2002). Whilst the majority of research involving hearing in poultry focuses on pathology in the inner ear of chickens, most aural problems diagnosed in commercial and backyard flocks involve the external ear.

Infectious diseases

Birds will frequently present with a caseous plug in the auditory meatus, which is indicative of bacterial infection. The diagnosis can be confirmed with cytology. The associated inflammation can cause considerable irritation and affected individuals may self-traumatize the side of their head on wooden posts or other rough surfaces (Figure 14.18). Topical medication is unlikely to resolve such lesions and surgical debridement followed by packing with antibiotic ointment or systemic antibiotics may be necessary.

Inflammation of the inner ear (or labyrinthitis) often leads to vestibular signs with birds circling and presenting with a head tilt. *Pasteurella multocida* is often the causative agent in such cases and the resulting suppurative

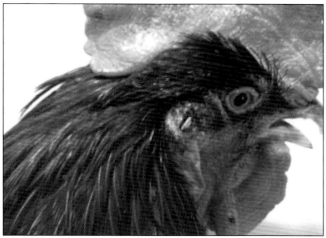

14.18 Crusting in and around the infected ear canal in a chicken.
(Courtesy of V Roberts)

reaction can be severe and very difficult to treat. Similarly, *Salmonella* species have been reported as causing otitis externa in turkey poults (Shivaprasad *et al.*, 2006). The clinical signs seen in affected birds include paralysis, opisthotonus, torticollis, blindness and meningitis. Newcastle disease can give rise to similar signs and should be high on the list of differential diagnoses in such cases. Systemic antibiosis and anti-inflammatory medication may be helpful in these birds; however, treatment is often unsuccessful and euthanasia may be the best option in terms of the animal's welfare if the signs persist and become severe.

Infection can also spread from the ear canal to cause osteomyelitis. This has been reported in partridges with *Ornithobacterium rhinotracheale* infection (Moreno *et al.*, 2009), although this organism more commonly causes lower respiratory tract disease in conjunction with other agents.

References and further reading

Baba T, Kawata T, Masumoto K and Kajikawa T (1990) Role of the Harderian gland in immunoglobin. A production in chicken lacrimal fluid. *Research in Veterinary Science* **49**, 20–24

Beckman BJ, Howe CW, Trampel DW *et al.* (1998) *Aspergillus fumigatus* keratitis with intraocular invasion in 15-day-old chicks. *Avian Disease* **38**, 660–665

Bencina D, Mrzel I, Rojs OZ, Bidovec A and Dovc A (2003) Characterisation of *Mycoplasma gallisepticum* strains involved in respiratory disease in pheasants and peafowl. *Veterinary Record* **152**, 230–234

Brach V (1975) The effect of intraocular ablation of the Pecten oculi of the chicken. *Investigative Ophthalmology* **14**, 166–168

Bradley FA, Bickford AA and Walker RL (1993) Diagnosis of favus (avian dermatophytosis) in Oriental breed chickens. *Avian Disease* **37**, 1147–1150

Curtis PE, Baker JR, Curtis R and Johnston A (1987) Impaired vision in chickens associated with retinal defects. *Veterinary Record* **120**, 113–114

DeMello LR, Foster TM and Temple W (1992) Discriminative performance of the domestic hen in a visual acuity task. *Journal of Experimental and Analytical Behaviour* **58**, 147–157

Dooling RJ, Fay RR and Popper AN (2000) *Springer Handbook of Auditory Research, Volume 13: Comparative Hearing in Reptiles and Birds*. Springer, New York

Droual R, Bickford AA, Walker RL, Channing SE and McFadden C (1991) Favus in a backyard flock of game chickens. *Avian Disease* **35**, 625–630

Dukes TW and Pettit JR (1983) Avian ocular neoplasia – a description of spontaneously occurring cases. *Canadian Journal of Companion Medicine* **47**, 33–36

Durham D, Park DL and Girod DA (2002) Breed differences in cochlear integrity in adult, commercially raised chickens. *Hearing Research* **166**, 82–95

Ehrlich D, Stuchbery J and Zappia J (1989) Morphology of congenital microphthalmia in chicks (*Gallus gallus*). *Journal of Morphology* **199**, 1–13

Glünder G, Hinz KH, Löhren U and Kaleta EF (1982) Torticollis in chickens caused by *Pasteurella multocida*. *Deutsche Tierarztliche Wochenschrifte* **89**, 34–36

Gover N, Jarvis JR, Abeyesinghe SM and Wathes CM (2009) Stimulus luminance and the spatial acuity of domestic fowl (*Gallus g. domesticus*). *Vision Research* **49**, 2747–2753

Green TC and Mellor DJ (2011) Extending ideas about animal welfare assessment to include 'quality of life' and related concepts. *New Zealand Veterinary Journal* **59**, 263–271

Huchzermeyer FW and Cooper JE (2000) Fibriscess, not abscess, resulting from a localised inflammatory response to infection in reptiles and birds. *Veterinary Record* **147**, 515–517

Landman WJ, Boeve MH, Dwars RM and Gruys E (1998) Keratoglobus lesions in the eyes of rearing broiler breeders. *Avian Pathology* **27**, 256–262

Lauber JK (1991) Review: avian models for experimental myopia. *Journal of Ocular Pharmacology* **7**, 259–276

Leavitt S and Ayroud M (1997) *Riemerella anatipestifer* infection of domestic ducklings. *Canadian Veterinary Journal* **38**, 113

Miles DM, Branton SL and Lott BD (2004) Atmospheric ammonia is detrimental to the performance of modern commercial broilers. *Poultry Science* **83**, 1650–1654

Miles DM, Miller WW, Branton SL, Maslin WR and Lott BD (2006) Ocular responses to ammonia in broiler chickens. *Avian Disease* **50**, 45–49

Montali RJ (1988) Comparative pathology of inflammation in the higher vertebrates (reptiles, birds and mammals). *Journal of Comparative Pathology* **99**, 1–26

Montiani-Ferreira F, Cardoso F and Petersen-Jones S (2004) Postnatal development of central corneal thickness in chicks of *Gallus gallus domesticus*. *Veterinary Ophthalmology* **7**, 37–39

Moreno B, Chacón G, Villa A *et al.* (2009) Nervous signs associated with otitis and cranial osteomyelitis and with *Ornithobacterium rhinotracheale* infection in red-legged partridges (*Alectoris rufa*). *Avian Pathology* **38**, 341–347

Nimmermark S, Lund V, Gustafsson G and Eduard W (2003) Ammonia, dust and bacteria in welfare-oriented systems for laying hens. *Annals of Agricultural and Environmental Medicine* **16**, 103–113

Nunoya T, Yagihashi T, Tajima M and Nagasawa Y (1995) Occurrence of keratoconjunctivitis apparently caused by *Mycoplasma gallisepticum* in layer chickens. *Veterinary Pathology* **32**, 11–18

Pandiri AK, Cortes AL, Lee LF and Gimeno IM (2008) Marek's disease virus infection in the eye: chronological study of the lesions, virus replication, and vaccine-induced protection. *Avian Diseases* **52**, 572–580

Pettigrew JD, Wallman J and Wildsoet CF (1990) Saccadic oscillations facilitate ocular perfusion from the avian pecten. *Nature* **343**, 362–363

Prashar A, Guggenheim JA, Erichsen JT, Hocking PM and Morgan JE (2007) Measurement of intraocular pressure (IOP) in chickens using a rebound tonometer: quantitative evaluation of variance due to position inaccuracies. *Experimental Eye Research* **85**, 563–571

Ritchey ER, Code K, Zelinka CP, Scott MA and Fischer AJ (2011) The chicken cornea as a model of wound healing and neuronal re-innervation. *Molecular Vision* **17**, 2440–2454

Saunders JC (2010) The role of hair cell regeneration in an avian model of inner ear injury and repair from acoustic trauma. *ILAR Journal* **51**, 326–337

Saunders JC, Duncan RK and Doan DE (2000) The middle ear of reptiles and birds. In: *Springer Handbook of Auditory Research, Volume 13: Comparative Hearing: Reptiles and Birds*, ed. RJ Dooling, RR Fay and AN Popper, pp. 13–69. Springer, New York

Schaeffel F, Hagel G, Eikermann J and Collett T (1994) Lower-field myopia and astigmatism in amphibians and chicken. *Journal of the Optical Society of America A. Optics, Image Science and Vision* **11**, 487–495

Shivaprasad HL, Cortes P and Crespo R (2006) Otitis interna (labyrinthitis) associated with *Salmonella enterica arizonae* in turkey poults. *Avian Diseases* **50**, 135–138

Shivaprasad HL and Korbel R (2003) Blindness due to retinal dysplasia in broiler chicks. *Avian Diseases* **47**, 769–773

Smittkamp SE, Colgan AL, Park DL, Girod DA and Durham D (2002) Time course and quantification of changes in cochlear integrity observed in commercially raised broiler chickens. *Hearing Research* **170**, 139–154

Thekisoe MM, Mbati PA and Bisschop SP (2004) Different approaches to the vaccination of free ranging village chickens against Newcastle disease in Qwa-Qwa, South Africa. *Veterinary Microbiology* **101**, 23–30

Torres RM, Merayo-Lloves J, Blanco-Mezquita JT *et al.* (2005) Experimental model of laser *in situ* keratomileusis in hens. *Journal of Refractive Surgery* **21**, 392–398

van Ginkel FW, Gulley SL, Lammers A *et al.* (2012) Conjunctiva-associated lymphoid tissue in avian mucosal immunity. *Developmental and Comparative Immunology* **36**, 289–297

Wilkinson JL and Hodos W (1991) Intraocular pressure and eye enlargement in chicks. *Current Eye Research* **10**, 163–168

Wood CA (1917) *The Fundus Oculi of Birds as Viewed by the Direct Ophthalmoscope*. Lakeside Press, Chicago

Yamashita T and Sohal GS (1986) Development of smooth and skeletal muscle cells in the iris of the domestic duck, chick and quail. *Cell and Tissue Research* **244**, 121–131

Chapter 15

Respiratory disorders

Michael Lierz and Ursula Heffels-Redmann

Respiratory disorders in backyard poultry tend not to be problems that affect single birds, but diseases that affect the whole flock. These disorders are most commonly caused by an infectious agent. Traditionally, backyard poultry are kept in a closed system in which only progeny from the existing flock, which are protected against circulating pathogens by maternally derived antibodies, maintain the population. Opening this system by the necessary introduction of new birds (new genetic material) may introduce respiratory pathogens into the flock. This may also occur when birds return from exhibitions and are reintroduced to the flock. Other sources of infection may include free-ranging birds, other farm animals, rodents, humans, foodstuffs and other materials being introduced to the environment.

For these reasons, an extensive clinical history is required. In severe cases, it might be useful to visit the holding not only to inspect the flock but also to review the environmental conditions. The examination procedure should follow the steps outlined in Figure 15.1. The clinical signs associated with the most common respiratory conditions are given in Figure 15.2, and Figure 15.3 details the possible differential diagnoses associated with lesions of the different parts of the respiratory tract. As the clinical signs are often not pathognomonic, necropsy of dead birds or diseased birds euthanased for diagnostic purposes followed by further laboratory tests is advantageous to make an aetiological diagnosis.

Step	Comments
Swabs of exudate for laboratory diagnostics (microbiology, parasitology, virology, polymerase chain reaction) *continued*	• Virology: transport in special media or buffered saline with antibiotics • Polymerase chain reaction: wet swabs without media or transport in RNA buffer (e.g. RNAlater) (for detection of RNA viruses only)
Endoscopy	Individual birds
Blood samples for serology	Serum or plasma should be separated from whole blood before transport for the detection of specific antibodies to pathogens. Two samples within a 14-day interval should be evaluated for titre increase
Necropsy	Freshly dead birds or diseased birds euthanased for diagnostic purposes
Tissue samples from abnormal sites (microbiology, parasitology, virology, polymerase chain reaction, histology)	See comments above for microbiology, parasitology, virology and polymerase chain reaction • Histology: samples in 10% formalin
Immunofluorescence	Fresh samples or samples at -20°C
Immunohistochemistry	Samples in 10% formalin or at -20°C

15.1 (continued) Examination procedure for poultry with respiratory disease.

Step	Comments
Inspection of the bird/flock from a distance	Special regard to general condition/morbidity, behaviour, breathing, respiratory sounds, head posture
Direct inspection of the bird (dead or alive)	Special regard to eye/conjunctiva, nose/nostrils, sinuses, surrounding skin and feathers, exudates
Palpation of nostrils	Exudates, crusts
Sinuses	Grade of filling, squeezing of exudates
Trachea	Form, weakness
Skin	Thickness, crusts
Swabs of exudate for laboratory diagnostics (microbiology, parasitology, virology, polymerase chain reaction)	• Swabs from birds in different disease phases to detect primary and secondary pathogens; rapid transport with cooling • Microbiology: swabs from nose, eye and trachea; transport in special media • Parasitology: fresh faeces and tracheal swabs

15.1 Examination procedure for poultry with respiratory disease. (continues) ▶

Condition	Clinical signs
Upper respiratory tract	
Conjunctivitis	Ocular discharge, epiphora, swollen eyelids
Rhinitis	Nasal discharge, sneezing, staining or discharge on the skin and feathers around the nares, frequent head shaking or yawning to dislodge discharge, plugged nares, open-beak breathing
Sinusitis	Buccal blow, infraorbital swelling
Lower respiratory tract	
Tracheitis and bronchitis	Dyspnoea, change in vocalization, breathing sounds, gasping, oral discharge, open-beak breathing, extended neck, deformed and weak trachea
Pneumonia and air sacculitis	Dyspnoea, tachypnoea, breathing sounds, open-beak breathing

15.2 Clinical signs associated with respiratory diseases in poultry.

BSAVA Manual of Backyard Poultry Medicine and Surgery. Edited by Guy Poland and Aidan Raftery. ©BSAVA 2019

Condition	Clinical sign										
	Conjunctivitis	Rhinitis	Sinusitis	Head oedema	Laryngitis	Tracheitis	Bronchitis	Pneumonia	Air sacculitis	Egg drop	Misshapen eggs
Infectious bronchitis		+	+			+	+			+	+
Infectious laryngotracheitis			(+)		+	+	(+)			+	
Avian metapneumovirus infection	+	+	+	+							
Newcastle disease (lentogenic)	+	+								(+)	
Avian paramyxovirus-2, -3, -6, -7 infection	+	+									
Low pathogenic influenza	+		+						+	+	+
Chlamydiosis	+	+	+					+	+		
Mycoplasmosis	(+)	+	+			+	+	(+)	+		
Ornibacterium rhinotracheale infection		+	+	+		+		+	+	+	+
Infectious coryza	+	+	+	+				(+)	(+)	+	
Turkey coryza		+				+					
Fowl cholera (acute)								+		+	
Fowl cholera (chronic)	+	+	+		+	+	+	+	+	+	
Anatipestifer disease (acute)	+	+	+						+		
Colobacillosis						+		+	+		
Aspergillosis								+	+		
Gapeworm					(+)	+	(+)				
Cryptosporidiosis	+	+	+			+		+	+		
Heat stress								+		+	
Vitamin A deficiency	+	+	+			+	+				

15.3 Differential diagnoses of respiratory diseases in poultry.

Infectious bronchitis

Infectious bronchitis (IB) or avian infectious bronchitis (AIB) is a worldwide, common, highly contagious, acute disease of the respiratory tract of chickens. It is caused by a coronavirus, which may also affect the urogenital tract. Coronaviruses genetically similar to infectious bronchitis virus (IBV) have been demonstrated in other bird species, including pheasants, turkeys, guinea fowl and peafowl. Whilst the pheasant coronavirus is associated with both respiratory and kidney disease, and the turkey coronavirus with enteritis, it is not clear whether the coronaviruses isolated from guinea fowl and peafowl were genuinely from these species or IBV strains transferred from commercial chicken farms and whether they cause disease in these particular species.

Epidemiology

Transmission of the virus occurs via aerosol (airborne disease) as well as by mechanical means such as contaminated feed trucks, visiting persons etc. Other bird species may also act as vectors for IBV. Chickens of all ages are susceptible to the disease. It is highly contagious and quick virus replication and shedding leads to a rapid spread of the virus within a flock. Following a short incubation time, clinical signs develop within 24–48 hours. The outcome of the infection depends not only on the virus type and dose, but also on the breed of chicken and the age of the bird at the time of infection. The disease is most severe in very young chicks and can be fatal. Although IBV passes through the birds of a flock within a short period of time, individual birds may remain infected, intermittently excreting the virus via the nose and faeces. This may result in the disease persisting within the flock over a long period of time. The tenacity of the virus outside the bird is low. It is susceptible to heat, lipid solvents and disinfectants.

Aetiology and pathogenesis

Avian IBV (the prototype virus of group 3 of the genus *Coronavirus* in the family Coronaviridae) is a round to pleomorphic virus particle approximately 120 nm in diameter with single-stranded RNA and an envelope with club-shaped spikes on its surface. Due to high mutation and recombination rates, the variability of the virus is large, leading to the occurrence of numerous serovars and genotypes with different virulence and tissue tropism. Currently, there is no uniform nomenclature for the existing IBV strains and types. In Europe, the so-called Massachusetts-type still dominates, but other strains such as D207, D274, D1466, 793B, Italy 2 and QX are also quite widespread. Differentiation of new subtypes is very important in the diagnosis process, as any vaccinated flock can be affected by another subtype due to the lack of cross-immunity.

Infection with IBV is initiated via the respiratory tract, where the virus replicates and produces typical lesions in the epithelial cells, followed by further dissemination and replication in the epithelia of the urogenital tract. Depending on the pathogenicity and tissue tropism, this can cause nephritis and/or salpingitis. In very young chicks this inflammation may cause severe damage of the oviduct and can result in the chickens being unable to produce eggs when they come into lay (up to 5% 'false layers'). The virus also grows and persists in the gastrointestinal tract, and results in similar inflammation. After recovery, a long-lasting immunity protects the birds against challenge with homologous, and to a certain extent also heterologous, serovars. The damage to the respiratory epithelium caused by IBV strains often predisposes young chickens to secondary infections with pathogenic bacteria such as *Escherichia coli* and *Mycoplasma* spp.

Clinical signs

Morbidity and mortality in flocks reduces as the birds age. The characteristic respiratory signs are gasping, sneezing, tracheal rales and nasal discharge; wet eyes and swollen sinuses can sometimes be seen (Figure 15.4). Chicks demonstrate more severe respiratory signs, which can be associated with depression and decreased feed intake. Mortality due to exhaustion or asphyxiation may reach 25%. In chickens older than 6 weeks of age, the clinical signs are less pronounced or even absent. After recovery from the respiratory phase, infection with nephropathogenic strains may induce wet droppings, increased water intake, impaired growth (especially in broilers) and mortality. In laying hens, the predominant clinical sign is a drop in egg production associated with a high proportion of eggs with a thin, rough and misshapen shell (typical transverse and longitudinal ribs). The albumin may also appear watery and the hatchability of the eggs can be reduced. The drop in egg production has a sudden onset and usually lasts up to 3 weeks,

depending on whether secondary infections occur. A return to the pre-infection level of egg production takes 6–8 weeks, but occasionally this is never attained.

Differential diagnoses

IB resembles other acute respiratory diseases such as Newcastle disease (lentogenic strains), influenza A (low pathogenic strains), infectious laryngotracheitis (slow spread, more severe signs) and infectious coryza (facial swelling). The reduced number of eggs and egg quality is similar to that seen with egg drop syndrome (EDS) virus, but with the latter condition the albumin is not affected.

Post-mortem findings

In the acute phase, catarrhal inflammation of the mucosal membranes of the trachea, bronchial tubes and, in younger chicks, the nose and sinuses can be observed. Pneumonic areas around the large bronchi and foamy air sacs may be observed in the lower respiratory tract. Over the course of the disease, exudates may become mucoid, often with yellow caseous deposits due to secondary infection. Kidney lesions are characterized by swelling and paleness, and the tubules and ureters are distended with urates. Involution of the oviduct may be observed in laying hens, as well as yolk material in the abdominal cavity, although it should be borne in mind that these signs can also be seen with other diseases that cause reduction in egg production. A contraction or obstruction of the oviduct may be seen in 'false layers' that can cause the development of oviduct cysts with enormous volumes of fluid (Figure 15.5).

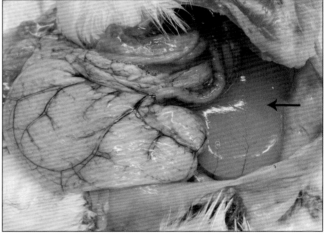

15.5 Post-mortem view of ovarian cysts (arrowed) in a laying hen due to infectious bronchitis.
(© Michael Lierz)

Laboratory diagnosis

The history, sudden-onset of illness of many birds, clinical signs and tissue alterations identified at post-mortem examination only allow a tentative diagnosis. Definitive diagnosis of IB can only be made by isolation of the virus in egg or tracheal ring culture, detection of virus antigen (immunofluorescence, antigen-capture enzyme-linked immunosorbent assay (ELISA)) or RNA (by reverse transcription polymerase chain reaction (RT-PCR)) or rising IBV antibody titres. The latter two methods are most commonly used. In the first days of disease, tracheal swabs or tracheal tissue collected at necropsy are the preferred

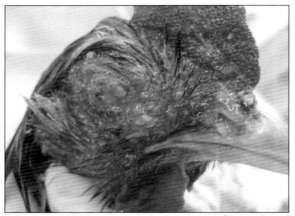

15.4 Severe sinusitis in a laying hen due to infectious bronchitis.
(© Clinic for Birds, Reptiles, Amphibians and Fish, JLU Giessen)

samples for detection of IBV-RNA. One week post-infection, cloacal swabs or caecal tonsils are more suitable samples. In cases that involve the urogenital tract, the kidney and oviduct should also be considered as sources for the detection of IBV. The RT-PCR should be performed in two steps. After detection of IBV-RNA, an identification of the genotype by PCR is recommended because of the large variation of circulating IBV strains, including circulating virus strains. The detection of rising specific antibodies against IBV in serum/plasma samples taken at 2-week intervals is possible in agar gel precipitation and ELISA (group specific antibodies) or haemagglutination inhibition and neutralization (serotype specific antibodies) tests. PCR as a diagnostic tool is recommended as it is far quicker. However, owners of backyard poultry often delay consulting a veterinary surgeon (veterinarian) and by the time the bird is examined the virus may have been eliminated, making a serological diagnosis advantageous.

Treatment

As causal treatment is not possible, intensive supportive treatment is essential. Optimizing ventilation and heat supply for young chicks is most important. Hygiene conditions should be improved and secondary bacterial infections should be treated with antibacterial drugs. Poor feed consumption may be improved by moistening of the feed. Individual birds should receive fluids and be force-fed until clinical signs reduce. Isolation of diseased birds may prevent further virus transmission.

Prognosis

The prognosis is usually good in backyard poultry as clinical signs reduce over time. In addition, with the treatment of secondary infections, mortality is usually low. However, the occurrence of 'false layers' can be a problem, as can the fact that newly hatched chicks become infected by the virus as it remains in the flock. Establishing a variable vaccination protocol usually overcomes these problems.

Prevention

Effective protection against IB can only be achieved by vaccination. For this purpose live vaccines containing virus of different grades of attenuation, as well as inactivated vaccines, are available. It is important to know that vaccines are based on different viral strains. Thus, protection is usually only achieved by a homologous vaccine. Vaccines should contain the strain of virus prevalent in the area or that has caused problems in the flock previously. Chicks are usually protected in the first weeks of life by maternal antibodies if the parents were vaccinated. However, in flocks with high infection pressure, the first vaccination with a highly attenuated strain (H120 = 120 passages in embryonated eggs) or a low pathogenic virus clone (Ma5) can be administered on the first day of life by spray or eye drop. Otherwise, the initial dose of the vaccine is given when the chick is 2–4 weeks old. Booster vaccinations with less attenuated strains (H52 or 793B) of one or more serovars should follow in intervals. The administration of vaccines with different serovars also induces a broad protection to strains of the virus that are not antigenically related. Vaccines can be administered via the oculonasal route or in drinking water. Before the beginning of the laying period, birds should be vaccinated with an inactivated vaccine (often combined with Newcastle disease) via subcutaneous injection to provide long-lasting

immunity to the individual and a high maternal antibody titre to their progeny. This principle should also be applied before sending birds to an exhibition. It should also be noted that because of the different coronaviruses in other backyard poultry, cross-immunity between species is questionable.

> **WARNING**
>
> Do not use less attenuated live vaccines in flocks with susceptible birds because of the risk of illness

Infectious laryngotracheitis

Infectious laryngotracheitis (ILT) is a worldwide viral respiratory disease that occurs in mild and severe forms, mainly in chickens. ILT has also been seen in pheasants and peafowl. The course of the disease may be acute or protracted. Turkeys and ducks may become infected and shed the virus, but do not usually develop clinical signs.

Epidemiology

The infectious laryngotracheitis virus (ILTV) is transmitted horizontally by virus-excreting birds, as well as via contaminated equipment and litter. Vertical transmission has not been proven. The virus spreads through the flock by direct or indirect contact. Although chickens of all ages are susceptible to the disease, the most severe and characteristic signs are seen in adult birds. Clinical signs are observed following 6–15 days incubation. After recovery, the virus persists in the ganglion of the trigeminal nerve and may cause recurrent infection. In the environment, the virus is fragile and easily destroyed by most disinfectants.

Aetiology and pathogenesis

ILTV is classified as Gallid herpesvirus-1, a member of the genus *Iltovirus* within the family Herpesviridae (subfamily Alphaherpesvirinae). This double-stranded DNA virus is antigenically homologous. Virus replication is limited to the epithelium of the respiratory tract, mainly the larynx and trachea, and results in more or less severe epithelial damage and haemorrhage. Viraemia has not been proven. The virus may persist in the trachea as well as the trigeminal ganglia, and intermittent virus shedding may occur up to 20 weeks post-infection.

Clinical signs

With severe infections, marked inspiratory dyspnoea with painfully doleful breathing sounds and expectoration of blood-stained mucus is characteristic (Figure 15.6). Birds demonstrate a penguin-like body posture. In laying hens this is associated with a drastic drop in egg production. Morbidity is high and mortality can reach up to 50% caused by sudden asphyxia or protracted by exhaustion after 1–2 weeks of illness. In mild cases, clinical signs include conjunctivitis, rhinitis, sinusitis and tracheitis. Generally, birds recover in about 2 weeks; however, in extreme cases recovery may take up to 4 weeks.

Differential diagnoses

The clinical signs of the severe form of ILT are quite reliable for diagnosis. Gapeworms may also be present in a

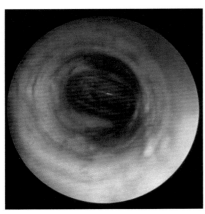

15.6 Endoscopic view of severe tracheitis due to infectious laryngotracheitis in a laying hen. Note the swollen, red appearance of the mucosa indicating inflammation.
(© Michael Lierz)

bloody tracheal exudate. Milder forms of the disease may be comparable with other respiratory diseases (see Figure 15.3) and diagnosis can only be confirmed by laboratory diagnostic tests.

Post-mortem findings

Gross lesions vary from clear mucus in the trachea to severe haemorrhage and/or diphtheritic changes in the larynx and trachea (Figure 15.7). Pneumonia and air sacculitis as well as haemorrhagic cloacal inflammation may sometimes be observed.

Laboratory diagnosis

Tracheal haemorrhage in severe cases makes ILTV the most likely diagnosis. Milder forms are similar to IBV, Newcastle disease and influenza A. The diagnosis can be confirmed by histopathology (intranuclear inclusion bodies) and/or demonstration of ILTV in embryonated egg or cell cultures, or by detection of viral DNA by PCR from respiratory or conjunctival exudates. Anti-ILTV antibodies can be detected approximately 7 days after infection by ELISA or virus neutralization test.

Treatment

There is no specific treatment; however, vaccination (see below) of an apparently still healthy chicken may be an appropriate measure to prevent further spread of the field virus within the flock. Providing vitamin A in the drinking water may enhance the local immune reaction. Antibiosis may be advisable for the control of secondary infections

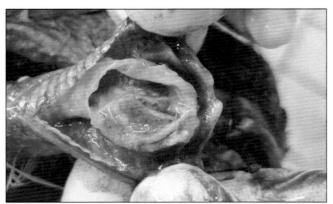

15.7 Post-mortem view of severe fibrinous tracheitis due to infectious laryngotracheitis in a laying hen. The mucosal membrane is completely coated with a diphtheritic membrane material.
(© Clinic for Birds, Reptiles, Amphibians and Fish, JLU Giessen)

caused by bacteria and fungi. Individual birds may require force-feeding and fluid therapy. In severe cases with blocked airways, an air sac breathing tube may need to be placed to allow the bird to recover.

Prognosis

In severe cases, the prognosis is poor. Euthanasia should be considered on animal welfare grounds. In mild cases, the prognosis is good for the individual as prevention of secondary infections, fluid therapy and appropriate nutritional support will help the bird to overcome the clinical signs. However, it should be borne in mind that birds, once infected, are lifelong carriers.

Prevention

Vaccination with attenuated live virus vaccines is possible. However, since vaccination results in latently infected carrier birds and is associated with the risk of the vaccine virus returning to virulence; it should only be used in geographical areas where the disease is endemic. The vaccine is most effectively administered by eye drop, but can also be given via drinking water or spray (avoid small droplet size because of the risk of illness due to deep penetration of the vaccine virus in the respiratory tract). The priming vaccination may cause slight conjunctivitis. Immunity develops 4–7 days following vaccination. Vaccination should take place twice at about 7 and 15 weeks of age to induce disease resistance for up to 12 months. An inactivated vaccine should be administered for the second vaccination. Maternally derived antibodies do not provide protection against infection, but also do not interfere with the vaccines, so vaccination can occur even at 1 day old in highly endangered chicks. Alternatively, a new vector vaccine (turkey herpesvirus with two ILTV glycoprotein genes) can be used.

In large flocks where only a small percentage of the chicks are clinically affected, all non-clinically affected birds should be vaccinated immediately by eye drop of an attenuated vaccine. The vaccine virus competes with the field virus at the receptors in the tracheal cells and prevents field virus infection in all non-infected birds. Thus, all birds in the potent period demonstrate clinical signs even after vaccination.

> **WARNING**
>
> Some pheasant species, especially Lady Amherst's, Eared, Glanz, Reeve's, Elliot, Argus and Monal, may react with severe disease following vaccination

Avian metapneumovirus infection

Diseases that are caused by avian metapneumoviruses (AMPVs) include turkey rhinotrachetitis, swollen head syndrome and avian rhinotracheitis.

Epidemiology

The primary natural hosts are turkeys and chickens of all ages. Pheasants, guinea fowl and Muscovy ducks are also susceptible to the disease, whilst geese, other ducks and pigeons appear to be refractory to the virus. Once introduced the virus spreads rapidly within a flock, as well as to neighbouring flocks in areas with intense poultry farming, by contact transmission from bird to bird or via contaminated items. Airborne spread, vertical transmission and transmission by migratory birds have been suggested but not yet proved.

Aetiology and pathogenesis

As members of the subfamily Pneumovirinae, family Paramyxoviridae, avian metapneumoviruses have a non-segmented, single-stranded RNA genome. Four subtypes are known:

- Subtypes A and B occur in Europe, Africa, Asia and South America
- Subtype C is present in turkeys in the USA
- Subtype D has only been detected in turkeys in France.

The virus is sensitive to lipid solvents and most disinfectants. Infection with AMPV alone induces only a mild rhinotracheitis combined with complete deciliation of the trachea. Poor management and concurrent infection with other respiratory bacteria, such as *E. coli*, *Bordetella avium*, *Ornithobacterium rhinotracheale*, *Mycoplasma gallisepticum*, *Chlamydophilia psittaci* or lentogenic Newcastle disease virus, significantly enhance the clinical signs, morbidity and mortality.

Clinical signs

In turkeys, typical clinical signs include snicking, rales, sneezing, nasal discharge, foamy conjunctivitis, head shaking, swollen infraorbital sinuses and submandibular oedema (Figure 15.8). In chickens, the infection is associated with swollen head syndrome, which is characterized by swelling of the periorbital and infraorbital sinuses, and can sometimes be complicated by central nervous signs such as torticollis, disorientation and opisthotonus because of secondary *E. coli* infection. Laying birds may experience up to a 70% drop in egg production associated with poor eggshell quality and peritonitis. Morbidity is usually high, whilst mortality may reach 50% in adult turkeys and 4% in chicks.

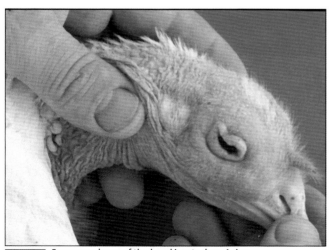

15.8 Severe oedema of the head in a turkey. Avian metapneumovirus is a likely cause.
(© Clinic for Birds, Reptiles, Amphibians and Fish, JLU Giessen)

Differential diagnoses

A wide range of viruses (paramyxovirus, influenza, infectious bronchitis viruses) and bacteria (*E. coli*, *B. avium*, *O. rhinotracheale* and *Mycoplasma* spp.) may cause clinical signs similar to those seen with AMPV infections. As bacterial infections can occur secondarily to AMPV infections, this may be the reason for the considerable diagnostic problems encountered. Direct or indirect identification of the virus in affected birds provides a definitive diagnosis.

Post-mortem findings

The main lesions recognized in turkeys are excess watery to mucoid exudates in the turbinates and trachea, which become purulent. The major gross lesions encountered in chickens include extensive yellow gelatinous to purulent oedema in the subcutaneous tissues of the head, neck and wattles. Similar lesions may be seen in pheasants.

Laboratory diagnosis

The clinical signs and gross lesions may suggest a presumptive diagnosis of AMPV infection, but the diagnosis has to be confirmed by detection of the causative agent. Virus isolation or genome detection by RT-PCR is only reliable if the samples are taken as early as possible after infection. The virus is only present for 6–7 days in the affected tissues. The most suitable samples for virus detection are ocular/nasal secretions and tissue scraped from the sinuses/turbinates of several birds with only mild or not yet developed clinical signs. Due to the difficulties with direct detection of the virus, indirect aetiological diagnosis by demonstration of specific antibodies is important. This is possible 7 days after infection by ELISA, indirect immunofluorescence or neutralization tests.

Treatment

Antibacterials should be used to reduce the severity of secondary bacterial infections.

Prognosis

The prognosis for chickens is usually good as the clinical signs decrease after several days. Treatment of secondary infections and supportive care is important. As the virus is usually eliminated from both the individual bird and the flock over time, long-term problems are not usually encountered. In turkeys, the prognosis may be poor as they develop more severe clinical signs.

Prevention

Besides biosecurity, the only way to protect against AMPV infection is vaccination. For this purpose both live attenuated and inactivated vaccines of subtypes A and B are available for use in turkeys and chickens. They provide protection not only from the homologous but also the heterologous subtype. Maternally derived humoral antibodies do not prevent young birds from developing disease after AMPV infection. For this reason, a course of two or three live virus vaccinations, starting as early as possible (e.g. in turkeys – spray on day 1, boosters at day 7–10 and at 4–6 weeks via drinking water), is recommended. In chickens, interference with the IBV vaccination may prevent the achievement of reliable immunity to AMPV.

Avian paramyxovirus infections

Ten serogroups of avian paramyxoviruses (APMV-1 to APMV-10) have been identified, of which Newcastle disease virus (APMV-1) is the most important pathogen for poultry. APMV-2 and APMV-3, as well as to a lesser degree APMV-6 and APMV-7, are known to cause disease in poultry.

Newcastle disease

Newcastle disease is also known as pseudo-fowl pest, pseudo-poultry plague, avian pest, avian distemper, Ranikhet disease, Tetelo disease, Korean fowl plague and avian pneumoencephalitis. As an epizootic disease, Newcastle disease is listed by the World Organisation for Animal Health (OIE), and as such is subject to international control policies.

Epidemiology

Newcastle disease is encountered worldwide and the vast majority of, if not all, birds become infected. In domestic avian species, chickens and turkeys are highly susceptible to the virus, with young chicks more susceptible than adults. Waterfowl have mainly asymptomatic infections and serve as a virus reservoir, as do many other wild birds. Newcastle disease virus varies widely in the type and severity of the disease it can produce (see Chapter 18). Velogenic (viscerotropic and neurogenic) strains cause a highly contagious, septicaemic peracute to acute disease associated with high mortality.

Clinical signs

Depending on the virus pathotype, host species, age of the host, environmental stress and co-infections with other microorganisms, the respiratory tract may be more or less involved in the disease pattern. After infection with velo-genic (highly pathogenic) strains, initial signs include oedema of the conjunctiva, as well as lethargy, inappetence and ruffled feathers (Figure 15.9). As the disease progresses, birds may develop severe dyspnoea and subcutaneous inflammation of the head and neck, often with cyanotic discoloration. These signs are often associated with enteritis and neurological signs and a dramatic fall in egg production (see Chapter 18). Mesogenic (medium pathogenic) strains usually cause acute respiratory catarrhal disease and are sometimes associated with nervous signs. Laying birds may show a reduction in egg production.

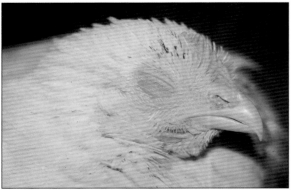

15.9 Severe general clinical signs, such as sleepiness and ruffled feathers, combined with sinusitis in a broiler chick caused by avian paramyxovirus infection.
(© Clinic for Birds, Reptiles, Amphibians and Fish, JLU Giessen)

Mortality rate is low (<10%). Lentogenic (low pathogenic) strains usually provoke signs only in young birds. Clinical signs may range from a mild to serious respiratory disease with coughing, gasping, sneezing and rales. Diagnosis and control measures are described in Chapter 18.

Other avian paramyxovirus infections

Epidemiology

Avian paramyxovirus type 2: APMV-2 (Yucaipa virus) infections cause a mild respiratory disease in chickens and turkeys, but latent infections are also common. Free-ranging passerine and imported psittacine birds are virus reservoirs. Transmission occurs horizontally via virus shed from the respiratory and gastrointestinal tracts of infected birds.

Avian paramyxovirus type 3: Natural APMV-3 (Wisconsin virus) infections in poultry are restricted to turkeys. In the absence of any wild bird host, it seems that this subtype can be introduced into a flock only by latently infected turkeys or by humans. The virus is transmitted horizontally.

Avian paramyxovirus type 6: Infections with the APMV-6 serotype occur rarely in turkeys causing respiratory signs, and are asymptomatic in ducks and geese.

Avian paramyxovirus type 7: The prevalence of APMV-7 in pigeons and doves suggests that they are the source of the virus seen in turkey flocks, occasionally causing a mild respiratory disease.

Aetiology and pathogenesis

The major characteristics of the avian paramyxoviruses are described in the section on Newcastle disease (see above). Differentiation between the serovars is possible using the haemagglutination inhibition test with specific antisera, although there are some cross reactions particularly between APMV-1 and APMV-3. Little is known about the pathogenicity of APMV-2 to APMV-10. Affinity to the respiratory tract seems to be common to all types, and it is assumed that virus replication is similar to that of APMV-1.

Clinical signs

Infection with APMV-2, APMV-3, APMV-6 and APMV-7 induce mild respiratory signs, especially in turkeys. Conjunctivitis and rhinitis with serous discharge are encountered most often. When complicated by other organisms, the clinical signs become more severe and include sinusitis, tracheitis, pneumonia and air sacculitis. In laying birds, the infection can be associated with egg production problems (increase in white shells, reduced number produced and decreased hatchability, but normal fertility). Morbidity may be high, but mortality is usually low.

Differential diagnoses

Differentiation between respiratory diseases with similar clinical and pathological signs (see Figure 15.3) is only possible by laboratory diagnosis.

Post-mortem findings

Depending on the phase of the infection, the character of the inflammation of the affected parts of the respiratory tract changes from catarrhal to fibro-purulent.

Laboratory diagnosis

As none of the clinical signs or lesions are typical, isolation of the aetiological agent is necessary for diagnosis. Swabs from the conjunctiva, nose or trachea of diseased birds, or samples of affected tissues from dead birds, should be sent to a diagnostic laboratory for virus isolation. Serotyping of a detected APMV using a haemagglutination inhibition test with monoclonal antibodies is recommended for a reliable diagnosis. Indirect diagnosis of an APMV infection is also possible by detection of an increase of specific antibodies in the haemagglutination inhibition test. The risk of a misdiagnosis because of cross reactions between the different APMV types can be eliminated by the use of control sera and antigens to all serotypes.

Treatment

In the case of secondary infection with bacteria, the use of antibiotics may be advisable. Birds should also receive supportive care as needed.

Prognosis

Whilst all APMV-1 infections are covered by law (see Chapter 26), infections with other subtypes are usually not regulated. With the exception of APMV-1, paramyxovirus infections only cause mild clinical signs, leading to a good prognosis when supportive care and antibiotics to control secondary infections are provided.

Prevention

Biosecurity measures may reduce the risk of virus introduction into the flock. APMV-3 oil emulsion vaccines are registered in Europe and the USA. Specific vaccines against the other APMV serotypes are not commercially available, but the production of a flock-specific vaccine may be reasonable in the case of valuable birds.

Avian influenza

Depending on their virulence and/or pathogenicity, avian influenza viruses cause different diseases.

High pathogenic avian influenza

High pathogenic avian influenza virus (HPAIV) provokes a highly lethal, systemic disease which is listed by the OIE and as such in most countries is a notifiable animal epidemic liable for control. Acute respiratory distress, gasping for air, purple discoloration of wattles, and sudden death may indicate HPAIV and should be kept in mind as a differential diagnosis.

Clinical signs that would be highly suspicious of HPAI when seen in multiple birds:

- Sudden deaths
- Swelling of the head, eyelids, comb, wattles and hocks
- Purple discoloration of the wattles, comb and legs
- Gasping for air (difficulty breathing)
- Coughing, sneezing and/or nasal discharge
- Stumbling or falling down

Low pathogenic avian influenza

Low pathogenic avian influenza virus (LPAIV) causes respiratory disease in poultry.

Epidemiology

Free-ranging (especially aquatic) birds are reservoirs for low pathogenic avian influenza viruses (LPAIVs), being latently infected and shedding the virus for long times without clinical signs. In backyard flocks, usually containing birds of different ages and species (including waterfowl), mutual infections are facilitated. Transmission of the virus is also possible by different vectors. Disease outbreaks often occur in autumn and winter due to the high multiplication rate of the virus in free-ranging birds when they assemble prior to migration and the high tenacity of the virus at low temperatures. At present, the H9N2 virus in chickens and the H6N strain in turkeys are of greatest importance. Influenza viruses from swine (H1N1) may also induce disease in chickens and turkeys.

Aetiology and pathogenesis

LPAIVs of all subtypes (H1 to H16) are only able to induce local infections. LPAIV subtypes H5 and H7 may mutate to HPAIV via circulation in poultry farms and therefore they are subject to international control policies (see Chapter 26).

Clinical signs

Clinical signs include reduced food and water intake, lethargy, respiratory signs (e.g. dyspnoea), conjunctivitis, sinusitis, cyanosis of the comb and wattle (rare) and temporary diarrhoea. In younger birds, the signs are more severe. Laying birds show a reduction in egg production combined with deformed, depigmented, thin-shelled eggs and a reduced fertilization rate. Morbidity is high, but the mortality rate is low. Birds recover within 3 weeks without returning to their previous performance level.

Differential diagnoses

The differential diagnoses include Newcastle disease (lentogenic virus), other paramyxoviruses, infectious laryngotracheitis, infectious bronchitis and avian metapneumovirus. Chlamydiosis, mycoplasmosis and other bacterial infections produce similar respiratory signs and reduction in egg production. Concurrent infection with other viruses and bacteria is common.

Post-mortem findings

At necropsy, fibrinous inflammation of the upper respiratory tract and air sacs with excess mucus in the larynx and trachea can be found. Fibrinous sinusitis (Figure 15.10) is usually present, with pancreatitis, nephritis, splenic hyperplasia and catarrhal enteritis (less frequently) observed later in the disease course. Laying birds may develop egg yolk peritonitis.

Laboratory diagnosis

Pharyngeal and/or cloacal swabs from living birds or tissues samples from the respiratory tract, proventriculus, kidney, caecum, tonsils, cloaca or bursa of Fabricus of dead birds may be used for the diagnosis of the virus either by isolation (embroynated eggs) or PCR. Differentiation of the virus subtype is very important due to legal aspects,

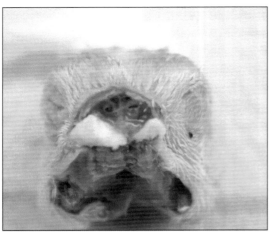

15.10 Fibrinopurulent sinusitis in a turkey chick due to a low pathogenic avian influenza virus infection.
(© Lierz & Hafez, FU Berlin)

and is achieved by a haemagglutination inhibition test or specific PCR. Antibodies specific to avian influenza may be detected by agar gel precipitation test, haemagglutination inhibition test or ELISA.

Treatment

Infection with LPAIV H5 and H7 is notifiable in most countries and the control measures implemented are based on the legal requirements of the respective national authorities. In all other cases, only treatment of secondary infections with antibiotics is possible to prevent losses. Individuals should receive appropriate supportive care.

Prognosis

The prognosis for a clinical cure of LPAIV is good as infection in a flock is usually self-limiting. However, it does recur, so vaccination in the case of non-H5/H7 subtypes via a flock-specific vaccine may be an option. As avian influenza viruses recombine, depopulation of the flock to prevent spreading the virus to other birds or risking mutation to HPAIV should be considered.

Prevention

As backyard poultry usually have contact with free-ranging birds, viral introduction is always possible and hard to prevent. Hygiene measures and separation of waterfowl from other poultry may reduce the risk of infection. In some countries, inactivated vaccines against H9N2 and H6N2 are commercially available. Flock-specific vaccines against other LPAIV subtypes may be also produced and administered.

Chlamydiosis

Avian chlamydiosis is a systemic disease in birds, which can also be transmitted to humans (see also Chapter 16). Formerly, the disease was termed psittacosis or parrot fever in psittacine birds and humans, and ornithosis in other birds. The disease is termed respiratory disease complex in cases of simultaneous infection with *O. rhinotracheale* and AMPV.

Epidemiology

Infection occurs worldwide in all poultry species and approximately 500 species of free-living and pet birds. Amongst poultry, disease outbreaks are more often observed in turkeys, ducks and geese than in chickens. Younger domestic birds are generally more susceptible to infection than older birds. However, undiagnosed infection is widespread amongst poultry and wild birds, with the pathogen being shed via respiratory tract exudates and in faeces. Stress may induce activation of the infection and an outbreak of the disease. Transmission occurs by inhalation of contaminated dry dust, in which the organism can survive for a long time. This pathogen can also infect humans and may cause severe, possibly fatal, disease. People in contact with infected birds are especially in danger. Vertical transmission is possible, but seems to occur only rarely.

Aetiology and pathogenesis

The infectious form of *Chlamydophila psittaci* (elementary body) is a small prokaryote that needs host cells for multiplication in a biphasic developmental cycle. There are eight known serovars with significant differences in virulence. Serovar C mainly occurs in waterfowl, whilst serovar D is seen in turkeys. Highly virulent strains cause acute epidemics in which 5–30% of the affected birds may die, whilst low virulent strains induce slowly progressive epidemics with <5% mortality when uncomplicated by concurrent infections (e.g. AMPV, *O. rhinotracheale*, *Salmonella* spp. and *Pasteurella* spp.). After infection by aerosol, replication of the pathogen begins in the epithelial cells of the upper respiratory tract and subsequently spreads to the epithelia and macrophages throughout the whole respiratory tract. Following septicaemia, chlamydiae appear in the epithelial cells and macrophages of various tissues, provoking vascular damage and increasing the response to inflammation.

Clinical signs

The highly virulent strains induce cachexia, anorexia, conjunctivitis (Figure 15.11), respiratory distress, excretion of yellow-green droppings and a decrease in egg production in laying birds. In birds infected with low virulent strains, the signs are less severe or even absent. Splenomegaly is commonly seen, even on radiography, and is sometimes accompanied by hepatomegaly.

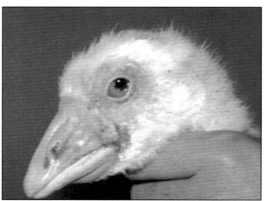

15.11 Severe conjunctivitis in a goose due to *Chlamydophila* infection.
(© Clinic for Birds, Reptiles, Amphibians and Fish, JLU Giessen)

Differential diagnoses

Due to the similar signs and lesions, pasteurellosis, colibacillosis, mycoplasmosis, avian influenza, turkey coryza, duck plague, salmonellosis and paramyxovirus infection have to be taken into consideration and excluded by detection of the pathogen.

Post-mortem findings

Depending on the virulence of the causative agent, different degrees of catarrhal to fibrinous conjunctivitis, sinusitis, rhinitis, keratitis, pneumonia, air sacculitis, pericarditis, hepatomegaly, splenomegaly, enteritis, and congestion of the kidneys, ovaries and testes can be observed. None of these clinical signs is pathognomonic for the disease, but in combination (especially conjunctivitis with splenomegaly) should always raise suspicion for chlamydiosis.

Laboratory diagnosis

Methods for diagnosing *C. psittaci* infections are:

- Direct visualization of the organism in stained (Stamp, Giemsa or Gieminez) smear samples (conjunctiva, liver)
- Isolation of the organism in cell or egg cultures
- Detection of the genome of the organism by PCR
- Detection of specific antigens by direct immunofluorescence, ELISA or immunochromatography
- Detection of specific antibodies by complement fixation, ELISA or indirect immunofluorescence tests.

Currently, the preferred and most commonly used detection method is PCR. Swabs from the conjunctiva, choana, pharynx or cloaca of live birds or tissue samples from the air sacs, spleen and liver of dead birds can be submitted for PCR. PCR also allows differentiation of *C. psittaci* from other *Chlamydophila* species, which may be important for epidemiological evaluation. Antibody detection alone is not reliable for a diagnosis, as it only shows is that the bird had contact with the pathogen.

Treatment

Due to its zoonotic potential, there may be regulations that have to be adhered to with regard to handling infected birds. When treatment is allowed, the flock should be treated with chlortetracycline via their feed (0.4 g/kg) for at least 42 days or enrofloxacin for 21 days (see Appendix 2). Affected birds should also be treated with systemic antibiosis. The effectiveness of the treatment with regard to eliminating carrier states should be checked following the course of medication. Supportive care is extremely important.

Prognosis

In severely diseased birds, the prognosis is very poor and the birds will die despite treatment. If the entire flock is treated immediately, the prognosis for the other birds is usually good (even though several more birds may die despite starting treatment). However, it needs to be borne in mind that birds may become carriers even after treatment, and that this may be a risk to other birds within the flock as infection does not confer lifelong immunity. Thus, testing each bird following treatment, separating those with positive results from those with negative results, and retreatment or

euthanasia of the positive birds is highly recommended. A flock is considered clear if all the birds have tested negative on two consecutive occasions (5 days apart).

Prevention

Prevention of infection in birds housed outside may be difficult. Avoidance of stress and reduction of dust in the house may be helpful.

Mycoplasmosis

The term mycoplasmosis refers to several worldwide occurring contagious diseases of the respiratory, musculoskeletal (see Chapter 18) and reproductive (see Chapter 17) tracts of poultry. These diseases are induced by *Mycoplasma gallisepticum* (chronic respiratory disease in chickens; infectious sinusitis in turkeys), *M. meleagridis*, *M. synoviae* and *M. iowae*. There are several more *Mycoplasma* spp. known to occur in poultry, but their role in respiratory diseases appears to be minor.

Epidemiology

Natural poultry hosts of *M. gallisepticum* and *M. synoviae* are chickens and turkeys, but pheasants, partridges, peafowl, quails, ducks and geese can also be infected. Turkeys are the only hosts for *M. meleagridis* and *M. iowae*, whereas *M. imitans* can be seen in ducks, geese and partridges. *M. gallisepticum* and *M. synoviae* are of greatest importance and are common in all kinds of backyard poultry. Sources of infection are latently and chronically infected birds. Transmission can be vertical and horizontal, and both ways directly from bird to bird (as well as via the semen) and indirectly by living or inanimate vectors, with transmission via aerosol being of special importance. Within a flock, the spread of the pathogen is normally slow. Outside of the host, *Mycoplasma* spp. can only survive for a few days, with some dying within hours.

Aetiology and pathogenesis

Mycoplasmas are very small prokaryotes that lack a cell wall. Due to their very small genome size, they rely on host cell metabolism and require special culture methods. The organisms enter the body via the mucosa of the conjunctiva and/or respiratory tract or are vertically transmitted. These organisms then attach to the epithelial cells and multiply. Some strains are able to enter tissues and may cause embryo death, as well as different apparent clinical diseases without other predisposing factors. Usually, the infection remains latent, due to the ability of mycoplasmas to 'hide' from the host immune system by mimicry (absorption or imitation of host cell structures) or due to the variation in antigen dominant membrane structures. They pave the way for infection with other pathogens (e.g. Newcastle disease virus, infectious bronchitis virus, infectious laryngotracheitis virus (and vaccine strains), *E. coli*, *Avibacterium paragallinarum*, other *Mycoplasma* spp., *Pasteurella* spp. and *O. rhinotracheale*), and clinical disease can only occur in the presence of these secondary pathogens. Disease is also possible following impairment of the host's defence system by stressors such as transportation, suboptimal environmental conditions and sexual maturation. Turkeys are usually more susceptible to disease than other poultry species.

Clinical signs

The respiratory form of the disease is associated with dyspnoea (which can be severe) and rasping sounds on breathing, as well as nasal discharge and swelling of the infraorbital sinus and eyelids, especially in turkeys. Often poor egg hatchability is seen and the embryos demonstrate curled toes or dwarfism (Figure 15.12).

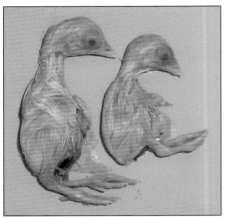

15.12 Dwarfism in a chick (right) compared with a normal chick (left) at the time of hatching due to a vertical *Mycoplasma* infection.
(© Michael Lierz)

Differential diagnoses

Mycoplasmosis has to be differentiated from other respiratory diseases with similar clinical signs (see Figure 15.3) by identification of the pathogen. Concurrent infections with other causative agents of respiratory diseases are likely.

Post-mortem findings

Gross lesions include catarrhal to fibrinous rhinitis, sinusitis, tracheitis, bronchitis and, in most cases, air sacculitis. Pericarditis and epicarditis only occur in cases complicated by secondary *E. coli* infection. Some degree of pneumonia may also be observed.

Laboratory diagnosis

Direct detection and identification of the *Mycoplasma* spp. is possible by cultivation on special media (Figure 15.13) followed by biochemical differentiation, direct immunofluorescence, and genus- and species-specific PCR.

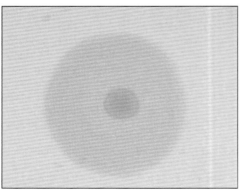

15.13 Fried-egg appearance of a *Mycoplasma* colony on a specific *Mycoplasma* agar after isolation.
(© Michael Lierz)

Detection of specific antibodies is also possible by serum plate agglutination, ELISA, indirect immunofluorescence and, in some strains, by a haemagglutination inhibition test. Due to the genetic relationship between *M. gallisepticum* and *M. imitans*, differentiation of these two strains requires special attention. Simultaneous infection with other pathogens is very common.

Treatment

Antibiotics, such as macrolides (e.g. tylosin), tetracyclines and fluoroquinolones, may be useful to reduce the severity of the clinical signs, but treatment does not eliminate the organisms from carrier birds. Treatment administered via drinking water is usually effective at reducing the clinical signs, but severely diseased birds should be treated individually, rather than as part of the flock.

Prognosis

The clinical prognosis for the flock is usually good. Treatment reduces clinical signs; however, it is nearly impossible to eliminate the pathogen from the flock and recurrence of the disease is likely eventually. For an individual bird, the prognosis depends on secondary infections and the severity of the disease. Severely affected birds may recover, but there is usually lower productivity. These animals also pose a risk to other birds, as they might be latently infected. In vulnerable birds, testing of each individual following treatment and removing any with positive results is expensive but may lead to eradication.

Prevention

Once introduced *Mycoplasma* infections may be difficult to eradicate from backyard flocks. Optimal environmental and nutritional conditions may prevent clinical outbreaks of the disease. Alternatively, vaccination with live or inactivated adjuvant vaccines is possible for *M. gallisepticum* and *M. synoviae*, but it should be remembered that if the flock is infected this may interfere with the vaccination.

Ornithobacterium rhinotracheale infection

Epidemiology

O. rhinotracheale has a worldwide distribution and causes an acute to subacute disease in turkeys and chickens. Natural infections occur not only in other farmed poultry (e.g. ducks, geese, pheasants, quails, partridges, guinea fowl), but also in many wild birds, which may serve as a source of infection. Transmission occurs mainly horizontally via direct contact or indirectly by living and inanimate vectors. Vertical transmission is assumed. Birds of all ages seem to be susceptible, although signs of disease are more severe in older animals.

Aetiology and pathogenesis

O. rhinotracheale is a Gram-negative, rod-shaped to pleomorph bacterium that grows best on blood agar under microaerobic or anaerobic conditions. As most strains are resistant to gentamicin this should be added to the media to reduce secondary growth of other bacteria. There are

18 known serovars (chickens: mainly serovar A; turkeys: serovars A, B and D). Infection of the mucosa of the respiratory tract induces exudative inflammatory lesions. The severity of the disease is influenced by synergistic interactions with other pathogens such as Newcastle disease virus, infectious bronchitis virus, *Mycoplasma* spp., AMPVs and *E. coli*, as well as by poor environmental conditions.

Clinical signs

Illness usually occurs at or during the end of the maturation period. Clinical signs are variable and initially include sneezing and nasal discharge, followed by oedema around the infraorbital sinus and dyspnoea of varying degrees. These clinical signs may be associated with depression, a decrease in egg production and an increase of commercially non-usable eggs. Mortality varies from 1–50%.

Differential diagnoses

Respiratory clinical signs associated with *O. rhinotracheale* are similar to those seen with numerous other bacteria, including *E. coli*, *P. multocida*, *Rimerella anatipestifer*, *A. paragallinarum* and *C. psittaci* (see Figure 15.3). A blood smear of a sample taken from the heart and stained with methyl blue can be examined to identify the bipolar staining associated with *P. multocida*, which is the main differential to *O. rhinotracheale*.

Post-mortem findings

The main lesions identified are pulmonary oedema, unilateral or bilateral consolidation of the lungs, pneumonia, pleuritic and air sacculitis with a foamy, white, yoghurt-like exudate (Figures 15.14 and 15.15).

Laboratory diagnosis

The history and clinical and pathological signs allow a presumptive diagnosis, which has to be verified by cultural isolation of the pathogen. In particular, differentiation from *P. multocida* is important. Suitable samples for laboratory analysis are tracheal swabs from live birds and tissue samples from the lungs and air sacs of dead birds. Specific antibodies can be tested by ELISA or agar gel precipitation test.

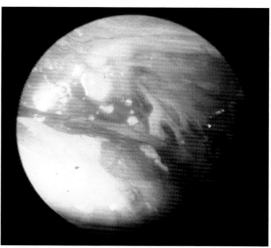

15.15 Endoscopic view of caseous material on the air sac membrane and liver capsule as a result of a bacterial infection. In such cases, *Ornithobacterium rhinotracheale* and *Pasteurella multocida* are the most likely pathogens.
(© Michael Lierz)

Treatment

As *O. rhinotracheale* can develop resistance to antimicrobials quickly, and there are significant differences in the susceptibility of the pathogen to antibiotics in different countries, it is essential to perform a sensitivity test before commencing treatment.

Prognosis

The prognosis for the flock is usually good and repeated treatment usually leads to reduction of clinical signs. However, in the individual bird, especially if it is chronically and severely affected, the prognosis is poor as the massive fibrinopurulent air sacculitis is usually difficult to treat, and a full recovery may not be possible.

Prevention

Strict biosecurity measures should be followed to prevent the introduction of *O. rhinotracheale*. Once endemic in a flock, especially multi-age flocks, eradication is very difficult. Live and inactivated vaccines for *O. rhinotracheale* are available. It is important to determine the serotype causing the infection, so that a vaccine containing a similar serotype is administered, as cross protection seems to be rare.

Infectious coryza

Infectious coryza is a highly contagious, acute respiratory bacterial disease of chickens.

Epidemiology

The disease occurs worldwide and chickens of all ages are susceptible; the disease is more severe in mature birds. Pheasants, quails and guinea fowl may also become infected, but turkeys and ducks appear to be refractory. As the tenacity of the pathogen is very low outside the body, the sources of infection are chronically diseased or latently infected carriers who transmit the bacteria via respiratory exudates either directly by contact with another bird or indirectly by vectors (particularly contaminated drinking water).

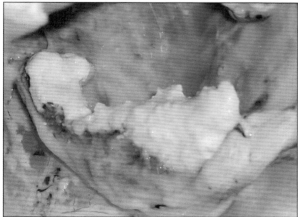

15.14 Post-mortem view of severe fibrinopurulent air sacculitis due to *Ornithobacterium rhinotracheale* infection. Note the presence of caseous material. A similar appearance is seen with *Pasteurella multocida* infection.
(© Lierz & Hafez, FU Berlin)

Aetiology and pathogenesis

Avibacterium paragallinarum (formerly known as *Haemophilus paragallinarum*) is the causative agent of infectious coryza. It is a Gram-negative, encapsulated, non-motile bacterium that typically needs a feeder bacterium (e.g. *Staphylococcus epidermidis*) to grow on blood agar plates. *A. paragallinarum* has a tropism to the cilia-covered epithelia of the upper respiratory tract but low invasiveness. Morbidity is high, and mortality is low. Only interactions with other primary or secondary pathogens may induce lesions in the lower respiratory tract (bronchi, lungs and air sacs) with an increase in mortality.

Clinical signs

The clinical signs of acute infection include clear-seromucoid to opaque-flocculated nasal discharge, conjunctivitis and collateral facial oedema. Birds sneeze with sticky nostrils, breathe with an open beak, shake their heads and wipe the exudate on to the feathers of their wings and back. Depression, reduced water and food intake and diarrhoea leads to growth retardation and reduction in egg production. In chronic cases, birds develop dyspnoea and the oedema extends to the wattle and eyes.

Differential diagnoses

A. paragallinarum has to be differentiated from other viral and bacterial primary and secondary pathogens (see Figure 15.3), but it should be noted that mixed infections occur regularly.

Post-mortem findings

During the acute phase of the disease, all chickens exhibit catarrhal to fibrinous rhinitis, conjunctivitis and sinusitis, as well as subcutaneous oedema of the face. Chronic complicated cases are characterized by the presence of bronchopneumonia and air sacculitis.

Laboratory diagnosis

Suitable samples for the detection of *A. paragallinarum* include swabs of exudate squeezed from the sinus of live birds and swabs of the deep sinus cavity obtained after sterile opening of the skin below the eyes of dead birds. The swabs should be placed in commercial transport medium to improve the viability of the pathogen. Identification of the bacterium is possible by cultivation and physiological and biochemical characterization or PCR.

Treatment

Various antibiotics and sulphonamides can be used for the treatment of *A. paragallinarum* infection. The choice of antimicrobial should be based on sensitivity testing. Following the end of the course of treatment, relapse may occur, and the carrier state cannot always be avoided.

Prognosis

The prognosis for both the individual bird and the flock is usually good when treatment is started immediately. More severely affected birds should be treated individually with the injection of antibiotics or sulphonamides, whilst others can be treated via medicated drinking water.

Prevention

If depopulation of the infected or recovered flock, cleaning and disinfection, and restocking after 2–3 weeks is not possible, then vaccination should be considered. A course of two subcutaneous injections, given 1–2 months apart, using an inactivated adjuvant vaccine leads to a serotype-specific immunity for approximately 9 months. However, this is limited to the availability of the vaccine in certain countries. Alternatively, a flock-specific vaccine can be used.

Turkey coryza

Turkey coryza (also known as bordetellosis) is a widespread, highly contagious respiratory disease of turkeys caused by *Bordetella avium*. This disease is seldom seen in chickens, quails and ducks.

Epidemiology

The turkey is the natural host of *B. avium*. The disease usually occurs in poults up to 6 weeks of age. Older turkeys, as well as chickens and ducks, only become ill following impairment of their immune systems by other infectious or non-infectious factors. Infection has also been encountered in geese, partridges and quails, as well as in wild birds. These birds, as well as a contaminated environment, may serve as the source of infection. Transmission within the flock is horizontally from bird to bird or via contaminated drinking water.

Aetiology and pathogenesis

B. avium is a Gram-negative, non-fermentative, motile, strictly aerobic bacillus. It has a tropism to the cilia-covered epithelia of the upper respiratory tract but low invasiveness. After adhesion to the cilia, the toxin produced by the pathogen induces dystrophic necrobiotic alterations of the mucosa of the upper respiratory tract, provoking catarrhal-fibrinous reactions in the affected bird. The second phase of the disease process is characterized by productive inflammatory repair processes. Systemic reactions to the infection may cause an impairment of the immune system, allowing infection by secondary pathogens such as *E. coli*, *M. gallisepticum* and *P. multocida*. Morbidity is high and mortality varies depending on the course of the disease and the presence of secondary infections.

Clinical signs

An abrupt onset of sneezing accompanied by watery and later turbid nasal and ocular discharge is suggestive of turkey coryza. Often the skin around the eyelids and nostrils, as well as the feathers of the wings, becomes crusted with tenacious, brownish exudates. Beak breathing, dyspnoea and altered vocalization in the second week of clinical signs are the result of mucus clots in the nose and upper trachea. Tracheal softening can be palpated through the skin in some birds.

Differential diagnoses

B. avium has to be differentiated from other viral (especially AMPV) and bacterial primary and secondary pathogens (see Figure 15.3), but it should be noted that mixed infections can also occur.

Post mortem-findings

With uncomplicated infections, gross lesions are restricted to the upper respiratory tract with nasal and tracheal exudates altering in character from serous to tenacious and mucoid during the course of the disease. Softening, distortion and dorsoventral compression of the trachea are highly suggestive of bordetellosis. Air sacculitis, bronchopneumonia and lesions in other organ systems are signs of complication of the disease by other pathogens.

Laboratory diagnosis

The suspected diagnosis should be confirmed by isolation of *B. avium* or a positive serological reaction (e.g. ELISA).

Treatment and prognosis

Treatment with antibiotics (e.g. tetracyclines) results in a variable improvement in the clinical signs, but recurrences can occur.

Prevention

Biosecurity measures and vaccination with a live mutant of *B. avium* vaccine (administered via spray, eye drop or orally) or an inactivated adjuvant vaccine (administered subcutaneously) are possible strategies for the prevention of bordetellosis in turkeys. Vaccination of breeding hens may be useful for the prevention of disease outbreaks in poults via the transmission of maternal antibodies.

Fowl cholera

Fowl cholera (also known as avian cholera, avian pasteurellosis and avian haemorrhagic septicaemia) is a contagious disease of domesticated as well as wild birds. It occurs as either a peracute to acute septicaemic disease (see Chapter 16) or as a chronic localized disease.

Epidemiology

Many birds are susceptible to fowl cholera. Amongst poultry, the disease occurs mainly in free-range turkeys, chickens, geese and ducks, with young mature birds affected most severely and most often. However, partridges and pheasants can be affected as well. Chronically infected but healthy carriers of the pathogen (e.g. convalescent birds, free-flying birds, rodents, cats, dogs, pigs, cattle, raccoons and insects) are the major source of infection. Transmission occurs via direct contact, via the air or indirectly via vectors such as people and equipment.

Aetiology and pathogenesis

Pasteurella multocida, a Gram-negative, non-motile, non-spore-forming, bipolar staining rod bacterium, is the causative agent of fowl cholera. The virulence of *P. multocida* varies from apathogenic to highly virulent. The entry points for the bacterium into the body are the mucous membranes of the upper respiratory and gastrointestinal tracts, as well as skin wounds (e.g. bite injuries). Highly virulent strains induce septicaemia followed by a systemic coagulopathy, with endotoxin production leading to shock and death within hours. Strains of lower virulence result in disease processes restricted to the respiratory tract or, following bacteraemia, is spread to other organ systems.

Clinical signs

The peracute disease causes sudden death in >50% of affected birds. Clinical signs of acute disease, including impairment of general condition, anorexia, mucous discharge from the nose and beak, dyspnoea, and cyanosis of the comb and wattles, often only become obvious a few hours prior to death. Chronic disease may follow the acute phase or result from infection with low virulent strains of the pathogen. The clinical signs here are generally related to localized infections and include tracheal rales, dyspnoea, nasal and ocular discharge, swelling of the sinuses, wattles, leg or wing joints, foot pads and sternal bursa, and torticollis. There may also be impairment of growth or egg production.

Differential diagnoses

The peracute and acute courses of fowl cholera resemble those of highly pathogenic avian influenza and Newcastle disease. In chronic cases, infection with *Mycoplasma* spp., *Mycobacterium tuberculosis*, *Streptococcus* spp. and *Staphylococcus* spp. have to be excluded.

Post-mortem findings

Acute disease is characterized by general hyperaemia associated with widespread petechial and ecchymotic haemorrhage, especially in the lung, subserosa and abdominal fat. Exudative pneumonia, hydropericardium and small necrotic foci in the swollen liver are also common. Chronic disease is generally associated with localized tissue lesions. The respiratory tract (all parts, including the sinuses and pneumatic bones) is very often involved. Pneumonia (hepatization of the lungs) and fibropurulent air sacculitis (Figure 15.16) are especially common findings in turkeys. The catarrhal-fibrinous-suppurative inflammatory alterations may also affect the musculoskeletal system (e.g. joints, bones, synovial tendon sheaths), skin, wattles and bursae, cerebral membranes, eyes, middle ears and oviducts.

Laboratory diagnosis

A presumptive diagnosis may be made from the clinical signs and findings at necropsy, but confirmation should be based on the isolation of *P. multocida*. Preferred samples for culture include swabs of the squeezed mucus from the nostrils or nasal cleft of living birds and specimens of

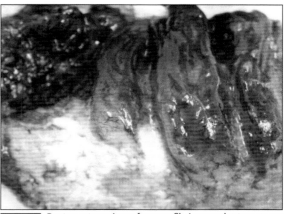

15.16 Post-mortem view of severe fibrinopurulent pneumonia with caseous material in the lung. In this case, *Pasteurella multocida* infection was confirmed as the cause.
(© Lierz & Hafez, FU Berlin)

the liver, viscera, bone marrow, blood from the heart and other localized lesions in dead birds. With imprints of liver and heart blood samples, a tentative diagnosis can be made by demonstrating the presence of bipolar organisms using Wright's stain.

Treatment

Treatment with sulphonamides and antibiotics is possible to reduce the severity of the clinical signs and mortality rate. Birds with acute disease should receive intensive treatment, including intravenous antibacterial drugs. The duration of treatment should be long (approximately 10 days), but it should be noted that recurrence of the disease may occur after cessation of treatment. As the infection regularly affects locomotion, the whole flock should be treated with a single dose of a long-acting antibiotic (e.g. chlortetracycline). This can be followed by a second injection 3 days later or, if the birds are already showing signs of improvement and are able to move, this dose can be administered via the drinking water. Parenteral drug administration is always preferred for acutely unwell birds.

Prognosis

The prognosis for birds with *P. multocida* infection is uncertain. Clinical signs in flocks are reduced by treatment, but recurrence is common after the cessation of medication. In individual birds, the prognosis depends on the lesions present as severely affected birds with pneumonia and air sacculitis seldom recover.

Prevention

Prevention of fowl cholera can be achieved by eliminating reservoirs of *P. multocida* and by excluding their access to the flock, combined with good management practices. Vaccination with commercially available live or inactivated adjuvant vaccines is possible, but should not be a substitute for good husbandry. Inactivated vaccines confer protection only against the homologous serovar, so confirmation of the isolate responsible for the infection is required. This information is also required if a flock-specific vaccine is to be produced.

Anatipestifer disease

Anatipestifer disease is a contagious, septicaemic disease seen in young ducks and geese, but it has also been reported in other poultry and wild bird species. It is caused by infection with the bacterium *Riemerella anatipestifer*. Anatipestifer disease is also known as new duck disease, duck septicaemia, anatipestifer syndrome, anatipestifer septicaemia and infectious serositis, as well as goose influenza and septicaemia anserum excudativa when it occurs in geese. Adult birds that shed the bacterium via the respiratory tract are the main source of infection. The disease may have a peracute, acute or chronic course. In the acute course, respiratory signs such as seromucous ocular or nasal discharge, mild dyspnoea, sneezing and listlessness are commonly seen. Catarrhal to fibrinous conjunctivitis, rhinitis, sinusitis and air sacculitis, accompanied by a general serositis, may be found on necropsy. As these changes may also be observed with other bacterial infections (e.g. *E. coli*, *P. multocida*, *C. psittaci* and *Salmonella* spp.), only the detection of *R. anatipestifer* is necessary for diagnosis of the disease (see also Chapter 18).

Colibacillosis

Colibacillosis (colisepticaemia) is an important, worldwide, systemic disease caused by avian pathogenic *E. coli* and can affect all birds (see also Chapter 16). In addition, localized forms restricted to single organ systems are also very common. Colibacillosis in the respiratory tract develops when *E. coli* colonizes the host following damage to the respiratory mucosa by infectious (e.g. IBV, Newcastle disease virus, including vaccine strains, AMPV and *Mycoplasma* spp.) and non-infectious (e.g. ammonia) agents. Lesions from the resulting disease, which is commonly called air sac disease, chronic respiratory disease (CRD), multi-causal respiratory disease or swollen head syndrome (SHS), are prominent in the trachea, lungs and air sacs, and are characterized by a serofibrinous inflammation. To confirm the diagnosis, isolation and identification of all involved pathogens are essential.

Aspergillosis

Avian aspergillosis is also known as fungal or mycotic pneumonia, pneumonomycosis and bronchomycosis. In young birds, the disease is often called brooder pneumonia. Less common manifestations of the infection are seen in the eye (see Chapter 14), brain, skin, joints and viscera.

Epidemiology

Many, if not all, birds are susceptible to aspergillosis. Sources of infection include litter, food (moist hay or straw), faeces, dust and incubators, as well as drinking and feeding systems in which fungal growth is promoted by the humid environmental conditions. Infection occurs by inhalation of the fungal conidia. In confined birds, morbidity and mortality may reach up to 50%; free-ranging birds are more resistant. Aspergillosis can also be acquired *in ovo* by penetration of the fungus through the eggshell during incubation.

Aetiology and pathogenesis

The main causative agents are members of the genus *Aspergillus*, particularly *A. fumigatus* and *A. flavus*. The spores of these organisms are able to survive in the environment for years. Aspergillosis occurs mainly in young birds, especially directly after hatching, and seldom in older animals, unless the bird's immune system has been depressed by factors such as poor environmental conditions, inadequate feed, other infectious diseases or long-term antibiotic treatment. The disease is characterized by exudative necrotizing and/or granulomatous inflammatory processes, primarily in the lower respiratory tract. *Aspergillus* spp. are able to produce mycotoxins that may induce invasive disease forms. Stress or other predisposing factors (e.g. immunosuppression) may allow the acute development of aspergillosis even without an increase in the number of spores in the environment.

Clinical signs

Young birds present high-grade dyspnoea and gasping, but usually no breathing sounds. With chronic disease, there are often only non-specific clinical signs such as weakness, loss of weight and apathy, whilst respiratory signs become obvious only shortly before death. In addition, ophthalmitis is often observed in young birds (see Chapter 14). Less commonly, central nervous system signs such as torticollis and lack of equilibrium, probably induced by mycotoxins, may be seen.

Differential diagnoses

The clinical signs of avian aspergillosis are non-specific and depend on the organ systems involved. Granulomatous lesions should raise suspicion for aspergillosis, but should be differentiated from those caused by tuberculosis and colibacillosis.

Post-mortem findings

At necropsy, catarrhal to fibrinous inflammatory lesions and/or yellowish grey, miliary to pie-sized granulomas are observed in the lungs and air sacs (Figure 15.17). In chronic cases, diffuse mycelia may cover the opaque and thickened air sacs. The brain, eyes, bones and other organs may also be affected. Sometimes mould growth is macroscopically visible.

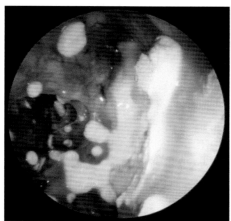

15.17 Endoscopic view of the air sac membranes coated with grey granulomas. Upon closer inspection, the mould appearance of the granulomas is clearly visible, indicating aspergillosis.
(© Michael Lierz)

Laboratory diagnosis

As *Aspergillus* spores are ubiquitous, the detection of the fungus alone on culture is not significant and can only be interpreted in combination with the clinical and pathological signs. The identification of fungal mycelium within tissue samples is possible by microscopic evaluation of a squeeze preparation after staining with ink or lactophenol blue. In live birds, a diagnosis can be made by endoscopy, as it facilitates direct visualization of the fungal growth. However, isolation of the fungus and histological demonstration of invasive growth is required for confirmation of the diagnosis.

Treatment

The main treatment measures include sanitation of the hatchery and house (removal of mouldy litter and food, daily cleaning and disinfection of food and water utensils), the addition of copper sulphate to the drinking water (1–3 g/l), and fumigation with thiabendazole or enilconazole. Oral or parenteral administration of antifungal drugs is useful in affected birds, but legislation regarding the use of pharmaceuticals in food-producing animals should be

reviewed before commencing any treatment (see Chapter 26). Voriconazole (10 mg/kg orally q12h for 3 weeks, followed by 10 mg/kg orally q24h for 3 weeks; repetition of this treatment regimen may be necessary) is the drug of choice; however, it is very expensive. Itraconazole is a good alternative antifungal drug. Treatment must be given for at least 3 weeks and this often has to be repeated two or three times. Inhalation of antifungal drugs may improve the prognosis.

Prognosis

The prognosis for the flock is poor. As environmental factors are the main cause of infection, they need to be identified and removed. Antifungal treatment is only possible for the individual bird (rather than for a flock) because it can take several weeks to complete the course of medication. The prognosis for the individual bird depends on the severity of the infection, but is always guarded. However, it should be noted that even severely affected birds can recover from the infection, although productivity usually remains low.

Prevention

All measures that reduce the environmental load of fungal spores are useful for the prevention of aspergillosis (e.g. dry feed storage, dry litter, sufficient ventilation, cleaning regimen and the use of disinfectants with an antifungal effect). In addition, repeated stressful events should be avoided, especially in chicks.

Gape

This disease is called 'gape' because birds gape or gasp due to heavy infestations of the nematode *Syngamus trachea*. It is also known as syngamosis.

Epidemiology

Infestations can occur in all species of birds (especially if eating worms) and chickens, turkeys, geese, guinea fowl, pheasants, peafowl, emus and quails are regularly infected. Transmission from bird to bird may occur directly by ingestion of embryonated worm eggs or larvae, or indirectly be eating paratenic hosts, particularly earthworms, in which gapeworm larvae may remain infective for as long as 4 years. For this reason, free-range birds are more often exposed to infection than those birds that are kept indoors.

Aetiology and pathogenesis

S. trachea is also called 'redworm' because of its noticeable red colour and 'forked worm' because of the formation of a 'Y-shape' as a result of the permanent copulation of the male and female worm. The prepatent period lasts 12–21 days. After infection, larvae migrate to the respiratory tract, either by penetration of the crop or oesophagus, or via the portal bloodstream, where they attach to the trachea, bronchi and bronchioles. Young birds are most seriously affected by the nematode, which can quickly obstruct the lumen of the upper airways due to its rapid growth, inducing severe dyspnoea and leading to suffocation.

Clinical signs

Stertorous and whistling breathing sounds in combination with a stretched neck and head, an open beak and head chucking may be observed.

Differential diagnoses

All respiratory diseases that present dyspnoea (see Figure 15.3) have to be excluded. Worms that are coughed up may look like bloody mucus and thus resemble the clinical signs seen with ILT.

Post-mortem findings

At necropsy, 'redworms' can be found attached to the trachea (males: 2–8mm; females: ≤36 mm). They induce lesions and nodules in the tracheal mucosa as an inflammatory reaction to the attachment of the worms.

Laboratory diagnosis

Clinical signs in combination with the detection of worm eggs (74–125 μm x 36–55 μm) in faecal samples using the flotation method confirms the diagnosis. In severe cases, adult worms may be seen in the oral cavity or, at necropsy, in the trachea, allowing confirmation of the diagnosis. In the individual bird, tracheoscopy allows rapid confirmation of the diagnosis.

Treatment

Treatment with flubendazole (1.8 mg/kg bodyweight for 7 days orally) is possible. Alternatively, fenbendazole, levamisole or ivermectin could be considered, depending on the restrictions regarding the use of these drugs in food-producing animals. In cases of recurrent disease occurring within cages placed on natural ground, the ground (up to 10 cm deep) should be changed. However, it should be borne in mind that reintroduction by free-ranging birds or earthworms usually occurs.

Prognosis

The prognosis is usually good for the flock and the individual bird, as treatment is usually successful. In heavy infestations with severe clinical signs, the airway may be blocked and worms can be removed via endoscopy to allow breathing and provide time for treatment.

Prevention

A dry run area and litter, as well as regular examination of the faeces for eggs (with treatment as required) is necessary for prevention.

Cryptosporidiosis

Cryptosporidiosis is an infection with a protozoan parasite that causes respiratory and/or gastrointestinal disease (see Chapter 16) in young chickens, turkeys, quails, ducks and geese.

Epidemiology

Cryptosporidium spp. are known to be prevalent worldwide in 30 species of domesticated, caged and wild birds, and seem to be of increasing importance. Infection of the respiratory tract results from aspiration or inhalation of oocysts, whilst infection of the gastrointestinal tract, cloaca and bursa of Fabricius results from the oral intake of contaminated feed or water. *Cryptosporidium* spp. oocysts can survive in a humid environment for a long period of time and are remarkably resistant to commonly used disinfectants, but are susceptible to heat and ultraviolet radiation.

Aetiology and pathogenesis

Two *Cryptosporidium* spp. that affect birds have been identified: *C. bayleyi* and *C. meleagridis*. They are small (4–7 μm) protozoa with a similar lifecycle to *Eimeria* spp. Following infection (only a few oocysts are necessary), multiplication takes place in the microvillus region of the respiratory, bursal and/or intestinal epithelial cells of the host, resulting in the development of thin- and (mainly) thick-walled oocysts. Thin-walled oocysts invade adjacent host cells, causing severe damage, whilst thick-walled oocysts are shed via the respiratory mucus or the faeces.

Clinical signs

Infection may cause clinical signs and growth retardation in young chickens, turkeys and quails, but does not usually induce clinical signs in ducks and geese. The severity of the respiratory signs (sneezing, swelling of the infraorbital sinuses, aggravated breathing), as well as the morbidity and mortality, can vary considerably. The intestinal clinical signs associated with *Cryptosporidium* infection are described in Chapter 16. The disease may be complicated by secondary infections.

Differential diagnoses

All infections with tropism to the epithelia of the respiratory and gastrointestinal tracts have to be considered. In cases that involve the bursa of Fabricius, cryptosporidiosis has to be differentiated from infectious bursitis and circovirus infection.

Post-mortem findings

Catarrhal-fibrinous conjunctivitis, sinusitis, tracheitis, air sacculitis and pneumonia may be found at necropsy. Alterations in the gastrointestinal tract may also be induced by the protozoan (see Chapter 16).

Laboratory diagnosis

Cryptosporidium spp. can be identified in faecal samples as well as in scrapings taken from the epithelia of the respiratory and gastrointestinal tracts that have been stained with carbol fuchsin or submitted for histological examination. Fresh faecal and respiratory tract samples should be collected and placed in 10% formalin or in an aqueous solution of 2.5% potassium chloride. Diagnosis is difficult because of the small size of the oocysts and their location at the brush border of epithelial cells. PCR for the detection of parasite-specific DNA is possible, but very few laboratories offer this service.

Treatment and prevention

Sanitation and disinfection by steam cleaning is recommended. In addition, the use of paramomycin and azithromycin (Molina-Lopez *et al.*, 2010) has been described, but the use of these drugs in food-producing animals may be limited due to national regulations.

Prognosis

The prognosis for the individual and the flock following treatment is poor. Severely affected birds are difficult to treat and usually do not fully recover.

Heat stress

Temperatures above the comfort zone (>28°C), especially in combination with high humidity (>80%) (e.g. due to warm weather, overcrowding in houses and transport boxes), can cause heat stress in poultry.

Aetiology and pathogenesis

As birds do not have sweat glands, they use non-evaporative cooling (radiation, conduction, convection) and evaporative cooling via the respiratory tract as a means of heat dissipation. Increasing the respiration rate decreases the carbon dioxide concentration in the blood and thus increases the pH. In turn, this reduces the amount of ionized calcium available for eggshell formation. Consequently, the number of thin-shelled eggs may rise in laying birds. In cases where this physiological system still does not prevent body temperature from rising, birds may die from respiratory, circulatory or electrolyte imbalances. The extent of losses from heat stress is influenced by the age of the bird, the maximum temperature, the length of time the high temperature lasts, the rate of temperature change and the relative humidity. In severe cases, massive losses may occur within a short time period.

Clinical signs

At environmental temperatures between 28 and 35°C birds relax their wings and hang them loosely at their sides to increase the body surface area over which heat can be lost. At the same time, the peripheral blow flow is increased. Environmental temperatures approaching body temperature (41°C) induce an increase in the respiration rate accompanied by open-beak breathing. Panting may lead to respiratory infections, as the natural filters in the nose are bypassed. Reduction of food intake causes growth retardation and a drop in egg production. If panting is not sufficient to reduce the body temperature, birds become listless, comatose and then die.

Post-mortem findings

The most prominent sign is cyanosis of the head and, occasionally, the legs. Right atrium hypertrophy with excessive blood accumulation, heart enlargement and hypertrophy of the right ventricle can also be observed. Congestion, oedema and hyperaemia are present in the lungs. The liver may be pale and yellow, whilst the kidneys may show signs of generalized oedema and haemorrhage in the subrenal capsule.

Laboratory diagnosis

The environmental conditions on site (high temperature, high stocking rate, inadequate transport) provide clear indications for heat stress. Nevertheless, swabs and tissue samples obtained from both diseased and dead birds should be tested for infectious agents, particularly to exclude HPAIV, Newcastle disease and fowl cholera.

Treatment and prevention

Free-range birds should be provided with access to shaded areas. Measures to reduce and prevent heat stress for birds housed indoors include:

- Increasing air circulation using ventilation equipment
- Cooling the air using sprinklers
- Spraying the roof with cool water
- Providing access to sufficient fresh and cool drinking water.

In areas with permanently high environmental temperatures, building insulation, roof overhangs to prevent sunlight from directly hitting the house, painting the house with white or aluminium paint to reflect heat, and fans and foggers are adequate means for heat stress prevention. In the individual bird, rapid cooling including use of cold intravenous infusions with isotonic 0.9% NaCl are lifesaving. Birds in recovery should receive broad-spectrum antibiotics as severe heat stress leads to immunosuppression and the open-mouth breathing enables respiratory tract infections.

Prognosis

The prognosis is usually good, except for birds that are already laying on the floor and are comatose.

Vitamin A deficiency

Vitamin A deficiency causes keratinization of the epithelia in glands and mucosa (see also Chapter 20). In the respiratory tract, the process begins with exudation of seromucoid watery clear to milky white caseous masses in the eyes, nose, sinuses, trachea and bronchi. It is difficult to differentiate this condition from infectious bronchitis and infectious coryza. Later in the disease process, the epithelium is replaced by a stratified squamous keratinizing epithelium, giving the surface a dry, dull and uneven appearance.

References and further reading

Aldous EW and Alexander DJ (2008) Newcastle disease in pheasants (Phasianus colchicus): a review. *The Veterinary Journal* **175**, 181–185

Bagust TJ, Jones RC and Guy JS (2000) Avian infectious laryngotracheitis. *Revue Scientifique et Technique* **19**, 483–492

Capua I and Alexander DJ (2009) *Avian Influenza and Newcastle Disease.* Springer, New York, USA

Capua I and Mutinelli F (2001) *Avian Influenza.* Papi Editore, Bologna, Italy

Cook JK, Jackwood M and Jones RC (2012) The long view: 40 years of infectious bronchitis research. *Avian Pathology* **41**, 239–250

De Wit JJ, Cook JK and van der Heijden HM (2011) Infectious bronchitis virus variants: a review of the history, current situation and control measures. *Avian Pathology* **40**, 223–235

Majó N and Dolz R (2012) *Atlas of Avian Necropsy.* Grupo Asís Biomedia, Zaragoza, Spain

Molina-Lopez RA, Ramis A, Martin-Vazquez S *et al.* (2010) Cryptosporidium baileyi infection associated with an outbreak of ocular and respiratory disease in otus owls (*Otus scops*) in a rehabilitation centre. *Avian Pathology* **39(3)**, 171–176

Pattison M, McMullin PF, Bradbury JM and Alexander DJ (2008) *Poultry Diseases, 6th edn.* Elsevier, Oxford, UK

Siegmann O and Neumann U (2012) *Kompendium der Geflügelkrankheiten, 7th edn.* Schlütersche Verlagsgesellschaft mbH, Hannover, Germany

Swayne DE (2008) *Avian Influenza.* Blackwell publishing, Ames, USA

Swayne DE (2017) *Diseases of Poultry, 13th edn.* Wiley-Blackwell Hoboken, New Jersey, USA

Williams SM, Dufour-Savala L, Jackwood MW *et al.* (2016) *A Laboratory Manual for the Isolation, Identification and Characterization of Avian Pathogens, 6th edn.* American Association of Avian Pathologists, OmniPress Inc., Madison, USA

Chapter 16

Gastrointestinal disorders

Richard Jackson

Gastrointestinal disorders in backyard poultry are incredibly common and, whilst there are many potential pathogens that can cause disease, the most common aetiology is poor husbandry.

Of all the management failures, an inappropriate diet is the most common. Poultry should be fed a commercial pellet or mash with perhaps a little corn given as a treat. Kitchen scraps certainly do not make good treats and can lead to crop and intestinal issues through the disruption of the normal flora of the digestive tract. Furthermore, it is illegal to feed kitchen scraps to any poultry in some countries, including the UK. See Chapter 5 for more information on nutrition for backyard poultry.

Contaminated water is also an important cause of disease. All animals should have access to clean fresh water; however, there are a surprising number of owners who do not change their birds' drinking water daily. In addition, most backyard flocks are also free ranging and so invariably have access to muddy puddles in their range area, which can harbour pathogens. Where possible, these areas should be either drained or filled in. Agricultural lime can be applied to the range to reduce pathogenic contamination.

Environmental stresses, such as being taken to a show or being rehomed, can allow the recrudescence of latent pathogens, both intestinal and otherwise, such as *Mycoplasma gallisepticum*.

Many gastrointestinal pathogens such as *Trichomonas* and *Salmonella* species can be carried by wild birds. Owners should therefore try to discourage wild birds where possible. Owners will often plant trees in their chicken runs to encourage their birds to range. Whilst tree cover certainly does encourage ranging behaviour, these trees will also attract wild birds to roost, which will then defecate on the ground below. Feeding poultry in the range area is an additional attractant for wild birds and pests and should be strongly discouraged.

Almost all pathogens are incapable of causing disease on their own and improving husbandry is often the best prevention of all for gastrointestinal disease.

Conditions of the oral cavity

During the clinical examination, it is always important to check the oral cavity for both foreign bodies and lesions. Whilst pathology of the oral cavity is relatively rare, two conditions worth bearing in mind are the 'wet form' of fowlpox and trichomoniasis.

Fowlpox
Aetiology, epidemiology and pathogenesis
Fowlpox is caused by a poxvirus. There are two forms of the disease:

- The cutaneous form ('dry form') of fowlpox is spread by mechanical transmission (e.g. by biting insects or through pecking-related wounds)
- The fibrinoproliferative form ('wet form') of fowlpox is caused by inhalation/ingestion of the virus (much rarer than via the mechanical route).

The virus has an incubation period of 4–10 days and is not highly infective. Its spread throughout a flock can therefore be slow.

Clinical signs
- Dry form: 'pocks' (papules, nodules and scabs) on featherless skin such as the comb or snood. Lesions begin as nodules and progress to scabs (Figure 16.1).
- Wet form: white nodules in the buccal cavity, which often progress to become more extensive caseous lesions. In extreme cases, these lesions can become diphtheritic. Such lesions can potentially cause inappetence and difficulty breathing.

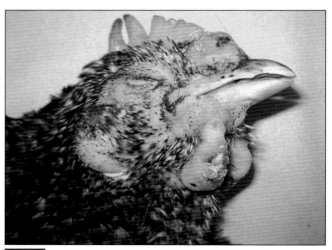

16.1 A 5-year-old Maran hen with the dry form of fowlpox.

Diagnosis

The discovery of lesions indicative of fowlpox (either during clinical examination or on post-mortem examination) implies the presence of the infection; virus isolation, histopathology or polymerase chain reaction (PCR) testing can then be used to provide a definitive diagnosis. Serology may also be used to provide a diagnosis retrospectively.

Treatment

There is no specific treatment for fowlpox and the majority of cases have an uneventful recovery. Practitioners should, however, ensure that in the 'wet form' of fowlpox the diphtheritic membrane does not obstruct the larynx and that the bird is kept both hydrated and nutritionally supported. Antimicrobials may be beneficial in such cases to control secondary bacterial infection. In the face of a local outbreak, a vaccination protocol can be implemented.

Prognosis

The prognosis is excellent for birds with the 'dry form' of the disease; lesions resolve in 2–8 weeks. For birds with the 'wet form' the prognosis is fair provided the larynx remains unobstructed.

Prevention

Prevention is based upon good hygiene and biosecurity. Like other poxviruses, the fowlpox virus can be difficult to remove from a holding. A live attenuated vaccine can potentially be given through cutaneous scarification, usually on the wing web. However, in the UK there is currently no authorized fowlpox vaccine. The pigeon pox vaccine is more readily available and offers some cross protection against fowlpox.

Differential diagnoses

Differential diagnoses for the 'wet form' of fowlpox include trichomoniasis and oral mycosis.

Trichomoniasis (oral canker, frounce, roup)

See Endoparasites.

Conditions of the crop and oesophagus

The crop is a region of the oesophagus found in poultry, located at the thoracic inlet and used to store food before it enters the proventriculus. The crop varies in its development depending on the species, with chickens having very well developed, large crops compared with waterfowl, in which the crop is poorly developed and is often difficult to locate. The crop can vary tremendously in size from a virtually undetectable sac with a few particles of food or stones present through to the size of an orange after feeding.

Many owners will contact veterinary surgeons (veterinarians) stating that their birds have an enlarged crop; however, provided that the bird is otherwise well, it is worth withholding food (not water) for a few hours to see if the crop reduces in size.

When a bird is presented with a chronically enlarged crop there are three potential causes:

- Sour crop
- Impacted crop
- Pendulous crop (especially in turkeys).

When clinically examining an enlarged crop, it should be gently palpated. One differentiating feature is the consistency of the contents; an impacted crop has hard contents whereas sour and pendulous crops usually have fluidic contents.

Sour crop (crop mycosis, thrush, moniliasis)
Aetiology, epidemiology and pathogenesis

Sour crop is caused by a disruption of the normal flora of the crop, leading to a fungal overgrowth of *Candida albicans*. Although this is most commonly a condition of the crop, it should be noted that other areas of the digestive tract may be affected. Whilst there is no single cause for sour crop, the main predisposing factors include an inappropriate diet, the use of antimicrobials and the presence of any disease that causes subnormal levels of gastrointestinal motility.

Although the condition is not contagious, it is likely that if one bird in a flock is exposed to the predisposing factors then more than one bird may go on to develop the condition.

Clinical signs

Affected birds are often dull and inappetent, with a large fluid-filled pendulous crop (Figure 16.2). Occasionally, these birds will have a yeast-like odour to their breath.

Post-mortem findings

On post-mortem examination the crop of affected birds will often have raised white circumscribed lesions, together with ulceration and mucosal necrosis.

Diagnosis

Diagnosis is usually based upon clinical signs; however, the crop contents may be aspirated using a feeding/crop tube and checked for the presence of *Candida*. It should be remembered that this organism is commensal and as such a few yeasts will be seen in a healthy bird but large numbers indicate an overgrowth.

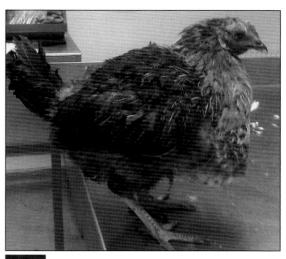

16.2 A 2-year-old hen with sour crop.

Treatment

There are several suggested treatments for sour crop. Traditionally, the recommended treatment was to invert the bird and massage its crop to empty its contents; however, this method carries a genuine risk of choking. The preferred method for treating this condition is to identify and treat/remove any predisposing factors and to reduce the crop using a crop tube.

Some clinicians advocate the use of oral probiotics to help re-establish the crop's normal flora. Owners may try to give live yoghurts to this effect and, whilst these do contain *Lactobacilli* bacteria, they should not be given as birds cannot digest dairy products. If probiotics are given they must be poultry-specific and dairy-free.

In the majority of cases these steps alone are sufficient; however, antifungal agents such as nystatin may be given at 100,000–300,000 IU orally, daily for 10 days. Many owners will use apple cider vinegar to improve the health of their bird's digestive system through acidification. Whilst there is evidence of a benefit to gastrointestinal health though acidification, in cases of sour crop it is unlikely that the decrease in pH will be sufficient to reduce the numbers of *Candida*.

Prognosis

The prognosis is good, providing the underlying causes are removed; however, repeat treatments may be necessary.

Prevention

Prevention is based upon ensuring an appropriate diet, along with avoiding excessive use of antimicrobials.

Differential diagnoses

Impacted crop and pendulous crop.

Impacted crop
Aetiology, epidemiology and pathogenesis

Crop impaction is most commonly caused by birds ingesting long grass, straw, plastic or string, which can physically obstruct the crop and proventriculus. However, in rare cases there may be underlying dysmotility of the gastrointestinal tract.

Clinical signs

Affected birds will have a large distended crop.

Post-mortem findings

The crop will often have a large matt of the offending material blocking the entrance to the proventriculus. This material may also block the proventriculus and ventriculus.

Diagnosis

The large distended crop with hard contents does not reduce after several hours of withholding food.

Treatment

The outcome with conservative treatment is poor and an ingluviotomy is recommended (Figure 16.3). The surgical technique for an ingluviotomy is described in Chapter 23. It is nearly impossible to ascertain how far distally the

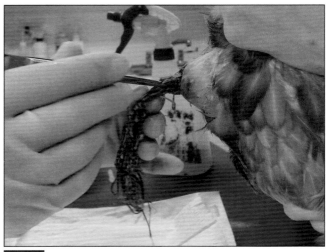

16.3 An ex-battery hen undergoing surgery for an impacted crop.

blockage extends and so it may subsequently be discovered that more invasive surgery into the proventriculus and/or ventriculus is necessary. Aftercare is very important in such cases to prevent the bird gorging and putting pressure on the wound. The bird should be given *ad libitum* water immediately after surgery and small amounts of food should be given little and often (every 2–4 hours).

Prognosis

The prognosis of such cases is highly variable. If there is an underlying motility disorder, the condition will likely return. In the case of foreign bodies after surgical intervention, provided that there is no further obstruction more distally in the gastrointestinal tract, then the condition should not return.

Prevention

Prevention of crop impaction involves restricting the access of birds to long grass, straw and plastic/string.

Differential diagnoses

Sour crop and pendulous crop.

Pendulous crop
Aetiology, epidemiology and pathogenesis

A pendulous crop is caused by a loss of tone of the crop wall and is most commonly seen in turkeys. It may be a sequel to chronic, subclinical crop impaction and over time escalates until the crop becomes so flaccid and pendulous that it is unable to empty without intervention. There is also thought to be a hereditary influence in turkeys.

Clinical signs and diagnosis

Affected birds will have a large pendulous crop that does not empty upon the withholding of food. Affected birds are often bright and will eat; however, they may lose body condition due to abnormal gastrointestinal tract function.

Treatment

As with an impacted crop, the outcome without surgery to resect the flaccid crop wall is poor. The ingluviotomy technique is described in Chapter 23. As with any ingluviotomy procedure, aftercare is very important to prevent the bird gorging and putting pressure on the wound. The bird should be given *ad libitum* water immediately after surgery and small amounts of food should be given little and often (every 2–4 hours).

Prognosis

The prognosis is guarded.

Prevention

As with the prevention of crop impaction, restricting birds' access to long grass, straw and plastic/string may help. If there is a suspicion of a genetic influence in a certain breeding line of birds, then these birds should not be bred from.

Differential diagnoses

Impacted crop and sour crop.

Capillaria (hairworm, threadworm)

See Endoparasites.

Conditions of the proventriculus and ventriculus (gizzard)

The proventriculus and gizzard are very difficult organs to examine clinically and, although abdominal palpation may be of use, radiography or endoscopy are the only practical diagnostic aids. Remember that the ventriculus can vary in size tremendously depending on the bird's diet, with birds fed exclusively on pellets/mash having a relatively small atonic ventriculus, whilst those with access to stones and grass have a large muscular ventriculus.

Proventricular and ventricular foreign bodies

Birds have a remarkable ability to ingest a whole range of foreign bodies of varying size.

Clinical signs

Foreign bodies of the proventriculus/ventriculus can lead to crop impaction (the crop fills once the ventriculus and proventriculus are full and it empties once they are empty), inappetence and weight loss.

Diagnosis

Diagnosis using radiography or endoscopy can be of assistance but it should be remembered when interpreting radiographs that small stones are a normal finding in this region of the gastrointestinal tract.

Treatment

Treatment involves surgical removal of the foreign body. The surgical approach to the proventriculus and ventriculus is detailed in Chapter 23.

Prognosis

The prognosis for such cases is usually favourable provided that intervention is prompt.

Prevention

Prevention is based upon keeping birds away from foreign bodies, including long grass and pieces of string.

Differential diagnoses

Impacted crop and intussusception.

Proventricular parasites

See Endoparasites.

Gizzard worms

See Endoparasites.

Endoparasites

Nematodes

A large number of nematodes can infect poultry (detailed below). These parasites can vary in their predilection site, from the crop right through to the caecum. The first important thing to remember with regard to nematodes is that many species can complete their lifecycles indoors and therefore worms are not solely an issue for free-ranging birds. Identification of eggs in faeces is discussed in detail in Chapter 10.

Capillaria (hairworm, threadworm)

Aetiology, epidemiology and pathogenesis: *Capillaria* is a genus of nematode worm with many different species, each of which varies in both its predilection site (from the crop through to the intestine) and in its intended host (*Capillaria* can infect all species of poultry). *Capillaria* spp. may use earthworms as intermediate hosts, although the parasite's lifecycle may also be completed directly. The worm is approximately 2 cm in length (range: 1.5–8 cm) and burrows into the mucosa, causing damage. The pre-patent period varies between 3 and 4 weeks.

Clinical signs: Affected birds are often inappetent and lose weight. In young birds, severe burdens can lead to death.

Post-mortem findings: The most common findings are inflammation and thickening of the affected region of the gastrointestinal tract. In severe cases the result is the formation of a diphtheritic membrane. Upon close inspection (often aided by a hand-held lens) the adult worms may be seen.

Diagnosis: Diagnosis can be based upon faecal worm egg counts where *Capillaria* eggs can be clearly identified by their elongated shape and bipolar plugs. However, where the worm burden is large, affected birds may show clinical signs before the adult worms are found.

Treatment: Due to their pathogenicity, the presence of any *Capillaria* eggs should constitute grounds for treatment. (See later for the treatment of nematodes.)

Prognosis: If treated in the early stages of infection the prognosis is excellent.

Prevention: See later.

Differential diagnoses: Other helminths may produce similar clinical signs. Similar post-mortem findings may be found with mycosis of the digestive tract and trichomoniasis.

Proventricular parasites

Aetiology, epidemiology and pathogenesis: There are several nematode species that can inhabit the proventriculus of poultry; these include *Tetrameres* spp., *Eustrongylides* spp., *Heterakis* spp., *Dispharynx* spp. and *Echinuria* spp. Proventricular worms are approximately 0.5 cm in length. They typically burrow into the proventricular wall and suck blood, causing inflammation, thickening, proventricular necrosis and anaemia. Many species have intermediate hosts such as insects, earthworms or crustaceans.

Clinical signs: Proventricular worms are rare and are only pathogenic in large numbers. Affected birds are often lethargic, lay fewer eggs, are anaemic and have diarrhoea. In severe cases death may occur.

Post-mortem findings: The main findings are inflammation, thickening and necrosis of the proventricular mucosa together with serosal haemorrhages. There may also be signs of anaemia (pallor of the carcass).

Diagnosis: Diagnosis is based upon faecal worm egg counts (to look for embryonated eggs with thick shells) or post-mortem findings.

Treatment: See below.

Prognosis: The outcome of such cases is usually favourable.

Prevention: See later.

Differential diagnoses: Other nematodes.

Gizzard worms

Aetiology, epidemiology and pathogenesis: There are several species of worm that can infect the gizzard of waterfowl; there is some evidence that other fowl can be infected by gizzard worms but this is thought to be rare. Most of these worms belong to the genus *Amidostomum*. These species are predominantly a problem for young birds, especially *Amidostomum anseris* in goslings. The pre-patent period is between 2 and 3 weeks.

Clinical signs: Infection causes affected birds to lose weight and in severe cases become anaemic with subsequent death being a real possibility.

Post-mortem findings: The worms burrow into the mucosa and feed on blood, leading to irritation and thickening of the gizzard wall.

Diagnosis: Diagnosis can be based on post-mortem findings of worms in the gizzard together with haemorrhage, thickening and necrosis of the gizzard mucosa. Faecal worm egg counts may be used to diagnose infection; the eggs are approximately 60 x 100 μm and have thin walls.

Treatment: See below.

Prognosis: The prognosis is good if detected early enough.

Prevention: See below.

Differential diagnoses: Other nematodes.

Ascaridia galli

Aetiology, epidemiology and pathogenesis: *A. galli* is a common nematode of backyard poultry. The adult worm infests the small intestine and can be up to 12 cm in length. Although this nematode can complete its lifecycle directly, it may also utilize an intermediate host such as the earthworm. The pre-patent period varies between 4 and 8 weeks.

Clinical signs: Although mild infections are asymptomatic, if the burden is sufficient then affected birds can lose weight, have reduced egg production, develop anaemia and, in severe cases, the worms can cause intestinal obstruction.

Post-mortem findings: The worms damage the intestinal mucosa and feed on blood, leading to irritation of the intestinal wall. The adult worms are large enough to be seen with the naked eye (Figure 16.4).

Diagnosis: Diagnosis can be based upon finding the adult worms on post-mortem examination or using faecal worm egg counts to look for oval smooth-shelled eggs.

Treatment: See below.

Prognosis: The prognosis is good.

Prevention: See below.

Differential diagnoses: Other helminths.

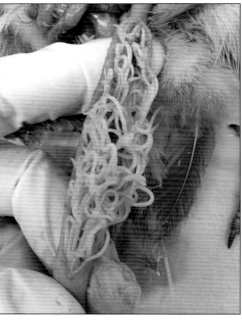

16.4

Ascaridia galli in a backyard chicken.

Heterakis species (caecal worms)

Aetiology, epidemiology and pathogenesis: *Heterakis* species are small worms measuring approximately 1.5 cm in length that can infect the caeca of all poultry species (Figure 16.5). This worm is generally considered to be non-pathogenic; however, *H. isolonche* infection in pheasants can result in typhlitis. Much more importantly *Heterakis* worms can carry the harmful protozoal parasite *Histomonas meleagridis*, which is primarily a pathogen of turkeys, though it is becoming more commonly reported in free-range chickens. The pre-patent period is approximately 4 weeks.

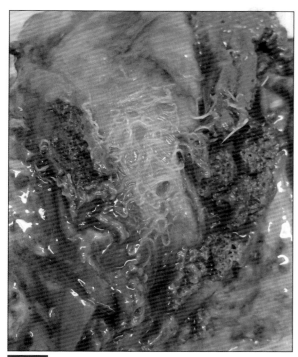

16.5 *Heterakis* worms in the caeca of a 6-month-old turkey.

Clinical signs: Infected birds are usually asymptomatic; however, *H. isolonche* may cause weight loss, diarrhoea and dullness in pheasants.

Diagnosis: Diagnosis can be based upon post-mortem findings of the worms in the caeca or using faecal worm egg counts (looking for oval smooth-shelled eggs). *H. isolonche* will cause typhlitis.

Treatment: See below.

Prognosis: The prognosis is good.

Prevention: See below.

Differential diagnoses: *H. isolonche* may cause similar caecal lesions to coccidiosis.

Treatment of nematodes in poultry

Flubendazole and fenbendazole are the only authorized anthelmintics for chickens in the UK. Flubendazole is administered in the food for 7 consecutive days at 30 ppm for chickens and geese and at 20 ppm for turkeys. Flubendazole can also be administered via the drinking water for 7 consecutive days to chickens at 1.43 mg/kg. Whilst flubendazole is only authorized for use in chickens, turkeys and geese, it is safe for other poultry species. Fenbendazole can be administered to chickens via the drinking water for 5 consecutive days at 2.5 mg/kg. It is recommended to repeat the treatment approximately a few weeks later in heavy infections, to take into account the pre-patent periods of worms.

Control of nematodes in poultry

Control of nematodes should be done using the results of regular faecal worm egg counts to determine if and when treatment is required. The number of worm eggs per gram of faeces at which worming should be carried out is

the subject of debate, with some authors suggesting the presence of any worm eggs as being grounds for worming (this is certainly the case with *Capillaria*); however, traditionally it has been recommended that only when the worm egg count (excluding *Capillaria*) exceeds 400 eggs per gram of faeces should worming take place. The sampling intervals should depend on the disease history of the holding and should be recommended by the veterinary surgeon.

Controlling helminth eggs in the poultry house requires good cleaning and disinfection. Pasture management can be difficult. Whilst rotating the pasture will reduce the egg burden, it ought to be remembered that some eggs are incredibly long-lived and they can be carried by intermediate hosts such as earthworms. Ultraviolet (UV) light is good at destroying eggs; keeping the pasture short will allow UV light to reach the soil, helping to destroy worm eggs. This, along with applying agricultural lime, will help control pasture burdens.

> **PRACTICAL TIP**
>
> Pasture rotation is essential to reduce the burdens of gizzard worms in goslings, together with keeping goslings away from adult waterfowl

Cestodes in poultry

Tapeworms (Figure 16.6) are uncommonly diagnosed as a problem in poultry and, even when present, they tend to be non-pathogenic. However, certain species such as *Davainea proglottina* can lead to weight loss, haemorrhagic enteritis, poor growth and inappetence. Like all tapeworms, those infecting poultry require intermediate hosts (usually insects). Diagnosis can be based upon finding either worms or gravid segments in faeces.

Traditional treatments and prevention aim to kill the intermediate host. There is no authorized treatment for cestodes in poultry; however, praziquantel has been reported to be of benefit when given at 10 mg/kg.

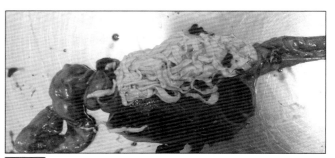

16.6 Occlusion of the gut in a red grouse with tapeworms.

Trematodes in poultry

Intestinal fluke species can occasionally cause disease in poultry (mainly waterfowl) and can lead to enteritis, weight loss, anaemia and emaciation. Like many other trematodes, snails act as intermediate hosts.

Diagnosis can be made by looking for fluke eggs in faecal samples or looking for flukes at post-mortem examination.

Treatment will involve the use of a suitable anthelmintic. There are no authorized anthelmintic treatments for fluke in poultry; however, the use of praziquantel at 10 mg/kg has been suggested.

Non-motile protozoa
Histomonas meleagridis (blackhead)

Aetiology, epidemiology and pathogenesis: *Histomonas* is a protozoal parasite that can cause disease in all poultry, excluding waterfowl. Turkeys appear to be highly susceptible, whilst chickens are relatively resistant to infection. The parasite is generally carried by *Heterakis gallinarum* (the caecal worm), although direct transmission through cloacal drinking has been documented.

Once in the caecum (usually via the *Heterakis* worm) the parasite invades the caecal mucosa causing typhlitis, potentially leading to a sulphur yellow diarrhoea. The parasite next crosses the coelomic cavity to the liver where it causes areas of focal necrosis in the liver.

Clinical signs: The most frequent sign is sudden death in birds. Those found alive will be dull, hunched up and have ruffled feathers. A sulphur yellow diarrhoea may be observed. A cyanotic head (hence the term 'blackhead') is a rare clinical feature.

Post-mortem findings: Caecal cores and ulceration, along with 'hobnail' liver lesions, are pathognomonic findings (Figure 16.7). Caecal worms will also likely be found.

Diagnosis: Due to the rapid progression of the condition, post-mortem examination is the best diagnostic option, with the liver lesions being pathognomonic.

Treatment: Treatment involves giving the birds metronidazole to destroy the protozoa along with flubendazole/fenbendazole to kill the caecal worms. The prohibition of the use of metronidazole in food-producing animals in the EU and elsewhere is particularly problematic in these cases. The use of tetracyclines combined with tiamulin for at least 5 days in food producing animals should be considered. Whilst this combination does not appear to have a direct action on the parasite, it does appear to control secondary infection and is the only practical option when the use of metronidazole is contraindicated. Moving the range area to lower exposure to the parasite may help. Oregano-based feed or water supplements have been anecdotally considered to be of use following

conventional treatment. (The use of oregano is widespread in commercial free range and organic layer systems in the UK.)

Prognosis: The prognosis of clinical cases is poor.

Prevention: Prevention is based upon successfully controlling the intermediate host *Heterakis gallinarum*. Ideally, turkeys and chickens should never share the same pasture because chickens are relatively resistant to *Histomonas* and can be carriers, whilst turkeys are very susceptible. Oregano-based supplements have been anecdotally used as a preventive measure in either feed or water.

Differential diagnoses: The liver lesions are pathognomonic; however, rotavirus and *Hexamita* can produce similarly yellow droppings.

Apicomplexans
Coccidiosis

Aetiology, epidemiology and pathogenesis: There are several species of coccidia (*Eimeria*) that can be found in poultry, each of which is host-specific. Furthermore, there are several species of coccidia that can infect any given species of fowl. Whilst these species of coccidia vary in both their predilection site and pathogenicity, for the purposes of diagnosis and treatment there is no real need to speciate them.

There are no maternal antibodies against coccidiosis found in the young chick. Therefore, young birds are vulnerable to clinical disease if the level of challenge is great enough.

Coccidiosis tends to be a flock problem and often the first birds in a flock to be infected do not show clinical signs but instead act as amplifiers, as large numbers of oocysts can be passed before natural immunity develops. Large numbers of oocysts can then build up in the environment, which go on to infect the rest of the flock, leading to clinical signs.

There are several species of coccidia that can infect a given species of poultry but only *E. tenella* is likely to be of concern in backyard chickens. Infection occurs through the ingestion of sporulated oocysts, which can sporulate in as little as 48 hours in warm (25–30°C) humid conditions. As the parasite undergoes several rounds of asexual reproduction followed by a round of sexual reproduction (to produce many more oocysts) the intestinal wall is damaged. This damage can lead to blood loss, bacterial overgrowth, necrotic enteritis, malabsorption and even septicaemia.

Clinical signs: Affected birds are often dull, inappetent (often the birds will flick the feed out of the feeders and on to the floor, as well as leaving behind whole wheat, due to abdominal pain), hunched up with ruffled feathers and have diarrhoea. In certain instances, the intestinal pathology is great enough to produce a bloody diarrhoea leading to anaemia, characterized by a pale comb and wattles (Figure 16.8). Acute infection can result in sudden death due to anaemia without any other clinical signs. Note that haemorrhagic droppings are not a finding in cases of coccidiosis in species other than chickens. Bloody droppings in turkeys are usually indicative of haemorrhagic enteritis.

Post-mortem findings: Post-mortem lesions vary depending on the species of coccidia involved. The most well known species of coccidia in chickens (*Eimeria tenella*)

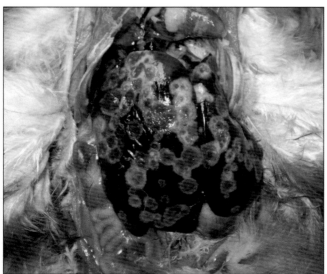

16.7 'Hobnail' liver lesions caused by *Histomonas meleagridis* ('blackhead').

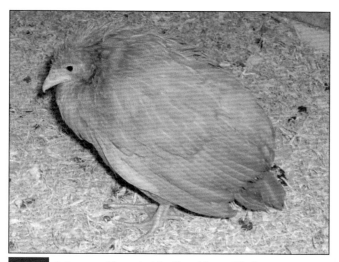

16.8 A depressed 6-week-old pullet with coccidiosis.

causes haemorrhagic caecal contents (Figure 16.9). Other species of *Eimeria* can cause milder lesions such as inflammation, petechiae (Figure 16.10), thickening of the intestinal mucosa, haemorrhage, white foci (schizonts) (Figure 16.11) and caseous intestinal contents. Where there is sufficient blood loss the carcass will be pale and anaemic.

Diagnosis: Diagnosis is often based upon clinical signs and history, with high faecal oocyst counts (>50,000 oocysts per gram of faeces) backing up clinical suspicion (Figure 16.12). Post-mortem findings may be diagnostic but in many instances they can be difficult to interpret, especially in mild cases. The preparation of wet smears of the mucosal intestinal surface in three locations (the duodenum, the jejunum near Merkel's diverticulum and the caecum) is recommended to look for both oocysts and schizonts.

Treatment: Treatment of coccidiosis involves two components:

- The first is to control the coccidiosis with an anticoccidial agent such as toltrazuril (given at 7 mg/kg in drinking water for 2 consecutive days) or amprolium, which can be given in drinking water for 5–7 consecutive days at 20 mg/kg

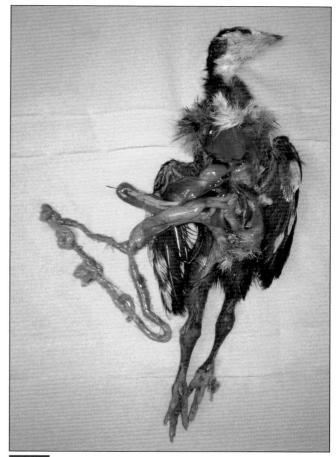

16.10 A 2-week-old Bronze turkey with coccidiosis.

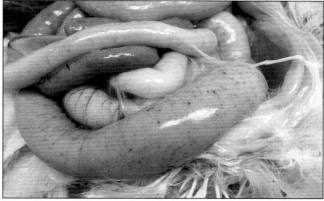

16.11 Petechial haemorrhages in the jejunum of a 4-week-old chicken.

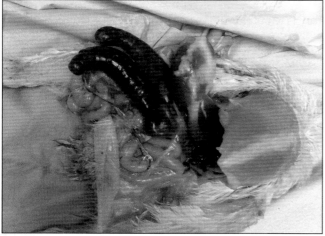

16.9 The blood filled caeca of a 4-week-old Hubbard chicken with coccidiosis.

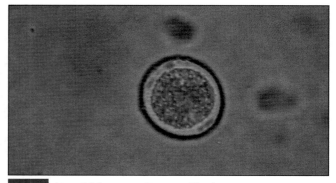

16.12 A coccidial oocyst at X40 magnification.

- The next is to control secondary bacterial growth concurrently using antimicrobials such as tylosin at 20 mg/kg or amoxicillin orally at 15 mg/kg. When coccidiosis damages the intestinal wall it can lead to secondary bacterial overgrowth manifesting itself as necrotic enteritis.

As for all conditions causing diarrhoea, nursing is very important to keep the bird hydrated and comfortable. Bedding must be kept dry to keep the birds comfortable and to slow down oocyst sporulation. Supplying extra heat to young birds with coccidiosis may be of use to encourage activity, including feeding and drinking.

Prognosis: The prognosis for early cases and the flock is good but for severely affected individuals treatment is often too late.

Prevention: Prevention of clinical coccidiosis but not of exposure is key because it is desirable for the birds to develop immunity.

- Good hygiene is the first step in preventing large numbers of oocysts persisting (for up to several years) in brooding houses between batches of birds. After removing the bedding, a detergent should always be used to remove dirt and grease, otherwise any disinfectant will be inactivated by organic material. Next, after letting the pen dry, owners must use a disinfectant with anticoccidial activity – *if a disinfectant does not state that it destroys oocysts then it should be assumed that it will not*.
- Once the birds are being reared, anticoccidial agents such as toltrazuril can be used preventively or an ionophore coccidiostat (such as lasalocid) can be given in feed. Note: *turkeys are highly sensitive to ionophore coccidiostats and doses safe for other species of poultry can be fatal to turkeys. Birds receiving ionophore coccidiostats such as monensin, salinomycin or narasin must not be given the bacteriostatic drug tiamulin as this combination is usually fatal.* All ionophore coccidiostats have the potential to cause mortality, due to myopathy, when fed at high levels. Tiamulin is thought to be competitively metabolized, leading to a toxic accumulation of the ionophore. Toltrazuril can be given concurrently with tiamulin.
- Reducing the rate of oocyst sporulation is also beneficial. Whilst heat cannot be removed from young birds, humidity can be reduced through regular topping up of the bedding especially in wet areas such as those around the drinkers.
- A live attenuated vaccine is available for chickens only and can be given in the first week of life. However, for the vaccination to be successful the environmental conditions must be conducive for the sporulation and cycling of the vaccine strains of *Eimeria*.
- Many practitioners will contemplate routine faecal oocyst counts of young birds in rear rather than using preventive treatment. However, if such monitoring is carried out then sampling needs to be done twice a week (between the ages of 2 and 12 weeks) and the birds may develop clinical signs before the results of such tests are known.

Differential diagnoses: Dysbacteriosis, *Salmonella* spp., endoparasites, rotavirus, histomoniasis, ulcerative enteritis, parvovirus (geese and Muscovy ducks), poult enteritis mortality syndrome, haemorrhagic enteritis, duck viral enteritis and *Hexamita*.

Cryptosporidiosis

Aetiology and epidemiology: Cryptosporidiosis is a relatively rare condition of poultry. The organism is predominantly spread via the faeco–oral route and can make its way into the bursa, the intestine and the respiratory tract.

Clinical signs: There are predominantly two species found in poultry: *C. meleagridis*, which causes diarrhoea (especially in turkeys) and *C. baileyi*, which can cause respiratory signs. Cryptosporidiosis in poultry is not zoonotic.

Post-mortem findings: Post-mortem examination may reveal increased mucus in the respiratory tract and in extreme cases pneumonia. Bursal atrophy may also be found.

Diagnosis: Diagnosis is based upon making faecal smears and staining them with Ziehl–Nielsen.

Treatment: There is no effective reported treatment, although supportive care and improving husbandry will help. In severe cases antimicrobials may be considered to control secondary bacterial infections.

Prognosis: The prognosis is fair.

Prevention: Prevention is based upon good hygiene and biosecurity. Note that the oocysts are highly resistant to disinfection and as such only an approved disinfectant should be used.

Differential diagnoses: Respiratory infection should be differentiated from infectious bronchitis, avian rhinotracheitis, Newcastle disease, avian influenza and *Mycoplasma* species.

Motile protozoal parasites
Trichomoniasis (oral canker, frounce, roup)

Aetiology, epidemiology and pathogenesis: Trichomoniasis is predominantly caused by the motile protozoal parasite *Trichomonas gallinae*. However, in pheasants, infection may be caused by *T. phasiani*; this species causes different clinical signs (see below).

T. gallinae tends to be an opportunistic pathogen (though it can be a primary pathogen) taking advantage of any damage to the oral, oesophageal or crop mucosa. The parasite may subsequently spread to the liver. *T. gallinae* is widely present in wild birds and can be spread through shared drinking water (not through the faeco–oral route). Pigeons are a commonly recognized source of the parasite.

Clinical signs: *T. gallinae* causes caseous oral lesions (Figure 16.13) (which are often described as 'yellow buttons'), causing affected birds to become inappetent and lose weight.

Post-mortem findings: The caseous lesions in the oral cavity may extend as far distally as the proventriculus. In certain cases, such caseous lesions may be found in the liver.

Diagnosis: Whilst clinical signs and post-mortem findings may be suggestive of infection, confirmation requires microscopic examination (X40) using warmed slides to look for motile flagellate protozoa (trichomonads are pear-shaped

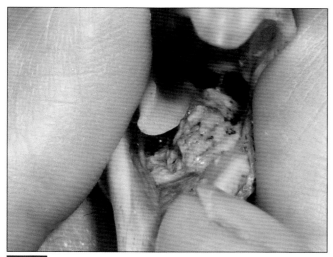

16.13 An ex-battery hen with oral canker.

and have four anterior flagella together with a protruding posterior axostyle). This must be done within minutes of sampling, before the parasite dies. Alternatively, PCR testing may be used.

Treatment: There is no currently authorized treatment in the UK. Due to concerns regarding the potential carcinogenic properties of metronidazole, the use of tetracyclines in food-producing birds for 5 days has been suggested although there is little documented evidence of their success. Since the organism can be spread through the drinking water, it is advisable to remove the affected bird from the flock and ensure all the birds in the flock have access to fresh clean drinking water.

Prognosis: The prognosis is guarded, even with the use of metronidazole.

Prevention: Prevention is based on ensuring poultry have continuous access to clean water and discouraging wild birds, namely pigeons, from frequenting the coop.

Differential diagnoses: The 'wet form' of fowlpox, mycosis and histomoniasis (liver lesions).

Trichomoniasis (in pheasants)

Aetiology and epidemiology: Trichomoniasis in pheasants is caused by *T. phasiani* and has a different presentation from *T gallinae*. *T. phasiani* is a commensal organism of the caeca of pheasants; however, large numbers can be indicative of disease. Infection is via the faeco–oral route.

Clinical signs: Affected pheasants often present with weight loss, inappetence and a frothy yellow diarrhoea (similar to *Hexamita*).

Post-mortem findings: The main finding is large distended caeca containing frothy yellow fluid. However, affected birds may have thin dark tacky carcasses with urate deposits in their ureters due to dehydration.

Diagnosis: As for trichomoniasis in other poultry (see above).

Treatment: There is no currently authorized treatment in the UK. The use of tetracyclines for 5 days has been

suggested for poultry that are considered as food-producing animals; however, their efficacy is variable, especially compared with metronidazole. As with all forms of diarrhoea, it is important to keep affected birds hydrated.

Prognosis: The prognosis is guarded.

Prevention: Prevention is based upon good hygiene ensuring the drinkers and feeders are as clean as possible. Preferably, they should be raised to reduce the chances of faecal contamination.

Differential diagnoses: *Hexamita*, blackhead, rotavirus and coccidiosis.

Hexamita (Spironucleus) meleagridis

Aetiology and epidemiology: *Hexamita meleagridis* is a motile protozoal parasite that is most commonly found in pheasants and partridges but can infect other domestic fowl, such as turkeys. The parasite, which is thought to be a commensal of the small intestine, can overgrow particularly in young birds undergoing stress to cause severe clinical signs.

Clinical signs: Affected birds are often dull (birds are often hunched up with ruffled feathers), dehydrated, have severe and rapid weight loss, are inappetent and have a frothy yellow diarrhoea.

Post-mortem findings: Post-mortem findings include: a thin carcass (prominent keel), dark tacky breast muscle and yellow frothy caecal contents (Figure 16.14).

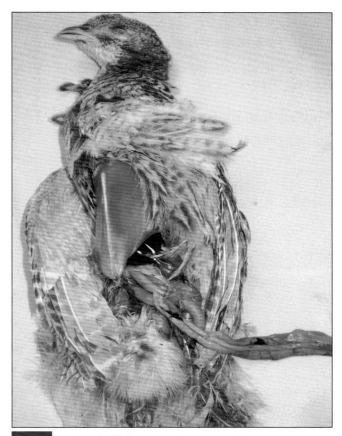

16.14 An 8-week-old pheasant with *Hexamita* infestation.

Diagnosis: Diagnosis is often based upon the finding of motile protozoa microscopically (X40 magnification) using freshly prepared wet smears from the small intestine. *Hexamita* organisms are leaf-shaped and have two nuclei, three pairs of anterior flagella and a pair of posterior flagella. Note, this requires the sacrificial euthanasia of a sick bird as the parasite will die rapidly after the bird dies, thus preventing identification.

Treatment: Treatment requires keeping affected birds adequately hydrated. For birds which may be classed as food-producing, treatment for 5 days with tetracyclines orally combined with tiamulin may be used predominantly to control secondary bacterial infections.

Prognosis: Effective treatment requires the bird to be kept well hydrated. The response to a combination therapy of tetracyclines and tiamulin is moderate.

Prevention: Prevention, as with all forms of diarrhoea, involves minimizing stress, and providing fresh clean drinking water together with an appropriate diet.

Differential diagnoses: Blackhead, coccidiosis and trichomoniasis.

Other conditions of the intestinal tract causing diarrhoea

Diarrhoea is a very common presentation in poultry in general practice. Due a varied diet and frequent contact with muddy puddles the droppings of free-range birds can vary considerably. This 'diarrhoea' is usually transient with no other obvious clinical signs.

Almost all of the conditions detailed below can lead to a secondary dysbacteriosis with an overgrowth of *Clostridium perfringens*.

Approach to diarrhoea in poultry
History-taking
When taking a history from an owner whose bird(s) has diarrhoea there are a number of important questions to ask.

- The age of the bird? Birds under 3 months are particularly vulnerable to coccidiosis.
- Is the bird eating and drinking normally?
- What is the bird being fed? Ask probing questions regarding treats.
- Has the bird been treated recently with any 'medication' (including anthelmintics)? There are many products widely available with no proven efficacy and no licensed products are effective against all intestinal parasites.
- What is the demeanour of the affected bird? Owners of pet chickens are usually very good at noticing behavioural changes.
- Is more than one bird affected? Remember poultry are flock animals and pathogens may be contagious.
- Clarify the onset, duration and progress of the condition.
- Ask the owner to describe the droppings or, ideally, examine a stool sample.

Clinical examination
Next, a thorough clinical examination should be carried out, paying particular attention to the bird's hydration status and checking the vent for pasting (vent pasting is a poultry keepers' term for adherent faecal material, usually diarrhoea, to the skin and feathers around the vent). Clinical examination of the digestive tract should start at the mouth, progressing to palpation of the crop and abdomen. The bird's temperature should also be taken. See Chapter 8 for more detail.

Faecal examination
Birds have two types of droppings:

- Caecal droppings, which should be caramel-like in appearance (Figure 16.15)
- Non-caecal droppings, which should consist of a firm brown material covered in a white urate cap from the urinary tract (Figure 16.16).

Care should be taken to differentiate diarrhoea from polyuria. Diarrhoea should be homogenous whereas polyuria often manifests as a normal dropping surrounded by fluid.

Next, rule in/out coccidiosis (there should be less than 50,000 oocysts/gram of faeces) and worms (there should be less than 400 eggs/gram of faeces; however, the presence of any *Capillaria* eggs is a cause for concern) through both the history and a faecal worm egg/oocyst count. Note that whilst blood in the droppings is most commonly related to coccidiosis in chickens or haemorrhagic enteritis in turkeys, there are several species of coccidiosis that do not produce bloody droppings.

If diet, worms and coccidiosis have been ruled out then PCR and faecal culture can be employed to look for specific viruses and bacteria. Figure 16.17 is a differential diagnosis list for diarrhoea in poultry.

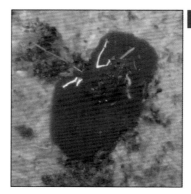

16.15 A normal caramel-like caecal dropping.

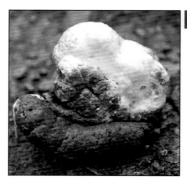

16.16 A normal dropping with a white urate cap.

Chickens	Turkeys	Waterfowl	Pheasants	Guineafowl	Peafowl
Age: 0–2 weeks					
Paratyphoid	Paratyphoid	Paratyphoid	Paratyphoid	Paratyphoid	Paratyphoid
Fowl typhoid	Fowl typhoid	Fowl typhoid	Fowl typhoid	Fowl typhoid	Fowl typhoid
Rotavirus	Rotavirus	Rotavirus	Rotavirus	Rotavirus	Rotavirus
Pullorum disease	Pullorum disease	Parvovirus (Muscovy ducks and geese only)	Pullorum disease	Pullorum disease	Pullorum disease
	Arizonosis	Duck viral enteritis			
	PEMS				
Age: 2–16 weeks					
Coccidiosis	Coccidiosis	Coccidiosis	Coccidiosis	Coccidiosis	Coccidiosis
Dysbacteriosis	Dysbacteriosis	Dysbacteriosis	Dysbacteriosis	Dysbacteriosis	Dysbacteriosis
Paratyphoid	Paratyphoid	Paratyphoid	Paratyphoid	Paratyphoid	Paratyphoid
Fowl typhoid	Fowl typhoid	Fowl typhoid	Fowl typhoid	Fowl typhoid	Fowl typhoid
Rotavirus	Rotavirus	Rotavirus	Rotavirus	Rotavirus	Rotavirus
Worms	Worms	Worms	Worms	Worms	Worms
Blackhead	Blackhead		Blackhead	Blackhead	Blackhead
Ulcerative enteritis	Ulcerative enteritis	Parvovirus (Muscovy ducks and geese only)	Ulcerative enteritis	Ulcerative enteritis	Ulcerative enteritis
Pseudotuberculosis	Pseudotuberculosis	Pseudotuberculosis	Pseudotuberculosis	Pseudotuberculosis	Pseudotuberculosis
	Hexamita	Duck viral enteritis	*Hexamita*		
Gumboro disease	PEMS		*Trichomonas phasiani*		
Infectious bronchitis	Haemorrhagic enteritis virus				
	Arizonosis				
Adults					
Worms	Worms	Worms	Worms	Worms	Worms
Dysbacteriosis	Dysbacteriosis	Dysbacteriosis	Dysbacteriosis	Dysbacteriosis	Dysbacteriosis
Fowl typhoid	Fowl typhoid	Fowl typhoid	Fowl typhoid	Fowl typhoid	Fowl typhoid
Blackhead	Blackhead	Duck viral enteritis	Blackhead	Blackhead	Blackhead
Chlamydophila	*Chlamydophila*	*Chlamydophila*	*Chlamydophila*	*Chlamydophila*	*Chlamydophila*
Pseudotuberculosis	Pseudotuberculosis	Pseudotuberculosis	Pseudotuberculosis	Pseudotuberculosis	Pseudotuberculosis
Tuberculosis	Tuberculosis	Tuberculosis	Tuberculosis	Tuberculosis	Tuberculosis
Brachyspira	*Hexamita*		*Hexamita*		
Infectious bronchitis			*Trichomonas phasiani*		
Lymphoid leucosis					

16.17 Differential diagnoses for diarrhoea. PEMS = poult enteritis and mortality syndrome.

Management of diarrhoea

In cases of diarrhoea without other clinical findings the best option is to monitor the bird closely over the next few days with a deterioration or failure to recover being grounds for further action. Management of diarrhoea as in all species primarily involves keeping the bird hydrated. There are several aniseed-based electrolytes available, which give a pleasant taste to the bird's drinking water and help maintain water intake and therefore hydration. In severe cases subcutaneous or intraosseous fluids may be required together with thermal and nutritional support (see Chapters 8 and 9).

Antimicrobials can be administered orally for a 3- to 5-day course. Traditionally, enrofloxacin has been extensively used in practice; however, this can damage the beneficial intestinal flora and raises issues regarding a suitable egg withdrawal period. There are two antimicrobials that this author has found to be of use for enteritis in poultry: tylosin at 20 mg/kg and amoxicillin at 15 mg/kg, either of which should be administered orally. Note that it is important to give antimicrobials treating intestinal dysbacteriosis orally so that they can act locally in the gut rather than systemically. Tylosin has a zero egg withdrawal and is the better choice for birds laying eggs for human consumption, whereas amoxicillin will necessitate an egg withdrawal in accordance with the cascade.

After antimicrobial therapy for diarrhoea or any other condition for that matter, probiotics should be considered.

Coccidiosis

See above.

Necrotic enteritis

Aetiology, epidemiology and pathogenesis

Necrotic enteritis is a rare condition of backyard poultry and is usually restricted to intensive broiler production. The condition is associated with an overgrowth of *Clostridium perfringens* (usually type A), which is an intestinal commensal. This overgrowth may be triggered by dietary factors, stress or intestinal mucosal damage. In most cases overgrowth is triggered by coccidiosis. The coccidia damage the intestinal mucosa causing the intestine to secrete protective mucus. However, as *Clostridium perfringens* is mucolytic, this excessive mucus secretion encourages clostridial overgrowth. This overgrowth causes toxic insults to the mucosa of the small intestine leading to the formation of a diphtheritic pseudomembrane.

Clinical signs

Affected birds are often hunched up with ruffled feathers, have diarrhoea and tend to be dehydrated. Acute cases may present as sudden death.

Post-mortem findings

The classical pathognomonic finding is a 'Turkish towel'-like diphtheritic pseudomembrane in the small intestine along with necrotic contents (Figure 16.18). The breast muscle is often dark and tacky due to dehydration. Affected birds often have enlarged gall bladders due to inappetence antemortem.

Diagnosis

Diagnosis is usually based upon post-mortem examination. Whilst cytology or bacteriology may be considered it is virtually impossible to differentiate harmless commensal strains from an overgrowth of a pathogenic strain.

Treatment

Treatment involves maintaining hydration, treating any under-lying coccidiosis and the use of oral tylosin at 20 mg/kg or amoxicillin at 15 mg/kg for 5 days to control the bacterial overgrowth.

Prognosis

Providing the condition is treated in reasonable time the prognosis is good for the flock but clinically affected birds often die.

Prevention

Prevention of the condition involves successfully controlling coccidiosis together with good husbandry.

Differential diagnoses

Coccidiosis and ulcerative enteritis.

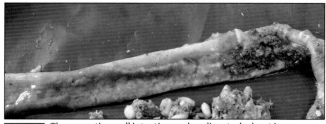

16.18 The necrotic small intestine and undigested wheat in a 3-week-old Ross chicken with necrotic enteritis.

Histomoniasis

See Endoparasites.

Haemorrhagic enteritis

Aetiology, epidemiology and pathogenesis

Haemorrhagic enteritis is a disease solely of turkeys caused by an adenovirus.

The condition affects young poults between 4 and 12 weeks of age when the levels of maternal antibodies have fallen sufficiently to allow for infection. Poor nutrition and husbandry will increase the likelihood and subsequent severity of such a condition. The virus predominantly damages the small intestine causing haemorrhagic lesions.

Clinical signs

Infection leads to affected poults being dull, hunched up (often with ruffled feathers) along with having a bloody diarrhoea. Acute blood loss can lead to anaemia and subsequent death. The virus is also immunosuppressive leading to poor growth and development of survivors.

Post-mortem findings

On post-mortem examination affected birds will have blood-filled haemorrhagic small intestines (Figure 16.19). Affected birds often have hepatosplenomegaly together with marbling of the spleen.

Diagnosis

While post-mortem findings and clinical signs are suggestive of infection, virus isolation, histopathology and retrospectively serology can be used for confirmation.

Treatment

Fluids and supportive care are essential to help birds through this condition. Whilst it is viral in aetiology, secondary bacterial enteritis is highly likely and, therefore, amoxicillin at 20 mg/kg orally per day for 5 days is recommended as part of the treatment plan.

Prognosis

The prognosis depends on the severity of the condition but the survivors may be stunted.

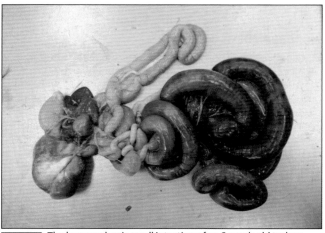

16.19 The haemorrhagic small intestine of an 8-week-old turkey poult with haemorrhagic enteritis.

Prevention

There are currently no authorized vaccines in the UK; vaccines are available in other countries. Good hygiene and biosecurity are essential.

Differential diagnoses

Coccidiosis.

Dysbacteriosis

Aetiology and epidemiology

Dysbacteriosis is a widely used vague term to describe a non-specific diarrhoea involving a disruption to the normal intestinal flora of birds. This may affect an individual bird or the entire flock.

This disruption is usually caused by either a poor/unbalanced diet or an underlying pathogenic agent such as coccidia or mycotoxins.

Clinical signs

Such birds often are presented with diarrhoea but are otherwise bright and alert with no other clinical signs. Severe cases may progress to necrotic enteritis.

Post-mortem findings

Affected birds often have watery intestinal and caecal contents with a pale flaccid distended intestine.

Diagnosis

Diagnosis is frequently based upon apparently healthy birds being presented with diarrhoea. Faecal cultures have been found to be of little use.

Treatment

In mild cases birds will often spontaneously recover. Probiotics may aid such a recovery. More chronic cases may respond to antimicrobials such as tylosin at 20 mg/kg or amoxicillin at 15 mg/kg orally for 5 days.

Prognosis

The prognosis is usually excellent. However, if there is an underlying problem that is not resolved the condition may reoccur.

Prevention

Prevention is based upon a good diet along with good hygiene and coccidial control.

Differential diagnosis

Brachyspira infection.

Brachyspira (intestinal spirochaetosis)

Aetiology and epidemiology

Brachyspira spp. (*B. pilosicoli* and *B. intermedia*) are a genus of anaerobic bacteria that have been known to cause diarrhoea in adult chickens (up to 20% of infected birds may have diarrhoea). The bacteria are usually transmitted by the faeco–oral route from infected birds.

Clinical signs

Affected birds often present with a frothy yellow diarrhoea together with mild weight loss and a drop in egg production. Such birds rarely appear unwell and the condition rarely leads to death.

Post-mortem findings

Post-mortem findings are usually non-specific but include frothy mustard-coloured caecal contents.

Diagnosis

Diagnosis is made on clinical signs confirmed by faecal cultures or PCR (which can be used for both confirmation and speciation).

Treatment and prognosis

Most affected birds will recover on their own but if the case is severe then a 5-day course of tiamulin at 25 mg/kg can be administered.

Prevention

Prevention is based upon good hygiene and biosecurity together with an appropriate diet.

Differential diagnoses

Dysbacteriosis.

Hexamita (Spironucleus) meleagridis

See Endoparasites.

Trichomoniasis

See Endoparasites.

Rotavirus

Aetiology and epidemiology

Rotaviruses can infect all species of poultry at all ages; however, they most frequently cause pathology in pheasants between 4 and 14 days of age.

The virus is spread via the faeco–oral route including the surface contamination of eggs leading to early infection of chicks.

Clinical signs

Infection can cause dullness, birds to be hunched up with ruffled feathers, inappetence, frothy yellow diarrhoea (Figure 16.20), dehydration and in some cases death.

Post-mortem findings

Post-mortem findings are usually restricted to distended caeca with frothy yellow contents.

Diagnosis

A diagnosis can be made using either enzyme-linked immunosorbent assay (ELISA) kits, polyacrylamide gel electrophoresis (PAGE) or by PCR.

Treatment

There is no specific treatment but maintaining hydration is crucial. Antimicrobials such as amoxicillin can be used orally at 15 mg/kg to prevent secondary bacterial infection.

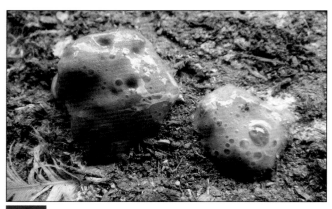

16.20 Frothy yellow droppings caused by rotavirus infection.

Prognosis

The prognosis is fair but surviving birds can be left stunted.

Prevention

Prevention is based upon good hygiene especially in relation to hatching eggs. There are no known authorized rotavirus vaccines for use in poultry.

Differential diagnoses

Dysbacteriosis, coccidiosis, blackhead and *Hexamita*.

Goose parvovirus (Derzsy's disease, goose/gosling plague)
Aetiology and epidemiology

Parvoviruses can infect both Muscovy ducks and geese with similarly devastating effects to those found with canine parvovirus. The virus is spread both horizontally and vertically.

Clinical signs

Vertical infection can initially cause poor hatchability. The clinical signs of infection are age-related with birds under 1 week of age showing difficulty breathing, inappetence, weight loss and almost certain death. Birds from 1 week up to 1 month will often have diarrhoea, weight loss, naso-ocular discharge, ascites, conjunctival swelling, a diphtheritic oral membrane and neurological signs. Older birds tend not to show clinical signs; however, they can excrete the virus for several weeks.

Post-mortem findings

Post-mortem findings include hepatosplenomegaly, pallor and enlargement of the heart, pericarditis, pulmonary oedema, pancreatic enlargement, perihepatitis, ascites and a catarrhal enteritis.

Diagnosis

Diagnosis is based upon clinical signs in young goslings and Muscovy ducklings. Whilst post-mortem findings can be suggestive of parvovirus infection, histopathology looking for intranuclear inclusion bodies can help support the diagnosis. Virus isolation can be used to confirm clinical suspicion.

Treatment

Treatment may be attempted in mild cases using fluid therapy and potentially antimicrobials to control secondary infection, but ultimately treatment outcomes are age-dependent. The virus is highly infectious and this will usually be a flock problem.

Prognosis

For affected birds under 1 week of age death is almost certain. Birds aged between 1 week and 1 month will have a guarded prognosis. For birds over 1 month old, the outlook is favourable.

Prevention

Prevention includes good hygiene and biosecurity. Vaccination of breeding stock can effectively control infection in their offspring through maternally derived antibodies.

Differential diagnoses

Duck viral enteritis, duck viral hepatitis and *Riemerella*.

Duck viral enteritis (duck plague)
Aetiology and epidemiology

Duck viral enteritis is caused by a herpesvirus. The virus is typical of herpesviruses in that it becomes latent in the trigeminal nerve. During the stress of the breeding season, wild migrating birds will shed the virus in their faeces leading to infection via the faeco–oral route and through cloacal uptake from contaminated water. This gives the disease a seasonal occurrence usually from April to June.

Clinical signs

The most common sign of infection is sudden death of birds in spring/summer. Birds observed alive may show systemic signs of illness including naso-ocular discharge, inappetence, neurological signs, photophobia, polydipsia and a watery (often haemorrhagic) diarrhoea.

Post-mortem findings

Post-mortem lesions include haemorrhages throughout the body (due to vascular damage), thymic oedema, inflammation of the gut associated lymphoid tissue, diptheresis of the oesophagus and vent, and necrosis and haemorrhage of the intestine (Figure 16.21).

Diagnosis

Diagnosis is based upon clinical signs, the time of year and confirmation is by PCR or virus isolation.

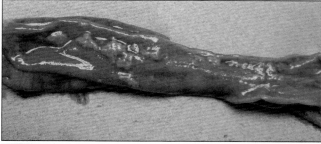

16.21 The necrotic mucosa of a 6-week-old duckling with duck viral enteritis.

Treatment

Treatment is based upon supportive care.

Prognosis

The prognosis is poor. Survivors will be latently infected and will intermittently shed the virus when immuno-compromised or stressed.

Prevention

Prevention is primarily based upon keeping wild waterfowl away. There are currently no commercially available vaccines in the UK but they are available in other countries.

Differential diagnoses

Duck viral hepatitis, coccidiosis and *Riemerella*.

Cryptosporidiosis

See Endoparasites.

Intussusception
Aetiology and pathogenesis

Intussusception is a relatively rare condition of poultry. As with all species it involves a portion of the intestine telescoping due to hypermotility and spasming of the intestine. Whilst there is no single cause there are several potential underlying contributing factors including hypermotility, hypocalcaemia, internal parasites and other intestinal pathogens.

Clinical signs

Affected birds may strain, be inappetent, have diarrhoea, be dull and in severe cases may go into shock and die. Many such cases have been reported along with rectal prolapses.

Post-mortem findings

The affected section of intestine will be telescoped and congested, together with ballooning due to a build-up of digesta proximal to the point of intussusception.

Diagnosis

Diagnosis is best made through diagnostic imaging. This should help differentiate the condition from intestinal foreign bodies.

Treatment

Surgical intervention is essential. The intussusception should be surgically reduced and, where necessary, resection of the relevant section of the intestine must be carried out. It is also important to identify and treat any underlying causes.

Prognosis

The prognosis is guarded.

Prevention

Prevention is based upon controlling contributing factors such as endoparasites.

Differential diagnoses

Intestinal foreign bodies.

Poult enteritis and mortality syndrome
Aetiology and epidemiology

Poult enteritis and mortality syndrome (PEMS) is a disease syndrome of turkey poults. The exact infectious agent responsible has yet to be determined, although it is thought to be caused by a virus and to be spread horizontally via the faeco–oral route.

Clinical signs

The condition causes a non-specific diarrhoea in young poults leading to weight loss, dehydration, inappetence, poor growth and, in severe cases, death. Clinical signs are most commonly seen in young turkeys between 1 and 3 weeks of age.

Post-mortem findings

Post-mortem findings tend to be non-specific but pale dilated intestines can be found.

Treatment

Supportive therapy should be used to nurse the birds through this infection.

Prognosis

The prognosis is moderate as surviving birds will be severely stunted.

Prevention

Prevention is based upon good hygiene and biosecurity.

Differential diagnoses

Rotavirus, dysbacteriosis and coccidiosis.

Reovirus (viral arthritis, tenosynovitis, malabsorption syndrome)
Aetiology and epidemiology

There are several serotypes of reovirus found in poultry, each of which is associated with a range of clinical signs (poor growth, tenosynovitis, enteritis and malabsorption). Transmission is primarily through the faeco–oral route; however, vertical transmission has also been documented. Whilst reoviruses have been detected in most species of poultry, they have only been associated with pathology in chickens and (to a lesser extent) turkeys.

Clinical signs

The clinical signs are dependent on the strain of reovirus involved but infection is most commonly associated with viral arthritis. Certain strains have been associated with enteritis, the passage of wholly or partially undigested feed, poor growth and inappetence.

Post-mortem findings

Findings are strain-dependent but may include tenosynovitis (Figure 16.22), gizzard erosion, enlargement of the proventriculus, catarrhal enteritis (often with partially undigested feed present) and a pale distended intestine.

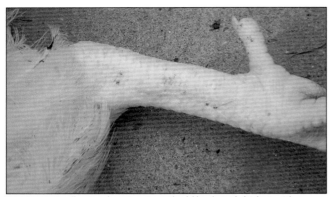

16.22 Swollen tendons in a 6-week-old backyard chicken with reovirus.

Treatment

There are no specific treatments recommended; however, supportive care should be given and antimicrobials may be of use in the event of secondary bacterial infections.

Prognosis

Affected birds will likely recover but may be stunted.

Differential diagnoses

Dysbacteriosis and rotavirus.

Pseudotuberculosis (yersiniosis)
Aetiology, epidemiology and pathogenesis

Yersinia pseudotuberculosis is a rare pathogen of domestic poultry with the majority of reported cases being in turkeys. The infection is spread primarily through the faeco–oral route and occasionally through cutaneous abrasions.

Once the organism gains entry into the body it enters the bloodstream to cause a bacteraemia and subsequently septicaemia. *This organism has zoonotic potential.*

Clinical signs

Infected birds usually die peracutely but in some birds the disease can have a chronic course with diarrhoea, weight loss and lameness being common clinical signs.

Post-mortem findings

On post-mortem examination hepatosplenomegaly and a congested bright red carcass (due to septicaemia) are the most common findings. Inflammation of the digestive tract and caseous tuberculosis (TB)-like nodules may be found in the bird's visceral organs.

Diagnosis

No post-mortem lesions are diagnostic and bacteriology is needed for confirmation.

Treatment

Treatment with antimicrobials based upon antimicrobial sensitivities may be of use in at-risk birds in a flock where the condition has been previously diagnosed.

Prognosis

The prognosis is poor for individual birds if clinical signs are already present.

Prevention

Prevention is based upon good hygiene and ensuring wild animals cannot defecate in the range as poultry will readily peck at anything (including animal carcasses).

Differential diagnoses

Escherichia coli, *Salmonella* spp. and avian tuberculosis.

Avian tuberculosis
Aetiology and epidemiology

Avian TB is caused by *Mycobacterium avium*. It is a relatively rare condition in non-aquatic fowl but is much more common in ornamental waterfowl and tends to infect older birds. The primary source of infection is through the faeco–oral route; however, the cannibalization of infected carcasses is an important additional route of infection.

Clinical signs

Once infected, the course of the infection is slow with it taking up to several months for clinical signs to develop. Avian TB leads to the formation of tubercle-like granulomas throughout the body. The clinical signs can be variable depending upon the location of the lesions but the most common finding is chronic weight loss. Affected birds may show lameness, yellowing of tissues due to hepatic damage, and diarrhoea.

Post-mortem findings

Post-mortem examination findings include a thin carcass with white/yellow/grey granulomas throughout the internal organs and bones.

Diagnosis

Diagnosis on live birds can be carried out using the tuberculin test. This involves injecting 0.05 ml of avian tuberculin intradermally into one wattle and checking the reaction site 48 hours later. The injected wattle should be compared with the uninjected wattle for comparison; any swelling in the injected wattle indicates a positive result. On post-mortem examination, suspected lesions can be stained to look for acid-fast bacteria.

Treatment

Treatment is not successful.

Prognosis

Due to the risk posed to other birds in the flock, euthanasia should be considered. Although rare, it should be remembered that *M. avium* has zoonotic potential.

Prevention

Prevention is based upon keeping wild birds away because faecal contamination of the soil and water (especially at the land–water interface) is an important risk factor for infection. It is also important only to buy new birds from reputable sources.

Differential diagnoses

Lymphoid leucosis, Marek's disease, *Salmonella* spp., yersiniosis and *Pasteurella multocida*.

Ulcerative enteritis (quail disease)
Aetiology and epidemiology
Ulcerative enteritis is a rare condition of young domestic fowl. Ulcerative enteritis was first reported in quails though the disease can occur in other poultry (except waterfowl).

The condition is caused by *Clostridium colinum*. Infection is via the faeco–oral route though exposure alone is unlikely to cause disease unless there are additional stressors such as coccidiosis or immunosuppressive disease.

Clinical signs
Infection usually leads to sudden death of birds in good condition but in some cases dullness and diarrhoea may be the main presenting signs.

Post-mortem findings
Post-mortem findings include ulceration of the intestine, occasionally with the formation of a pseudomembrane. Affected birds may have splenomegaly and large areas of focal hepato-necrosis.

Diagnosis
Whilst post-mortem lesions are not pathognomonic, they are suggestive. Bacterial culture is required for a definitive diagnosis.

Treatment
Treatment involves treating/removing any stressors, maintaining the bird's hydration status and using antimicrobials such as amoxicillin for 5 days at 15 mg/kg orally.

Prognosis
If detected early enough the prognosis is good on a flock level but is guarded at an individual level.

Prevention
Prevention involves controlling underlying factors such as coccidiosis and immunosuppressive agents together with good hygiene and biosecurity.

Differential diagnoses
Coccidiosis, necrotic enteritis, blackhead and *Salmonella* spp.

Salmonella enterica subspecies Arizonae (Arizonosis)
Aetiology and epidemiology
S. Arizonae is predominantly a pathogen of young turkeys (under 5 weeks of age). Infection is mostly through the faeco–oral route; however, both venereal and vertical transmission are possible. The mortality varies but can be as high as 90%. Survivors can become latent carriers and as such will invariably remain potential sources of infection for other birds in the flock. Rodents and wild birds have also been implicated in its transmission. Note that *S.* Arizonae has zoonotic potential and cases in the UK are reportable to the Animal and Plant Health Agency (APHA).

Clinical signs
Clinical signs include dullness, huddling, enteritis (leading to vent pasting), nervous signs (torticollis) and blindness.

Post-mortem findings
Lesions are non-specific but include septicaemic signs (a reddened congested carcass, inflamed liver (with necrotic foci), inflamed spleen and inflamed kidneys), peritonitis, yolk sac infection, typhlitis (caseous caecal cores; Figure 16.23) and ophthalmitis.

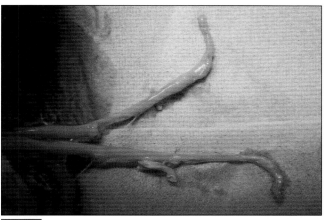

16.23 Caseous caecal cores caused by *Salmonella* Arizona infection.

Diagnosis
Diagnosis is usually tentative based upon the clinical signs but bacteriology is necessary for a definitive diagnosis.

Treatment
Treatment may be attempted based upon bacterial culture and sensitivity.

Prognosis
The prognosis is poor.

Prevention
Prevention of infection is through good hygiene and the control of rodents. If sourcing new birds, these should be free from infection. The use of probiotics and/or continuous use of organic acids in feed or water may reduce the likelihood of a flock becoming infected.

Differential diagnoses
Escherichia coli and other *Salmonella* species.

Salmonella enterica subspecies Gallinarum (fowl typhoid)
Aetiology and epidemiology
S. Gallinarum is a rarely isolated but pathogenic *Salmonella* that infects all poultry species of all ages. The bacteria are shed in the droppings from latently infected birds. Infected hens can transmit the pathogen vertically. Vermin and fomites have been implicated in the epidemiology of fowl typhoid. As with all *Salmonella* species, *S.* Gallinarum is reportable in the UK.

Clinical signs

Vertical transmission results in poor hatchability. Those birds that do hatch are often weak showing signs of dyspnoea and a yellow/white diarrhoea. Adult birds may appear depressed (hunched up with ruffled feathers), have respiratory signs diarrhoea, pale comb and wattles, they are pyrexic and show weight loss.

Post-mortem findings

Findings include septicaemic signs (a bright red congested carcass, an enlarged, friable, congested, inflamed liver (Figure 16.24; often with a bronze hue), an enlarged spleen and inflamed kidneys), catarrhal enteritis (often with bilious staining), miliary necrosis (of the liver, intestine, heart and pancreas) and pericarditis.

Diagnosis

Diagnosis is based upon bacteriology as clinical signs and post-mortem lesions are not diagnostic.

Treatment

Treatment is based upon using antimicrobials and supportive therapy.

Prognosis

The prognosis is moderate with between 10 and 50% of birds dying. Most survivors will remain carriers.

Prevention

Prevention is based upon good hygiene and biosecurity along with controlling pests and sourcing new stock from disease-free flocks. Serology and bacteriology can be used to identify carriers. There are currently no authorized vaccines in the UK. The use of probiotics and/or continuous use of organic acids in feed or water may reduce the likelihood of a flock becoming infected.

Differential diagnoses

Escherichia coli, other *Salmonella* species and *Pasteurella multocida*.

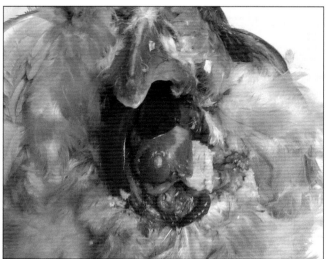

16.24 The emaciated septicaemic carcass of a 4-year-old backyard hen with fowl typhoid. Note the inflamed liver.

Salmonella enterica subspecies Pullorum (bacillary white diarrhoea, pullorum disease)

Aetiology and epidemiology

S. Pullorum is a pathogenic *Salmonella* of poultry (rarely waterfowl). The bacteria are predominantly transmitted vertically from infected hens through the egg meaning the disease is mostly one of young chicks. This subspecies of *Salmonella* has zoonotic potential and is reportable in the UK.

Clinical signs

Vertical transmission will cause poor hatchability. The chicks that do hatch are often weak and depressed (huddling with drooped wings). The digestive and respiratory systems are also infected leading to a white diarrhoea and respiratory distress. Infected chicks can then go on to infect their flock mates.

Post-mortem findings

Findings are non-specific but may include retained infected yolk sacs, septicaemic signs (a bright red congested carcass, inflamed liver (occasionally with haemorrhage), enlarged spleen and inflamed kidneys), peritonitis, caseous caecal cores, pericarditis and widely distributed necrotic foci.

Diagnosis

Diagnosis is often based upon bacteriology as post-mortem findings are non-specific.

Treatment

Antimicrobial therapy can be attempted to save affected chicks. Treatment will not eliminate the pathogen and only suppresses it. As such, it is unlikely the owner would want such carriers to remain in the flock.

Prognosis

Prognosis is poor; mortality can be variable from zero in birds over 1 month of age up to 100% in younger birds.

Prevention

Prevention is based upon careful sourcing of new birds from disease-free flocks (bacteriology and serology can be used to detect carriers) along with good hygiene and pest control to keep out disease. The use of probiotics and/or continuous use of organic acids in feed or water may reduce the likelihood of a flock becoming infected.

Differential diagnoses

Escherichia coli and other *Salmonella* species.

Paratyphoid (salmonellosis)

Aetiology and epidemiology

Whilst *S.* Gallinarum and *S.* Typhimurium are two host-specific pathogens of poultry, there are other *Salmonella* species that can cause health problems for flocks and these are collectively covered by the term 'paratyphoid'.

Some of these species are zoonotic and all are reportable to APHA in the UK.

Most *Salmonella* species are spread by fomites, latently infected carriers, vertical transmission, rodents, wild birds and contaminated feed/water.

Clinical signs

Clinical signs are mostly restricted to young birds. Vertical transmission can lead to poor hatchability. Young chicks that do become infected are often dull and huddled up and with faecal pasting around the vent due to diarrhoea. Blindness can occur due to ocular lesions. Nervous signs are common in ducklings.

Post-mortem findings

Post-mortem findings include yolk sac infection, septicaemic signs (a reddened congested carcass, inflamed liver, enlarged spleen and inflamed kidneys), widespread necrotic foci, pericarditis, peritonitis, haemorrhagic enteritis, caseous typhlitis and ocular lesions.

Diagnosis

Diagnosis is based upon bacteriological isolation.

Treatment

Treatment with antimicrobials or organic acids in drinking water may be attempted; however, survivors are likely to be carriers.

Prevention

Prevention is based upon purchasing new birds from disease-free flocks, controlling vermin, wild birds and flies along with restricting the movement of fomites. Always ensure clean feed is sourced (commercial mash and pellets are routinely tested).

Competitive exclusion using probiotics (especially for day-olds) and the use of in-feed or in-water organic acids may also be considered.

Differential diagnoses

Escherichia coli and other *Salmonella* species.

Diseases primarily affecting other body systems but which may also be associated with diarrhoea

Escherichia coli

Aetiology, epidemiology and pathogenesis

E. coli is a normal commensal organism of the avian intestine with little or no harmful effects. However, there are several pathogenic serovars. Isolating *E. coli* on faecal culture does not mean it is the cause of diarrhoea.

Yolk sac infection (omphalitis) is discussed in more detail in Chapter 21 but in general terms is associated with poor hatching egg and incubator hygiene. Likewise, peritonitis caused by *E. coli* is usually secondary to respiratory pathogens that damage the mucociliary escalator allowing commensal organisms free access to the poorly vascularized air sacs where they can go on to cause peritonitis.

There is little evidence to suggest *E. coli* is a cause of diarrhoea in poultry.

Clinical signs

Yolk sac infections (chicks) manifesting in dullness and poor growth and peritonitis (in laying adults) manifesting in dullness, enlargement of the abdomen and the cessation of laying.

Post-mortem findings

Post-mortem lesions include septicaemia in birds of all ages (congested reddened carcasses, inflamed liver, enlarged spleen and inflamed kidneys), yolk sac infection in chicks (Figure 16.25), pericarditis, air sacculitis (mostly in adults), salpingitis (in laying females) and peritonitis.

Diagnosis

Bacterial culture is used to confirm *E. coli*.

Treatment

E. coli can be treated with antimicrobials when systemic.

Prognosis

The outlook is poor for affected birds.

Prevention

Prevention is based upon good hygiene (particularly of hatching eggs) and control of any underlying respiratory disease.

Differential diagnoses

Salmonella species and *Pasteurella multocida*.

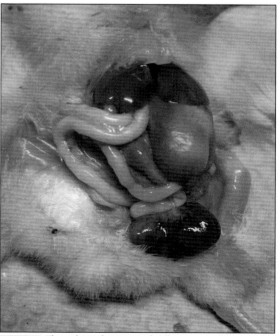

16.25 The enlarged congested yolk sac in a 4-day-old chick with yolk sac infection.

Mycotoxicoses

Whilst all commercially manufactured poultry feed should have maximum legally defined levels of fungal toxins, many owners with a few birds who buy a 20 kg bag of feed may find it becoming stale when they get to the end of it. This is a more common problem in warm and humid climates. If a bag of feed becomes contaminated, the mould will often be visible on the surface and food should be discarded should evidence of any such growth be identified.

Clinical signs

There is a plethora of potential mycotoxins all of which can produce rather non-specific signs. In almost all cases the birds are reluctant to eat and young growing birds tend to have a reduced growth rate. Laying hens will often stop laying. Any eggs laid often show poor hatchability. Many mycotoxins lead to anaemia and immunosupression. Mycotoxins can lead to diarrhoea due to irritation of the digestive tract. In addition, certain mycotoxins have specific additional lesions.

- Ergotism tends to result in cutaneous lesions of peripheral tissues such as the comb, wattles and feet. The lesions often begin as vesicles and progress through to scabs.
- Ochratoxin can cause renal damage leading to polydipsia and polyuria (owners may report this as diarrhoea) and dehydration.

Post-mortem findings

Trichothecene toxins are often caustic and can lead to focal necrosis of the digestive system. This is noticeable mostly on the oral mucosa where ulcers may be seen.

Diagnosis

Mycotoxin assays are expensive and testing can be unreliable due to uneven distribution of the mycotoxins in the food.

Treatment

If there is any doubt as to the quality of the feed it should be replaced immediately (this is the cheaper option) and the birds treated symptomatically.

Prevention

Prevention is based upon buying in an appropriate amount of feed and keeping it free from moisture. There are mycotoxin absorbers available to buy as feed additives.

Differential diagnoses

Chicken anaemia, gumboro disease, rotavirus, poult enteritis and mortality syndrome (PEMS) and dysbacteriosis can all produce some of the signs associated with mycotoxins.

Chlamydophila psittaci (ornithosis, psittacosis, chlamydiosis)
Aetiology and epidemiology

C. psittaci is a rare pathogen of backyard poultry but can occasionally infect domestic fowl especially turkeys.

Wild birds are the most common source of infection with the bacteria being shed in the faeces and respiratory secretions of carriers. Once infected, a bird will likely be a lifelong carrier of the disease.

Clinical signs

Infected birds may be asymptomatic (especially chickens). However, affected birds may be pyrexic, have respiratory distress, naso-ocular discharge, dullness, inappetence, a green diarrhoea (Figure 16.26), weight loss and a lack of egg production. Nervous signs may be seen in ducklings.

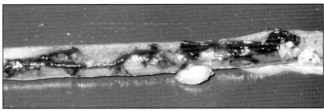

16.26 The bile-stained intestinal contents of a 2-year-old turkey that presented with green diarrhoea due to chlamydiosis.

Post-mortem findings

Post-mortem findings include pericarditis, pneumonia, air sacculitis, serositis, hepatomegaly and splenomegaly (both may have areas of necrotic foci/focal necrosis).

Diagnosis

Whilst clinical signs can be suggestive, PCR testing (from cloacal swabs), histopathology (of the heart, spleen, liver and kidney) to stain for elementary bodies or retrospectively paired serology samples are necessary for a definitive diagnosis. Note, detecting asymptomatic carriers is very difficult.

This is a potential zoonosis and in some countries it is a legal requirement to report all cases to the authorities.

Treatment

Treatment involves a prolonged course of doxycycline (45 days at 40 mg/kg).

Prognosis

The prognosis of such cases is guarded because even a prolonged course of antimicrobials is no guarantee of elimination of the organism.

Prevention

Prevention involves purchasing new birds from a disease-free source and keeping wild birds away.

Differential diagnoses

Escherichia coli and *Pasteurella multocida*.

Erysipelas
Aetiology and epidemiology

Erysipelothrix rhusiopathiae is predominantly a soil-based bacterium, which most commonly infects poultry on holdings with pigs. The bacteria tend to enter the body via abrasions.

Clinical signs

Infection causes septicaemia often leading to sudden death in turkeys. In less acute cases in turkeys and in infection in other poultry, clinical signs may include dullness and diarrhea; turkeys may have swollen, congested, cyanotic snoods.

Post-mortem findings

On post-mortem examination, peracutely infected birds may have no gross lesions. In the acute form affected birds may have septicaemic signs (a congested reddened carcass, an enlarged congested friable liver (often with mottling) and an enlarged congested spleen) together with widespread petechiation of the carcass. A catarrhal enteritis and thickening of the proventriculus and ventriculus can also occur. In chronic cases endocarditis and polyserositis/synovitis may also be found.

Diagnosis

Diagnosis is based upon history and clinical signs with bacterial culture providing a definitive diagnosis.

Treatment

Treatment with penicillin is the most common course of action as the majority of isolates are penicillin sensitive; however, the exact choice of treatment will be based upon bacterial sensitivities.

Erysipelothrix rhusiopathiae is a zoonotic disease.

Prevention

Prevention involves keeping poultry separate from sheep and pigs. A commercial vaccination is available, requiring two initial doses followed by annual boosters.

Differential diagnoses

Escherichia coli, *Pasteurella multocida*, *Salmonella* species and Newcastle disease.

Pasteurella (fowl cholera/pasteurellosis)
Aetiology and epidemiology

P. multocida is a relatively infrequent pathogen of poultry with turkeys being the most susceptible species followed by pheasants then waterfowl. Chickens are relatively resistant to infection. It is traditionally thought of as a disease of mature birds. The bacteria are often carried by wild birds, recovered domestic fowl and possibly rodents.

Clinical signs

Peracute infection leads to sudden death. Acute infection can lead to respiratory distress, a naso-ocular discharge, cyanosis, anorexia, a white watery diarrhoea (which subsequently becomes bile stained and mucoid) and dullness.

In chronic cases there may be caseous abscesses of the comb, wattles and joints, torticollis, respiratory signs and salpingitis. In turkeys a necrotizing dermatitis has also been reported.

Post-mortem findings

In acute cases findings include septicaemia (congestion of the carcass, an enlarged congested liver (often with focal necrosis), an enlarged congested spleen and congested kidneys), pneumonia (mostly in turkeys), increased mucus throughout the digestive tract and widespread petechiae.

In chronic cases lesions include caseous lesions of the comb and wattles, arthritis, endocarditis, pneumonia (usually in turkeys), sinusitis, salpingitis and peritonitis.

Diagnosis

Diagnosis of pasteurellosis requires confirmation by bacterial culture as post-mortem lesions are only suggestive.

This organism has zoonotic potential and is notifiable in many countries. Virulence varies with the strain of the organism and it is thought that there are avian and mammalian specific strains.

Treatment

Treatment with antimicrobials may help improve clinical signs.

Prognosis

A complete recovery is rare and treatment will not eliminate *Pasteurella* from the flock.

Prevention

Prevention is based upon biosecurity, hygiene and careful sourcing of new stock. A commercial vaccination is available, which requires two initial doses followed by annual boosters.

Differential diagnoses

Escherichia coli, *Salmonella* species and *Erysipelothrix*.

Avian influenza (bird flu, fowl plague)
Aetiology and epidemiology

Avian influenza is a rare but highly contagious notifiable disease caused by an orthomyxovirus (for a more in-depth description see Chapter 15). Wild birds are thought to be the main vector for the virus since waterfowl appear to be asymptomatic carriers. The disease is often spread via the faeco–oral route but aerosol transmission can also occur.

Clinical signs

The virus varies in both virulence and serotype causing a whole range of clinical signs varying from mild sneezing through to very dull hunched up birds with respiratory distress and cyanosis. In severe cases sudden death may be the only presenting sign. Diarrhoea and neurological signs may also be observed.

Post-mortem findings

Post-mortem lesions are not pathognomonic but may include cyanosis of the head, congestion of the carcass, sinusitis, tracheitis, air sacculitis and enteritis.

Diagnosis

Diagnosis requires virus isolation or PCR (by the Animal and Plant Health Agency (APHA) in the UK, under the World Organisation for Animal Health (OIE) guidance).

Treatment

There is no effective treatment but treatment of secondary infections with antibiotics may reduce losses. In most countries this condition is notifiable and treatments and control measures may be controlled according to the legal requirements of the relevant authorities.

Prevention

Prevention is based upon hygiene, biosecurity and discouraging the presence of wild birds. In some countries commercial vaccines are available.

Differential diagnoses

Infectious laryngotracheitis, *Mycoplasma* species, avian rhinotracheitis, Newcastle disease and infectious bronchitis.

Newcastle disease (avian paramyxovirus type 1, fowl pest)

Aetiology and epidemiology

Avian paramyxoviruses are found with varying pathogenicity. Strains showing sufficient virulence can be classed as Newcastle disease as determined by the APHA according to OIE guidelines. Suspected cases are notifiable in many countries (see Chapters 15 and 18 for greater detail).

Like avian influenza, the virus is spread by fomites and shed by migrating birds (especially waterfowl, which may be asymptomatic carriers). Strains of the virus will vary in both virulence (being classed as lentogenic, mesogenic or velogenic) and tissue tropism (with the strains being classed as pneumotropic, viscerotropic or neurotropic).

Clinical signs

Clinical signs vary and may include respiratory signs, nervous signs, dullness, an emerald green diarrhoea, sudden death, weight loss, a drop in egg production and poor egg shell quality.

Post-mortem findings

Post-mortem lesions are often non-specific but gastrointestinal tract lesions may include haemorrhage of the digestive tract especially the proventriculus (Figure 16.27), caecal congestion together with focal mural necrosis of the intestine and gut associated lymphoid tissue.

Diagnosis

Diagnosis is based upon virus isolation or PCR.

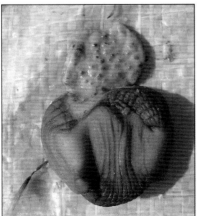

16.27 Proventricular haemorrhage caused by Newcastle disease.

Treatment

There is no specific treatment; however, antimicrobials may help control secondary bacterial infections. This is a notifiable disease in many countries including the UK.

Prevention

Prevention is based upon hygiene, biosecurity and discouraging the presence of wild birds. Vaccination can also be carried out using both live attenuated and killed vaccines.

Differential diagnoses

Infectious laryngotracheitis, *Mycoplasma* species, avian rhinotracheitis, avian influenza and infectious bronchitis.

Infectious bronchitis virus

Although infectious bronchitis virus is not a cause of diarrhoea, it is included here because the related polyuria is often reported by owners as being diarrhoea.

Aetiology and epidemiology

Infectious bronchitis virus is a coronavirus, which, as its name suggests, causes respiratory disease. However, it also affects the cells of the reproductive tract (leading to poor egg shell quality) and the kidneys (causing nephropathy).

Clinical signs

Such birds can present with respiratory signs, a drop in egg production and pale eggs (which have poor shell quality). Kidney damage can result in polydipsia and polyuria, which many owners will report as diarrhoea. The virus is spread via the faeco–oral route and can be carried on fomites.

Post-mortem findings

Pathological lesions include visceral gout, urate deposits in the kidneys, tracheal inflammation and air sacculitis. Birds may have secondary peritonitis and salpingitis (in laying hens).

Diagnosis

Diagnosis can be made retrospectively using serology (paired samples are best) or using PCR. Remember, like all coronaviruses infectious bronchitis viruses mutate frequently meaning there are several serotypes.

Treatment

Treatment is based upon maintaining hydration and potentially using antimicrobials to prevent secondary bacterial infection (*E. coli*).

Prognosis

The prognosis is variable with formerly vaccinated birds having a good rate of recovery; however, unvaccinated birds may succumb to renal failure or respiratory pathology.

Prevention

Prevention is based upon biosecurity and vaccination. There are several serotypes to protect against with varying levels of cross-protection.

Differential diagnoses

Infectious laryngotracheitis, *Mycoplasma* species, avian rhinotracheitis, Newcastle disease and avian influenza.

Gumboro disease (infectious bursal disease)
Aetiology, epidemiology and pathogenesis

Gumboro disease is a birnavirus that attacks the bursa of Fabricius (chickens only). Infection tends to occur from 3–6 weeks of age when levels of maternal derived antibody (MDA) have fallen. The virus causes bursitis followed by bursal atrophy. The infection will damage B-cells causing immunosupression. The bursa should have atrophied by 4 months leaving older birds refractory to infection. The virus is shed via the faeces and can survive in the environment for several months.

Clinical signs

In acute cases, birds will be dull, hunched up (with ruffled feathers) along with having a white diarrhoea. Many of these birds will rapidly die. In cases where the MDA levels are high the birds will show poor growth and an increased predisposition to other diseases.

Post-mortem findings

Post-mortem examination will often reveal bursae filled with pus or blood, regarded as pathognomonic for this condition.

Diagnosis

Whilst post-mortem findings are diagnostic in acute cases, for birds with subacute infection serology, bursal histopathology or PCR testing can be used to confirm clinical suspicion.

Treatment

Treatment involves supportive care and potentially using antimicrobials to control secondary bacterial infection.

Prognosis

The prognosis is variable depending on the levels of MDA present.

Prevention

Prevention is based upon vaccinating the parents, typically with a live vaccine at approximately 28 days followed by a killed vaccine at 16 weeks to provide adequate levels of MDA. This should be followed by live vaccination of the chicks at approximately 28 days.

Differential diagnoses

Infectious bronchitis and coccidiosis.

Marek's disease
Aetiology, epidemiology and pathogenesis

Marek's disease is caused by a herpesvirus. The virus is shed in the dander from feather follicle epithelium of infected birds and is inhaled by young chicks (typically in their first 10 weeks of life). After initially replicating in the pneumocytes, the virus goes on to infect the lymphocytes, initially causing immunosuppression and subsequently tumours (usually after several months). In the 'acute form' the tumours form in the visceral organs; in the 'classical form' the tumours form in the nervous system leading to paralysis (see Chapter 18).

Clinical signs

Whilst Marek's disease is classically known for causing paralysis of the limbs, the associated immunosuppression can predispose birds to many pathogens of the enteric system and therefore give rise to diarrhoea (often such cases respond poorly or transiently to treatment).

Post-mortem findings

Post-mortem findings include sciatic nerve enlargement, hepatosplenomegaly and tumours throughout the visceral organs.

Diagnosis

Diagnosis can be carried out using feather samples for PCR or by using histopathology of suspected lesions.

Treatment

There is no treatment.

Prognosis

The neoplasia is always fatal.

Prevention

Prevention is based upon reducing stress in young chicks, keeping them separate from older (potentially infected) birds and potentially vaccinating them with a live attenuated vaccine at 1 day old. Note that the vaccine is only effective if hygiene and management standards are high.

Differential diagnosis

Lymphoid leucosis and reticuloendotheliosis.

Lymphoid leucosis
Aetiology, epidemiology and pathogenesis

Like Marek's disease, lymphoid leucosis causes both immunosuppression and neoplasia. However, unlike with Marek's disease, the nervous system is spared from neoplastic invasion.

Lymphoid leucosis is caused by a retrovirus and is transmitted via biting insects, needles and vertically. Not all exposed birds succumb to the infection.

The tumours often form in the visceral organs (including the intestine) and in some cases will form in the bones of the legs (see Chapter 21).

Clinical signs

Affected birds show weight loss, poor growth and an increased susceptibility to other infections (including gastrointestinal infections). If the tumours invade the bones the legs may become bowed.

Post-mortem findings

Post-mortem lesions include neoplastic invasion of the visceral organs but histopathology will be required to differentiate lymphoid leucosis related tumours from those caused by Marek's disease (Figure 16.28).

Diagnosis

Diagnosis is based upon histopathology or serology.

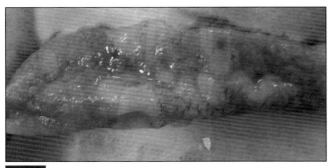

16.28 Intestinal lymphoma in a 6-month-old Maran hen.

Treatment

There is no treatment.

Prognosis

The tumours are eventually fatal.

Prevention

Prevention is based upon sourcing disease-free stock, controlling biting insects and using sterile needles when blood testing.

Differential diagnoses

Marek's disease and reticuloendotheliosis.

Reticuloendotheliosis (lymphoid tumour disease)

Aetiology and epidemiology

Reticuloendotheliosis is caused by a retrovirus infection of poultry leading to the formation of tumours in the visceral organs. The virus has also been suggested to be the cause of lymphomatous tumours in pheasants. The virus is spread mostly via the faeco–oral route but can be transmitted vertically.

Clinical signs

Affected birds may be asymptomatic; however, clinical signs may include diarrhoea, weight loss and poor growth.

Post-mortem findings

Post-mortem findings are of visceral tumours and occasionally inflammation of the digestive tract.

Diagnosis

Virus isolation, serology and histopathology can be used to diagnose the condition.

Treatment

There is no treatment.

Prevention

Prevention involves sourcing disease-free stock.

Differential diagnoses

Marek's disease and lymphoid leucosis.

The inappetent bird

The inappetent bird can be a rather challenging patient. In general terms, most birds will eat unless they are very unwell; however, some birds can become fussy eaters, refusing to eat until offered their preferred foods.

History-taking

- What is the bird fed? Ask probing questions regarding treats.
- How long has the bird been inappetent?
- Has the bird any other clinical signs such as weight loss or diarrhoea?
- Is the bird drinking normally? Large fowl hens in lay should drink 200 ml/day and non-laying birds should drink 50 ml/kg/day.
- Are any other birds in the flock affected?
- When was the bird last treated for internal parasites or have the faeces been evaluated for internal parasites recently? Was an appropriate treatment used at the correct dose?

Clinical examination

Next, a thorough clinical examination should be carried out. The oral cavity should be checked for foreign bodies, trichomoniasis and fowlpox. If trichomoniasis is suspected, then wet smears can be prepared and examined immediately (at X40 magnification under the microscope).

Check the crop for enlargement. If the crop is firm and the bird hasn't eaten in the preceding few hours, then crop impaction is possible and as such surgery may be necessary. It should be noted that a clinician needs to be familiar with a normal filled crop. Many normal crops are commonly misdiagnosed as impacted by inexperienced veterinary surgeons who are often led by an owner's diagnosis.

If the crop has fluid contents, then use a crop tube to aspirate a sample for cytology. Large numbers of *Candida* may indicate sour crop, whilst small numbers are a normal finding.

Check the body condition of the bird, paying attention to the pectoral muscles.

Check the bird for distension of the coleomic cavity. This could indicate bacterial peritonitis, ascites, obesity, neoplasia or the enlargement of the internal organs. Abdominocentesis can help differentiate between peritonitis and other causes of ascites; however, it should be noted that in some cases of peritonitis the pus is too thick to be aspirated. Check the bird for diarrhoea and faecal soiling around the vent (vent pasting), which is suggestive of diarrhoea.

Take a faecal sample and carry out faecal worm egg counts/coccidial oocyst counts. Worm egg counts of >400 eggs/gram or the presence of any *Capillaria* eggs indicate that treatment is necessary. Coccidial oocysts of >50,000 are likely to be significant.

If the bird is drinking and is otherwise normal it would be beneficial to withhold food and offer it again after 24 hours.

If the bird is still inappetent, not drinking or is hunched up with ruffled feathers then blood samples for haematology and biochemistry (see Chapter 10) to look for liver and kidney disease should be taken together with the employment of diagnostic imaging (see Chapter 11).

Veterinary public health

Backyard poultry tend to be classed as both pets and food-producing animals and there is a real risk of zoonotic infection for owners. The two main pathogens of concern are *Salmonella* species and *Campylobacter*.

Campylobacter

Traditionally, *Salmonella* was considered the most important zoonotic infection, but with the advent of vaccines and increased control due to legislative changes, *Campylobacter* has now replaced *Salmonella* as the main organism of public health concern in poultry.

Epidemiology

As far as poultry health is concerned, *Campylobacter* is considered to be non-pathogenic. Whilst there have been anecdotal reports of vibrionic hepatitis in poultry caused by *C. jejuni*, this has not yet been proven.

The main reason for concern about *Campylobacter* is its ability to cause gastroenteritis in humans. The infection is not thought to be readily transmissible between humans; poorly cooked poultry meat remains the main source of infection.

Campylobacter can be carried by both domestic fowl and mammals. It is thought the disease is spread predominantly via the faeco–oral route and through drinking contaminated water. Pests such as rodents and flies are also important vectors.

The disease is not thought to be transmitted vertically so eggs are not a source of infection for humans.

Owners coming into contact with poultry droppings (especially children not washing their hands) is likely to be the main source of infection among poultry keepers.

It is essential that everyone who comes into contact with pet chickens washes their hands correctly.

Some poultry owners will fatten birds for the table and, whilst there is no legislative control, it is important that during slaughter and dressing they minimize faecal contamination of the carcass. Good kitchen hygiene and thorough cooking are essential.

Diagnosis

Faecal cultures may be used to diagnose *Campylobacter*.

Treatment

Where cases of *Campylobacter* have been diagnosed owners should take extra care when handling birds and keep children and immunosuppressed people away. It is questionable as to whether or not erythromycin should be used to control this commensal organism in infected flocks.

Prevention

A better approach than treatment is to ensure good hygiene and husbandry together with vermin and fly control to reduce the chances of birds becoming infected in the first place. Those fattening birds should observe good hygiene at slaughter and dressing. All owners should observe good personal hygiene.

Salmonella Enteritidis and Typhimurium

Epidemiology and pathogenesis

S. Enteritidis and *S.* Typhimurium are considered the most important poultry derived species involved in human cases of salmonellosis. Whilst neither are of consequence for infected poultry they can cause gastrointestinal disease in humans. Routine testing, competitive exclusion (probiotics), use of organic acids in feed or water and vaccination have been used to reduce the prevalence of these species in poultry in many parts of the world.

When birds older than 1 month of age are infected, the majority of birds will clear this infection within 60 days. However, a small number of animals remain carriers and act as reservoirs within a flock. If young chicks are infected the bacteria has a large free intestine to colonize leading to a much more difficult challenge for the body to clear.

S. Enteritidis can also be transmitted vertically and as such can be transmitted to humans through egg consumption. For owners with pet chickens, unwashed hands are another source of infection. For owners that eat their own poultry, poor kitchen hygiene and faecal contamination of carcasses can lead to infection.

Infection can get into a flock from infected animals including domestic fowl, wild birds, vermin, flies and of course fomites. Whilst in the past feed was an important source of infection for poultry there is now legislation in force that reduces the risk from this source.

Diagnosis

Diagnosis is by bacterial culture and subsequent serotyping.

Treatment of an outbreak

In flocks whose eggs are being sold for human consumption, upon the detection of either *S.* Enteritidis or *S.* Typhimurium, egg sales must be halted immediately. In such circumstances, slaughter of the flock followed by good cleaning and disinfection should be recommended.

Where the affected birds are pets, owners must be advised not to consume the eggs. There are a number of potential approaches to such birds depending on the owners' expectations. Some owners will wish to euthanase the flock and 'start again' with vaccinated birds. If an owner is keen to keep the birds, then there are a number of options:

- Test the birds and remove all carriers
- Test the birds and retest a few months later (at least 60 days later) to ensure any birds that initially tested positive have now cleared the infection, together with checking that none of the birds that initially tested negative have become positive. Any birds testing positive twice are likely to be potential carriers and should be removed
- Any new birds being added to knowingly positive flocks should be vaccinated prior to coming on to the holding (both live attenuated and killed vaccines are available)
- Antimicrobial therapy has been suggested; however, it is unlikely to completely eliminate the bacteria from affected birds
- Control rodents and flies on affected holdings to prevent the spread of the bacteria.

Prevention

Aside from good personal and kitchen hygiene, probiotics given to 1-day-olds may act as competitive excluders and can be used to help reduce *Salmonella* carriage by birds

(Nakamura *et al.*, 2002). The use of organic acids in feed or drinking water can reduce the chances of infection.

All new birds added to a flock should come from reputable disease-free sources.

Vaccines are available in both live and inactivated forms. Vaccination should be initiated before the birds come into lay and boosted annually.

In the UK, keepers with more than 350 laying hens or those wishing to sell their eggs through local shops must register with the *Salmonella* National Control Programme via the APHA, which will involve routine monitoring.

References and further reading

Calnek B, Barnes HJ, Beard C, Reid W and Yoder H (1991) *Diseases of Poultry, 9th edn*. Wolfe Publishing Limited, London

Nakamura A, Ota Y, Mizukami A *et al.* (2002) Evaluation of aviguard, a commercial competitive exclusion product for efficacy and after-effect on the antibody response of chicks to *Salmonella*. *Poultry Science* **81**, 1653–1660

Pattison M, McMillin P, Bradbury J and Alexander D (2007) *Poultry Diseases, 6th edn*. Elsevier, Philadelphia

Taylor M, Coop R and Wall R (2007) *Veterinary Parasitology, 3rd edn*. Blackwell Publishing, Oxford

Welchman D (2008) Diseases in young pheasants. *In Practice* **30**, 144–149

Chapter 17

Reproductive and laying disorders

Aidan Raftery and Richard Jones

Reproductive disease is common in birds but appears overrepresented in backyard poultry especially among female birds. This is most likely a result of the genetic selection pressures that have been in place for centuries, with the goal of maximizing egg production for human consumption. Of the poultry covered in this manual, chickens and ducks are the most commonly presented for reproductive disease.

The ancestors of domesticated chickens (the Red Jungle Fowl) and ducks (the Mallard duck) have defined breeding seasons during which they lay 8–12 eggs per clutch, which may be replaced if lost to a predator, for example. Therefore, they will generally produce a maximum of 24 eggs per year. Following the breeding season, the oviduct involutes and may undergo 'repair' until the following year. Modern commercial chickens and ducks are able to lay all year round (although moulting and winter months may reduce the rate) and are easily capable of producing 300 eggs per year. This 'chronic' ovulation and laying activity results in the high incidence of inflammatory, neoplastic and infectious diseases of their reproductive tracts.

Disorders of the female reproductive tract

Salpingitis

Salpingitis or inflammation of the oviduct is the most common cause of mortality in commercial poultry and is associated with a wide variety of infectious agents. It is a very common presentation at veterinary surgeries for both ducks and chickens.

Aetiology and pathogenesis

Predisposing factors include age, malnutrition, obesity, high rates of egg laying or history of reproductive disorders (e.g. yolk coelomitis). Salpingitis may be septic or non-septic. *Escherichia coli* is the most common infectious cause. There are certain serotypes of *E. coli* that are regarded to be primary pathogens of the hen's reproductive tract. However, other bacteria, such as *Streptococcus*, *Mycoplasma*, *Actinobacter*, *Corynebacterium*, *Salmonella* and *Pasteurella*, have been implicated as potential causes. Viral infections such as infectious bronchitis virus and Newcastle disease virus (as well as bacteria such as *Mycoplasma* spp.) may damage the mucosa allowing invasion of secondary

bacterial pathogens leading to salpingitis. Salpingitis can also be secondary to diseases of the ovary, such as cystic ovarian disease, oophoritis and neoplasia.

Salpingitis commonly leads to an impacted oviduct. A lack of eggs often just means none laid; the ovary may continue ovulating every 25 hours resulting in an impacted oviduct, which is distended with a mass of caseated material or with misshapen soft-shelled eggs. On surgery it is common to find the oviduct packed with an amorphous mass of adhered shell-less egg material. The oviduct will not be functioning so shells will not be formed and the oviduct will not be contracting to expel the eggs.

Yolk coelomitis is a common sequela to salpingitis as the ovary may continue to ovulate and, due to the lack of normal peristaltic movements of the oviduct, some of the ova may end up in the coelomic cavity leading to a yolk coelomitis when they break up.

Oviduct prolapse is also a potential sequela due to prolonged contractions to expel an egg or a mass of eggs that may be adherent to the wall of the oviduct. Oviduct torsion can occur due to the build-up of material in the oviduct with its contractions increasing the risk. Oviduct rupture is a relatively common sequela to oviduct impaction secondary to salpingitis. This usually results in a dramatic deterioration in the bird as a consequence of the yolk coelomitis that is caused by the amorphous mass of egg material that leaks into the coelomic cavity.

Clinical signs

Clinical signs of salpingitis are often non-specific and include weight loss, fluffed plumage, anorexia and lethargy. There may also be a flaccid vent with cloacal discharge.

Malformed eggs may be passed (soft-shelled, an abnormal shape or blood-streaked). If a cloacal discharge is present it may resemble scrambled egg.

Non-septic salpingitis will generally result in vague signs of illness and can be a chronic condition, whereas birds with a septic salpingitis are usually clinically very ill. In addition to the clinical signs already mentioned, the coelomic space may be distended and a distended oviduct may be palpable per the cloaca.

Diagnosis

Radiography should confirm the presence of a coelomic mass but the presence of coelomic fluid will reduce the value of radiography.

Ultrasonography is more helpful and will identify an enlarged oviduct. Ultrasonography may also confirm whether the condition is complicated by oviduct rupture. Ultrasonography may detect a retained right oviduct, which some believe may predispose the bird to salpingitis.

Cloacal endoscopy can also help confirm salpingitis. The clinician may be able to insert an endoscope into the oviduct, but it is usually difficult to visualize due to the difficulty of creating an air space when a salpingitis is present.

Cytology of any discharge from the cervix and of any abdominal fluid aspirated will help differentiate between septic and non-septic salpingitis. If cytology points towards a septic salpingitis then a culture and sensitivity test will help with the treatment plan. Cytology samples collected from the coelomic cavity will help identify whether there is an ongoing yolk coelomitis.

Treatment

Treatment for salpingitis depends on the underlying cause. Anti-inflammatories are a very important part of the treatment as inflammation is a major component of the pathology. Meloxicam is the most commonly used anti-inflammatory drug. Septic salpingitis will require antibacterial drugs. If there is significant coelomic fluid present, draining as much fluid as possible will usually result in significant relief for the bird and provide diagnostic samples. Supportive care as needed is very important to support the bird whilst the medication starts to work and the condition starts to resolve. Supportive care includes parenteral fluids, thermal support, nutritional support and analgesia. This is covered in detail elsewhere in this manual and is a vital part of the treatment. It is also important to try to prevent further ovulations, which will just cause further complications. Deslorelin, a gonadotropin-releasing hormone agonist, is the most common drug used for this purpose. Repeated deslorelin implants may be necessary for the long-term management of some cases. Some cases of salpingitis require surgical intervention for resolution of the condition but this has to be balanced with the chance of a successful outcome. Coeliotomy will also allow a definitive diagnosis and full evaluation of associated structures. Salpingohysterectomy is a long complicated surgical procedure that will require intensive postsurgical management (see Chapter 23).

Abdominocentesis

Conditions such as yolk coelomitis and neoplasia can cause an accumulation of fluid. Free fluid may be collected for cytology, culture and biochemical analysis. There are five peritoneal cavities in which fluid can accumulate, depending on the site of pathology (see Chapter 2).

The intestinal cavity lies in the midline and contains the gastrointestinal tract, the gonads, and the left oviduct; this is where fluid accumulates when associated with reproductive disease.

Removing the fluid will give the bird significant temporary relief.

1. Restrain the bird firmly in a standing position.
2. Slightly tip the bird forwards.
3. Pluck overlying feathers, if necessary.
4. Aseptically prepare the skin on the midline at the level of the umbilicus.
5. Insert a small-gauge needle (21–27 G) or a Teflon i.v. catheter through the skin and muscle, directly in at the level of the umbilicus to avoid the liver cranially.
6. It is not uncommon for the needle to become blocked with clots of yolk material.

Deslorelin – a gonadotropin-releasing hormone (GnRH) agonist

Deslorelin is a non-steroidal, peptide-based contraceptive GnRH agonist implant that mimics overproduction of GnRH, thereby suppressing function of the pituitary–gonadal axis. Production of follicle stimulating hormone (FSH) and luteinising hormone (LH) decreases and, as a result, ovulation is prevented (Ubuka and Bentley, 2011).

- The implant is inserted subcutaneously or intramuscularly.
- A 4.7 mg implant suppresses ovulation in most chickens for an average of 161 days (5–7 days before suppression).
- A 9.4 mg implant suppresses ovulation in most chickens for an average of 385 days (2–3 days before suppression).
- Weight loss of 10–25% is seen due to involution of the reproductive tract.
- Moulting is often seen after implantation, which is normal with a cessation in laying.
- Use of deslorelin has been found to significantly reduce the incidence of ovarian cancer in chickens (De Matos, 2013).

There are significant differences in the effects between species; however, there is as yet no information on the response to deslorelin implants in the other poultry species covered in this manual. Differences in GnRH receptor subtypes is probably the reason for the different responses seen across avian species.

Veterinary surgeons can find more information on this drug on the European Medicines Agency website. It is the responsibility of the prescribing clinician to decide if this is the appropriate drug in the given situation, and to provide withdrawal periods for eggs and meat for the situation in which it is being used

---

Yolk coelomitis
Aetiology and pathogenesis

Yolk coelomitis occurs when the infundibulum fails to engulf the ovum, when reverse peristalsis stops the egg entering the oviduct, or if there is an oviduct rupture due to salpingitis. Yolk coelomitis has also been called egg yolk peritonitis, yolk peritonitis, ectopic ovulation and ectopic eggs.

Any disease of the ovary, such as cystic ovarian disease, oophoritis and neoplasia, can lead to yolk coelomitis. The tissues surrounding the ovary help funnel ovulated ova into the infundibulum so any pathology of these tissues (abdominal air sac, proventriculus and the ventriculus) will predispose to ectopic ovulations as will any adhesions affecting the infundibulum.

Once in the coelomic cavity the ovum breaks up. Yolk is a very irritating substance to the serosal surfaces so the result is a sterile yolk coelomitis. It is a very common condition and in most cases is self-resolving with supportive treatment. Clinical signs seen in mild cases are non-specific.

If the condition is reoccurring with several ectopic ovulations, then more severe clinical signs will be seen as it develops into a potentially fatal condition.

Clinical signs

Clinical signs can include anorexia, depression, abdominal swelling, ascites and dyspnoea. There is usually cessation of egg laying. Deformed or soft-shelled eggs may sometimes be passed if the condition is secondary to a salpingitis. Birds with severe ascites are often seen to stand with a wide-based penguin-like stance (Figure 17.1).

Diagnosis

This is based on a history of supporting clinical signs. Often, an irregular distended oviduct is palpable either externally or more commonly by digital examination per cloaca. Yolk coelomitis causes a severe inflammatory response with a profound leucocytosis in many cases on haematology. A biochemistry screen will give information about concurrent and secondary disease processes. Radiography is often of limited value in cases of yolk coelomitis, with ultrasonography providing more useful information. Coelioscopy is contraindicated if there is significant coelomic fluid present due to the risk of fluid entering the air sacs and the bird potentially drowning. Abdominocentesis will give significant relief to the bird and will yield potentially diagnostic samples for cytology and for culture and sensitivity testing.

Treatment

Treatment depends on the severity of the clinical signs. Appropriate doses of non-steroidal anti-inflammatory drugs (NSAIDs) are the most important treatment in mild cases. Septic yolk coelomitis will require appropriate antibacterial therapy, ideally based on culture and sensitivity testing, but the predominant bacteria seen on cytology will help with the initial choice. Draining ascitic fluid will provide immediate relief (see above). It is not uncommon for the bird's bodyweight to be reduced by 25% following removal of the ascitic fluid. Preventing further ovulations is an important part of the treatment plan. Deslorelin will result in cessation of ovulations in a high percentage of

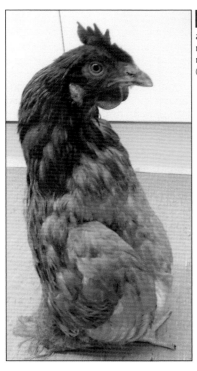

17.1 This bird with severe ascites has adopted an upright stance to relieve pressure on its respiratory tract.
(Courtesy of Ian Brown)

hens (see above). Some cases may need to be managed by repeated deslorelin implants. There is as yet no research in ducks or the other poultry species covered in this manual to establish its efficacy in these species. Many cases will require a salpingohysterectomy together with the removal of the yolk material from the coelomic cavity.

Complications

Pancreatitis, splenitis, yolk-thromboembolic disease, hepatitis, nephritis and coelomic adhesions are all possible complications, with coelomic adhesions the most common secondary problem.

Egg binding and dystocia

Failure of an egg to pass from the level of the uterus/shell gland is most commonly due to salpingitis; usually the clinical signs are associated more with the salpingitis than the retained egg/ovum and treatment should be directed at the salpingitis and its cause. Many hens presented with an acute illness will also have an egg passing down the reproductive tract that may be misdiagnosed as egg binding. Any bird with suspected egg binding should have a full clinical examination to rule out other causes of the clinical signs.

Aetiology and pathogenesis

Where there is a mechanical obstruction to the passage of an egg such as a stricture of the vent (more commonly seen in ducks) or some other mechanical obstruction such as neoplasia or granulomas, this is more correctly called dystocia. A very large or misshapen egg can also occasionally cause dystocia. Nutritional insufficiencies, especially vitamin D3 deficiencies and calcium phosphorus deficiencies/imbalance (see Chapter 20), and pelvic/spinal trauma are also possible causes of egg binding/dystocia. The severe life-threatening signs of egg binding seen in small psittacines such as budgerigars and lovebirds are not seen in poultry as their larger size means that the nerve compression and vascular compromise does not occur. See Chapter 11 for reference radiographs of normal egg laying in a chicken.

Clinical signs

Hens with dystocia/egg binding will usually have been found in the nest box. They may have a wide stance and be seen to have episodes of straining.

Diagnosis

A complete history including diet and laying activity may often suggest a pathogenesis and on physical examination an entire, damaged or malformed egg may be palpated, which would increase the likelihood of dystocia as the diagnosis. Cloacal prolapse can occur as a complication of dystocia and as a result of any condition that causes excessive staining. See Chapter 23 for information on dealing with a cloacal prolapse.

Radiography may reveal pathology that has caused the dystocia. Ultrasonography can also provide useful information and may help identify oviduct changes as well as other abnormalities in the coelomic cavity.

Treatment

In cases where the cause is nutritional, the egg may often pass if the hen is provided with supplemental heat, subcutaneous calcium gluconate 10% (50 mg/kg) and oral/subcutaneous fluids (Figure 17.2). More depressed and shocked patients require intravenous (Figure 17.3) or intraosseous fluids and analgesia (see Chapter 22). In some cases, antimicrobials will be needed.

If possible, the tissues surrounding the egg should be lubricated and then applying gentle pressure may result in egg expulsion. The patient should be placed in a warm humid oxygenated environment, for example a commercial brooder or veterinary intensive care unit (Figure 17.4). If there is a prolapse the tissue should be identified (if a prolapse of the oviduct has occurred, thick 'longitudinal folds' will be apparent in comparison to the relatively smooth texture of the cloacal mucosa), moistened and cleaned. See Chapter 23 and below for information on dealing with a cloacal prolapse. Oviduct prolapses may need a salpingohysterectomy (see also Chapter 23).

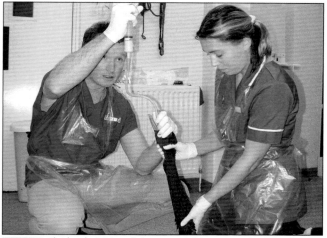

17.2 Fluids administered via gavage tubing using a lamb feeder tube.

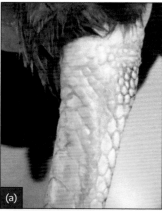

(a)

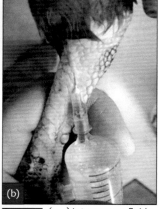

(b)

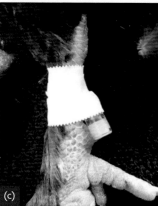

(c)

17.3 (a–c) Intravenous fluids administered into the medial metatarsal vein.

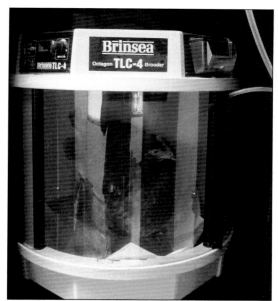

17.4 A dyspnoeic chicken is placed in a warm, humid environment with oxygen supplementation (in this case a commercially available intensive care/brooder unit).

If oviposition has not occurred within 6 hours of treatment (depending on the condition of the bird), then a further evaluation under general anaesthesia is generally indicated. With the bird in dorsal recumbency and with the benefits of the now relaxed musculature, the cloaca is lubricated and carefully examined with the aid of cotton-tipped applicators. The egg is palpated through the abdominal wall, and gentle pressure applied behind the egg directed caudally and slightly ventrally towards the vent. Care is required to avoid breaking the egg, which may result in a prolapse or cause damage to internal viscera. With gentle pressure the egg should become visible at the uterovaginal sphincter and with continued steady pressure and using lubricated cotton-tipped applicators to gently ease back the mucosa and dilate the sphincter, the egg may be expelled intact. If the egg does not become visible at the sphincter, this may be a due to adhesion to the oviduct wall secondary to oviduct disease, torsion of the oviduct or oviduct rupture resulting in ectopic eggs.

In the case where an egg is just visible at the uterovaginal opening but reasonable pressure has not resulted in expulsion of the egg, ovocentesis (the aspiration of egg contents using a large bore needle) may be attempted (Figure 17.5). The needle is inserted into the visible tip of the egg and, using a 20 ml syringe, the contents are aspirated with gentle pressure simultaneously applied to the egg externally. Due to the presence of the shell membranes internally, the egg will collapse into a 'cigar' shape, which is ideally removed in its entirety with gentle traction using a pair of haemostats or tissue forceps. As many shell fragments as possible should be removed, although if becoming traumatic it is best to lubricate the area using warm saline (keeping fluid volumes low to prevent flushing up the oviduct and into the body cavity causing a peritonitis) via a crop tube or canine urinary catheter, allowing them to pass naturally.

Finally, if the above are unsuccessful and the egg is lodged in the oviduct, surgical exploration is indicated to remove it and to evaluate the underlying pathology (see Chapter 23).

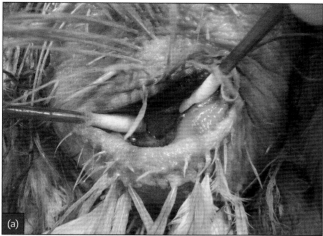

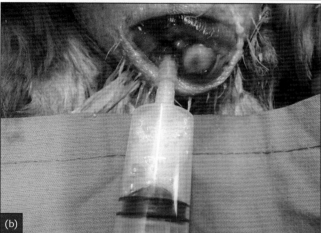

17.5 Ovocentesis is performed by (a) identifying and exposing the egg at the uterovaginal opening using lubricated cotton tipped applicators and (b) inserting a large bore needle into the exposed shell and aspirating the contents.

Cloacal/oviduct prolapse

Prolapse of the cloaca and/or oviduct can occur secondary to a variety of disease states, including salpingitis, oviduct impaction, oviduct torsion, cloacitis/cloacoliths, obesity, intestinal inflammation/endoparasitism, malnutrition, spinal disease, neoplasia (Figure 17.6) and occasionally dystocia. It is imperative that the underlying cause is ascertained and addressed prior to the instigation of therapy. Radiography, endoscopy, ultrasonography, faecal parasitology, haematology and biochemistry screens may all be of value.

The cloaca and oviduct are the most commonly prolapsed tissues but any part of the oviduct, intestines or even an intussusception may be prolapsed. Exposed tissues are susceptible to trauma, devitalization and infection, and should be kept moist and clean with warm sterile flushes. Often, cannibalistic behaviour by other flock members results in significant damage prior to presentation and in severe cases euthanasia should be considered on humane grounds. However, acute cloacal prolapses carry a fair prognosis with appropriate management.

Historically, a variety of techniques have been described to prevent prolapse reoccurring following reduction (see Chapter 23).

Concurrent medical therapy should include antibiosis, analgesia and agents to attempt to temporarily prevent further laying. If treated promptly, the prognosis for a prolapse is good.

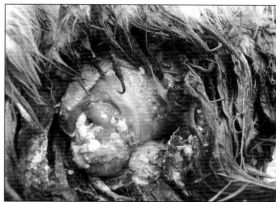

17.6 Cloacal prolapse can occur secondary to dystocia, normal egg laying or a variety of disease states affecting the reproductive tract including neoplasia.

Egg problems
Soft-shelled eggs

Soft-shelled or misshapen eggs (Figure 17.7) can occur as a result of dietary calcium deficiency. This is, however, very rare in birds fed a complete layer pellet. Infections involving the shell gland can also cause soft or misshapen eggs with infectious bronchitis (see Chapter 15) being a common cause in chickens. The occasional strangely shaped or soft-shelled egg may, however, just be due to the beginning or the end of lay. Soft-shelled eggs are quite common in older birds, especially in high production as they come out of lay. Other stressors including bullying can result in a similar phenomenon.

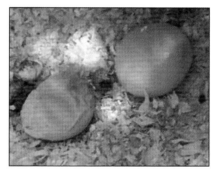

17.7 Soft-shelled or misshapen eggs can occur due to malnutrition or infection of the shell gland.
(Courtesy of Gary Mounfield)

Egg drop syndrome

Egg drop syndrome (EDS) is caused by an adenovirus infection in laying hens and is characterized by an initial loss of shell pigmentation followed by the production of soft-shelled and shell-less eggs in otherwise apparently healthy birds. There is no decrease in egg numbers; however, some of the affected eggs may be eaten, giving the impression of a fall in production. The natural hosts for EDS virus are ducks and geese, who are asymptomatic carriers. Chickens of all ages and breeds are susceptible. In general, cases of EDS can be distinguished from Newcastle disease and influenza virus infections by the absence of 'clinical illness' and from infectious bronchitis (IB) by the absence of ridges and misshapen eggs sometimes seen with IB infection. Virus isolation can be a problem due to transient excretion of the virus. The haemagglutination inhibition test using red blood cells is the preferred diagnostic test in unvaccinated flocks; however, spread is slow so it is important to only test birds producing affected eggs. There is a vaccine available, which is given before the point of lay.

Blood/meat spots

These may occur within the egg and, although generally harmless, are an aesthetic problem. These can arise if a cockerel is running with the hens, with resulting fertile eggs, or arising from pin point haemorrhages from the oviduct mucosa due to trauma or inflammation.

Egg eating

This vice is where birds break and eat either their own or the eggs of their flock mates. It may develop as a consequence of poorly designed nest boxes where eggs are prone to breakages or due to suboptimal nutrition, or 'boredom' due to lack of foraging opportunities. Once this habit occurs it can be difficult to break. A possible solution is to ensure eggs are collected as soon as possible and to scatter a number of table tennis balls in the run as 'non-productive' decoys. See Chapter 19.

Neoplasia

Laying hens are known to spontaneously develop ovarian and uterine cancer and are therefore used extensively as a model to elucidate disease aetiologies and pathogenesis in humans. Similar to humans, four types are observed in hen ovarian tumours including serous, endometroid, mucinous and clear cell or mixed carcinomas. Uterine adenocarcinoma (Figure 17.8) is the most commonly encountered tumour of the reproductive tract. Neoplastic cells are shed from tumours in the oviduct into the abdominal cavity. They implant on the ovary, pancreas, and other viscera and produce multiple hard yellow nodules. They may block lymph return and result in ascites. The incidence increases with age, and this tumour may be a frequent cause of death in hens over 2 years of age. Leiomyoma of the broad ligament is an oestrogen-induced hypertrophy of the smooth muscle of the broad ligament. It is benign and is generally an incidental finding at necropsy. Marek's disease has been known to induce lymphoid tumours of the female reproductive tract and adenomas and granulosa cell tumours are also described in the literature.

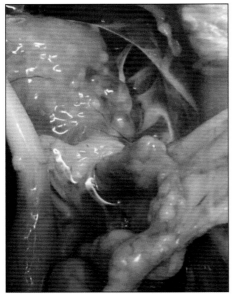

17.8 Uterine adenocarcinoma in a laying hen. Neoplastic cells are shed from tumours in the oviduct into the abdominal cavity. They implant on the ovary, pancreas and intestine producing multiple, hard, yellow nodules as shown.
(Courtesy of Alan Wren)

Egg retention, abdominal swelling, ascites and cloacal prolapse are common sequelae to reproductive tract neoplasms. Radiography and ultrasonography can be useful although an enlarged ovary or oviduct creates an image similar to that seen when uncalcified eggs are present, and therefore definitive diagnosis requires histopathological examination of surgical or endoscopy/ultrasound-guided biopsy samples (see Chapters 10 and 11). Excisional surgery, if possible, is the treatment of choice (see Chapter 23) although deslorelin implants have been used in the management of such lesions in other species (see above).

Oviductal cystic hyperplasia

In such cases the entire oviduct may be dilated with a white or brown mucoid fluid, creamy masses and secondary cysts. Cysts can occur due to improper formation of the left oviduct or from adhered lips of the infundibulum. The ovary in affected birds may also have cystic changes suggesting an endocrine abnormality. Progressive abdominal distension, ascites and subsequent respiratory distress are the most common clinical changes. Palpation, radiography and ultrasonography may reveal the distended oviduct although endoscopy and coeliotomy are required for a definitive diagnosis. Abdominocentesis (Figure 17.9) and GnRH agonist therapy may be useful in the short term but salpingohysterectomy is necessary for long-term management (see Chapter 23).

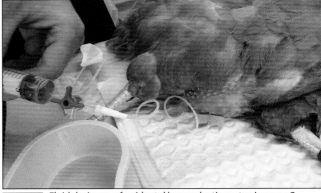

17.9 Fluid drainage of oviductal hyperplastic cyst using a 23 G butterfly catheter and three-way tap.

Infectious diseases affecting the reproductive tract in poultry

- Avian influenza virus
- Infectious bronchitis virus
- Newcastle disease virus
- Pasteurellosis (fowl cholera)
- Marek's disease
- Egg drop syndrome

Infectious diseases affecting the embryo in poultry

- Avian encephalomyelitis
- Fowlpox
- *Chlamydophila psittaci*
- Infectious bronchitis
- Infectious laryngotracheitis
- *Mycoplasma gallisepticum*
- Newcastle disease

Disorders of the male reproductive tract

Infertility

Infertility in the cockerel can be due to senility, obesity, anatomical or chromosomal abnormalities, or disease. Some breeds may have such 'voluminous' feathers that copulation is impossible and trimming or removing feathers around the vent may be indicated. Vent feathers may also become matted together with mud/faecal material thus preventing copulation; however, this is usually indicative of some additional disease process. Multiple cockerels may compete and prevent access to the hens.

After a detailed history on husbandry practices and nutritional status, further investigations of infertility in a flock would include cloacal bacteriology, cytology and histology, and endoscopic examination of the reproductive tract with testicular biopsy as appropriate (see Chapter 12).

Orchitis

Infection of the testes can arise following cloacitis, renal disease or via haematogenous spread. The most commonly found bacteria in orchitis are *E. coli*, *Salmonella* and *Pasteurella*.

Prolapsed phallus (Anseriformes)

This is generally a problem in sexually mature drakes. It is suggested that the aetiology of this condition is traumatic, because the incidence of this disease is higher under conditions where the drakes have to mate with the females out of water. Medical management involves gentle cleansing and reduction of prolapsed tissue and systemic use of appropriate analgesics, NSAIDs and in some cases antimicrobials. Often stay sutures are required to keep the phallus in place but some cases will require amputation of the phallus (see Chapter 23). Implantation with deslorelin may be an adjunct therapy in such cases in an attempt to temporarily reduce libido.

Neoplasia

Marek's disease has been known to induce lymphoid tumours of the testes and testicular teratomas and Sertoli cell tumours have also been described. Radiography and ultrasonography may identify an abnormal shape but an endoscopy biopsy will be required for a definitive diagnosis.

Incubation

Successful incubation and hatching require intensive management and veterinary surgeons are often called on by the poultry keeper to investigate problems associated with incubation, hatching, and chick growth and development.

Incubation can be natural where the female parent bird incubates the eggs, or sometimes broody hens are used to incubate eggs other birds (chickens or sometimes even from other species), or artificial where eggs are incubated using mechanical incubators.

Natural incubation

The female parent bird incubates her own eggs in all the species covered in this manual. She uses heat from her body to maintain the eggs at a constant temperature over the incubation period. There is an area of skin ventrally that is well supplied with blood vessels at the surface to facilitate the transfer of heat to the eggs. Ducks and geese pluck out the feathers that would normally insulate this area to line their nest. In other species the overlying feathers are usually shed. Broody hens will incubate any eggs that vaguely resemble their own and are often used to incubate eggs from other hens or even from different species. The nest is best positioned close to ground level to prevent any unfortunate accidents when the hatchlings are emerging. A small coop is ideal as it also allows the female and the chicks some safety and privacy if she is to raise them. She will need to leave the nest from time to time, but these periods will be brief, and unless she is quite young and/or flighty, she is not likely to abandon the nest unless she has cause to, for example due a predator attack.

The biggest benefit of hatching eggs naturally is that the female bird does all the work and incubation problems associated with inappropriate temperature and humidity are rare.

The downsides of natural incubation, however, include:

- Timing or even occurrence of broodiness in a particular bird cannot be controlled
- The bird will stop laying eggs whilst she is brooding, and will not start laying again until her young are well developed (that could mean as many as 4 months without eggs from this bird)
- There is a limit to the number of eggs one bird can hatch and raise
- Not all birds make good mothers; some can be clumsy and break the eggs they are supposed to be hatching, others will ignore their new hatchlings, and some may even peck at and attack them.

Artificial incubation

Successful artificial incubation depends on numerous parameters including temperature, humidity, airflow in the incubator or hatcher, vibration and egg rotation. Appropriate egg rotation or turning is required to prevent embryo adhesion to shell membranes. In natural incubation the eggs will be turned or rotated as often as every half hour. Inadequate turning in artificial incubation will result in early 'dead in shell', malposition or late dead in shell embryos. Good quality commercial incubators will turn eggs at different rates on mechanical rollers with 10 turns per day being the average. A minimum of five manual turns per day is required on machines without an automated turning facility. Several types of incubator are available for the incubation of poultry eggs. Incubators with a heating element on top without ventilation are inexpensive but have a relatively poor hatch rate. Automated incubators ventilated by warmed circulated air are a better choice especially if equipped with a slow turning roller mechanism. With such machines the eggs are 'rolled' every 2 hours with the actual turning process taking an hour (Figure 17.10). This avoids sudden vibrations, which is especially important during the first half of incubation. Good incubator hygiene is also vital for breeding success. The warm moist incubation environment encourages bacterial and fungal growth. It is preferable to only choose clean eggs to incubate. If soiled eggs have to be incubated, then they should be washed using an egg wash solution following the manufacturer's instructions. It is important that the temperature of the cleaning solution

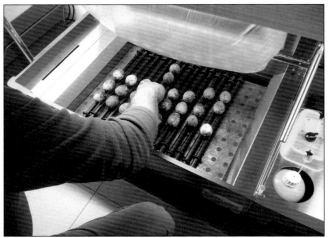

17.10 Modern incubator systems use a series of timed rollers to gently turn the eggs, with appropriate heat provided topically by a warm-air-filled latex bag simulating the brooding behaviour of a hen.

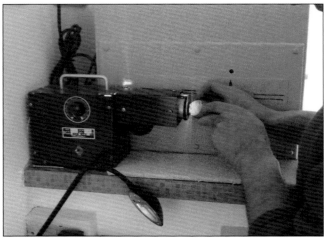

17.11 An egg is candled using a focused light source to monitor embryonic development.

is 'warmer' than the egg: the egg is porous and if the liquid is colder than the egg, any bacteria in the pores may be 'sucked' into the egg resulting in contamination and infection of the developing embryo. It must also be remembered that all solutions will remove the outer cuticle from the egg leaving them more vulnerable to microbial contamination. Discard any cracked and misshapen eggs.

Nest hygiene

Nest hygiene is also an important but often overlooked consideration. If the nest site is dirty there will be a soup of potential pathogens waiting to infect the egg as it cools. As soon as the egg is laid it cools and draws air in through the pores, and if large numbers of potential pathogens are present they are drawn in, so by the time the egg is collected it may have already been infected.

In order to synchronize incubation and hatching, provided the egg has not been warmed up, the eggs from most poultry species can be stored in trays sharp end down at a temperature of approximately 10°C for up to 2 weeks. The embryo is thus placed into 'suspended animation' until incubation of a batch begins and therefore hatching can be synchronized.

The incubation period for different poultry species varies from 21 to 28 days (see Chapter 4). Incubation temperatures also vary between the species, from 37.4 to 37.8°C, with relative humidity 40–55% depending on the species for the incubation period, increasing to approximately 65% for the last 3 days before hatching.

Embryo development

Artificially incubated eggs can be 'candled' using a focused light source in a darkened room to monitor development (Figure 17.11). The first signs of fertility are blood vessels radiating uniformly from the embryo in a branching pattern from days 3–5. Eggs with clear yolks showing no signs of blood vessels or development by day 7 are either infertile or early 'dead in shell' and should be removed. Mortality during the first 7 days is more commonly due to poor incubation technique but can be due to egg-borne infection, contamination or genetic abnormalities. Some causes of early embryonic death during artificial incubation include improper handling, excessive or insufficient temperature/humidity, excessive vibrations, improper egg turning or poor ventilation and build-up of carbon dioxide.

For successful incubation and hatching, poultry eggs must lose 13–16% (depending on the species) of fresh egg weight in water between laying and pipping. If humidity is too high, there will be too little water loss, leading to a generalized oedema resulting in unretracted yolk sacs, and the chick often drowns on the internal pip. When the humidity is too low there will be excessive weight loss and poor bone mineralization due to impaired calcium metabolism. These chicks will be weak and dehydrated after hatching. Water (thus weight) loss of an incubated egg is dependent on the humidity of its environment and therefore inappropriate weight loss can be managed by its manipulation. During this period of weight loss an 'air cell' develops at the rounded end of the egg. If the humidity is too high the air cell will be small; if it is too low the air cell will be too large.

Hatching

Hatching is the time of greatest embryo mortality. Hatching has four stages: drawdown; internal pip; external pip; and emergence from the egg.

Drawdown (Figure 17.12) is when the air cell expands and extends down one side of the egg. This occurs approximately 24–48 hours prior to the internal pip.

The gaseous exchange needs of the embryo are no longer met by the chorioallantoic circulation resulting in the onset of hypoxia and hypercapnia, and carbon dioxide levels rise, causing the hatching muscle in the neck to

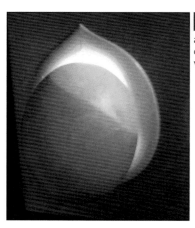

17.12 In this case drawdown is apparent with the air cell now occupying 20–30% of the egg volume.

twitch and move the head, forcing the egg tooth through the chorioallantoic membrane into the air cell (internal pip). This is a crucial moment as the chick now changes from chorioallantoic to pulmonary respiration. It is at this point when if weight loss has been insufficient pulmonary oedema will prevent effective gaseous exchange from the lungs and death can occur from asphyxiation. Once internal pip has occurred, the egg no longer needs to be turned.

As the lungs begin to function, cheeping vocalizations will be heard from within the egg. Movements of the abdominal musculature, which occur as a consequence of breathing, cause the yolk sac to be retracted into the chick's abdomen. With subsequent breaths the carbon dioxide levels within the air cell rise and the hatching muscle again begins to twitch causing the egg tooth to penetrate the shell (external pip). It is important that the humidity in the hatcher is sufficient to prevent the chick from drying up whilst still in the egg. The chick needs to be able to rotate inside if it is to be able to break the egg shell all the way round. If the air around the egg is too dry the chick becomes sticky and may adhere to the egg membranes preventing a successful hatch. Once the chick has broken through the circumference of the shell it still needs to push its way out by rupturing through shell membranes. These membranes break with ease if moist but if allowed to dry out become extremely tough and again can prevent successful hatching. The time between internal and external pipping is typically 24–48 hours (range 3–72 hours). There may not be any further pipping for 24–48 hours, with continued vocalizations, and retraction of the yolk sac. The vessels of the chorioallantois also regress at this point with blood transferred to the chick via the umbilicus.

Assisted hatching can be attempted if no progress has been made following initial external pip after a period of approximately 12 hours. In such cases, a small hole is made over the air cell and gently widened by removing small pieces of shell using fine forceps. The membranes can be moistened to aid visualization of active vessels and, if found, action suspended until they have constricted as fatal haemorrhage can result from iatrogenic trauma. Radiosurgery bipolar forceps can be useful to control bleeding in such cases. If the chick is removed from the egg too early the yolk sac may not have retracted.

Embryo and chick mortality

In artificial incubation, poor temperature control, malposition (the 'normal' chicken embryo develops with its head beneath the air cell and tucked under its right wing), inadequate moisture loss, infection and incorrect turning can all contribute to embryonic mortality prior to hatching. Therefore, every apparently infertile egg or dead in shell egg should be necropsied. Candling cannot distinguish early embryonic deaths from infertile eggs and the presence of fertility is an important criterion when proceeding with a diagnostic programme in avian reproduction. The majority of eggs for necropsy will fall into two distinct age groups: embryonic death at 3–5 days of incubation and death perihatching. Early embryonic mortality is generally associated with improper incubation temperature, jarring, inbreeding and chromosomal abnormalities. Deaths at the end of incubation are usually associated with hatching and the stressful period of switching from chorioallantoic to pulmonary respiration. Factors including improper incubation humidity, temperature and turning and malpositions are thought to be the leading causes of late embryonic death in poultry.

Necropsy technique

All eggs should ideally be candled prior to necropsy to determine the best point for entering the egg. This also permits the correlation of candling with necropsy findings. Eggs should be weighed, measured and external shell characteristics (shape, size, external deposits, cracks or thinning) should be noted. Pip marks should be evaluated for turning direction, location and size. Chicks normally pip anti-clockwise as seen from the round end of the egg. Samples may be obtained at this point for microbiological examination (providing death has been identified early and therefore they are not too rotten for meaningful bacteriology) by swabbing the shell with an alcohol wipe, making a hole into the shell with a hypodermic needle and inserting a swab.

The egg should be supported in an 'egg cup' and opened over the air cell with sharp scissors to expose the shell membranes, which are examined for abnormalities. The hole in the egg is enlarged using forceps. If a small embryo or no embryo is identified, the contents of the egg can be poured into a sterile Petri dish. If a well developed embryo/chick is present, the position of the air cell with respect to the egg, orientation of the embryo/chick as a whole within the egg, and position of the beak in relation to the air cell should be evaluated. The 'normal' chicken embryo develops with its head below the air cell and tucked under its right wing. Causes of malpositions include turning problems, position in the incubator (and resulting temperature discrepancies), oxygen deprivation, excess carbon dioxide, lack of embryo vigour and delayed development. Specific malpositions have been traditionally described in poultry but there are almost endless varieties of malpositions that may occur with varying success rates for hatching.

Chick embryo malpositions
- **Malposition 1:** Head between the thighs; failure of the chick to lift and turn its head in the middle of the last trimester; completely lethal; incidence increased by high incubation temperature
- **Malposition 2:** Head in the small end of the egg; chick is upside down in the egg; hatchability decreased by 50%; incidence increased by incorrect incubator egg orientation and low temperature
- **Malposition 3:** Head is under the left wing; chick rotates its head to the left as oppose to the right; usually lethal; incidence increased by incorrect incubator egg orientation, temperature and suboptimal parenteral nutrition
- **Malposition 4:** Beak is away from the air cell; upward turned egg tooth is not near the air cell but the rest of the embryo is normally positioned; slightly reduced hatchability; incidence increased by incorrect incubator egg orientation/ inappropriate turning
- **Malposition 5:** Feet over head; usually lethal
- **Malposition 6:** Head over the right wing; slightly reduced hatchability; incidence may be increased by parental malnutrition

---

If a well developed chick is present it should undergo a full necropsy and tissues shoule be retained for histopathological examination.

Care of hatchlings

Galliformes and Anseriformes are precocial species with well developed and fully functional eyes and musculo-skeletal systems from hatching. As soon as they are dry, newly hatched chicks are able to ambulate and find food for themselves. They do, however, require careful management in the first few weeks of life. Day-old chicks need thermal support and need to be protected from draughts whilst ensuring adequate ventilation. This can be achieved using a large plastic storage container with ventilation holes drilled in the sides (ideally it should be approximately 2 ft high to avoid older chicks escaping or perching on the sides) with a suspended infrared heat lamp, which can be raised or lowered to alter ambient temperature as required. For the first week of life they require an air temperature of 32–35°C, for the second approximately 29–32°C and going down approximately 3 degrees per week until they are ready to make the transition to outside. It is important, however, to monitor the behaviour of the birds when managing the temperature. If chicks are all crowded together directly under the heat source, they are cold and the height of the heat lamp should be lowered to increase the temperature. If they are around the edges of the brooder, avoiding the heat and each other, the lamp should be raised to decrease ambient temperature. If the lamp is suspended towards one end of the brooder this will provide a temperature gradient so they can choose their comfort zone.

An appropriate absorbent substrate is important to maintain a hygienic environment and avoid problems such as splay leg, which may occur due to a slippery surface. Dust-extracted pine shavings are commonly used as a brooder substrate. Cedar shavings should be avoided as the aromatic oils can irritate the chicks' delicate respiratory mucosa.

Feeding

A good quality commercial starter crumb (approximately 20% protein) and water offered *ad libitum* will provide all the chicks' nutritional needs from day 1 to 6–8 weeks when they can be weaned on to grower pellets (see Chapter 5). Careful consideration must be given as to how food and water are provided; open dishes can easily become contaminated with faeces and in the first few days of life pose a possible drowning risk. Commercial chick feeders and drinkers are recommended (Figure 17.13).

Roosting poles

Roosting poles in the form of 10 mm wooden dowels about 150 mm off the ground (adjusted as necessary depending on species and breed) may be supplied for the gallinaceous species as most will naturally seek and are comfortable in an elevated position. This will also hopefully prevent the chicks from perching on and thus contaminating feeders.

Common paediatric problems

Unretracted yolk sac

The yolk sac provides the young bird with nourishment and maternal antibodies during the first 1–2 days of life. It should be retracted into the body during the last stages of incubation and then is completely absorbed. Sometimes, the yolk sac does not retract fully, usually due to sub-optimal incubation conditions (e.g. hyper- or hypothermia, incorrect humidity, infection or any condition resulting in a weak bird during the hatch). In this situation the bird should be placed on a clean towel within the hatcher and the umbilicus bathed gently with chlorhexidine or povidone–iodine scrub. In some cases, using a moistened cotton-tipped applicator, the yolk sac can be gently eased back into the abdomen although reoccurrence is common. In such cases the exteriorized portion of the yolk sac can be 'tied off' at the umbilicus using 4/0 monofilament suture material or haemostatic clip and removed (Figure 17.14). The prognosis for such cases is guarded. See Chapter 23 for a more detailed discussion of omphalectomy (surgical excision of the yolk sac). These birds will require intensive care in the form of subcutaneously administered and oral fluids, antimicrobials and nutritional support (see Chapter 8). The inguinal fold is a preferred site for subcutaneous administration of fluids although only small volumes can be given by this route.

Infection of the yolk sac within the abdomen most commonly occurs due to temperature variations during incubation. Inflammation of the naval may occur with poor incubation hygiene or with bacterial contamination of the egg. Usually *E. coli* or staphylococci are the causal organisms. Immediate disinfection of the naval after hatching using povidone–iodine solution is recommended. An infected naval appears inflamed, progressing to a large reddened area on the abdomen. Within hours it can develop a blue/green colour as the infection involves the

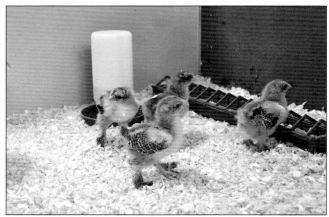

17.13 Chick feeders and drinkers are preferred to open dishes, which are easily contaminated by faecal material.
(Courtesy of Andy Cawthray of ChickenStreet)

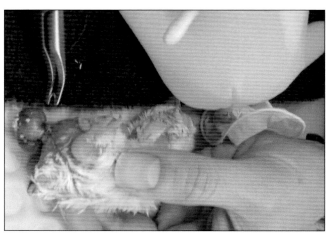

17.14 Application of haemostatic clip to an unretracted yolk sac prior to removal in a newly hatched chick.

retracted yolk sac and then liver, progressing to a fatal septicaemia. Aggressive fluid and nutritional support and antibiotic therapy is indicated in such cases but even with early recognition and therapy prognosis is poor.

Developmental abnormalities

Deformities of the extremities may be genetic, or related to incubation technique or infection.

Crooked or bent toes

Crooked toes sometimes occur at the time of hatching (see Chapter 18). For a successful outcome it is important to initiate treatment as soon as possible. Delaying treatment for a few days will result in irreversible joint deformities. Treatment involves straightening the toe and applying a tape splint, which only needs to be left in place for 5–7 days.

Splay leg

Many theories are put forward as potential causes of splay leg (Figure 17.15a), including suboptimal nutrition, hyperthermia or inappropriate substrate (e.g. newspaper or another slippery surface). It may also occur in chicks struggling to get around with a number of crooked toes (see above). Treatment involves a 'hobble brace'. It can be made from plaster tape or from a small rubber band with a knot tied in the centre (Figure 17.15b). It must be fitted snug enough to prevent splaying whilst allowing the chick to walk. The response to treatment is good if treatment is initiated early; most only require a brace for up to 48 hours. If there is no improvement in 48 hours, then the prognosis is poor.

Curled toes, tarsometatarsal shortening and hock osteodystrophy

These conditions have been described in association with *Mycoplasma* infection in chicks and turkey poults (see Chapter 18).

Angel wing

See Chapter 24.

Enteritis

Infectious enteritis in chicks can be caused by a number of infectious aetiologies including *Salmonella*, *Escherichia coli*, rotavirus and coccidiosis with suboptimal hygiene (incubator and/or housing) and overcrowding being possible predisposing factors. For further details on diagnosis and management see Chapter 16. Rectal prolapse may arise secondary to chronic intestinal inflammation and may be managed by gently lubricating and replacing prolapsed tissue whilst addressing the primary cause.

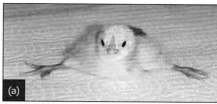
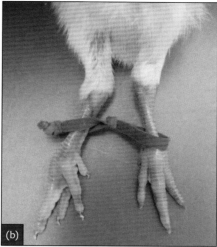

17.15 (a, b) Splay leg in chicks can be addressed using a rubber band 'hobble' as shown.
(Courtesy of John Squire)

References and further reading

De Matos R (2013) Investigation of the chemopreventative effects of deslorelin in domestic chickens with high prevalence of ovarian cancer. *Proceedings of the 1st International Conference on Avian, Herpetological and Exotic Mammal Medicine*, p. 90. Wiesbaden, Germany, April 20–26, 2013

Joyner KL (1997) Theriogenology. In: *Avian Medicine Principles and Applications*, ed. BW Ritchie, GJ Harrison and LR Harrison, pp. 748–804. Wingers Publishing Inc., Lake Worth, Florida

Keller KA, Beaufrere H, Brandao J *et al.* (2013) Long-term management of ovarian neoplasia in two cockatiels. *Proceedings of the 1st International Conference on Avian, Herpetological and Exotic Mammal Medicine*, p. 302. Wiesbaden, Germany April 20–26, 2013

King AS and McLelland J (1984) *Birds: Their Structure and Function*. Bailiere Tindall, Eastbourne

Roberts V (2009) *Diseases of Free Range Poultry*, 3rd edn. Whittet Books Ltd, Cambs

Straub J and Zenker I (2013) First experience in hormonal treatment of sertoli cell tumors in budgerigars (*M. undulates*) with absorbable extended release GnRH chips (Suprelorin®). *Proceedings of the 1st International Conference on Avian, Herpetological and Exotic Mammal Medicine*, pp. 299–301. Wiesbaden, Germany, April 20–26, 2013

Ubuka T and Bentley GE (2011) Neuroendocrine control of reproduction in birds. In: *Hormones and Reproduction of Vertebrates*, ed. D Norris and KH Lopez, pp. 1–25. Academic Press, Cambridge, Massachusetts

Vegad JL, Kolte GN and Shukla RR (1979) An ovarian condition with multiple cystic follicles in a hen. *Veterinary Record* **105**, 19

Wilson HR, Neuman SL, Eldred AR and Mather FB (2003) Embryonic malpositions in broiler chickens and bobwhite quail. *The Journal of Applied Poultry Research* **12**, 14–23

Chapter 18

Neurological and musculoskeletal disorders

Deborah Monks

Musculoskeletal and neurological diseases are extremely common in poultry and often cause similar signs. This chapter provides a synopsis of the common diseases encountered in veterinary practice (for basic problem-solving algorithms, see Appendix 1). Although there is a paucity of published information regarding the treatment of pet and small hobby poultry, referenced information regarding commercial birds has been extrapolated to provide the clinical tools for the poultry patients seen in general practice. Legislative guidelines regarding the medication of food-producing animals must still be followed.

Neurological diseases

Marek's disease

Epidemiology, aetiology and pathogenesis

Marek's disease, also known as polyneuritis, neurolymphomatosis, transient paralysis, acute leucosis, neural leucosis and grey eye, is a common and contagious condition of chickens. Pheasants, turkeys and quail can also be affected. Marek's disease is caused by a herpesvirus, which is very resistant in the environment, and infects chicks shortly after hatching. Vertical transmission does not occur. Several distinct syndromes have been recognized:

- Classic Marek's disease
- Acute Marek's disease
- Chronic Marek's disease
- Ocular lymphomatosis
- Cutaneous leucosis
- Transient paralysis.

The incubation period varies but can be as short as 8 days. The virus enters via the respiratory tract and then spreads to the lymphoid organs within 24–36 hours. B and T lymphocytes experience cytolytic infection, leading to transient or permanent immune suppression. Lymphoid and reticulum cell hyperplasia results in gross splenomegaly. The virus is also incorporated into the feather follicular epithelium, which is the only site of complete viral replication within the body. This occurs regardless of host immunity, viral strain or infection outcome.

If the host immune system can control the infection, the latent phase follows, in which the virus is present within lymphocytes but without tumour growth or cytolytic changes. Viral shedding continues indefinitely. Genetically resistant birds can maintain this phase permanently. In progressive infections, there may be a second cytolytic phase, which occurs in the lymphoid tissue aggregations around the body. The final, lymphoproliferative phase, in which tumours comprising neoplastic inflammatory and non-neoplastic immune cells develop, occurs in genetically susceptible or immunosuppressed birds. This can occur as early as 3 weeks following infection.

Clinical signs and post-mortem findings

- The clinical signs of the **classic form** include asymmetrical limb paralysis (Figure 18.1) and the development of pale visceral tumours, leading to depression, weight loss, pallor, diarrhoea, anorexia and death. At necropsy, the nerves are often swollen, discoloured and have lost their cross-striations. Subtle lesions can be detected by comparing contralateral structures. Nerves and tumours are found to contain neoplastic lymphocytes on histopathological examination. Dyspnoea and crop dilatation may be seen when the vagus nerve is involved.
- The **acute form** of the disease is characterized by death in young unvaccinated birds following 24–72 hours of depression and stupor.
- The **chronic form** of the disease can lead to immune suppression and worsening of current diseases due to lymphocyte impairment, bursa of Fabricius atrophy and thymic atrophy.

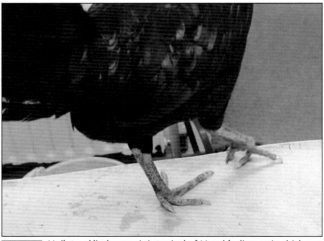

18.1 Unilateral limb paresis is typical of Marek's disease in chickens. (© J Chitty)

- With **ocular lymphomatosis**, lymphocytic infiltration of the iris leads to grey discoloration, pupillary irregularity and blindness.
- **Cutaneous leucosis** defines lymphocytic feather follicle infiltration. The end result of altered cholesterol metabolism can be atherosclerosis in some chickens.
- **Transient paralysis** is a non-neoplastic syndrome caused by vasogenic cerebral oedema, and is associated with flaccid paralysis of the limbs or neck for 24–48 hours. Birds can recover but often go on to die from classic visceral tumours a number of weeks later. Some birds develop persistent neurological disease with tics and torticollis.

Differential diagnoses

The differential diagnoses for the neurological and musculoskeletal signs of Marek's disease are viral arthritis, avian encephalomyelitis, joint infections, rickets due to calcium or vitamin D deficiency, musculoskeletal trauma, riboflavin and thiamine deficiency and Newcastle disease. Reticuloendotheliosis (caused by a retrovirus) results in similar clinical signs, namely stunted growth, diarrhoea, leg weakness and visceral tumours. The retrovirus can be a contaminant of Marek's vaccines, but can also be transmitted horizontally.

Laboratory diagnosis, treatment and prognosis

A presumptive diagnosis can be made on histopathology, using samples obtained from characteristic lesions. In some countries, feather or leucocyte polymerase chain reaction (PCR) tests are available, but the PCR needs to be specifically designed to differentiate vaccine-derived virus from wild-type (Nair, 2018). There is no effective treatment for this disease, and the prognosis is grave. In recovered transient paralysis cases, birds often relapse with the classic form of the disease at a later date.

Prevention

The only effective means of disease control is vaccination, which must take place before or just after hatching as early immunity is vital. Commercial birds are often vaccinated, into the egg, in automated systems on day 18 of incubation. Although the virus is inactivated by a number of disinfectants, complete environmental decontamination is unrealistic as the virus can persist for several months. In contaminated litter and a temperature of 4°C, viral persistence can last for years. Vaccinated birds can still shed virus into the environment (Nair, 2018).

Newcastle disease

Epidemiology, aetiology and pathogenesis

Newcastle disease rarely occurs in backyard poultry, but is of tremendous economic and commercial significance to the poultry industry. It is a notifiable disease in many countries, including the UK, and it is a legislative requirement to report any suspicious cases to the appropriate governmental agency.

Newcastle disease is caused by a paramyxovirus and is associated with respiratory, neurological and gastrointestinal signs. There is a high mortality rate. Chickens are the most susceptible species, although ducks, geese and wild waterfowl can harbour infection. Spread of the virus occurs via movement of wild birds, fomites or via windborne spread of infectious litter and debris. Although the virus can be found in eggs, affected hens usually cease egg production and vertical transmission is not common.

Epidemics can occur via the spread of virulent virus by wild birds, especially waterfowl. In countries with endemic avirulent or lentogenic strains, wild strains can mutate to virulence. The virus enters the body via ingestion or inhalation and replicates at the site of introduction during the incubation period, which lasts 2–15 days. Viraemia only occurs with velogenic and mesogenic viruses, and replication begins in other organs. Lentogenic viruses multiply on epithelial surfaces. A second viraemia follows and the virus begins to be excreted from both the respiratory and gastrointestinal tracts.

Clinical signs and post-mortem findings

Avirulent infections cause no noticeable clinical signs, whereas lentogenic strains cause subclinical or mild respiratory signs. Respiratory signs predominate with mesogenic infection, which has a low mortality rate. Velogenic strains are characterized by high mortality and are either viscerotropic (the bird shows gastrointestinal signs) or neurotropic (the bird shows respiratory and nervous signs).

There is usually a marked reduction in egg production. Young birds infected with velogenic, mesogenic and lentogenic strains show dyspnoea, tachypnoea, coughing, sneezing and cyanosis of swollen combs and wattles. Both viscerotropic and neurotropic velogenic strains cause muscle tremors, paralysis of the limbs, ataxia, circling, opisthotonus and torticollis. Birds surviving the viscerotropic form of the disease may have green or bloody diarrhoea, but mortality can approach 100%. Neurotropic forms tend to have lower mortality without diarrhoea.

In peracute cases, gross lesions may be absent at necropsy. With neurotropic infection, the trachea will have severe haemorrhagic inflammation but the presence of free luminal blood is rare. In viscerotropic cases, there may be marked cervical oedema with haemorrhage in the trachea, proventriculus and gizzard, as well as in other focal intestinal lymphoid tissues (e.g. Peyer's patches and caecal tonsils). Lesions progress to become ulcerative over time. Generalized petechial haemorrhage may be seen on the serosal surfaces.

Differential diagnoses

The differential diagnoses for Newcastle disease include Marek's disease, avian influenza, acute fowl cholera, infectious laryngotracheitis, the diphtheritic form of fowlpox, coryza, avian encephalomyelitis virus and intoxications.

Laboratory diagnosis

Clinicians should collect serum, cloacal and tracheal swabs for submission to the appropriate governmental agency. Further information about the legal requirements in the UK in relation to Newcastle disease can be found on the Defra website.

Prevention

Good hygiene and biosecurity with protection from wild waterfowl is advisable. Although vaccinations are available, they provide short-term (10–12 week) immunity and are used only in the event of an outbreak and at the behest of the government. Newcastle disease virus is highly susceptible to lipid-containing detergents.

Equine viral encephalitis

Outbreaks of equine viral encephalitis have mainly been recorded in pheasants, although turkeys, ducks and partridges have also been affected. Chickens are experimentally susceptible. This disease is notifiable, although no infections have ever been diagnosed in the UK. The disease is maintained in native reservoirs (often birds) and spread by biting insects, although transfer can occur within a flock via open skin lesions due to conspecific aggression. After entry, the virus multiplies locally and then becomes viraemic. Multiplication occurs in target organs, followed by a secondary viraemia. Target organs vary according to the virus, but can include the central nervous system, liver and the gastrointestinal tract.

Clinical signs vary and include depression, severe enteritis, leg paralysis, torticollis, tremors and mortality of up to 100% in pheasants. Young chickens show depression, paralysis and high mortality, although the main lesion is myocarditis. Surviving birds may show ascites and right ventricular failure. Differential diagnoses include Newcastle disease, avian influenza, avian encephalomyelitis, paramyxovirus 3, turkey coronavirus and turkey rhinotracheitis virus. If equine viral encephalitis is suspected, governmental guidelines regarding diagnostic testing of blood and brain tissue samples should be followed. There is no treatment.

Avian encephalomyelitis

This disease, often called epidemic tremor, is caused by a hepatovirus, family picornavirus. It causes ataxia and tremors in chickens, pheasants and turkeys less than 3 weeks of age. Older birds rarely show clinical neurological signs, although a reduction in egg production and hatchability may be seen. The virus can be transmitted both horizontally and vertically. With horizontal transmission, the virus is ingested and initially multiplies in the intestine, before causing a viraemia and spreading to the central nervous system. The incubation period is at least 11 days. With vertical transmission, signs occur within the first week following hatching. The virus is quite environmentally resistant and is shed for up to 2 weeks post infection.

Surviving birds may have ocular changes, including buphthalmos, lens opacities and pupillary paralysis, as well as permanent neurological impairment. At necropsy, white lymphocytic infiltration of the ventricular muscles may be the only gross sign. Disseminated non-purulent encephalomyelitis and ganglioneuritis may be seen microscopically. There is never peripheral nervous system pathology. Differential diagnoses include Newcastle disease, equine viral encephalitis, rickets, vitamin deficiencies (vitamins A, B2 and E), toxicities and *Dactylaria* infection. Diagnosis is via histopathology, serology and, occasionally, isolation. There is no treatment. The commercial poultry industry controls this disease by vaccinating breeding stock, to generate maternal antibodies in the chicks.

Enterococcus

Enterococcus species are Gram-positive facultative anaerobic cocci and generally cause two distinct clinical syndromes in chickens and turkeys.

- The **acute, septicaemic syndrome** is associated with lethargy, depression, diarrhoea, fine head tremors, a reduction or cessation in egg production, and pale combs and wattles (Figure 18.2). Fibrinous pericarditis, perihepatitis and air sacculitis may also be seen.
- The **chronic form** is associated with head tremors, lameness, depression and weight loss.

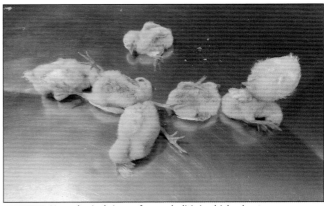

18.2 Neurological signs of encephalitis in chicks due to *Enterococcus* infection.
(© Professor Amir Noormohammadi, University of Melbourne)

The main differential diagnoses are other bacteria that cause septicaemia, including *Escherichia coli*, *Salmonella*, *Staphylococcus*, erysipelas and fowl cholera. The diagnosis is confirmed by demonstrating the presence of the bacterium in affected tissues. Antibiotics are likely to be useful early in the disease course, but resistance can occur. Penicillin, tetracyclines, erythromycin and nitrofurans can be used, although culture and sensitivity testing is advisable.

Botulism

Botulism, also known as limber neck and Western duck sickness, is caused by the toxin produced by *Clostridium botulinum*. The toxin causes ascending flaccid paralysis in waterfowl, chickens, turkeys and pheasants. Droopy wings, neck and eyelids are common as the disease progresses, and death results from respiratory and cardiac failure. *C. botulinum* is a spore-forming, Gram-positive, anaerobic bacterium that produces a range of exotoxins, which block nerve impulses at the peripheral cholinergic nerve receptors. It is present in the gastrointestinal tract of many bird species. It was thought that preformed toxin was ingested, after being concentrated by maggots feeding on decaying bird carcasses or multiplying in the gut of aquatic crustaceans that had died under conditions of oxygen depletion, which correlates with epidemiological findings that outbreaks tend to occur in stagnant or poorly oxygenated water bodies during warm weather. Recent work implies that clinical intoxication can also occur from absorption of toxin produced within the gastrointestinal tract (toxico-infection). The incubation period ranges from hours to 2 days, depending on the dose of toxin.

Differential diagnoses in mild cases include Marek's disease, intoxication from other sources and spinal or other musculoskeletal problems. In waterfowl with more severe signs, fowl cholera, lead poisoning and other poisons need to be considered. The diagnosis is made on clinical suspicion without any gross or microscopic lesions, and confirmed with a mouse bioassay and serum from the affected animals. Treatment is supportive (see Chapter 8) and aspiration pneumonia must be avoided. Antibiotics may be used to reduce further toxico-infection and specific antitoxins can be used. Prevention is by regular removal of carcasses and contaminated litter, aeration of water bodies (in the case of waterfowl), control of flies to reduce the number of maggots.

Anatipestifer disease

Anatipestifer disease, also known as pasteurellosis, new duck disease, duck septicaemia, goose influenza and infectious serositis, is caused by the Gram-negative bacterium *Riemerella anatipestifer* (previously called *Pasteurella* and *Moraxella*). Primarily a septicaemic disease of domestic ducks and geese, it has previously caused problems in domestic turkeys as well. Infection is via inhalation and through open skin wounds. There are some reports of transmission via biting arthropods. It can also be transmitted by faecal contamination of the environment. The incubation period is 2–5 days. Mortality is 5–75% in young animals.

Clinical signs include head and neck tremors, lethargy, ataxia, reluctance to walk, dyspnoea, incoordination, oculonasal discharge, green diarrhoea and hyperexcitability. Survivors can be stunted. A generalized fibrinous serositis is noted on necropsy, with occasional meningitis, purulent synovitis or arthritis. Differential diagnoses include any cause of bacterial arthritis or septicaemia, such as duck viral enteritis, duck viral hepatitis, fowl cholera, chlamydiosis and coccidiosis. The diagnosis is confirmed by identification of the organism along with characteristic lesions. Appropriate antibiotics include sulpha drugs, enrofloxacin, penicillins, lincomycin and spectinomycin. Prevention is best achieved with good biosecurity and hygiene. Vaccination is also possible.

Dactylariosis

This is a rare fungal disease caused by *Dactylaria*, which leads to encephalitis in young turkeys and chickens. It can occur in epidemic proportions and is spread via environmental contamination; litter is a common fomite. Clinical signs include loss of balance, incoordination, tremors, torticollis, paralysis and death. At necropsy, there are cerebellar and cerebral lesions, possibly in association with pulmonary granulomas. Diagnosis is via histopathology and fungal culture. Treatment has not been documented, but systemic antifungal medication could be tried. Control is via hygiene and removal of contaminated litter.

Mycotoxicosis

Certain fungal species produce toxins, which may or may not be associated with visible mould production. These toxins are ingested, usually from feed, and a variety of clinical signs can result (Figures 18.3 and 18.4). Disease can be subtle and clinical signs are not pathognomonic. All poultry are susceptible, although the degree of susceptibility varies. The list of differential diagnoses is extensive. A presumptive diagnosis is made on the basis of the clinical signs and history, although histopathology may be useful. A definitive diagnosis involves the identification of the toxin in the feed, which can be difficult. Removal of the source of the toxin is the most appropriate treatment and antifungal medication is not helpful after intoxication has occurred. Improved husbandry to reduce concurrent immunosuppression and exposure to other diseases assists in reducing disease.

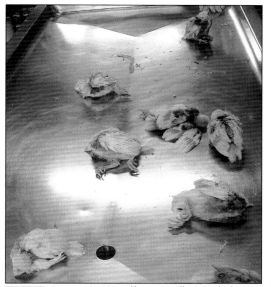

18.4 Mycotoxicosis and/or aspergillosis in chicks. Note the similar presentation to chicks with *Enterococcus* infection (see Figure 18.2). A post-mortem examination and histopathology are often required to differentiate the aetiology.
(© Professor Amir Noormohammadi, University of Melbourne)

Mycotoxin	Source	Signs
Fusarochromanone	*Fusarium* spp.	One particular species can be involved with tibial dyschondroplasia; can also be immunosuppressive
Fusaric acid and fusarocin	*Fusarium verticillioides*	Thiamine deficiency (which can manifest as neurological signs)
Ergotism	*Claviceps* spp. on cereal grains	Signs depend on which species of *Claviceps*; vesicular dermatitis of the head; necrosis of the beak, comb and toes; reduced feed intake; diarrhoea; reduced growth rate; poor feathering; loss of coordination; inability to stand; nervousness (triticale ergot only)
Fumonisins	*Fusarium verticillioides*	Black adherent diarrhoea; reduced feed intake and growth rate; reduced egg production; lameness; increased mortality
Trichothecenes	Common soil and plant fungi	Caustic and radiomimetic effects; necrosis of the oral mucosa and skin; reduced growth; bloody diarrhoea and gastrointestinal haemorrhage; haemorrhage; non-specific nervous signs; hepatonecrosis and haemorrhage; decreased bone marrow and immune function
Moniliformin	*Fusarium verticillioides* and other spp.	Cardiotoxic; nephrotoxic; haemorrhage; may resemble spiking mortality of broilers when in conjunction with other toxins
Zearalenone	*Gibberella zeae*	Oestrogenic activity; reduction in egg production with normal fertility and hatchability
Aflatoxin	*Aspergillus* spp.	Carcinogenic; hepatotoxic (reduced growth, inappetence, depression); may show nervous signs, including ataxia, convulsions and opisthotonus terminally
Ochratoxins, citrinin and oosporein	*Penicillium* spp., *Aspergillus* spp. and *Chaetomium* spp.	Nephrotoxic (polyuria, gout, death)

18.3 Mycotoxins and their associated clinical signs.

Hexamitiasis

Hexamitiasis is caused by the protozoan parasite *Hexamita meleagridis* and leads to catarrhal enteritis in young turkey poults. Affected birds can have terminal convulsions with coma. The diagnosis is usually confirmed by demonstrating the presence of the organism in samples of watery diarrhoea. There is no registered effective treatment.

Spiking mortality of chickens

This is a condition in which young broiler chickens show acute mortality after exhibiting neurological signs of tremor, paralysis and coma. Typically seen in 1–2 week old birds in good body condition, it is thought to be caused by a combination of altered food intake, a physical stressor and, possibly, a virus. Affected birds may be dehydrated with mild enteritis and mucoid droppings. Hypoglycaemia is present. The diagnosis is made via the characteristic signalment, signs and necropsy lesions. Treatment involves minimizing stressors and supplementing the flock with electrolytes and glucose. Prevention hinges around the avoidance of physical stressors, avoidance of breaches in food supply and avoidance of breaches in hygiene.

Bone, cartilage and joint diseases

Viral arthritis

Viral arthritis is a debilitating disease caused by an avian reovirus. There are different strains causing different syndromes. It occurs mainly in chickens, although turkeys may also show signs. The virus is mainly transmitted horizontally and is shed from the intestinal and respiratory tracts of affected animals. Ingestion or inhalation of the virus results in primary local multiplication, followed by viraemia and secondary multiplication in other organs. Entry through broken skin of the feet is possible. The incubation period varies but is at least 1 day. The virus is shed for prolonged periods of time and is quite hardy within the environment. Clinical signs include lameness, stunted growth and swelling of the hock joint, gastrocnemius tendon and digital flexor tendons. The gastrocnemius tendon may rupture. Serous, sanguineous or purulent joint effusions may be seen, as well as tendon sheath pathology, damage to the articular cartilage and an enlarged proximal metatarsal diaphysis. There is usually concurrent myocarditis present.

The differential diagnosis includes bacterial arthritis (*Mycoplasma synoviae*, *Staphylococcus*, *Salmonella*, *Riemerella anatipestifer* and other bacteria). Diagnosis rests on suggestive clinical signs and lesions, although virus isolation, reverse transcription polymerase chain reaction (RT-PCR) or serology may be helpful. Given the frequency with which reoviruses are seen in poultry, simple demonstration of the presence of the organism is not sufficient for a diagnosis. Commercially, affected individuals are euthanased and preventive measures (including vaccination) instituted. Protection is required at day 1 post hatch, so breeding hens are vaccinated in order to provide maternal antibodies to the chick. It is unlikely that non-commercial birds will be vaccinated; therefore, quarantine of young birds from contaminated environments is suggested. There is an age-related resistance to disease, beginning after 2 weeks, so protection of young birds until this time is advisable.

Bacterial arthritis

There are a number of bacteria that can cause joint or peri-articular infections. These usually occur secondary to septicaemic events. Differential diagnoses include viral arthritis, trauma or any of the pathogenic bacteria described below. Atypical or unusual bacterial infections of the soft tissue can also occur. When treating bacterial arthritis, antibiosis should ideally be based on culture and sensitivity testing. Effective treatment should include analgesia; non-steroidal anti-inflammatory drugs (NSAIDs) are a good choice for this purpose.

Staphylococcal arthritis

Staphylococcus aureus (and some other *Staphylococcus* species) is a common poultry pathogen and is very resistant in the environment. The bacteria enter the body through compromised epithelial or mucosal surfaces. Subsequent bacteraemia allows the bacteria to lodge in the joints and bones, leading to arthritis, peri-arthritis, synovitis and osteomyelitis. Predilection sites include the proximal tibiotarsus and femur, and there may be femoral head necrosis. The minimum incubation period is 48–72 hours. Clinical signs of bacterial arthritis include lameness, reluctance to walk, drooping of wings, ataxia and swollen joints. Laboratory diagnosis is via the demonstration of Gram-positive dividing cocci on joint tap cytology or positive growth on bacterial culture. Appropriate antibiotics include penicillins, tetracyclines, sulphonamides, lincomycin and spectinomycin. Preventive strategies include reducing trauma (no overstocking of birds, good flooring and safe equipment), reducing immunosuppression from stress and concurrent diseases, and improving hygiene to reduce bacterial load.

Mycoplasmosis

Mycoplasma spp. are small bacteria lacking a cell wall that cause a range of respiratory, reproductive and musculoskeletal problems in poultry. (The section below covers only those organisms that cause musculoskeletal problems.) Commercially, specific pathogen-free breeding flocks are created via antibiotic treatment of eggs.

Mycoplasma meleagridis: This is a specific pathogen of turkeys and is the cause of 'crooked neck'. *M. meleagridis* is antigenically different to other avian *Mycoplasma* spp. Although the main clinical sign is a low level air sacculitis, vertical transmission can result in tarsometatarsal chondrodystrophy (see Figure 18.6), hock swelling, sternal bursitis and synovitis, cervical vertebral deformity and stunted growth. Horizontal transmission is via aerosol, although fomites can be important. Tylosin is often used to control the clinical signs, whilst lincomycin and spectinomycin have been shown to be effective in water. However, it should be remembered that bony or cartilaginous pathology may persist past resolution of the bacterial infection.

Mycoplasma synoviae: Most commonly seen as a relatively low level upper respiratory tract infection, this species of *Mycoplasma* can cause infectious synovitis in chickens and turkeys. Ducks, geese, guinea fowl and pheasants can also be infected. The bacteria enter the body via the respiratory tract, but may subsequently become systemic. Vertical transmission is important. The incubation period is usually 11–21 days. Clinical signs include a pale comb, emaciation, leg weakness, sternal bursal enlargement, enlarged footpads and hock joints with swollen synovial membranes and tendon sheaths, and hepatosplenomegaly with concurrent renomegaly. In chronic infections, chondrodystrophy, stunted growth and damage to the articular surfaces can be seen. A presumptive diagnosis can be made of the basis of the clinical signs. The diagnosis is confirmed by isolation of the organism from infected fluid or tissues (this is much more sensitive in acute infections). Fluorescent antibody staining, PCR (more sensitive) and serology can also be used to confirm the diagnosis. Antibiotics can be used for individual cases, although there is some resistance to erythromycin.

Mycoplasma iowae: This *Mycoplasma* species is also specific to turkeys and can cause acute tenosynovitis. Mainly seen after experimental inoculation, haemorrhage, swelling, tendon fibre degeneration and fibrosis have been recorded. Vertical transmission usually results in egg death. Horizontal transmission is possible but not rapid.

Other bacteria

Many bacteria that cause septicaemia lead to arthritis and osteomyelitis as sequellae. *Escherichia coli* can cause arthritis and synovitis in conjunction with other clinical signs including air sacculitis, pericarditis, perihepatitis, hepatosplenomegaly with granulomas, peritonitis, enteritis, cellulitis, salpingitis and omphalitis in young birds. The incubation period is 3–5 days.

Fowl cholera, caused by *Pasteurella multocida*, is a significant disease leading to multiple syndromes in a number of bird species, including waterfowl, turkeys and chickens. Infection is via the oronasal route and the incubation period is usually 5–8 days. The bacterium is not very resistant to disinfection but can persist in soil. Other animals may also act as reservoirs. Clinical signs range from those of acute septicaemia (depression, anorexia, cyanotic and swollen face and wattles, sudden death) to diarrhoea, oculonasal discharge and coughing. Lameness and purulent arthritis with swollen joints can also occur. The diagnosis is confirmed by the demonstration of morphologically consistent Gram-negative bacteria on impression smears, cytological aspirates and bacterial culture. Sulphonamides, tetracyclines, penicillins, erythromycin and streptomycin have all been used to control the clinical signs, although relapse is common. Prevention is via good hygiene and biosecurity. Vaccination has also been used.

Infections with *Salmonella* spp. (particularly *S. pullorum* and *S. gallinarum*) in chickens and turkeys can cause blindness and arthritis. There is a predilection for the stifle and elbow, and some strains of *Salmonella* may exhibit tropism for these areas. Treatment with antibiotics may be helpful, but birds remain carriers (see Chapter 16 for further details).

Chronic infections with *Enterococcus* spp. can also result in fibrinous arthritis or tenosynovitis and osteomyelitis, as well as necrotic myocarditis, valvular endocarditis, and fibrinous perihepatitis and pericarditis. *Enterococcus cecorum*, in particular, has been associated with vertebral abscesses and arthritis (Dolka *et al.*, 2017).

Dyschondroplasia

Although often called tibial dyschondroplasia due to the predilection for the proximal tibiotarsus, this condition also occurs in the femur, tarsometatarsus and proximal humerus. Clinically, an abnormal mass is encountered below the growth plate, which corresponds to a core of persistent pre-hypertrophic cartilage that has neither matured nor ossified. The condition is exacerbated when there is a reduced calcium:phosphorus ratio, and has been variously associated with copper deficiencies, nutritional

deficiencies (including cysteine and homocysteine), certain antibiotics (zinc bacitracin and salinomycin) and some seeds (rapeseed, sorghum and soybeans). Recent research implicates the underlying pathophysiology as poor vascularization of the of the tibial growth plate cartilage (Huang *et al.*, 2018).

Many birds are asymptomatic, but others will show signs of lameness, stilted gait and bowing of the legs. When present in the proximal femur, the femoral head may be fractured or the femoral neck altered. Reducing the growth rate assists in reducing the incidence, as lesions are more severe in heavier birds. Fasting the birds overnight will reduce the flock incidence without necessarily reducing the growth rate. An inappropriately alkaline diet may worsen the signs (by reducing the calcium matrix within the bone). The differential diagnoses for disorders of the cartilage, growth plate and ossification include infectious synovitis, valgus/varus deformity, chondrodystrophy, rickets, infectious arthritis, ruptured ligaments and a rotated tibia. There is no medical treatment. Prevention is aimed at genetic selection, correct calcium, phosphorus and vitamin D supplementation, and ensuring that the acid–base balance within the diet is appropriate.

Chondrodystrophy

Whereas tibial dyschondroplasia manifests as a plug of unossified cartilage within the growth plate, birds with chondrodystrophy tend to manifest with short, widened leg bones. Distortion of the hock is also seen and may be accompanied by perosis (gastrocnemius tendon movement from the trochlear groove). This condition has been reported in chickens, ducks and turkeys, and may appear grossly similar to valgus/varus deformity. Chondrodystrophy has been associated with nutritional deficiencies in manganese, choline, zinc, pyridoxine, biotin, folic acid and niacin (Figure 18.5). In turkeys, there may also be a genetic deficiency in galactosamine production.

Nutrient	Results of deficiency
Biotin	See Figure 18.10
Calcium	A cartilaginous plug may form and resemble dyschondroplasia
Choline	Turkeys are especially sensitive to choline deficiency. Haemorrhage in joint, then swelling of hock; metatarsal rotation then slipped Achilles tendon; reduced growth rate
Folic acid	See Figure 18.10
Magnesium	Thickened bone cortex; often associated with severe hypocalcaemia; epiphyseal plate normal; reduced growth rate. Affected birds convulse when disturbed and may die from dyspnoea
Manganese	Often oedema; clinical signs of *in ovo* deficiency not resolved with post-hatch supplementation; reduced growth rate
Niacin	See Figure 18.10
Pantothenic acid	See Figure 18.10
Phosphorus	Often ascites (effects of rib malacia on respiration); death from right ventricular failure
Pyridoxine	See Figure 18.10
Vitamin D (rickets)	Shortening of mandible and maxilla; bending of long bones and fractures; reduced growth rate; poor feathering
Zinc	Increased haematocrit; reduced growth rate; poor feathering; dermatosis

18.5 Nutritional deficiencies involved in chondrodystrophy.

Clinically, lameness, hock swelling, slipping of the gastrocnemius tendon with a shallow trochlea, shortened or rotated bones (especially the tibiae) and shortened beaks (in embryos) may be seen (Figure 18.6). The differential diagnoses for disorders of cartilage, growth plate and ossification include infectious synovitis, dyschondroplasia, valgus/varus deformity, rickets, infectious arthritis, ruptured ligaments and a rotated tibia. The diagnosis is confirmed by examination of the gross lesions, histopathology and analysis of the food. Prevention is best achieved by feeding a balanced, nutritionally complete diet. However, it should be borne in mind that lesions may persist, even after the diet has been corrected. There is new research that suggests artificial incubation with diurnal lighting regime of 16 hours light:8 hours of darkness can reduce the incidence of growth plate related issues (van der Pol *et al.*, 2017).

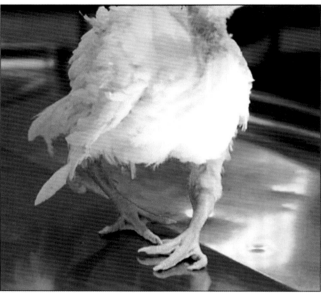

18.6 Chondrodystrophy in a turkey secondary to *Mycoplasma meleagridis* infection.
(© Professor Amir Noormohammadi, University of Melbourne)

Valgus/varus deformity

Birds with this condition present with twisted and crooked legs, along with long bone distortion, usually at <1 month old. The intertarsal joint is most commonly affected in chickens, whilst turkeys often have varus deformity of the stifle as well. The pathophysiology of this condition is obscure, although irregular vascular supply of the growth plate, delayed cortical bone differentiation and submicroscopic lesions due to nutritional deficiencies have been proposed. It is possible that valgus and varus deformities have different aetiologies.

Reducing the growth rate reduces the incidence, although this may be purely due to lower bodyweight, not improved bone ossification. The condition is worsened with reduced exercise and poor flooring. Valgus deformity is most common, often bilateral and chronic, and may be associated with displacement of the gastrocnemius tendon. The differential diagnoses for disorders of the cartilage, growth plate and ossification include infectious synovitis, dyschondroplasia, chondrodystrophy, rickets, infectious arthritis, ruptured ligaments and rotated tibia. Apart from corrective osteotomy in the individual bird, there is no treatment.

Osteochondrosis

This is a focal degenerative lesion of the growth plate and may be associated with trauma, mechanical forces or bacterial infection. This condition is rare in poultry. When seen, it often manifests as cervicothoracic vertebral malformation in broilers (which differs from the *Mycoplasma meleagridis* infection causing cervical osteochondrosis in turkeys), as well as changes in the femoral head and antitrochanter of broiler chickens and turkeys. There are rarely clinical signs.

Spondylolisthesis

This condition involves ventral dislocation of the fourth thoracic vertebra and causes posterior paralysis. Affected birds sit on their hocks with their feet raised, although they may become laterally recumbent. Diagnosis is via palpation, although radiography may assist in the individual bird. Flock control can be achieved by slowing the growth rate, either via feed restriction or genetic selection.

Spraddle legs

This condition is associated with high humidity during incubation and slippery flooring in the brooder after hatching. It causes the legs to splay laterally from the coxofemoral joint and may not manifest until 2–3 weeks of age, although it can be seen just after hatching. The differential diagnoses for disorders of the cartilage, growth plate and ossification include infectious synovitis, dyschondroplasia, valgus/varus deformity, chondrodystrophy, rickets, infectious arthrtitis, ruptured ligaments and rotated tibia. Treatment of advanced cases may be futile, but early treatment may be more successful (see Chapter 24). Early treatment involves improving the flooring and hobbling to keep the legs in a normal position as the bird grows.

Crooked neck

This condition is caused by cervical vertebral osteodystrophy as a result of *Mycoplasma meleagridis* infection. It is rarely seen today.

Rotated tibia

This condition, which is seen in turkeys, broiler chickens and guinea fowl, is poorly understood. It manifests as a rotational deformity of the tibiotarsus and can be unilateral or bilateral. The exact aetiology is uncertain, although genetics, nutritional and management factors may be involved. The main differential diagnosis is valgus/varus deformity. There is no sex predilection.

Bacterial chondronecrosis and femoral head necrosis

Although the terminal presentation of this syndrome involves osteomyelitis caused by a range of opportunistic bacteria, the initial lesion is one of avascular necrosis of the chondrocytes in the growth plates in broiler chickens. The disease is worsened by poor flooring, which increases the mechanical load on these areas. Concurrent immune suppression worsens the clinical severity of the disease, as do nutritional deficiencies leading to chondrodysplasia and poor bone quality. An initial bacteraemia is thought to allow bacterial seeding of growth plates and then infection becomes established. *Staphylococcus aureus* is most commonly involved, although *Escherichia coli*, other staphylococci and enterococci are seen less frequently.

Proximal femoral and tibiotarsal growth plates are most commonly involved, although the fourth thoracic vertebra may also be affected. When the leg is affected, reduced hip flexion, lameness and using wings as 'crutches' during ambulation may be seen. If the lesion involves the spinal column, leg paresis or paralysis may follow. The differential diagnoses include spinal trauma, synovitis, viral arthritis and spondylolisthesis. The diagnosis is based on the signs seen at necropsy (Figure 18.7), histopathology and isolation of the organism by culture. Lesions not grossly visible at necropsy may account for up to 60% of conditions. In a live bird, radiography may be more sensitive and culture of joint fluid may be attempted (although sensitivity may be poor). Should the condition be diagnosed in a live bird, judicious antibiotic usage may be initiated in order to sterilize the lesion, but the skeletal changes are likely to be progressive. Further treatment focuses on controlling inflammation and pain. Prevention is via hygiene (including fomites), by providing firm and stable flooring and by controlling the growth rates of heavy breeds. New research shows that artificial incubation incorporating a lighting regime of 16 hours light:8 hours of darkness reduced the incidence of bacterial chondronecrosis compared with a 24 hour lighting regimen (van der Pol *et al.*, 2017).

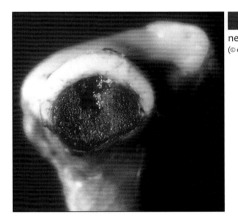

18.7 Femoral head necrosis.
(© of Shane Raidal)

Epiphysiolysis

The condition is usually seen incidentally at necropsy. Separation of the epiphysis mimics apparent dislocation or epiphyseal fracture. Predisposing conditions include chondrodystrophy, rickets, bacterial or viral arthritis, osteomyelitis (Figure 18.8) and trauma. Histopathology may help confirm the diagnosis. No treatment is required as this condition is normally only discovered on post-mortem examination.

Degenerative joint disease

This condition affects the coxofemoral, stifle and inter-tarsal joints of mainly adult male turkeys and broiler chickens, but may also be seen in the spine of laying hens. Erosion and thinning of the articular cartilage results in subchondral bone exposure, cartilage flaps, osteophytes and periarticular fibrosis. Pain and lameness are seen as a result. The pathogenesis is not completely clear, but excessive growth rates, physical trauma and other genetic factors may be involved. Commercially, there is no treatment and prevention is aimed at controlling growth rates

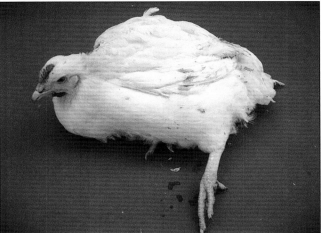

18.8 Hen with osteomyelitis. Without a thorough examination and potentially radiographs of the affected area, this condition cannot easily be differentiated from Marek's disease, viral arthritis, joint infections, rickets due to calcium or vitamin D deficiency, musculoskeletal trauma, riboflavin and thiamine deficiency, reticuloendotheliosis and Newcastle disease.
(© Professor Amir Noormohammadi, University of Melbourne)

and providing a safe environment. In pet birds, treatment is aimed at controlling pain and joint inflammation (NSAIDs will accomplish both) and providing an easily accessible environment.

Osteomyelitis complex of turkeys

This is a syndrome, diagnosed at necropsy, of young male turkeys, in which green discoloration of the liver is associated with arthritis, synovitis, abscessation and osteomyelitis (particularly of the proximal tibia). Many different bacteria are involved; however, the condition is thought to be due to failure of the bird's immune system rather than bacterial pathogenicity. In live birds, clinical signs can include lameness, depression and weight loss. Haematological assessment may show an inflammatory leucogram, and the physical examination and radiography may increase the index of suspicion for the disease. Judicious antibiotic use could be trialed in a pet bird. Supplementation of the diet with vitamin D3 reduced the incidence of the syndrome in an experimental model (Huff *et al.*, 2000). Prevention is aimed at ensuring optimal hygiene to reduce bacterial infection.

Osteoporosis

Osteoporosis (also known as cage layer fatigue) is a condition of decreased normal skeletal mineralization, usually secondary to insufficient weight-bearing activity. It is responsible for up to 30% of fractures in commercial poultry. Clinical signs include fractures of the ischium, humerus and keel, spinal fractures leading to paralysis, fractures of other bones and paresis caused by exposed spinal nerves from bone loss around the spinal column. At necropsy, thin bone cortices and parathyroid gland enlargement are seen. With the calcium demands of egg laying, there is continuous remodelling of medullary bone. In hens with heavy egg production, it seems that they start to metabolize structural as well as medullary bone in order to satisfy the calcium requirements. This eventually thins the bony cortices. Genetic selection for high egg production, poor nutrition and reduced weight-bearing exercise worsens the incidence. Good nutrition is not protective. Once the bird increases the amount of weight-bearing exercise (e.g. moving from a cage to free-range conditions), bone strength will improve by day 20. The best prevention is to provide ample exercise and a nutritionally balanced calcium replete diet, and to only select moderate egg producing birds as pets.

Spontaneous bone fractures

Spontaneous fractures are seen in laying hens secondary to osteoporosis, as well as in meat-type poultry. Fractures may be completely spontaneous or associated with handling or transportation. Poor bone quality due to lack of exercise, poor nutrition or excessive growth rates predisposes birds to spontaneous fractures. In addition, genetic selection for increased bodyweight with minimal corresponding skeletal weight may contribute to the incidence of these fractures. Commercially, there is no treatment. In pet birds, fractures may be surgically repaired, although a thorough assessment of the implant-holding ability of the adjacent bone may need to be undertaken. Prevention is by gentle handling of birds, providing a safe environment, controlling excessive growth rate and providing appropriate nutrition.

Angel wing

Angel wing, also known as flip wing, airplane wing, dropped wing, slipped wing or crooked wing, is most commonly seen in large waterfowl. It can be unilateral or bilateral. Affected birds have a valgus rotation of the carpal joint or metacarpal bones, giving dorsolateral rotation of the primary flight feathers when the wing is held at rest. A rapid growth rate seems to be the cause, with calcification of the bones lagging behind the weight-bearing requirements of the rapidly feathering distal wing. Diagnosis is via physical examination and early treatment by bandaging the wing into a normal position is usually curative (see Chapter 24 for further information). If possible, growth rates should be slowed.

Soft tissue disorders

Ligament failure and avulsion

Ligament failure and avulsion can be caused by trauma, in particular to the capital femoral ligament, and there is likely to be a genetic predisposition to this condition. Many other ligaments are also affected, including those in the intertarsal joint and the stifle. Grossly, stretching, rupture or avulsion can be seen. Older, heavier birds are more susceptible to the condition. In a live bird, the diagnosis is made following a physical examination, including range of movement palpation of the affected joints. Apart from gentle handling and a low impact environment, there is minimal prevention possible. Although the prognosis is poor, if only a single ligament is involved, surgery may be attempted. With multiple ligament involvement, the prognosis is hopeless.

Crooked toes

This condition manifests as shortening of the flexor tendons and there is the possibility of a heritable component. Poor flooring, brooding with infrared lighting, pyridoxine deficiency and some toxins will worsen the

condition. A differential diagnosis is riboflavin deficiency. For information on treatment, the reader is referred to Chapter 24.

Ruptured gastrocnemius tendon

This condition occurs in fast-growing heavy-bodied birds. The clinical signs of a ruptured gastrocnemius tendon include a dropped hock, inability to move and a palpable swelling in the tendon. Birds often sit on their hocks, with the toes pointing ventrally. Histopathologically, there may be inflammation due to viral arthritis or staphylococcal or other bacterial osteomyelitis or cellulitis. However, it can also be non-inflammatory and often occurs in the non-vascularized part of the tendon. Differential diagnoses include reovirus infection, *Staphylococcus* infection, spinal cord injury and tibial dyschondroplasia. Prevention is via good husbandry and avoiding high impact locomotion.

Bumblefoot

Bumblefoot, also known as pododermatitis, plantar dermatitis, contact dermatitis or plantar abscess, is a cause of significant concern in commercial poultry (Figure 18.9). Mainly seen in meat-type chickens and turkeys (as well as backyard poultry), wet litter is the predominant risk factor in the commercial industry. Leaking drinking vessels, high environmental humidity, poor ventilation and excessive stocking rates all worsen the litter moisture content, leading to an increase in lesions. Wood shaving substrates are least associated with problems. Heavier birds appear more susceptible to the condition. Genetics may play a role, although the challenge is to select for resistance to pododermatitis, whilst leaving bodyweight and growth rates relatively unaffected. Hock burns and breast blisters are associated with this condition. Dietary deficiencies in biotin, riboflavin, methionine and cysteine have been implicated in increasing the incidence of bumblefoot in commercial flocks.

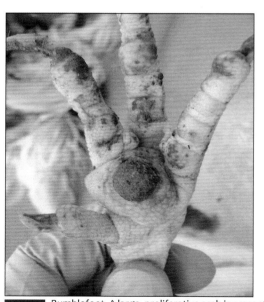

18.9 Bumblefoot. A large, proliferative scab is present centrally in the palmar aspect of the foot. There is surrounding swelling, and removal of the scab is likely to reveal a caseous core. If the tissue is very unhealthy, bleeding can be minimal, but as healing begins, debridement is likely to result in more bleeding. Bandaging is often required, to keep the lesion clean, to remove pressure from the healing tissue and to provide haemostasis.
(© Professor Amir Noormohammadi, University of Melbourne)

Once there is a breach in the integument, bacteria can enter and cause a range of infections, leading to cellulitis, tendonitis and osteomyelitis. Staphylococcal bacteria are often involved. A classification scheme for pododermatitis in raptors has been developed that provides veterinary surgeons (veterinarians) with a treatment plan and guide to prognosis. This classification scheme has been extended to other species with good results.

- **Class I lesions** carry a favourable prognosis, as there is no evidence of infection. The lesions generally respond to conservative husbandry changes, including altering perching surfaces or substrates, and the application of topical emollients (e.g. petroleum jelly). Emollients utilize fats and lipids to establish a protective barrier on the surface of the skin. This oily layer of lipids traps water in the stratum corneum (the outermost layer of the epidermis) and thus protects the skin.
- **Class II lesions** carry a good prognosis as infection is localized. Such lesions respond well to surgery, as the total affected area is easily resected and epidermal defects are characteristically small, and hence the architecture of the weight-bearing structures of the plantar aspect of the foot is maintained intact. This class of lesions will generally not respond to conservative treatment.
- **Class III lesions** traditionally carry a good to guarded prognosis as infection is well established and structural changes have affected the foot. Some can be treated as for Class II lesions; however, the majority should be treated by complete surgical removal of all affected tissue, followed by first intention healing.
- **Class IV lesions** carry a guarded to poor prognosis as infection is harboured in and affects deeper vital structures, making surgical debridement difficult or impossible. In view of the chronicity, pockets of encapsulated infective tissue are often present, which results in recurrence if not cleared.
- **Class V lesions** carry a poor to hopeless prognosis and may require euthanasia.

For information on medical treatment, see Chapter 13 and for the surgical approach, the reader is referred to Chapter 23.

Myopathies in meat-type chickens and turkeys

There are a number of myopathies seen in meat-type chickens and turkeys. Mainly discussed in terms of economic importance for meat quality and processing, these myopathies stem from localized muscle ischaemia from muscle growth outstripping vascular supply. As such, these are likely to be painful and constitute a welfare problem, as well as an economic one.

The most well known of these is Oregon disease, also known as green muscle disease and deep pectoral myopathy, is a syndrome of ischaemic necrosis of the deep pectoral muscles in meat-type chickens and turkeys. Clinical signs include swollen, pale, deep pectoral muscle masses and facial oedema. As the lesions progress, necrosis leads to a green discoloration and finally to scarring or friable muscle. It is thought that swelling in the muscle after exercise leads to vascular infarction from blood vessel constriction caused by a limited ability of the overlying fascia to accommodate the swelling. There is no

treatment. Prevention focuses on reducing high impact pectoral limb activity and changing handling techniques. There may be merit in breeding for an improved pectoral blood vessel supply.

As growth rates of meat-type poultry continue to increase, other myopathies are being identified at slaughter. These include 'white striping', 'wooden breast' and 'spaghetti' meat (Maiorano, 2017). There is no treatment, and pre-mortem diagnosis is likely to be difficult.

Shaky leg syndrome

This is a condition affecting turkeys, which may be associated with tendon injury. Birds show signs of pain with shaking of the legs whilst standing or just after rising. The aetiology is unknown and there are no visible signs at necropsy. For pet birds, anti-inflammatory and/or analgesic drugs may be appropriate, if legislation permits. Prevention hinges on gentle handling and appropriate housing.

Nutritional disorders
Vitamin B deficiency

Figure 18.10 provides information on the results of B vitamin deficiencies (Figure 18.11) and the response of birds to supplementation.

Calcium tetany

Whereas chronic calcium deficiency causes skeletal problems, an acute deficiency presents differently. Mainly seen in broiler breeds, clinical signs include lethargy, tremors, paralysis and death from cardiorespiratory failure. Diagnosis is made on clinical signs, ionized serum calcium levels, lack of other lesions and response to treatment. Treatment is supplementation with calcium and vitamin D. Prevention is best achieved via good nutrition and avoiding excessive supplementation (see also Chapter 20).

Vitamin E deficiency

There are three main syndromes that are seen with vitamin E deficiency:

- **Encephalomalacia** causes ataxia, paresis (but not paralysis), contraction and relaxation of the legs, and retraction (and sometimes lateral rotation) of the head (Figure 18.12). It is usually seen between days 15 and 30 following hatching. Chickens tend to show evidence of encephalomalacia, whilst turkey poults show lesions of poliomyelomalacia
- **Exudative diathesis** or subcutaneous oedema is seen in association with selenium deficiency. Lesions are associated with abnormal capillary permeability and an abnormal stance may be seen due to fluid pooling between the pelvic limbs
- **Muscular dystrophy** is seen in older birds when vitamin E deficiency occurs in conjunction with sulphur amino acid deficiencies. Grossly, white streaks in the muscle are seen (Figure 18.13). Chickens and turkeys may show particularly severe lesions in the ventriculus and myocardium.

The diagnosis of these three conditions is via clinical signs, histopathological lesions and response to medication.

Nutrient	Results of deficiency	Response to supplementation
Thiamine (vitamin B1; see Figure 18.11)	Anorexia; weight loss; leg weakness; unsteady gait; blue comb in adults; stargazing posture due to anterior neck muscle paralysis; toe flexors and leg extensors fixed	Respond in a few hours to injectable supplementation; response is diagnostic
Riboflavin (vitamin B2)	Slow growth rate; weak, emaciated with good appetite; diarrhoea; curled toes; may walk on hocks; leg paralysis; wings droop; dry harsh skin; show myelin degeneration of sciatic and brachial nerves; turkey poults have dermatitis of shanks and feet, and crusting of oral commissures	Good response if early stages; when chronic, improvement of curled toe deformity is unlikely; treatment: two 100 µg doses followed by restoration of adequate nutrition
Nicotinic acid (niacin, vitamin B3)	Chondrodystrophy (enlargement of hock joint) in chicks, ducklings and poults; Achilles tendon rarely slips from condyles; oral inflammation; poor feathering; diarrhoea	Supplementation pointless in advanced cases; avoid excess as decreased bone cortex thickness and strength
Pantothenic acid (vitamin B5)	Similar to biotin deficiency; dermatosis; broken feathers; chondrodystrophy; poor growth and emaciation; hypertrophied liver with atrophic spleen; viscous ocular exudate; death; in embryo, subcutaneous oedema and haemorrhage	Reversible if not too advanced by oral or injectable supplementation
Pyridoxine (vitamin B6)	Depressed appetite; poor growth; chondrodystrophy; jerky, nervous movements when walking; often have convulsions leading to death	Cause deficiency in collagen fibres and lead to osteoarthritis and chondrodystrophy
Biotin (vitamin B7)	Chondrodystrophic with parrot beak; reduced size; crooked tibia; shortened/twisted tarsometatarsus; associated with fatty liver and kidney syndrome; may be involved with sudden death syndrome; dermatosis around feet and beak/eyes	Supplementation will prevent clinical signs
Folic acid (vitamin B9)	Poor growth; extremely poor feathering; anaemia; chondrodystrophy; feather depigmentation; increased embryonic mortality	After single intramuscular injection, haematology and growth rate back to normal within 1 week
Cobalamin (vitamin B12)	No specific signs but slow growth, mortality and reduced egg size and hatchability	Single intramuscular injection improves hatchability within 1 week

18.10 Vitamin B deficiency syndromes.

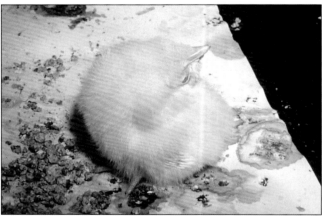

18.11 Classic stance of a chick with thiamine deficiency.
(© Professor Amir Noormohammadi, University of Melbourne)

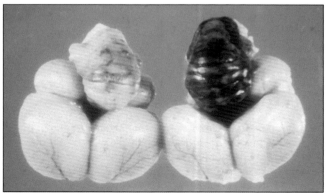

18.12 Brains of chickens with vitamin E deficiency.
(© Shane Raidal)

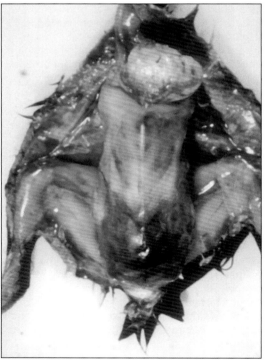

18.13 White muscle disease as a result of vitamin E deficiency.
(© Shane Raidal)

If vitamin E and selenium are supplied early in the course of the disease, exudative diathesis and muscular dystrophy should be reversible. The response of birds with encephalomalacia will vary. Differential diagnoses include encephalomyelitis, toxicities and other nutritional deficiencies. Further information on these conditions can be found in Chapter 20.

References and further reading

Animal Health Australia (2014) *Disease strategy: Newcastle disease (version 3.3)*. Animal Health Australia, Canberra

Berg C (1998) *Foot-pad dermatitis in broilers and turkeys*. Doctoral dissertation. Department of Animal Environment. Available at: http://pub.epsilon.slu. se/1514/1/Lotta_Berg_Avhandling.pdf

Dolka B, Chrobak-Chmiel D, Czopowicz M and Szeleszczuk P (2017) Characterization of pathogenic *Enterococcus cecorum* from different poultry groups: Broiler chickens, layers, turkeys, and waterfowl. PLoS ONE **12**:e0185199

Huang S, Rehman MU, Qiu G *et al*. (2018) Tibial dyschondroplasia is closely related to suppression of expression of hypoxia-inducible factors 1α, 2α, and 3α in chickens. *Journal of Veterinary Science* **19**, 107–115

Huff GR, Huff WE, Rath NC and Balog JM (2000) Turkey osteomyelitis complex. *Poultry Science* **7**, 1050–1056

Ley DH, Marusak R, Vivas E, Barnes HJ and Fletcher O (2010) *Mycoplasma iowae* associated with chondrodystrophy in commercial turkeys. *Avian Pathology* **39(2)**, 87–93

Maiorano G (2017) Meat defects and emergent muscle myopathies in broiler chickens: implications for the modern poultry industry. *Scientific Annals of Polish Society of Animal Production* **13**, 43–51

McMullin P (2004) *A Pocket Guide to Poultry Health and Disease*. 5M Publishing, Sheffield

McNamee PT and Smyth JA (2000) Bacterial chondronecrosis with osteomyelitis ('femoral head necrosis') of broiler chickens: a review. *Avian Pathology* **29(4)**, 253–270

Muir WM and Aggrey SE (2003) *Poultry Genetics, Breeding and Biotechnology, 4th edn*. CABI Publishing, Wallingford, Oxon

Nair V (2018) Hot topics in avian pathology: Marek's disease. *Avian Pathology*, doi: 10.1080/03079457.2018.1484073

Olsen J (1994) Anseriformes. In: *Avian Medicine: Principles and Application*, ed. GHBW Ritchie, pp. 1237–1275. Wingers Publishing, Lake Worth, Florida

Ritchie B (1995) *Viruses: Function and Control*. Wingers Publishing, Lake Worth, Florida

Saif Y (2008) *Diseases of Poultry*. Blackwell Publishing Professional, Ames, Iowa

Shepherd EM and Fairchild BD (2010) Footpad dermatitis in poultry. *Poultry Science* **89(10)**, 2043–2051

Smith K (1997) Angel wing in captive reared waterfowl. *Journal of Wildlife Rehabilitation* **20**, 3–5

van der Pol CW, van Roovert-Reijrink IAM, Aalbers G, Kemp B and van den Brand H (2017) Incubation lighting schedules and their interaction with matched or mismatched post hatch lighting schedules: Effects on broiler bone development and leg health at slaughter age. *Research in Veterinary Science* **114**, 416–422

Wideman RF and Prisby RD (2012) Bone circulatory disturbances in the development of spontaneous bacterial chondronecrosis with osteomyelitis: a translational model for the pathogenesis of femoral head necrosis. *Frontiers in Endocrinology (Lausanne)* **3**, 183

Wise D (1975) Skeletal abnormalities in table poultry – a review. *Avian Pathology* **4**, 1–10

Useful website

Defra
www.gov.uk/guidance/newcastle-disease

Chapter 19

Behavioural disorders

John Chitty

The majority of behavioural problems do not represent actual disease, but rather the expression of normal behaviours (see Chapter 3) in what may be an altered or inappropriate place. In the majority of cases, it is a failure to understand the needs of the bird and its normal behaviours that leads to husbandry that is more likely to promote problematic behaviours. This is particularly the case in birds rescued from intensive laying situations where normal behaviours may not have been able to develop or previously learned behaviours are no longer appropriate.

The majority of behavioural problems can be prevented by:

- Provision of a large enclosure with:
  - Adequate foraging opportunity
  - Adequate grooming opportunity
  - Adequate feeding and watering space/stations and laying boxes
  - Protection from the actual and perceived incursion of potential predators
- Establishing the correct social structure for each species (see Chapter 3)
- Correct means of introducing new individuals
- Establishing a daily routine and encouraging birds into night-time accommodation using positive reinforcement.

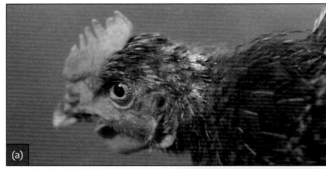

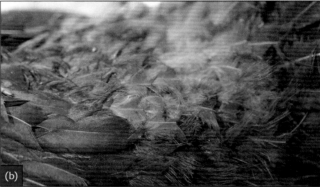

19.1 (a) New feather growth behind the head. (b) Broken feathers on the dorsum above the tail. In both cases, the location is highly suggestive of feather plucking by other birds.
(© J Chitty)

Feather destruction

Feather destructive disorders are not seen in poultry to the extent that they are encountered in parrots. It is also highly unusual for birds to peck at and destroy their own feathers (which must be distinguished from feather eating, see below). The vast majority of cases, therefore, are caused by other birds pecking at the feathers (Figure 19.1). The areas typically affected include the head, dorsum and vent region (including the abdominal area). Rarely, feather damage may be caused by the bird rubbing against wire or solid surfaces if they are pruritic. Broken feathers located at the end of the wings may be due to roosting next to and rubbing on wire. Previous nutritional problems or systemic disease may result in stress or fret marks on growing feathers that may break off at a later date.

The underlying cause is generally an exaggerated formation of the pecking order, with over-aggression from one or more birds towards at least one other. It is not rare for many birds to be affected. In some cases, all the birds

in the flock may be affected to a greater or lesser extent. In most of these instances, just one or two birds may be responsible for all of the pecking.

In other cases of feather destructive disorders, there may be an underlying disease, with birds pecking at ectoparasites or at a reddened vent following scour or a partial prolapse.

Clinical approach

When investigating feather destructive cases, the clinician needs to examine the affected bird as well as assess the overall health of the flock. Figure 19.2 details some of the points that should be addressed as part of this examination.

If the cause is determined to be behavioural in origin, then the problem may be resolved using an 'ABC'

History and examination of an individual bird with feather damage

- Overall clinical picture
- Health, feeding and laying history
- Presence of ectoparasites
- Which feathers are damaged? Does this suggest rubbing or pecking?
- Is the vent swollen or slack?
- Are there stress/fret marks present on intact feathers? If so, does their position tally with breakage position on the damaged feathers?
- Skin assessment – are there any lesions present? If so, these can be investigated as in other species using cytology (e.g. acetate strip samples), skin scrapes and culture (see Chapter 13)

History and examination of the flock

- How many birds are affected?
- Are all the birds affected to the same extent?
- Has there been any recent additions to the existing flock?
- Is a cockerel present?
- Have any aggressive interactions between the birds been observed? Is a potential aggressor identifiable?

19.2 Points that should be addressed as part of the investigation into feather destructive disorders.

approach (see the *BSAVA Manual of Canine and Feline Behavioural Medicine* for further information):

- Antecedents: pecking order not firmly established or maintained; there may be over-aggression in social interactions
- Behaviour: excessive pecking may result in damaged plumage
- Control:
  - Re-establish and maintain the pecking order (see below)
  - Reduce the likelihood of antisocial interactions. The majority of these interactions occur at specific locations, often where there is increased competition (e.g. for food, water or roosting). Providing additional feeders and drinkers, as well as ensuring that there are more laying/roosting boxes than there are birds will greatly reduce antisocial interactions
  - Encourage dust bathing and foraging (see below).

Prevention

Prevention of feather destructive disorders is largely by maintaining good health of the birds and a healthy pecking order, as well as providing adequate space and resources to reduce competition.

Vent pecking and cannibalism

To a large extent, vent pecking is an extension of feather pecking (see above). However, the consequences are far more severe and can often result in death of the affected bird. These birds are frequently cannibalized after death and it can be extremely difficult to determine whether the damage around the vent occurred ante or post mortem. Finding a dead bird with the vent portion of the body pecked out should raise suspicion for this type of behaviour. However, it should also be borne in mind that similar findings can be seen where there is a predator problem (especially rats and stoats) and this needs to be investigated as a matter of urgency. In general, where there is a behavioural problem, birds are affected one at a time; whereas predator attacks often result in several bodies each night.

Vent pecking can become habit-forming and known vent peckers should be removed from the flock. The underlying reasons for this type of behaviour are similar to those described for feather plucking. A frequently trigger is diarrhoea or partial prolapse, resulting in vent protrusion and creation of a 'bullseye' target for pecking. This is often enhanced in laying birds that have fewer feathers around the vent.

When this type of behaviour occurs, affected birds should be thoroughly assessed for any underlying causes and flock faecal parasitological checks should be performed to reduce the likelihood of further target formation. Otherwise, the behavioural 'ABC' approach is very similar to that described for feather pecking (see above), although the urgency of the situation is somewhat greater. The wounds of affected birds should be treated in a similar manner to other granulating open wounds (see Chapter 13). Severely affected individuals may need to be removed from the flock to prevent the bird from being a victim of further attack.

Head pecking

In some cases, head pecking may occur in groups of female ducks or geese. Eye injuries are possible but unusual, and it is rare to see much physical damage (unlike in poultry). Where one bird is 'driven off' food, additional feeding and drinking sites can be used to reduce intragroup competition. Extra roosting sites should also be provided as needed.

Establishing and maintaining a pecking order

A pecking order is formed and maintained in a group of hens. Once formed, it is normally stable and is controlled by the presence of a cockerel (see Chapter 3). However, should problems with aggression arise within the flock, the following should be attempted in order to reduce antisocial interactions:

- Keep the flock as stable as possible with minimal introductions or removal/reintroduction of individual birds
- If removal from the flock is essential (e.g. for treatment), always remove and reintroduce birds in pairs or trios so there is never an individual that is displaced
- Perform introductions gradually and, ideally, on 'neutral territory'. There will inevitably be some aggressive interactions, but these should be observed to ensure that they are not excessive. New birds should ideally be introduced in pairs. If an individual is to be introduced, it should be kept separately with a single bird from the original flock (following the quarantine period), and then both birds should be introduced to the main flock at the same time
- Keep a single cockerel with the flock
- Birds that are 'antisocial' and persistently aggressive need to be removed from the flock. Many of these aggressive behaviours do appear to be habit in some birds. In the author's experience, such birds can do well when placed in a new flock with similar birds or in a trio with another hen and a cockerel.

Eating feathers or foreign bodies

Eating feathers and other foreign material has been shown to be pica (a compulsive craving for non-food substances) and the result of a behavioural disorder. Importantly, it is a behavioural disorder that is learned by others and is passed on to chicks (Morishita *et al.*, 1999). The root cause appears to be lack of foraging and stress. The main consequence is crop and/or ventricular impaction with excess fibre or feathers (see Chapters 16 and 23 for the treatment of impaction). Treatment of the behaviour is difficult, as once established it can be hard to reduce the habit. Provision of increased foraging opportunities (see below) may help, as will removal of the preferred material for ingestion as soon as possible from the enclosure. Stress should also be minimized by:

- Maintaining a routine
- Reducing excessive changes in the environment
- Careful management of the flock structure.

Affected birds should not rear their own chicks and should not be paired with other birds for breeding, in order to 'dilute' the problem. These birds should not be kept in isolation, but rather non-breeding groups.

Prevention

Prevention is by provision of better foraging opportunities.

Cockerel crowing

One of the most common queries to the author's clinic regards preventing cockerels from crowing. As discussed in Chapter 3, this is normal behaviour but can be disruptive to owners and their neighbours, especially in the summer months when crowing at first light can begin very early in the morning and during the breeding season when birds may crow all day. The best means of avoidance is to not keep a cockerel. However, this does mean that it is harder to maintain flock pecking order and that breeding is not possible.

If a cockerel has been obtained and crowing is causing a problem, there are a number of options:

- Remove the cockerel
- Utilize light levels to reduce crowing – birds generally do not crow at night, so providing a lightproof house for overnight accommodation means that the cockerel can be let out and allowed to crow only at a reasonable hour of day. This is the best approach in the author's experience. Some suggest using housing with a low roof so that the bird cannot extend its neck to crow. However, light levels seem to be more crucial and space restriction may result in welfare problems. In addition, if the day length cycle is adjusted so that the bird is only let out for 6 hours a day, the cockerel may go 'out of season' for a period of time
- Deslorelin implants – the use of these implants has been discussed. However, anecdotal reports suggest a very variable response

---

Encouraging foraging and grooming

In accordance with the Five Freedoms, birds should have the opportunity to express natural behaviours, including foraging and grooming.

- A dust pit should be provided to allow dust bathing (Figure 19.3).
- Access to rain should be provided – this appears to assist with plumage maintenance and birds do appear to 'enjoy' light rain exposure, often choosing to get wet than to stay in the dry.
- Feed should be scattered rather than provided in a bowl or hopper to encourage foraging. In some situations this may encourage vermin, especially rodents, so it is vital not to provide excessive amounts of food and to combine this with appropriate vermin control measures.
- Housing with a natural grass substrate rather than bare earth or concrete should be provided.
- Within the parameters of a good balanced diet (see Chapter 5), a variety of food items including invertebrates, and natural vegetation should be provided. (For backyard poultry, the easiest way to achieve this may be to allow the bird free access to an enclosed garden.) Kitchen scraps must never be used for feeding as this is illegal in the EU. However, a variety of feeds may be purchased specifically for the birds, e.g. potato peelings may be used, as long as they are not a by-product from the kitchen.

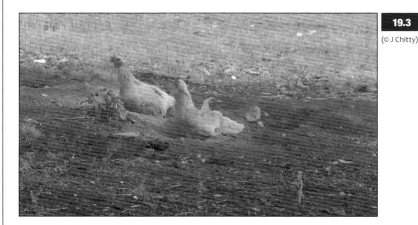

19.3 Provision of a dust bath enables normal grooming and foraging behaviours.
(© J Chitty)

- Surgical castration – this is possible but technically extremely difficult, carries a significant risk and is illegal in farmed birds in the UK (see Chapter 26). In addition, it is impossible to remove all testicular tissue and there is a high chance of it redeveloping within 6–12 months. It is often noted that castrated birds show reduced male secondary sexual characteristics but may still continue to crow. Castration is therefore not recommended.

It should be noted that chemical caponization is no longer performed and that devoicing is illegal in the UK (see Chapter 26), as well as being fairly ineffective at preventing crowing.

Peacock screaming

This problem is very similar in nature to crowing in cockerels. However, captive peafowl are rarely restrained or housed at night, so the problem is much more difficult to control. The major problem occurs in spring/summer each year when young males disperse to form new territories and then call for females. Naturally, these new territories tend to be formed in other people's gardens! As with cockerels, the birds call from first light. The only way to control this problem is to capture and remove the offending bird. However, this is much easier said than done as peafowl are notoriously flighty.

Training and catching peafowl

Another frequent enquiry at the author's practice concerns the capture of peafowl, either because of excessive noise or so that the bird can be taken to the veterinary practice for treatment. As these birds are very nervous and flighty, they are not easily captured once loose in a garden. The most common request is for chemical immobilization, either by dart gun or in the feed. Neither route is recommended as peafowl are usually fairly impervious to low levels of sedative agents. Even if a successful dose is administered, there is a serious chance of injury to the bird as it will be uncoordinated and unable to fend for itself if not captured immediately.

It is better to encourage birds into a restricted space using food bait. This may take time, but is relatively simple as most peafowl are fed by owners. The birds can gradually be fed closer to a pen or stable such that they may be trapped inside at some point. Importantly (unless the need for veterinary attention is urgent), birds should not be trapped the first time they enter the pen, otherwise the positive reinforcement effects are lost.

Prevention

Prevention is achieved in a similar manner to training/catching peafowl, in that young birds are fed in a pen into which they can be enclosed at night.

Spur damage in cockerels

Damage from the spurs of cockerels is common in both males and females (Figure 19.4). In the case of male–male aggression, this can be prevented by never housing two male birds together. However, it should be recognized that

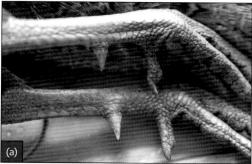
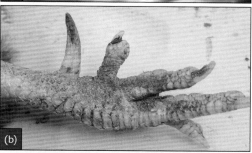
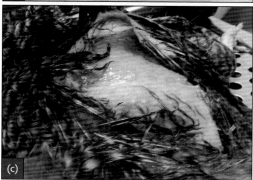
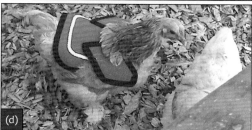

19.4 (a) Spurs of a male pheasant. These are of a size and sharpness that should be expected in poultry. (b) Spurs of a cockerel. Note that these are much longer and sharper than the spurs of the male pheasant in (a), which is why damage is more likely when the bird mates or fights. The spurs in this bird are by no means extreme for captive poultry. (c) Spur damage caused during mating. (d) Poultry 'saddle' to help reduce mating injuries.
(© J Chitty)

mistakes do occur as sexing is not easy in young birds. The problem is controlled by removing one of the male birds.

Cockerel damage to hens is also seen; this is usually where the spurs of the cockerel are dug into the flanks of the hen during copulation, sometimes causing deep wounds. This is the result of spurs being especially long in some species and/or individuals as a result of selective breeding. The wounds heal surprisingly well (see Chapter 13). Prevention is by removing or trimming/blunting spurs (see Chapter 7). If a male is particularly vigorous during mating and causes damage even after the spurs have been shortened, replacement of the bird should be considered. Some cockerels have a preferred hen; in these cases, the hen can be protected using a poultry 'saddle'.

Aggression during mating in ducks

Aggression problems may be seen in ducks. Typically, this is male to female aggression and occurs during the breeding season when females may be mobbed by multiple male birds. Injuries around the neck may be seen, and some females may even be drowned when over-vigorous mating occurs on the water. The worst offenders appear to be male mallards or mallard crossbreeds. Treatment involves removing females from the group of male birds. Wounds can be treated in a conventional manner (see Chapter 13). Prevention is by ensuring that only single male birds are kept with females (either in pairs or in a group).

Aggression towards people or other species

Aggression towards other species is reported in many poultry breeds, including pheasants, turkeys, geese and swans. As well as people, birds will attack all potential predators, especially dogs. This behaviour is commonly utilized when employing geese for guarding. The main problems concern guarding of territory and of mates and/or young. There is no real solution to this problem, other than avoidance. Breeding season times should be known and the birds disturbed as little as possible during these periods. Territories should be formed and fenced off to reduce incursion into these areas, as well as enable better protection of visitors or members of the public.

Broodiness

Hens, particularly Bantams, may become broody. This is a natural behaviour where, instead of laying eggs in nesting boxes for collection, a bird will remove herself to an isolated location (or use the nesting box provided) and attempt to incubate a clutch. Some hens may gather eggs from other birds as well. A broody hen should be lifted off the eggs twice daily and taken to the food and water bowls so that she can feed before returning to incubate the eggs.

Simply removing the eggs and bringing the hen back to the flock will rarely eliminate the behaviour. Instead, the nest should be located and once the 'normal' clutch size is reached, the eggs should be replaced with dummy eggs. These dummy eggs can be removed at the end of the incubation period (approximately 28 days) and the hen returned to the flock. If there are problems reintegrating the bird, the steps described earlier may be followed (see above). In some instances, the hen may be permitted to brood fertile eggs, even of different species.

In semi-commercial flocks, persistently broody hens may need to be replaced. Traditionally, in an attempt to get a valuable breeding hen out of broodiness, the bird may be removed from the nest and placed in a wire-based cage (with food and water provided). The wire base of the cage comprises narrow mesh which prevents the feet and legs from slipping through but allows air circulation underneath the hen. This 'cooling' effect is believed to help bring the hen out of broodiness. However, the success of this method (and the many others advocated) is low; most hens eventually come out of broodiness on their own.

Egg damage

Some hens will damage their own and other birds eggs. In the author's experience, this is particularly prevalent when soft-shelled eggs are being laid. It is important to distinguish egg damage from occasional 'clumsy damage', vermin damage (e.g. by rats) and soft/thin-shelled eggs that break on laying. To assist in this task, any damaged eggs should be 'pieced together' to determine what is missing. It is also useful to assess the pattern of when and how many eggs are damaged.

Various causes of egg damage have been proposed:

- Dietary insufficiency – in the author's experience, this is particularly prevalent when soft-shelled eggs are being laid. In these cases, the calcium and vitamin D content of the diet should be investigated (see Chapters 17 and 20)
- Excess light in the nesting box – this can be easily checked and corrected
- Too little space or overcrowding in the nesting box – nesting boxes should be of an adequate size for the bird being housed. There should be a nesting box for each bird, plus a couple of 'spare' boxes to reduce competition
- Height of the nesting boxes – it has been suggested that if the nesting boxes are too low, eggs can be seen and attract the egg-damaging bird
- Lack of foraging opportunity (see above).

Escape

Escaping is not, in itself, a behavioural problem, although it may certainly represent a failure in management. In some cases, it may simply represent an inadequacy in enclosure design. However, for territorial species such as poultry, peafowl and most waterfowl, there should be little inclination to leave the home territory and, therefore, escape may represent the presence of stressors within the enclosure such as:

- Male–male competition and/or aggression
- Dispersal of young male birds
- Presence of an aggressive hen
- Inadequate food and/or foraging opportunities
- The presence of potential predators or vermin
- Inadequate space within the enclosure.

Most escapes can be prevented not only by using fully enclosed pens and/or wing clipping birds (see Chapter 7), but also by providing for the birds' behavioural needs in the first instance. By providing for the birds' behavioural needs, not only does this allow larger, less enclosed spaces to be used, but also results in better fulfilment of the Five Freedoms for these birds.

References and further reading

Horwitz D and Mills D (2009) *BSAVA Manual of Canine and Feline Behavioural Medicine, 2nd edn*. BSAVA Publications, Gloucester

Morishita T, Aye P and Harr B (1999) Crop impaction resulting from feather ball formation in caged layers. *Avian Disease* **43(1)**, 160–163

Chapter 20

Nutritional disorders

Keith Warner

Nutritional disorders are most likely to be seen in rapidly growing birds or those laying a lot of eggs. Nutritional requirements in laying birds are greater, as there is an increased consumption of nutrients to support egg production. As small scale production tends to include more traditional, lower egg producing breeds and management systems, deficiencies should be relatively infrequent, as long as birds are fed solely on a commercially produced balanced diet, correct for their age and production status (see Chapter 5). However, there is also a significant chance that birds kept as pets may be housed in an environment with external sources of food, be fed 'treats' in addition to their normal food ration or, in more extreme cases, be fed an inappropriate diet in entirety.

Investigations of nutritional disorders should initially assume a less than ideal diet, and obtaining a thorough history from the owner with regard to feeding is essential. It is important to enquire specifically about treats (type, frequency and volume), as many owners will not consider these to be part of the diet of the bird. In fact, feeding kitchen waste is often considered good, ethical practice in the modern family looking to minimize waste. However, in the UK it is illegal to feed kitchen scraps to pet poultry (see Chapter 26); similar legislation may apply in other countries.

On-site visits, investigation of the environment and nutritional supply can be valuable in determining whether nutritional deficiencies should be included in the differential diagnosis list. It is also worth remembering that inappropriate foodstuffs can be toxic (see Chapter 5 for a list of toxic plants). In addition, rapid changes in diets may have grave effects on the effectiveness of the bird's alimentary tract, especially where high protein foods (e.g. those intended for cats) are accessed.

The breed and history of the bird can be important factors. Whilst there is no specifically recognized signalment, commercial layer breeds and birds used previously in commercial layer systems will have the genetic potential for high egg production. These birds are very dependent on good quality nutrition.

Approaches to treatment

In many cases, where nutritional imbalances occur, the exact identification of the deficiency is difficult to ascertain through clinical examination as the clinical signs tend to overlap. When presented with birds with a suspected nutritional disorder, the mainstay of the advice should be to feed a commercial diet. Treatment and/or supplementation for nutritional inadequacies may come too late for some individuals, but changing to an appropriate diet and/or the use of vitamin or mineral preparations can often reverse the decline in the majority of birds.

There are a variety of multivitamin preparations available that can be added to drinking water at the recommended rate. These can be used instantly to start correcting any suspected problem. An advantage of these preparations is that they generally contain sugars in some form, so also provide energy and drive the birds to drink, which will help with the dehydration that is very commonly seen in sick birds.

There are no injectable vitamin preparations marketed for birds. Dosages of injectable solutions are typically calculated on the same dose per bodyweight rate as the target species for the particular preparation.

Perosis

Perosis (or chondrodystrophy) can be seen in growing birds whose diet is deficient in manganese, choline, nicotinic acid, pyridoxine, biotin or folic acid. It is characterized as an anatomical deformation of the leg bones in young birds, caused by retarded growth of the long bones, a widening of the tibiometatarsal joint, with twisting or bending of the distal end of the tibia and the proximal end of the metatarsus. If severe, it can lead to slipping of the gastrocnemius muscle tendon from its condyles. Clinically, it manifests as impaired locomotion because of lateral and posterior malposition of the leg.

Vitamin A deficiency
Epidemiology

Most adult birds have over 2 months' store of vitamin A in the liver and, therefore, to encounter vitamin A deficiency (also known as nutritional roup) requires long-term dietary inadequacy. For this reason, it is unlikely that the condition will be seen in a bird fed on a commercial diet, although all species of poultry can be affected if their diet is deficient. Nutritional roup is also unlikely to be seen in chicks hatched from eggs laid by a dam fed on a commercial diet, as vitamin A reserves are passed to the chick via the yolk sac. Chicks are more likely to show signs and the condition will develop much quicker if they are hatched from eggs laid by vitamin A deficient hens.

Clinical signs

Since vitamin A is involved in mucus production, clinical signs typically affect the eyelids, nose and oesophagus. Nasal and ocular crusting may be seen, sometimes to the extent that the eyelids are stuck together. Affected birds may also exhibit poor growth rates and have poor feathering. Vitamin A deficient chicks may exhibit ataxia. Older birds present with pale combs and wattles.

Differential diagnoses

The differential diagnoses include:

- Ocular and nasal signs – mycoplasmosis, infectious coryza and fowl cholera
- Ataxia – vitamin E deficiency and Newcastle disease
- Combs and wattle pallor – anaemia.

Post-mortem findings

Plaques in the mouth, pharynx and oesophagus are the most common finding on post-mortem examination. These plaques are often secondarily infected with bacteria. The eyelids can be inflamed and stuck together with a thick, sticky exudate. Excessive white crystalline urate deposits may be seen in the kidneys and ureters.

Laboratory diagnosis

Laboratory assay of the vitamin A content of the liver confirms the diagnosis.

Treatment

Multivitamin preparations for use in water are available, which contain vitamin A, if supplementation is required.

Prevention

Prevention is via providing correctly formulated commercial feeds.

Vitamin B deficiencies

Thiamine

Pathogenesis and epidemiology

Thiamine (vitamin B1) is involved in the Krebs cycle (also known as the citric acid cycle or the tricarboxylic acid cycle). Deficiency causes intermediates of carbohydrate metabolism to build up and leads to polyneuritis, resulting in impaired digestion and general weakness. The onset of clinical signs in adult birds typically occurs 3 weeks after the start of feeding a thiamine deficient diet.

Clinical signs

Lethargy, inappetence and head tremors are seen with a mild thiamine deficiency. Birds may be presented recumbent, with flexed legs and a retracted head, due to paralysis

of the anterior neck muscles. Progression leads to lateral recumbency, with the head still retracted, decreased temperature and respiratory rate and convulsions.

Differential diagnoses

The differential diagnosis for thiamine deficiency is Newcastle disease.

Post-mortem findings

Testicular degeneration, heart atrophy and severe anorexia are found on post-mortem examination.

Treatment and prognosis

Mildly affected birds that are able to eat can be fed a commercial diet and be given oral multivitamin preparations containing thiamine at the standard dosage. It may be worth considering drenching (directly and carefully administering by pouring down the throat) affected birds using a multivitamin solution in a 10 ml syringe. Severely anorexic birds will not eat unless force-fed or thiamine is injected. Dosages of injectable thiamine need to be scaled by weight compared with the target species.

Riboflavin

Pathogenesis

The epithelium and myelin sheaths are most affected by riboflavin (vitamin B2) deficiency. Birds may not actually have a low amount of riboflavin in the diet, but it may be antagonized by substances such as mycotoxins, so feed storage and fungal/mycotoxin contamination may be a problem.

Clinical signs

Affected birds are most likely to be presented as chicks with 'curled toe paralysis', as the sciatic nerve is most often involved. The birds stand with a clenched foot and, hence, on the dorsolateral aspect of the toes (Figure 20.1). If they are seen to move, these birds may also be wing walking. On closer inspection, 'clubbed down' may be seen (Figure 20.2). This is present immediately after hatching and is where the feather does not break the sheath and therefore has the appearance of a club. When determining whether a bird has a riboflavin deficiency, it should be remembered that clubbed down can also be seen to a

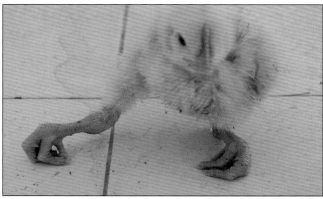

20.1 A chick showing 'curled toe paralysis' as a result of riboflavin deficiency.
(Image by Lucyin, licensed under CC BY-SA 3.0 (https://creativecommons.org/licenses/by-sa/3.0/deed.en))

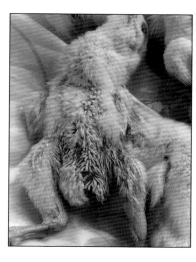

20.2 A chick with 'clubbed down' as a result of riboflavin deficiency. The feather has not broken through the feather sheath, resulting in the appearance of a club.

certain degree in normal chicks. Adult hens affected by riboflavin deficiency have decreased egg production with decreased embryo vitality in breeding hens.

Differential diagnoses

The differential diagnoses include infectious lameness and bumblefoot.

Post-mortem findings

Clubbed down, clenched feet and abrasions from wing walking may be seen in chicks on post-mortem examination. In hens, the liver may be enlarged with an excessive fat content.

Treatment and prognosis

Affected chicks may spontaneously recover as the requirement for vitamin B2 rapidly decreases with age. Coprophagia is beneficial in accessing more riboflavin as the microbes of the large bowel synthesize the vitamin and therefore excessive cleaning of the litter by owners should be discouraged.

Treatment with a potent riboflavin source can result in a rapid recovery, as long as the condition is not too long-standing. The use of injectable vitamin B2 at a scaled dose compared with the target species can be considered for individual birds. Multivitamin preparations containing riboflavin for use in water are available.

Niacin
Pathogenesis and epidemiology

Niacin (vitamin B3) is the vitamin component of coenzymes involved in the metabolism of fat, protein and carbohydrate. All species of bird at any age are susceptible to this condition, although some authors state that a marked deficiency cannot occur in chickens without a deficiency in its precursor, the amino acid tryptophan.

Clinical signs

Niacin deficiency is most likely to be seen as leg bowing in growing turkeys, ducks and pheasants due to chondrodystrophy and therefore may be difficult to distinguish from rickets and other mineralization problems. However, with niacin deficiency, the gastrocnemius tendon rarely slips from its condyles, unlike with perosis (see above).

The long bones are often shorter in length than normal, and a marked swelling of the tibiotarsal joint may be seen. Reduced feed consumption and reduced bodyweight gain can also be seen. Dermatitis and poor feathering may be a feature that can help distinguish niacin deficiency from other conditions (Scott et al., 1982).

Differential diagnoses

The differential diagnoses include vitamin D3 deficiency and rickets.

Post-mortem findings

The post-mortem examination may reveal bowed, possibly shortened legs, inflammation and a dark-coloured tongue and oral cavity in chicks. Dermatitis may also be seen.

Treatment and prognosis

The active form of nicotinic acid is sometimes used for its effect on the nicotinic receptors in the central nervous system (CNS), in an attempt to calm birds and decrease the incidence of feather pecking. This product can also be used for the treatment of vitamin B3 deficiency. The product should be added to the drinking water at the standard dose for an initial 5 days, whilst a balanced diet is introduced. The prognosis is guarded for large birds with severe bowing of the legs, and the welfare of the bird should be assessed before attempting treatment.

Pantothenic acid
Epidemiology

All groups of poultry may be affected by a deficiency in pantothenic acid (vitamin B5).

Clinical signs

The major lesions associated with vitamin B5 deficiency in poultry affect the skin, adrenal cortex and nervous tissue (Scott et al., 1982). The embryo can be affected by subcutaneous haemorrhage and oedema. Clinical signs in chicks are very similar to those seen with biotin deficiency and include dermatitis of the skin around the eyes and beak, as well as lesions to the feet. Dermatitis around the eyes and beak is more likely to be seen with external parasites or poxvirus (see Chapter 13). Growth retardation and poor plumage quality with broken feathers has been reported and long-term deficiency can lead to the eyelids sealing closed with a viscous discharge.

Differential diagnoses

The differential diagnoses include biotin deficiency, mite infestation and footpad dermatitis.

Post-mortem findings

The post-mortem examination may reveal liver hypertrophy and yellow discoloration of the liver.

Treatment and prognosis

Treatment of pantothenic acid deficiency includes changing to a commercial diet and use of multivitamin solutions in the drinking water. For severely affected birds, injectable preparations for other species can be used and the dose adjusted according to the weight of the bird.

Pyridoxine

Pathogenesis and epidemiology

All types and ages of poultry with a dietary deficiency in vitamin B6 can be affected. Vitamin B6 is involved in the formation of several neurotransmitters, and is essential for normal brain development and function.

Clinical signs

Along with many other deficiencies, pyridoxine (vitamin B6) deficient chicks show retarded growth, dermatitis and poor feathering. More specifically, they may develop nervous signs. Initially, the chicks become very excitable, but as the condition progresses, the birds begin to tremble and their movement becomes jerky. Chicks have been reported to run aimlessly with dropped wings and a lowered head. Further progression leads to convulsion and death through exhaustion.

A chronic deficiency can lead to perosis. Unilateral crippling may be seen or one or two middle toes may be bent inwards at the middle joint.

In adults, vitamin B6 deficiency leads to inappetence and decreased egg production with reduced hatchability. Involution of the oviduct, ovary, testes, combs and wattles can be seen. Specific blood changes are recorded with vitamin B6 deficiency. A mild deficiency leads to microcytic, normochromic polycythaemia, whilst severe deficiencies cause microcytic, polychromatic, hypochromic anaemia. Deficient chicks also show decreased immunoglobulin M and immunoglobulin G immunological responses. A marked increase in serum iron content and a marked decrease in serum copper levels are seen. Vitamin B6 deficiency has been associated with gizzard erosion, which can also be caused by adenovirus infection and feed contamination with histidine or gizzerosine (e.g. associated with a spoiled fish meal).

If the deficiency is corrected, hens may undergo a short moult of around 2 weeks' duration and then return to lay.

Differential diagnoses

The differential diagnoses include *Enterococcus* infection, other nutritional deficiencies, Newcastle disease and avian encephalopathy.

Post-mortem findings

The post-mortem examination may reveal gizzard erosions and bent toes.

Treatment and prognosis

A balanced diet supplemented by a multivitamin solution helps the birds to recover. They will respond better if removed from stress, so separating them from flockmates and providing a warm dry environment is also advisable during the recovery phase. Some affected birds may need to be euthanased for welfare reasons.

Biotin

Pathogenesis and epidemiology

Biotin (vitamin B7) is a water-soluble B-complex vitamin (vitamin B7/vitamin H/coenzyme R). It is involved in gluconeogenesis, as well as the manufacture of fatty acids and amino acids. Most feeds contain biotin, but the bioavailability varies widely. For instance, biotin is 100% available from maize, but just 5% available from wheat.

Biotin deficiencies in poultry lead to reduced growth, as well as skin and, on occasion, bone lesions. Birds with a lower metabolic activity have a lower demand for biotin and, therefore, deficiencies are less likely in slow-growing traditional breeds kept as pets compared with fast-growing breeds. Due to the higher requirement at the time, biotin deficiency is most likely to be encountered in growing birds and is less common after maturity.

A reduced growth rate will only be noticed in fast-growing birds (typically commercial breeds reared for meat production) and, in extreme cases, a deficiency in biotin will lead to mortality due to fatty liver haemorrhagic syndrome (see Chapter 21). However, as most backyard chickens do not have an enormous energy requirement, this syndrome, which manifests as sudden death, is rarely seen. Biotin is also an important factor in the Krebs cycle (also known as the citric acid cycle or the tricarboxylic acid cycle) and disruption of this cycle results in the laying down of excessive fat in the liver and kidneys.

Clinical signs

The most common manifestations of biotin deficiency in backyard poultry affect skin integrity and sometimes result in bone lesions. The first sign of deficiency is dermatitis affecting the skin around the eyes and beak, as well as the feet. Crusty skin lesions are commonly seen around the beak and eyelid commissures (Figure 20.3). However, it should be remembered that dermatitis around the eyes and beak is more likely to be seen with external parasites or poxvirus (see Chapter 13). Care should also be taken not to confuse foot lesions with footpad erosion or podo-dermatitis caused by exposure to wet and soiled bedding. In these cases, damage to the sole of the foot is caused by maceration of the skin from persistent dampness and chemical and/or physical burn from faecal material. Chicks hatched from eggs laid by biotin deficient dams may have bent and shortened bones.

Differential diagnoses

The differential diagnoses include mite infestation, poxvirus infection and vitamin B5 deficiency.

Post-mortem findings

A fatty liver and/or kidneys with interstitial fat found on post-mortem examination of birds that have died suddenly is very suggestive for fatty liver haemorrhagic syndrome.

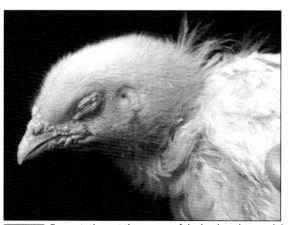

20.3 Encrustations at the corner of the beak and around the eyes in bird with biotin deficiency.
(Courtesy of Professor C Whitehead)

Treatment and prognosis

Changing to a proprietary diet for the type of bird being kept should resolve most mild problems over time. Chicks with stunted growth and any lame birds may need to be euthanased on welfare grounds.

Folic acid

Epidemiology

Poultry are the most susceptible of any farmed livestock to the effects of folic acid (folacin, vitamin B9) deficiency. Folic acid is necessary for cell multiplication and macrocytic anaemia may result from the cessation of erythrocyte formation in the bone marrow (Schweigert et al., 1948).

Clinical signs

Non-specific clinical signs are typically seen with folic acid deficiency, including poor food intake, poor growth and lethargy. These signs are most likely to be seen in growing birds, although any age of bird may be affected. Perosis with similar signs to niacin deficiency may be seen. In cases of severe deficiency, anaemia may develop, resulting in a pale comb and mucous membranes. Poor feather development and pigmentation can also occur. Turkeys may also develop spastic cervical paralysis where the neck is stiff and extended.

Differential diagnoses

The differential diagnoses include niacin deficiency and other causes of anaemia (particularly older birds with organ failure).

Post-mortem findings

The post-mortem findings are non-specific.

Treatment and prognosis

A commercial diet should be fed and oral multivitamins can be administered to initiate the treatment. Severely affected birds may need to be euthanased on welfare grounds. Poults usually die 2 days after the onset of clinical signs unless folic acid is administered.

Cyanocobalamin

Epidemiology

Adult birds are able to tolerate cyanocobalamin (vitamin B12) deficiencies for a prolonged period of time (2–5 months of deficiency may be necessary to deplete stores to a clinically significant level), so birds fed a balanced commercial diet are unlikely to suffer from this condition.

Clinical signs

Vitamin B12 deficiency in growing birds can result in poor growth, decreased feed intake, nervous disorders and defective feathering. It is also associated with perosis (see niacin deficiency) and anaemia may be seen. Adult birds are usually asymptomatic and maintain their bodyweight and rate of egg production. In these cases, poor hatchability and a high level of embryonic death are the most likely clinical signs (Squires and Naber, 1992; Zhang et al., 1994). Embryonic death tends to occur at 17 days. Egg size may be affected, with cyanocobalamin deficiency leading to reduced egg size (Scott et al., 1982).

Differential diagnoses

The differential diagnoses include infectious bronchitis, which can cause eggshell abnormalities and niacin deficiency.

Post-mortem findings

Common findings on post-mortem examination include gizzard erosion and fatty deposits in the heart, liver and kidney. Embryos appear haemorrhagic with oedema, may have a fatty liver, an enlarged and irregular heart and pale or yellow kidneys. Perosis and thigh muscle atrophy may also be seen (Olcese et al., 1950).

Treatment and prognosis

Both oral and injectable multivitamin products often contain vitamin B12 and can be used for treatment of deficiency. These multivitamin products should be used alongside a commercial diet.

Vitamin D3, calcium and phosphorus deficiencies

Epidemiology and pathogenesis

A total calcium deficiency and phosphorus imbalance should be rare in birds fed a commercial diet. However, imbalances can easily occur in birds fed a home ration of treats and kitchen waste, or where there has been overuse of grit/eggshell or tonics. Indoor reared birds can have problems utilizing dietary calcium, partly due to the lack of ultraviolet (UV) light to stimulate vitamin D3 production.

Vitamin D3 is probably the most commonly recognized deficiency/imbalance in commercial poultry. Vitamin D3, calcium and phosphorus are all metabolically linked. Thus, the diet has to not only provide sufficient calcium and phosphorus but also to provide them in the correct ratio (approximately 1.5–2 Ca:1 P). In addition, the bird needs sufficient circulating vitamin D3 to absorb and utilize both these minerals properly. Laying birds are particularly susceptible to deficiencies as during lay they are constantly utilizing medullary bone as a temporary store of calcium.

Clinical signs

In growing birds, clinical signs are likely to be caused by abnormal mineralization of the bones, leading to 'bendy bones' (e.g. rickets) or tibial dyschondroplasia. In adult birds (especially laying birds), deficiency may lead to osteoporosis, which can be seen as spontaneous fractures, or neurological signs associated with spinal compression. Misshapen bones due to remodelling can lead to an unusual stance or gait. Secondary joint effusions are also seen due to the abnormal strain placed on the joints. This most commonly affects the hocks, especially in large birds such as turkeys. Soft-shelled or thin-walled eggs and bone fractures may be encountered, along with paralysis, if there is spinal compression. This condition is known as cage layer fatigue.

Post-mortem findings

Soft, pliable bones are found on post-mortem examination. The bones have thin medullary walls and seem to be readily fractured; the tibia should break with a noticeable crack even in birds as young as 7 days old. For rickets to be diagnosed, rachitic rosaries (enlarged costochondral junctions) must be seen. The bones, especially the tibio-tarsus, may be misshapen and a clear joint exudate may be noted (especially in the hock joint). Tibial dyschondro-plasia, seen as plugs of cartilage in the proximal tibia, is the most commonly seen manifestation of deficiency in fast-growing meat birds. A milder form of this condition also occurs, where the affected tibial growth plate is un-even across the cut surface (Figure 20.4).

Treatment and prognosis

Overt vitamin D3 deficiency should be rare in birds allowed access to the outdoors, owing to synthesis when exposed to UV light. Vitamin D3 supplementation in water, along with provision of a commercial diet, should effectively treat any mild manifestation of the condition. Bones will re-mineralize, although misshapen bones will probably not correct in shape. Multivitamin preparations generally do not contain enough vitamin D3 for treatment of deficiencies, but specific D3 preparations are avail-able. In high producing laying birds, an added source of calcium, such as oyster shell, can be used along with D3 and a commercial diet when poor shell mineralization is noted.

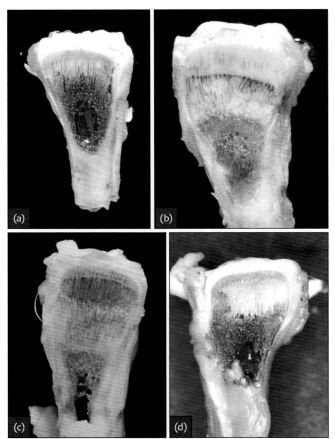

20.4 (a) A normal growth plate showing the usual spatial relationship between the proliferative and hypertrophic zones. (b) A growth plate showing a large increase in the relative size of the proliferative zone as a result of a calcium/vitamin D deficiency. (c) A growth plate showing a proliferative zone of relatively normal thickness and a hypertrophic zone of increased thickness due to a phosphorus deficiency. (d) A growth plate showing a large accumulation of avascular cartilage from the region between the proliferative and hypertrophic zones due to tibial dyschondroplasia.
(Courtesy of Professor C Whitehead)

Prevention

Vitamin D3 supplementation in water is part of many inten-sive broiler and turkey rearing programmes and can be considered in indoor breeding and rearing situations.

Calcium tetany

Epidemiology

Calcium tetany is due to an acute onset hypocalcaemia and is most likely to occur during periods of peak calcium mobilization such as the onset of lay. The signalment and history may be suggestive of calcium tetany.

Clinical signs

The clinical signs associated with sudden onset hypo-calcaemia include paralysis, panting, lethargy and sudden death. Cyanosis of the comb may also be seen.

Differential diagnoses

The differential diagnosis for calcium tetany is avian influenza.

Post-mortem findings

Lung congestion and a shelled egg in the shell gland may be found on post-mortem examination.

Treatment and prognosis

For mild cases where birds are eating and drinking, dietary calcium supplementation via the provision of oyster shell grit is beneficial. Vitamin D3 supplementation aids in calcium absorption. For more severe cases, calcium injec-tions could be considered. It should be borne in mind that excess calcium administration to birds at inappropriate life stages (e.g. during rearing) can be injurious and can cause, for example, renal damage.

Vitamin E deficiency

The role of vitamin E is closely linked to that of selenium and to a certain extent they can substitute for each other. Deficiencies of either will lead to the same clinical signs. Vitamin E and selenium are involved in the normal devel-opment of skin and muscles. Deficiencies have been reported in chickens, turkeys and ducklings. Three main syndromes are recognized and are usually seen in chicks rather than adults:

- Exudative diathesis
- Muscular dystrophy
- Encephalomalacia.

Clinical signs
Exudative diathesis

The clinical signs of exudative diathesis result from plasma leakage caused by a marked increase in capillary permea-bility. There may be blue, green or black skin discoloration of the affected areas, typically the breast and wings.

Chicks may be apathetic, inappetent and have a much reduced level of activity. An abnormal stance (i.e. the legs too far apart) owing to muscle weakness may be seen.

Muscular dystrophy

The clinical signs of muscular dystrophy include weakness and poor thrift. This condition may overlap with exudative diathesis. Muscular dystrophy occurs when vitamin E deficiency is accompanied by a methionine or cysteine (sulphur amino acid) deficiency. The condition is most prevalent in the breast musculature and is most severe at around 4 weeks of age.

Encephalomalacia

Encephalomalacia (also known as 'crazy chick disease') leads to haemorrhage in the cerebellum, which results in ataxia, incoordination and torticollis. The head may be twisted such that the bird is standing but the top of the head is resting on the floor (Figure 20.5).

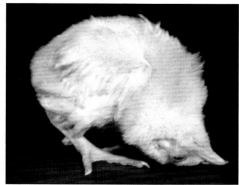

20.5 A chick with encephalomalacia ('crazy chick disease') showing abnormal head twisting as a result of a vitamin E deficiency.
(© UK Crown)

Differential diagnoses
Exudative diathesis

The differential diagnoses for exudative diathesis include chick anaemia virus, necrotic dermatitis and gangrenous dermatitis.

Encephalomalacia

The differential diagnoses for encephalomalacia include Newcastle disease, vitamin A deficiency and bacterial infection (e.g. enterococcal meningitis).

Post-mortem findings
Exudative diathesis

The post-mortem examination findings are characterized by profuse subcutaneous oedema, possibly followed by haemorrhage, generally affecting the breast and under the wings. Affected areas of skin can appear blackened or have a blue–green discoloration. The muscles may also appear pale.

Muscular dystrophy

The post-mortem examination may reveal pale 'striping' of the muscles (e.g. breast, thighs, ventriculus and myocardium).

Encephalomalacia

Cerebellar haemorrhage is found on post-mortem examination; although the lesions are not grossly apparent, histological examination confirms the diagnosis.

Treatment and prognosis

Vitamin E deficiency is unlikely in birds fed a commercial diet. For mild to moderate cases, the administration of vitamin E via drinking water should be effective in treating the deficiency. If not treated with vitamin E and/or selenium, affected chicks usually die within 2–6 days. Severely affected chicks are unlikely to recover and should be euthanased.

References and further reading

Moses MA and Aiello SE (2016) *The Merck Veterinary Manual, 11th edn*. Merck & Co. Inc., New Jersey

Olcese O, Couch JR, Quisenberry JH and Pearson PB (1950) Congenital anomalies in the chick due to vitamin B12 deficiency. *Journal of Nutrition* **41**, 423

Pattison M, McMullin P, Bradbury J and Alexander D (2007) *Poultry Diseases, 6th edn*. Elsevier, Philadelphia

Scott ML, Nesheim MC and Young RJ (1982) *Nutrition of the Chicken*. Scott & Associates, New York

Schweigert BS, German HL, Pearson PB and Sherwood RM (1948) Effect of the pteroylglutamic acid intake on the performance of turkeys and chickens. *Journal of Nutrition* **35**, 89

Siddons RC (1978) Nutrient deficiencies in animals: folic acid. In: *Handbook Series in Nutrition and Food: Section E – Nutritional Disorders, Volume 2*, ed. M Rechcigl Jr., p. 132. CRC Press Inc., Florida

Squires MW and Naber EC (1992) Vitamin profiles of eggs as indicators of nutritional status in the laying hen: vitamin B12 study. *Poultry Science* **71**, 2075

Zhang MY, Jia JS, Qin JH and Zhao YL (1994) Improvement of hatchability by treatment of hatching eggs with vitamin B12 during incubation. *Poultry Husbandry and Disease Control* **5**, 21

Chapter 21

Systemic, haematological and circulatory disorders

Kevin Eatwell and Jan Dixon

There are a wide variety of infectious agents that can cause systemic disease in poultry, many of which are not common in backyard birds (Figure 21.1). Biosecurity and hygiene is important and further information can be obtained in Chapter 7. A typical clinical presentation is a weak and collapsed bird, and systemic diseases are important conditions to rule out.

Disease	Species affected				
	Chickens	*Turkeys*	*Ducks*	*Pheasants*	*Guinea fowl*
Malabsorption syndrome	Yes	No	No	No	No
Avian leucosis sarcoma virus	Yes	Yes	No	Yes	Yes
Reticuloendotheliosis virus	Yes	Yes	Yes	Yes	No
Lymphoproliferative disease	No	Yes	No	No	No
Chicken anaemia virus	Yes	No	No	No	No
Inclusion body hepatitis	Yes	Yes	No	No	No
Hydropericardium-hepatitis syndrome	Yes	No	No	No	No
Big liver and spleen disease	Yes	No	No	No	No
Marble spleen disease	No	No	No	Yes	No
Haemorrhagic enteritis	No	Yes	No	No	No
Turkey haemorrhagic enteritis	No	Yes	No	No	No
Turkey viral hepatitis	No	Yes	No	No	No
Duck viral hepatitis	No	No	Yes	No	No
Avian infectious hepatitis	Yes	No	No	No	No
Streptococcus bovis septicaemia	Yes	Yes	Yes	Yes	Yes
Arizona disease	Yes	Yes	No	No	No
Tick-related anaemia	Yes	Yes	Yes	Yes	Yes
Ulcerative colitis	Yes	Yes	No	Yes	No
Favus	Yes	Yes	No	No	No
Red mites	Yes	Yes	Yes	Yes	Yes
Northern mites	Yes	No	No	No	No
Leucocytozoonosis	Yes	Yes	Yes	Yes	Yes
Capillaria	Yes	Yes	Yes	Yes	Yes
Proventricular or gizzard worms	No	No	Yes	No	No
Flipover	Yes	No	No	No	No
Dissecting aneurysm	No	Yes	No	No	No
Ruptured aorta	No	Yes	No	No	No
Fatty liver haemorrhagic syndrome	Yes	Yes	Yes	Yes	Yes
Visceral gout	Yes	Yes	Yes	Yes	Yes
Omphalitis	Yes	Yes	Yes	Yes	Yes
Starve outs	Yes	Yes	Yes	Yes	Yes

21.1 Systemic diseases of poultry, indicating the species affected.

Viral diseases

Malabsorption syndrome

This condition is also known as runting and stunting syndrome, infectious runting, pale bird syndrome and infectious stunting syndrome.

Aetiology and pathogenesis

This is an infectious syndrome seen worldwide, which can result in 5–90% runted and stunted chickens, and is most commonly encountered in poults. It is thought to have a multifactorial viral aetiology, as many viruses including calicivirus, enterovirus, parvovirus, reovirus and rotavirus have all been isolated from infected flocks, but none of these can individually cause the disease. Pathology can be found in the small intestine, pancreas and proventriculus, which implies that there are several different viral combinations involved in the production of the clinical signs.

Clinical signs

Birds up to 1 week old are stunted, have a hunched posture, exhibit coprophagia and have a mucoid diarrhoea, which causes faecal material to build up on the feathers and skin around the vent (vent pasting). There is poor feather development, with retained down and broken wing feathers. Some birds will be lame at 2–4 weeks of age due to secondary encephalomalacia. The birds may also be anaemic and pale. Severely affected chicks remain small and tend to gradually fade away, even though they may seem to be active initially. Euthanasia of birds that are obviously runted and stunted should be considered, but they may survive given supportive care.

Post-mortem findings

The post-mortem examination demonstrates small birds with pale subcutaneous fat. The intestine may be distended with poorly digested food or watery mucoid fluid. The pancreas may be affected in chickens >3 weeks old. It will be small, hard and pale, whilst the proventricular wall may be thickened and overlying pale lobules. There may be ulceration and haemorrhage of the mucosa around the oesophageal junction or proximal gizzard.

Osteodystrophy can be seen in stunted birds >2 weeks old, which means that the femoral head will separate easily from the femur when the hips are disarticulated. It should be noted that the femoral head separation will show a rough, red physis, which is not due to femoral head necrosis or bacterial osteomyelitis. The long bones may be pliable or easily broken. Secondary encephalomalacia with haemorrhage in the cerebellum can be seen in 3–6-week-old stunted birds.

Laboratory diagnosis

The diagnosis is based on clinical signs (runted, active birds with slow feather development and poor growth throughout the flock) and post-mortem examination findings.

Treatment and prevention

Antibiotics may have some effect on the diarrhoea, but will not cure the condition. If antibiotics are to be given these should ideally be based on the culture and sensitivity of the *Escherichia coli* isolates or based on sensitivities typical for *E. coli* isolates. Long-term supplementation of vitamins and trace elements may reduce the severity of the clinical signs.

Prevention is based on good early management and hygiene, with an all in/all out policy, if possible, together with good cleaning and effective disinfection between groups of birds in each enclosure. Hatchery hygiene is also important; faecal contamination of hatching eggs will allow transmission of disease. Temperature control is important for the chicks for the first few weeks, from hatching through transfer and into rearing. Management is important in both the treatment and prevention of the disease. Draughts should be eliminated, the floor temperature should be correct for the age of the birds, and the floor should be covered with clean, shallow, dry litter. Feed analysis should be carried out to eliminate mycotoxins (such as aflatoxins, ochratoxins, citrinin, ergot toxins, patulin and fusarium toxins), which may be encountered if the feed is damp. Specialized laboratories offer mycotoxin tests, which are commercially available. Interpretation of this analysis can be difficult, since mycotoxins are rarely evenly distributed throughout the feed and are usually concentrated in small patches.

Avian leucosis sarcoma virus

Aetiology and pathogenesis

There are three avian retroviruses (lymphoid leucosis, erythroid leucosis and myeloid leucosis) responsible for diseases worldwide in chickens, pheasants, turkeys and guinea fowl; they have also been encountered in other species, including partridges and quail. These retroviruses are usually absent from commercial strains of poultry (e.g. Ross, Cobb, Hyline), but may be found in rare breeds. Birds showing signs of chronic ill thrift may be found to have slow-growing tumours within internal organs, whilst other avian leucosis sarcoma viruses (ALSVs) result in tumours within days or weeks.

Clinical signs and transmission

ALSV has various subtypes that cause myeloid, erythroid and lymphoid leucosis with fibrosarcomas, haemangiosarcomas, nephroblastomas and osteopetrosis tumours. Subclinical infection with ALSV may occasionally cause lower egg production and slower growth rates, so this disease is of importance in commercial flocks.

- **Lymphoid leucosis** is seen in layers around 20 to 36 weeks of age.
- **Erythroid leucosis** and myeloid leucosis (ML) are both sporadic, although occur more commonly in broiler breeds (at 25 to 55 weeks of age).

ALSVs are transmitted either vertically through the egg or horizontally between in-contact birds. Some breeds are genetically resistant (e.g. Fayoumi). Chicks that are congenitally infected are permanently viraemic, with immunotolerance of the ALSV, and do not produce antibodies. Affected birds shed the virus and infect any eggs. Most chicks are infected by horizontal transmission between young birds and so develop antibodies, without viraemia, but may occasionally shed virus to their eggs.

Post-mortem findings

The post-mortem examination may reveal a variable anaemia, an enlarged cherry-red liver and an enlarged spleen caused by infiltrating lymphoblasts. Diffuse or nodular creamy white tumours of the liver, spleen, kidneys, eyes or the visceral surfaces of flat bones (e.g. ribs, skull, pelvis, sternum) may also be seen. Osteopetrosis is rare, but can result in thickened long bones and excess bone formation at the diaphysis. Tumours of the bursa of Fabricus may metastasize to the liver and spleen.

Laboratory diagnosis

As the clinical signs are non-specific, the diagnosis rests on the post-mortem examination findings and virology. Histology of several birds may be required to differentiate these conditions from Marek's disease. Virus isolation and enzyme-linked immunosorbent assays (ELISAs) are available for ALSV.

Treatment and prevention

Control is based on virus eradication from the breeding adults, to produce birds that are ALSV-free, together with high standards of hygiene and flock management.

Reticuloendotheliosis virus

Aetiology and pathogenesis

This is another retrovirus that can cause development of B and T cell lymphomas in older birds or a runting syndrome in juvenile turkeys, chickens, ducks, pheasants, geese and Japanese quail. It is relatively rare in the UK, but in other countries tumours can be found sporadically in turkeys and less commonly in other species. The method of transmission can be horizontal between birds or vertical through the egg. Turkey stags can transmit the virus to their progeny. Infection has also occurred via contaminated Marek's disease and fowlpox vaccines, as well as through mosquito vectors.

Clinical signs

Birds with functional reticuloendotheliosis virus (REV) strains may develop runting with abnormal feathering and, occasionally, paralysis. The non-specific clinical signs that result in tumours in older birds need to be differentiated from Marek's disease, ALSV and lymphoproliferative disease in turkeys.

Post-mortem findings

On post-mortem examination, widespread changes may be evident. The spleen, kidneys and liver can be enlarged and mottled. In older birds, pale, white or yellow-white tumours can be seen in multiple organs, including the spleen, liver, pancreas, intestines, proventriculus, heart, kidney, lung, pectoral muscles, other skeletal muscles, thymus, subcutaneous tissues and coelomic cavity. These tumours can be confirmed with histopathology.

Laboratory diagnosis

Virus isolation and/or serology are required to confirm REV infection. The virus is sporadic and may not be associated with clinical signs.

Treatment and prevention

Horizontal transmission is more important than vertical transmission so high standards of hygiene and flock management can help to reduce clinical cases. Ultimately,

control is based on virus eradication from the breeding adults with the young being raised in isolation. Birds for export are generally required to be REV free.

Lymphoproliferative disease

Aetiology and pathogenesis

Lymphoproliferative disease virus (LPDV) affects turkeys but is rarely found in the UK. It is caused by a retrovirus, which is transmitted horizontally. There is an increased susceptibility in the first few weeks of life, with most cases occurring between 7 and 18 weeks of age.

Clinical signs

Affected birds may be dull, with sudden death in up to 20% of the flock. Affected birds are often anaemic.

Post-mortem findings

The post-mortem examination reveals an enlarged pale pink marbled spleen, together with a moderately enlarged liver with miliary grey/white foci. Miliary or diffuse tumours of visceral organs may also be seen with enlarged nerves.

Laboratory diagnosis

The diagnosis is made based on gross post-mortem findings, with histopathology and virus isolation used to confirm the presence of the infection.

Prevention

Control of LPDV is possible only by eliminating infected turkey strains from the flock, as each line varies in their susceptibility to the disease.

Chicken anaemia virus

Chicken anaemia virus (CAV) is also known as infectious anaemia, anaemia–dermatitis syndrome and blue wing disease.

Aetiology and pathogenesis

This is now an uncommon disease, as many adult birds are immune to CAV. It is caused by a circovirus. The virus is passed vertically from the parents to the chicks, but the chicks will be protected if the parents have been previously exposed to the virus. Birds >2 weeks old are able to produce antibodies to the virus, which protects their future chicks.

Clinical signs

Infected chicks <2 weeks old may be seen to be anaemic and haemorrhagic with secondary dermatitis. The virus causes general immunosuppression. Death occurs at 10–14 days old.

Post-mortem findings

The post-mortem examination may show anaemic chicks with pale bone marrow and thymus atrophy. A presumptive diagnosis is often based on post-mortem appearance and histopathological lesions. Confirmation requires detection of the virus or viral DNA in the thymus or bone marrow via polymerase chain reaction (PCR) techniques.

Prevention

Serology on the breeding parents can be undertaken. If the adult birds have no immunity to CAV there is a risk of vertical transmission of the disease to the offspring. If this is the case, then a commercial vaccine can be administered that reduces the risk of disease in juvenile birds.

Inclusion body hepatitis

Aetiology and pathogenesis

Inclusion body hepatitis (IBH) is caused by an adenovirus (fowl adenovirus, virus FAdV). It is found in various species, including chickens, turkeys, pigeons and parrots, and can be isolated from both healthy and diseased flocks. The virus is widespread and can be transmitted both horizontally and vertically.

Clinical signs

IBH can be seen in poults between 2 and 7 weeks old and is characterized by a sudden increase in mortality over 3–4 days, which then subsides. Generally, mortality is up to 10% of the flock, although it may reach up to 30% in severe outbreaks. In some cases, mortality will continue for 3 weeks. The birds may be dull, huddled together and have a slower growth rate. Affected birds may also be anaemic and jaundiced.

Post-mortem findings

On post-mortem examination, a swollen pale liver (Figure 21.2) is found with general organ haemorrhage and bone marrow depletion. Hepatitis and pancreatitis are identified on histopathology. It is unclear whether the adenovirus can result in immunosuppression alone or only in association with another infection such as CAV or infectious bursal disease (IBD). Retroviruses have also been identified in affected birds.

Laboratory diagnosis

Virus isolation from cloacal swabs or post-mortem tissue samples is possible to confirm the diagnosis. Serology is available, but is little used due to the widespread nature of avian adenoviruses.

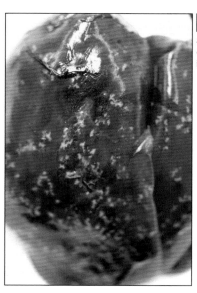

21.2 Typical gross post-mortem appearance of the liver in a chicken affected with inclusion body hepatitis.

Prevention

The virus is generally resistant to disinfectants. Good hygiene and avoiding immunosuppression in birds are important to reduce the risk of clinical disease.

Hydropericardium-hepatitis syndrome

This condition is also known as infectious hydropericardium or Angara disease.

Aetiology and pathogenesis

Hydropericardium-hepatitis syndrome is caused by an adenovirus (FAdV). There has only ever been one outbreak in Europe (in 2002), with other outbreaks seen in Central and South America, India, Iraq and Kuwait.

Clinical signs

The disease is similar to inclusion body hepatitis, but can cause mortality of up to 70%. The condition is found in 3–5-week-old broilers. Affected birds are dull, stunted with ruffled feathers and produce yellow mucoid droppings.

Post-mortem findings

The post-mortem examination may reveal hepatitis, hydropericardium and bursitis. Histopathology can aid a presumptive diagnosis.

Laboratory diagnosis

Virus isolation from post-mortem tissues can be used to confirm the diagnosis.

Prevention

Inactivated vaccines have been developed in countries that have the disease for use in local outbreaks. Spread of the virus is horizontal, so reducing the movement of people between farms has been important in reducing the transmission of the disease. Good hygiene, particularly with reference to water provision, is important to reduce transmission. Hydropericardium-hepatitis syndrome is often found with IBH in combined outbreaks.

Big liver and spleen disease

Aetiology and pathogenesis

This condition is caused by an avian hepevirus and is found both in poults and laying hens. The route of transmission is horizontal, typically via the faecal–oral route. Disease is caused by immune complexes forming in the tissues.

Clinical signs

Clinical signs are seen in birds over 24 weeks old and include pale, dull birds, soiled vent feathers, premature moulting and increased mortality. There is a 3–4 week drop in egg production and then a subsequent 5 weeks taken for full recovery.

Post-mortem findings

An enlarged spleen, possibly with pale foci, together with an enlarged liver, possibly with subcapsular haemorrhage, are seen post mortem.

Laboratory diagnosis

The post-mortem presentation can be typical for this condition, but the diagnosis is best confirmed by antibody or antigen-based ELISA serology. A reverse transcription polymerase chain reaction (RT-PCR) is also available. The virus occurs naturally in chickens, so it can be difficult to determine whether the virus was the primary problem. Virus propagation is not yet possible, so it may be difficult to confirm the disease.

Prevention

There is no specific treatment for this condition, so prevention is based on biosecurity and house hygiene. Particular attention should be paid to reducing faecal contamination of drinking water.

Marble spleen disease
Aetiology and pathogenesis

This disease is seen in pheasants and is caused by an adenovirus (genus *Siadenovirus*). The disease is widespread and endemic. It is transmitted via the faecal–oral route. Pheasants >1 month old are resistant.

Clinical signs

The adenovirus causes an acute respiratory disease in pheasants, which is characterized by dyspnoea, asphyxiation, depression and death. Morbidity can approach 100% of the flock. Mortality is commonly 2–3%, but can reach 15%. Secondary bacterial infections as a result of immunosuppression have also been noted.

Post-mortem findings

On post-mortem examination, an enlarged mottled spleen and pulmonary congestion may be evident. Histopathology of tissue samples confirms tertiary bronchi filled with fibrin and haemorrhage, as well as generalized vascular congestion and focal necrosis. Characteristically, splenomegaly with lymphoreticular hyperplasia and lymphoid necrosis occur. Basophilic (magenta-coloured) intranuclear inclusions may be found in a variety of tissues, including the spleen.

Laboratory diagnosis

The condition can be confirmed by PCR and agar gel diffusion should this be required.

Treatment and prevention

Antibiotics may be used to control secondary infections; if possible, the choice of antibiotic should be based on susceptibility profiles from post-mortem cases. Good biosecurity, and the use of vaccines administered in water when the bird is 1 month old, can confer lifelong protection. Haemorrhagic enteritis vaccines intended for use in turkeys should not be used for pheasants because the avirulent isolates in the turkey vaccines are typically virulent in pheasants. Vaccines should not be administered to birds exhibiting signs of illness.

Haemorrhagic enteritis
Aetiology and pathogenesis

This disease is seen in turkeys, generally 6–12 weeks of age, and is caused by a similar virus to marble spleen disease of pheasants. The disease is endemic and widespread. Turkey poults under 3–4 weeks of age are resistant to infection due to age-related resistance or, more commonly, the presence of maternally derived antibodies. Transmission is horizontal via the faecal–oral route.

Clinical signs

The clinical signs can include depression, pallor and bloody droppings in outbreaks involving virulent serotypes. Acute mortality can be up to 60%, with an average of 10–15% over a 2-week period. Birds that survive the acute phase experience a transient immunosuppression related to the lymphotropic, lymphocytopathic nature of the virus. This often manifests in the form of secondary bacterial infections, which may lead to a second peak in mortality.

Post-mortem findings

Gross congestion and occasional intraluminal haemorrhage in the proximal small intestine are evident on post-mortem examination. The spleen is usually enlarged, friable and can be mottled white unless there has been extensive haemorrhage. Histopathological changes seen in the intestine include congestion, haemorrhage and necrosis of the epithelium. Basophilic intranuclear inclusions can be found in the lymphocytes and macrophages from a variety of tissue samples, predominantly the spleen where lymphoreticular hyperplasia and lymphoid necrosis are noted.

Laboratory diagnosis

The diagnosis often rests on the clinical signs and typical gross port-mortem examination findings, but can be confirmed by PCR or agar gel diffusion.

Treatment and prevention

Virulent outbreaks of haemorrhagic enteritis have been successfully treated and controlled by the subcutaneous injection of antiserum obtained from recovered flocks. Controlling secondary infections is important and should be based on antibiotic susceptibility profiles for locally obtained *Escherichia coli* isolates. Good biosecurity and vaccination (which confers lifelong immunity) can be used for prevention, but should not be administered to birds showing signs of illness. Vaccines intended for use in turkeys must be used.

Turkey haemorrhagic enteritis
Aetiology and pathogenesis

Turkey haemorrhagic enteritis is caused by an adenovirus. It usually results in an acute enteritis in 6–12-week-old turkeys. The virus is transmitted horizontally between birds. Turkeys tend to develop antibodies and immunity between 8 and 19 weeks old.

Clinical signs

In acute cases, severe bloody droppings are seen 5–6 days post infection, with up to 60% sudden death. Variation in the virulence of the virus can lead to chronic disease with far less mortality.

Post-mortem findings

On post-mortem examination, the birds are found to be pale with haemorrhage and mucosal slough seen throughout the duodenum and, possibly, as far as the caecum in severe cases.

Treatment and prevention

Biosecurity is important to prevent horizontal transmission between birds and flocks. Prevention of acute cases is based on providing a clean, dry rearing house with dry feed and clean water at the correct temperature for the age of the birds. Vaccination is available in some countries.

Turkey viral hepatitis

Aetiology and pathogenesis

This is an acute contagious disease seen in turkeys caused by a picornavirus. It is seen in the USA, Canada, Italy and the UK. Birds affected are usually less than 6 weeks old. It is generally a subclinical condition and thus is only diagnosed during a routine post-mortem examination.

Clinical signs

The birds are depressed and anorexic with increased mortality, which can be precipitated by stress. There is high morbidity and low mortality, with the infection lasting 1–2 weeks. Infection in laying turkeys may reduce fertility. Birds greater than 6 weeks of age are more resistant to disease and mortality is rare.

Post-mortem examination

On post-mortem examination, there will be 1–2 mm of pale multifocal necrosis on the surface and deeper in the parenchyma of the liver.

Laboratory diagnosis

Electron microscopy of post-mortem tissues is required to confirm the presence of a picornavirus.

Treatment and prevention

There is no effective treatment or control method.

Duck viral hepatitis

Aetiology and pathogenesis

There are three forms of hepatitis attributed to three different viruses (adenovirus, astrovirus and picornavirus), which cause variable mortality in 2-day-old to 7-week-old birds. Ducks greater than 7 weeks old are immune to infection. These viruses are widespread and resistant in the environment, without any cross-protection between each virus. They are transmitted horizontally via ingestion from contaminated equipment, people and vehicles. The more common and internationally widespread of the three viruses is duck hepatitis virus (DHV) type 1, which is a member of the Picornaviridae from the new genus *Avihepatovirus*.

Clinical signs

The peracute infection may result in the sudden death of ducklings in good condition, with opisthotonus and mortality that may reach over 90%. Typically, these ducklings are less than 3 weeks of age. In an endemic area, the mortality rate may only be 5–10%.

Post-mortem findings

On post-mortem examination, an enlarged liver is found with petechial and ecchymotic haemorrhage. Older ducklings are likely to have secondary bacterial septicaemia and occasionally renal lipidosis.

Laboratory diagnosis

Bacterial septicaemia and duck viral enteritis are important differential diagnoses for this condition. Feed analysis is recommended to eliminate mycotoxin involvement. The diagnosis is confirmed by virus isolation from tissue samples obtained during the post-mortem examination as no other serological tests are available.

Treatment and prevention

Given the high and acute mortality rate there are few treatment options. However, it is possible to vaccinate ducks with a live attenuated DHV type 1 virus.

Bacterial diseases

Avian infectious hepatitis

Avian infectious hepatitis is also known as vibrionic hepatitis. Major differentials include avian leucosis/sarcoma virus (ALSV), histomoniasis, ulcerative enteritis, fowl cholera and typhoid.

Aetiology and pathogenesis

This condition is a slow onset disease of adult chickens, which is caused by *Vibrio*-like bacteria; subsequently identified as *Campylobacter jejuni*. It was seen regularly in the 1950s and 1960s and began to re-emerge in 2003. The bacteria are transmitted horizontally by faecal contamination. It is resistant in the environment and to many disinfectants, although morbidity is low. Birds remain carriers for months and disease is precipitated by stress.

Clinical signs

Birds are dull and not feeding, with diarrhoea and weight loss. The may be pale or jaundiced with a scaly comb.

Post-mortem findings

The post-mortem examination may reveal focal hepatic necrosis in 10% of the affected birds, which may also have a cauliflower-like 'spotty liver' with haematocysts under the capsule. Increased pericardial and perihepatic fluid can be seen.

Laboratory diagnosis

The diagnosis relies on the history of the bird, the lesions identified during the post-mortem examination and the isolation of the infective agent from bile samples using standard culture techniques.

Treatment and prevention

Treatment with antibiotics such as erythromycin (0.25 g/l of drinking water for 5 days), tiamulin (25 mg/l of drinking water for 5 days) or enrofloxacin (100 mg/l of drinking water daily for 5 days) may help to reduce mortality. In smaller numbers, parenteral treatment can be considered. Good hygiene and biosecurity will help to prevent this infection. To reduce the chance of infection, it is best to restock with birds that are confirmed to be free of disease. Stress should be reduced by ensuring that there is always access to feed and water, as well as the correct light and temperature in the house.

Streptococcus bovis septicaemia

Aetiology and pathogenesis

Streptococci and enterococci can cause septicaemia and localized infection in chickens, turkeys, ducks, pigeons and other birds. Diseases associated with streptococcal infections in poultry are relatively uncommon, but septicaemia caused by *S. bovis* is more common in ducks, pigeons and, occasionally, turkeys. Streptococci and/or enterococci have been isolated from birds with endocarditis, omphalitis, cellulitis, conjunctivitis, arthritis, osteomyelitis and amyloid arthropathy. Spread can be vertical via the egg or horizontal by oral or respiratory secretions.

Clinical signs

Birds may be dull, pale or cyanotic with ruffled bloody feathers around the head. Others may be lame or weak. Sudden death can occur. In chickens, the infection is more common in adult birds and mortality may reach 50%. In ducks, young birds are more commonly affected.

Post-mortem examination

The post-mortem examination may reveal a congested bird with a mottled spleen and a dark liver (which may have multifocal necrosis). *Streptococcus bovis* is commonly found in the intestinal tract of the pigeon, but not in other species.

Laboratory diagnosis

The clinical signs and lesions identified during the post-mortem examination are of a non-specific septicaemia, so a blood culture and antibiotic sensitivity testing is required to confirm the disease. A high white blood cell count may be identified on haematology, which may indicate the need for presumptive antibiotic therapy.

Treatment

Culture and sensitivity testing of tissue samples obtained during the post-mortem examination can aid antibiotic selection. Typical agents used in the face of *S. bovis* septicaemia include amoxicillin (15–20 mg/kg q24h for 3–5 days). This can be given orally or parenterally.

Arizona disease

Aetiology and pathogenesis

This disease is caused by the bacterium *Salmonella arizonae* (previously known as *Arizona hinshawii*) and is seen in turkeys and chickens. It is of main concern in North America, but has been isolated in other countries. It is not currently present in the UK. Mortality is 10–50% in young birds; older birds are asymptomatic carriers. Transmission is vertical through the egg and horizontal through faecal contamination of the environment by long-term carriers.

Clinical signs

Birds may be dull, huddled together and may have pasty diarrhoea, blindness with a deep opacity in the eye, nervous signs and paralysis. The ocular and nervous signs may be suggestive of arizonosis in the clinical setting.

Post-mortem findings

The post-mortem examination may reveal general signs of septicaemia with characteristic caseous plugs in the caeca, retinitis with a caseous disc or exudate covering the retina.

Laboratory diagnosis

The clinical signs and post-mortem findings are of a non-specific septicaemia, so isolation and identification methods specifically for *Salmonella* spp. are necessary. The ovary is an important site to obtain cultures at post mortem.

Treatment

The injection of antibiotics such as sulphonamides or fluoroquinolones at the hatchery is used in some countries. Eradication from the breeder population is possible with strict nest and hatchery hygiene to reduce faecal contamination of the eggs.

Tick-related anaemia

This condition is also known as spirochaetosis.

Aetiology and pathogenesis

Borrelia anserina is transmitted by the *Argas persicus* tick, which is found in North Africa, the Middle East and Asia. These ticks are also present in the USA, but disease is uncommon. The disease is not present in Europe. The spirochaete can infect a variety of birds, most commonly young fowl.

Clinical signs

Clinical signs may include anorexia, fever, depression, anaemia, cyanosis of the head, bile-stained droppings and, occasionally, paralysis before death.

Post-mortem findings

On post-mortem examination, there may be an enlarged mottled spleen and liver due to ecchymotic haemorrhage.

Laboratory diagnosis

The spirochaete can be seen on blood smears.

Treatment

Penicillins such as amoxicillin (15–20 mg/kg orally or parenterally daily for 3–5 days) and other antibiotics are very effective. Tick control will also help to reduce the incidence of infection. Vaccines have been developed, but as there are many serotypes, they can only be used locally.

Ulcerative enteritis

Aetiology and pathogenesis

This condition is caused by *Clostridium colinum* and affects chickens, turkeys, pheasants, guinea fowl and other birds, but not waterfowl. This strain of *Clostridium* is found worldwide, most commonly in chickens and turkeys that are between 4 and 10 weeks old. It causes up to 10% mortality in affected birds, but causes 100% mortality in Bobwhite quail. Immunosuppression due to other agents (e.g. CAV, IBD and coccidiosis) may result in clinical disease in conjunction with overcrowding and poor hygiene.

Clinical signs

The birds will be dull and huddled together. They may also be anorexic and have watery droppings.

Post-mortem findings

The post-mortem examination may reveal a haemorrhage duodenitis with small ulcers throughout the gastrointestinal tract (Figure 21.3). These ulcers gradually coalesce to penetrate the serosa, causing peritonitis. The liver may have necrotic foci and there may be haemorrhagic splenomegaly.

Treatment

Good hygiene and management is essential to control the disease.

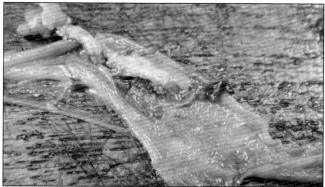

21.3 Ulcerative duodenitis in the intestine of a quail viewed during the post-mortem examination.

Fungal diseases

Favus

This condition is also known as scaly/white comb.

Aetiology and pathogenesis

Favus is caused by *Microsporidium gallinae* and is usually seen only in backyard chickens and, occasionally, in turkeys. It tends to affect just one bird, although it is slowly transmitted horizontally in the environment.

Clinical signs

White scaly lesions are seen on non-feathered skin (i.e. the comb, wattles and shanks) with superficial invasion of the skin.

Laboratory diagnosis

The diagnosis is confirmed by histopathology or fungal culture (which may be difficult), but in many cases treatment is based on the clinical presentation.

Treatment

Topical antifungals such as enilconazole or itraconazole are commonly prescribed for individual birds. Affected birds should be isolated for treatment and the environment should be disinfected. For further information, the reader is referred to Chapter 13.

Parasitic diseases

Red mite and northern mite infestations

Aetiology and pathogenesis

Red mites (*Dermanyssus gallinae*) (Figure 21.4) and northern fowl mites (*Ornithonyssus sylviarum*) are commonly seen blood-sucking ectoparasites (see Chapter 13 for more information). Levels of infestation increase during the spring,

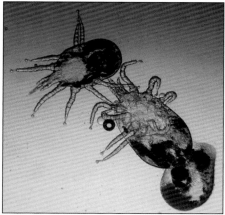

21.4 Microscopic image of red mites (*Dermanyssus gallinae*) from a chicken coop.

as the environmental temperature rises with life cycles being completed in 2 weeks. Red mites are found in the dark cracks and crevices of the house, so are seen more easily at night with the aid of a torch. Red mites are commonly located around the nest boxes and cause irritation to the birds when they are laying. Northern mites are similar to red mites, but live only on the bird.

Clinical signs

Birds will lose weight and are commonly seen with feather loss over the breast due to pruritus. There is a drop in egg laying and streaks of blood may be seen on the eggs. Affected birds may also appear dull with dirty tail base feathers. In severe cases, birds are weak, collapsed and anaemic. Death can result from anaemia with heavy infestation.

Treatment

Eliminating red mites can be difficult as both the birds and the environment require treatment; longer term environmental control can be used to avoid any egg withhold times in less severe outbreaks. Cleaning the house regularly will help control mite numbers and rotation of the type of environmental treatment is important to avoid resistance. Diatomaceous earth can be used in dust baths, as well as dusted around the nest boxes and the rest of the house, and causes desiccation of the mites that come into contact with it. Birds can be individually treated with a pyrethrum powder or topical ivermectin. Further discussion of the treatment and prevention of mites is given in Chapters 7 and 13.

Leucocytozoonosis

Aetiology and pathogenesis

This disease has been described in ducks, geese, turkeys and chickens and is caused by various *Leucocytozoon* spp. throughout the world. The protozoa are spread by blood-feeding vectors such as blackfly (*Simulium* spp.) found near fast-flowing rivers and midges (*Culicoides* spp.) seen in damp and dirty conditions. The parasites develop in the salivary glands of the vector and are transmitted by inoculation during feeding. The condition has not been reported in poultry in the UK, but has been the cause of fatal outbreaks in captive psittacine birds, owls and raptors exposed to vectors in outdoor aviaries. Chronic subclinical infections provide a source of infection, allowing epidemic outbreaks during the summer.

Clinical signs

Birds are inappetent, weak and anaemic, leading to death.

Laboratory diagnosis

Gamonts can be demonstrated in a blood smear to confirm disease.

Treatment and prevention

Control is via limiting exposure to the vectors by screening poultry houses. Prevention of infection is possible using pyrimethamine (1 ppm) and sulfadimethoxine (10 ppm) in feed. Treatment of individual birds has not been reported; however, in other species, pyrimethamine at a dose of 0.5 mg/kg orally q12h for 4 days or melarsomine at a dose of 0.25 mg/kg i.m. q24h for 4 days has been used (subject to prescribing regulations).

Capillaria
Aetiology and pathogenesis

Capillaria are the smallest and most pathogenic of the gastrointestinal nematodes. Different species of *Capillaria* are found in different sections of the gastrointestinal tract, including the oesophagus and the crop. These nematodes affect chickens, guinea fowl, turkeys, geese, pheasants and other birds.

Clinical signs

Severe disease can lead to weight loss and weakness in older birds, whilst in young birds with intestinal *Capillaria* bloody diarrhoea, anaemia and death may be seen.

Laboratory diagnosis

Faecal screening for *Capillaria* is an important diagnostic tool in the sick bird. Routine screening is also advised.

Treatment

Treatment with a licensed product is advised. More details on gastrointestinal nematodes can be found in Chapter 16.

Proventricular or gizzard worms
Aetiology and pathogenesis

Amidostomum anserii can cause ulceration at the isthmus between the gizzard and proventriculus margin in ducks and geese. Proventricular worms are less commonly encountered than other nematodes.

Clinical signs

The clinical signs associated with the presence of proventricular worms include weight loss, anaemia and weakness, particularly in young goslings.

Laboratory diagnosis

Routine screening is recommended.

Treatment

Regular deworming with licensed products such as fluben-dazole is advised if there is an ongoing problem. The reader is referred to Chapter 7 for details on preventive measures.

Miscellaneous systemic conditions
'Flipover'

Flipover is also known as a heart attack or sudden death syndrome.

Aetiology and pathogenesis

This condition was first diagnosed over 50 years ago and results in the sudden death of fast-growing poults, with up to 2% of the flock being affected. The affected birds will be large and healthy with full crops and over 70% of cases are cockerels. Only rapidly growing breeds appear to be affected.

Clinical signs

Death is peracute following a brief attack where the bird flaps its wings briskly and then dies, typically on its back. Mortality is most common in birds 1–3 weeks old, but can be seen in animals from 3 days to 3 months old.

Post-mortem findings

The post-mortem findings are non-specific and other cardiac conditions such as endocardiosis (Figure 21.5) may be identified during the examination.

Laboratory diagnosis

The cause of the condition is not clear, but it may possibly be due to an electrolyte and/or metabolite imbalance. A separate condition has been recognized in Australia in breeding broilers as they come into lay which is due to hypokalaemia.

Treatment and prevention

Altering management practices to reduce stress (e.g. reducing high intensity light and overcrowding) will help reduce mortality.

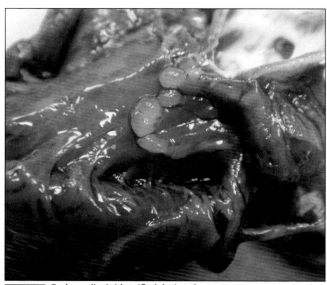

21.5 Endocardiosis identified during the post-mortem examination of a chicken.

Dissecting aneurysm or ruptured aorta

Aetiology and pathogenesis

Fast-growing male turkeys greater than 6 weeks old may bleed to death from a ruptured aorta. Turkeys of either sex may die from cardiac tamponade following rupture of the left atrium. Mortality is most commonly seen in birds 3–4 months old. These conditions are caused by systemic hypertension, which may also be associated with copper deficiency and rapid growth.

Clinical signs

The healthy turkey is found on its back with pale skin and possibly blood in its mouth.

Post-mortem findings

The post-mortem examination may reveal haemorrhage and a large clot in the ruptured aorta (with a longitudinal split between the external iliac and sciatic arteries), in the thoracic aorta dorsal to the heart or in the atrium, in the case of younger birds.

Prevention

Dissecting aneurysms and aortic rupture can be prevented by reducing the growth rate of the bird.

Fatty liver haemorrhagic syndrome

Aetiology and pathogenesis

Fatty liver haemorrhagic syndrome is seen in older layers of heavier breeds during hot weather, particularly if caged.

Clinical signs

Most cases are subclinical, but a fall in egg production and an increase in sudden death may be seen.

Post-mortem findings

The post-mortem examination may reveal that the liver is friable and putty coloured due to the increased fat content. Massive liver haemorrhage with swollen, pale kidneys and a large amount of abdominal fat may be seen. In subclinical cases, subcapsular haemorrhage, old haematomas and blood clots, with necrosis and other sites of recent minor haemorrhage, may be identified.

Laboratory diagnosis

Imaging such as radiography, ultrasonography or CT assessment may confirm hepatomegaly. Diagnosis in the live bird is dependent on histopathology of the liver. A biopsy sample can be obtained during surgery or coelioscopic examination (see Chapters 12 and 23 for details of these techniques). Histology reveals hepatocytes distended with fat globules that will eventually rupture the cell, together with inflammation, necrosis and regeneration.

The anticipated normal level of lipid in the liver can vary depending on the breed of bird, age and reproductive status. Although a fatty liver does not actually cause fatty liver haemorrhagic syndrome, it does predispose to haemorrhage and therefore is more common in heavier, older birds. Haemorrhage occurs as a result of trauma to a friable liver.

Treatment

Fatty liver haemorrhagic syndrome is a multifactorial condition. Birds are often fed an *ad libitum* high-energy diet, containing, in particular, high levels of corn, which may lead to obesity. Low linoleic acid and selenium levels exacerbate this condition. High temperatures result in less activity in caged birds that have little room to exercise and this will lead to increased stress levels. Thus, providing a balanced diet is of the utmost importance. Should a diagnosis be confirmed in a live bird, treatment is based on increasing activity, dietary modifications and hepatic support. Treatment for hepatic lipidosis includes anabolic steroids and levothyroxine sodium, both of which increase the catabolism of fat. Amino acids (e.g. carnitine and methionine) can also be administered to encourage fat metabolism.

Visceral gout

This condition is also known as avian urolithiasis, acute toxic nephritis, renal gout, kidney stones, nutritional gout and nephrosis.

Aetiology and pathogenesis

Visceral gout results from the accumulation of uric acid and its subsequent deposition in the tissues. This is essentially the result of end-stage renal disease and can be due to many inciting causes such as obstruction of the ureters, renal damage and dehydration. Other causes include infectious diseases, nutritional problems, electrolyte imbalances and toxins.

- Visceral gout following dehydration is observed in newly hatched chicks following overheating or being kept in the hatchery too long.
- A high-calcium, low-phosphorus diet in immature pullets can cause serious kidney damage. All calcium and phosphorus levels in the feed provided should follow recommendations for the age and variety of bird.
- Vitamin A deficiency over a long period of time can cause damage to the lining of the ureters, but is unusual.
- Diets that increase urine alkalinity can also contribute to gout mortality in pullets and layers.

Clinical signs

Chickens with renal damage can continue to be productive until less than a third of the kidney remains functional. This makes the diagnosis difficult, as there are minimal clinical signs until the point of sudden death.

Post-mortem findings

The post-mortem examination may reveal chalky white urate deposits in the renal tubules and on the serous layers of the heart, liver, mesentery, air sacs and peritoneum. In acute disease, these are not calcified, whereas, in more chronic cases, calcification can lead to these structures being evident radiographically. There is compensatory enlargement of any remaining normal kidney tissue in an attempt to maintain renal function.

Laboratory diagnosis

The evaluation of renal parameters on a biochemistry panel should be regularly performed (see Chapter 10) and any elevation in blood uric acid levels should prompt further investigation of renal pathology and function. In most cases, this will involve a coelioscopic examination and renal biopsy (see Chapter 12). Visceral urate deposits can also be easily visualized on endoscopy. Dystrophic calcification of damaged tissues can occur and this can be seen radiographically.

Treatment and prevention

Serial monitoring of uric acid levels is important. If high uric acid levels are identified, then treatment with allo-purinol (at a dose of 10 mg/kg orally q24h) should be insti-gated. This treatment may be lifelong. Allopurinol prevents the production of uric acid by inhibiting xanthine oxidase. Other agents that may be used include rasburicase, which converts existing uric acid to allantonin. Prevention of visceral gout centres on controlling all possible predis-posing problems, including correcting any dietary imbal-ances and providing a clean and constant water supply.

Omphalitis
Aetiology and pathogenesis

Omphalitis (yolk sac infection) arises due to contamination of the yolk sac with microbes (typically bacteria such as coliforms, *Staphylococcus*, *Streptococcus* and *Proteus*) from when the chick hatches.

Clinical signs

Chicks within the first few days of life may be presented as small, dull, hunched birds because of a yolk sac infection (Figure 21.6). These birds are often called 'non-starters'. Mortality peaks at around 5–7 days of age, although it can be seen from day 1. Any species can be affected.

Post-mortem findings

If the chick dies or is euthanased, a post-mortem examina-tion should be encouraged to enable samples to be col-lected for bacterial culture and to confirm the diagnosis. The post-mortem examination may reveal the yolk sac to be inflamed (Figure 21.7) and foul-smelling. Signs of septi-caemia may be present throughout the chick (e.g. an inflamed liver or spleen).

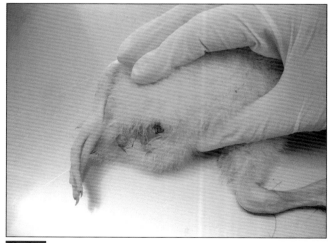

21.6 External appearance of a chick with omphalitis.

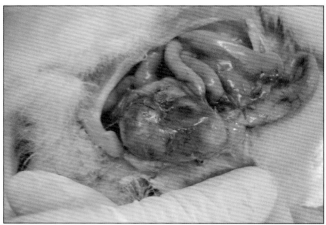

21.7 The post-mortem examination revealed that the yolk sac was discoloured, inflamed and had a foul odour.

Treatment

Affected chicks do not respond to medication with anti-biotics and thus surgical intervention (see Chapter 23 for information on omphalectomy) or euthanasia should be considered. Parenteral antibiotics should be administered to these cases. However, medical management with anti-biotics such as lincomycin and spectinomycin in the drinking water (marketed as a combination product at the dose rate of 227 mg/l and 555 mg/l of drinking water) or amoxicillin (15–20 mg/kg) daily for 3–5 days may improve the chances of survival of any mildly affected chicks and help protect the health of any other chicks in the flock. Culture and sensitivity testing should be undertaken, but antibiotics need to be initiated as soon as the problem has been identified.

Prevention

To help reduce yolk sac infections, only clean, unwashed eggs should be incubated and the brooding environment should be cleaned between flocks. Fresh, dry shavings should be provided and drinking water should be treated regularly with a commercially available water sanitizer to reduce contamination.

'Starve outs'
Aetiology and pathogenesis

'Starve out' occurs at around 4 days of age if the chick has not started eating. The yolk sac provides nutrition for the first 24 hours of a chick's life, after which it should start eating. If the chick does not eat, it will gradually fade away.

Clinical signs

The crop and its contents are easily palpated when the bird has consumed chick crumb. If the chick has not started to eat, it will be small, dull and have an empty crop.

Post-mortem findings

The post-mortem examination may reveal that the chick is dehydrated with tacky, dry subcutaneous tissues and dark muscles. White urate deposits may be visible throughout the kidneys due to dehydration. Litter or bedding may be present in the crop, which is otherwise empty. A soft, fatty liver and enlarged gallbladder may be identified.

Treatment and prevention

To encourage chicks to begin eating and drinking, fresh, dry feed and clean water should be readily accessible. Chicks also need to be kept at the correct temperature and humidity for their species, with sufficient light (>40 lux) to encourage feeding. It may be beneficial to add electrolytes to the drinking water (e.g. Solulyte) to facilitate rehydration. Crop feeding should be undertaken, alongside fluid therapy, for any chick that has become ill and not started to feed, whilst husbandry practices are corrected. Emergency care is discussed in Chapter 8.

References and further reading

Pattison M, McMullin P, Bradbury J and Alexander D (2007) *Poultry Diseases, 6th edn*. Elsevier, Philadelphia
Saif YM (2008) *Diseases of Poultry, 12th edn*. Wiley-Blackwell, Oxford

Useful information

The Poultry Health Course, the Pirbright Institute
https://www.pirbright.ac.uk/events/poultry-health-course

Chapter 22

Anaesthesia and analgesia

Steve Smith

Historically, birds were thought to be unable to feel pain because they fail to demonstrate the typical signs. Unfortunately, this is something that is still echoed today in some older texts and on internet forums. However, in the last 20 years, evidence-based avian studies have shown nociception in birds is similar to that in mammals, and has been demonstrated by anatomical, functional and biochemical studies. As veterinary surgeons (veterinarians), we accept that backyard poultry feel pain. Anaesthesia and analgesia must be used carefully to alleviate suffering and reduce stress in patients. Backyard poultry are prey species and susceptible to the negative effects of excessive stress. There are numerous procedures (e.g. radiography, blood sample collection) where anaesthesia may be used to simply reduce the stress associated with handling, even though the procedure is not painful. Chickens are the main focus of this chapter, but the techniques can apply equally to other species of backyard poultry, and specific differences will be highlighted where relevant.

Requirements for anaesthesia

Anatomical and physiological considerations

Successful anaesthesia depends on an understanding of avian anatomy, physiology and pharmacology, with the pulmonary and cardiovascular systems being most important. The scope of this chapter does not allow full explanation of comparative avian anatomy (see Chapter 2), but some clinically relevant points are highlighted and readers are directed to the References and further reading for more information.

Pulmonary system

Birds have two distinct functional pulmonary components: those responsible for ventilation (airways, air sacs, thoracic skeleton and muscles of respiration) and those involved in gaseous exchange (lungs). The opening of the trachea (glottis) is located at the base of the tongue, therefore more cranial than in mammals, and is not protected by an epiglottis. The trachea comprises complete tracheal rings, so cuffed endotracheal (ET) tubes should not be used in order to avoid inadvertent tracheal necrosis and stricture formation as the result of excessive cuff inflation. The avian trachea is generally longer and wider than a comparably sized mammalian trachea, so the overall resistance is similar. However, this creates a larger dead space, which is compensated for by a relatively lower respiratory frequency. Sound is produced by the syrinx at the level of the tracheal bifurcation in the cranial body cavity. This means that ventilation can produce sound and this does not suggest oesophageal intubation as may be suspected in a mammal. There are a variable number (7–9) of avascular air sacs (that may include one clavicular and one or two cervical, craniothoracic and abdominal air sacs) that act as bellows to the lung. These air sacs do not participate in gaseous exchange or accumulate anaesthetic gases.

Muscular activity is required to drive respiration. During inhalation, air moves down the trachea, bypassing the paleopulmonic parabronchi (main lung area) via aerodynamic valves, and through the neopulmonic parabronchi into the caudal air sacs. When the bird exhales, air moves back through the neopulmonic parabronchi and into the paleopulmonic parabronchi, where 75–80% of gaseous exchanges takes place (the remaining 20–25% occurs in the neopulmonic parabronchi). During the next inhalation, the exhaled air continues through the paleopulmonic parabronchi and passes into the cranial air sacs, and on the second expiration it exits via the trachea. Therefore, it takes two respiratory cycles for air to be moved through the avian respiratory system. During intermittent positive pressure ventilation (IPPV), it is possible for the direction of gas flow is the lung to be reversed, but this does not affect efficiency. The lung tissue comprises an intricate intercapillary anastomosing network that firmly anchors the air capillaries to the blood capillaries, in a cross current gaseous exchange arrangement, forming the rigid lung that has a constant volume during all phases of ventilation. These factors explain how the pulmonary system of a bird is 10 times more efficient than that of a mammal (O'Malley, 2005), and why birds are more sensitive to the effects of inhalational anaesthesia.

Cardiovascular system

Birds have a four-chambered heart that, compared with a similar sized mammal, is relatively larger, has a greater stroke volume, a lower heart rate and higher cardiac output. The avian heart receives a higher density of both sympathetic and parasympathetic fibres and appears more sensitive to catecholamine-induced arrhythmias. Birds have a renal portal system, which is controlled by a valve in the external ileac vein that is innervated by cholinergic and adrenergic nerves. Adrenaline (epinephrine) causes this valve to relax, directing blood into the central circulation rather than to the renal parenchyma.

Planning, risk management and owner counselling

Natural instinct often makes birds mask signs of illness until late in the disease process, when rapid decompensation can easily occur. This, coupled with their unique anatomical and physiological adaptations, means that birds are often regarded as high-risk patients. However, knowledge and understanding of avian anatomy and physiology, thorough pre-anaesthetic evaluation and preparation, careful monitoring and rapid intervention can help to avoid most complications. Owners should be fully informed of the risks involved, including the presence of undetected diseases that may unexpectedly increase the anaesthetic risks.

Physical examination

Every patient should undergo a thorough physical examination prior to anaesthesia (see Chapter 8). Quiet observation of the bird in the cage or carrier is essential to assess demeanour, posture, breathing and general awareness of the environment. Auscultation of the heart, lungs and air sac system should be performed and the keel should be palpated to assess overall body condition, as well as nutritional and hydration status. An accurate bodyweight should be obtained for subsequent dosage calculations. If a bird is very sick, depressed or dyspnoeic then some clinicians elect to anaesthetize the patient prior to extensive clinical examination to avoid excessive stress before anaesthesia.

Acclimatization

Poultry are often social and confident birds and should be allowed time to acclimatize to the hospital environment prior to anaesthesia. This allows stress levels (and circulating catecholamines) to reduce following clinical examination, making subsequent anaesthesia safer and allowing any further signs of disease to become apparent.

Fasting

The need to withhold food from chickens prior to anaesthesia remains debatable. Arguments against fasting are that birds have a high metabolic rate and will rapidly become hypoglycaemic. However, a chicken with a full crop will also be at risk of regurgitation and aspiration during anaesthesia and recovery. In addition, an empty stomach reduces the weight of coelomic viscera on the respiratory system. A reasonable approach is to withhold food long enough for the upper gastrointestinal tract (especially the crop) to be empty, which is likely to be 2–6 hours unless there is a specific problem affecting motility. Often birds will already have had food withheld for this time period, and the crop can be palpated to check for contents. In urgent situations where fasting is not possible and the crop is full, the bird can be held upright for anaesthesia induction with a finger placed just below the mandible to close the oesophagus. Water should be provided until immediately prior to anaesthesia.

Preparation

Every procedure should be carefully planned and all required equipment must be organized, on hand and ready to use before beginning to handle the bird. All medications should be drawn up ready for administration and emergency drugs should be pre-calculated (and even prepared in syringes) to avoid time-wasting in the event of an emergency. The author finds it useful to simply run through the whole procedure, step-by-step, out loud, whilst checking everything is ready for the procedure.

Premedication

Premedication is not commonly administered in birds since the potential benefits are normally outweighed by the stress of handling for administration. There may be some benefit to the anaesthetic-sparing effects of opioids as premedication. Atropine is often suggested to reduce salivary secretion, but it can also thicken the already viscous tracheal mucus. The use of midazolam, intranasally, as a premedication is increasing in popularity. If sedatives or tranquilizers are used, they should not excessively delay recovery or cause disorientation.

General anaesthetic protocols

Inhalational anaesthesia

For backyard poultry, inhalational anaesthesia is simple, relatively safe, effective and generally considered the method of choice. Inhaled agents offer several advantages for patient management:

- Rapid induction and recovery, especially when agents with low blood solubility are used (i.e. isoflurane and sevoflurane)
- Faster control of anaesthetic depth
- Improved oxygenation due to the use of oxygen as the carrier gas
- Recovery that is not dependent on metabolic or excretory pathways, which may be altered or impaired in the diseased bird.

Inhalational anaesthesia uses the concept of minimum alveolar concentration, which is defined as 'the alveolar concentration of anaesthetic gas that prevents muscular movement in response to a painful stimulus in 50% of patients'. This allows the relative potencies of anaesthetics to be compared and provides a guide to what percentage of the agent needs to be delivered. However, as birds do not have an alveolar lung, a more applicable term may be **minimum anaesthetic concentration** (MAC). The principle volatile agents available in veterinary practice are isoflurane and sevoflurane. Some of the more important properties of each agent are described here, but for more detailed information the reader is referred to Hall *et al.* (2001).

Summary of inhalational anaesthetic protocol for a chicken

1. Carefully plan the anaesthetic protocol. Prepare all equipment and medication needed (including provision of fluids, warmth and emergency drugs).
2. Perform a pre-anaesthetic examination (if appropriate).
3. Induce anaesthesia (using a mask) with 5% isoflurane in 100% oxygen after a 15–20 second period of pre-oxygenation.
4. Perform endotracheal intubation with a non-cuffed ET tube.
5. Maintain anaesthesia using 1.5–2.5% isoflurane, using reflexes and monitoring aids to maintain the bird at the appropriate anaesthetic depth.
6. Recover the bird, which should be wrapped gently in a towel until able to wriggle free and stand unaided.

Anaesthetic agents

Isoflurane: This is currently the most widely used anaesthetic agent in birds. Isoflurane has a low blood:gas partition coefficient (solubility), which means it has rapid induction and recovery qualities. Only around 1% is metabolized in the body, with the remainder being exhaled. Isoflurane is known to have a pungent odour and can be irritant to respiratory mucosa, but this effect appears mild in poultry. It causes cardiovascular and respiratory depression similar to that seen in mammals. MAC is reported as 1.3–1.44% in bird species. Induction of anaesthesia with isoflurane should be carried out at 5% and clinical experience suggests maintenance requires 1.5–2.5%, despite the reported MAC being lower. Isoflurane is the author's inhalational agent of choice for backyard poultry anaesthesia.

Sevoflurane: This produces dose-related respiratory depression and cardiovascular effects similar to that of isoflurane. It does possess an even lower solubility than isoflurane, suggesting slightly quicker induction and recovery. Five percent of sevoflurane is metabolized in the body. One significant difference with sevoflurane is that it is non-irritant to respiratory passages, so induction of anaesthesia is not complicated by discomfort or breath-holding. MAC in chickens is reported as 2.2%, but induction of anaesthesia is carried out at 8% and maintenance usually requires 3–5% sevoflurane. Sevoflurane is reported to be degraded by carbon dioxide absorbents to Compound A, which is nephrotoxic to rats. Toxicity has not been reported in human anaesthesia, and is unlikely to be a problem in birds because few avian patients are large enough to require a re-breathing circuit that contains soda lime. In birds, the potentially faster induction and recovery times are not strongly supported in the literature, and are not clinically significant to the author.

Halothane: This agent should not be used in avian anaesthesia as it sensitizes the heart to catecholamine-induced arrhythmias. This leads to spontaneous cardiac and respiratory arrest in birds, leaving little hope of successful resuscitation. With isoflurane and sevoflurane, there is a delay between respiratory and cardiac arrest, allowing successful intervention should they occur, making both agents preferable to halothane. In many countries, halothane is now unavailable as its use has been superseded by isoflurane and sevoflurane.

Nitrous oxide: Although rarely practiced, nitrous oxide can be used as an adjunct to inhalational anaesthesia in birds. It is not potent enough to induce anaesthesia on its own; however, it does allow for a reduction in isoflurane levels required for maintenance. Nitrous oxide is often associated with rapid diffusion into closed gas-filled spaces, but since the avian air sacs freely communicate with the respiratory system, the use of nitrous oxide is not contraindicated. The main limitation to nitrous oxide use in birds is the frequent presence of subclinical respiratory disease. Thus, the author prefers to use 100% oxygen as the anaesthetic carrier gas in order to maintain maximum oxygenation.

Equipment

Inhalational anaesthesia requires specific equipment, such as an oxygen source, vaporizer, breathing circuit and effective scavenging mechanism, which is standard in most veterinary practices. Small or paediatric non-breathing systems (such as the modified Ayres T-piece (Figure 22.1) are required for maintenance of anaesthesia. These are ideal for birds weighing <5 kg because they offer minimal resistance to patient ventilation. The inherent resistance of rebreathing circuits makes them impractical for avian anaesthesia. Gaseous flow rate should be based on an estimation of tidal volume and minute volume, then subject to the circuit factor. Tidal volume in chickens is approximately 20 ml/kg (King and McLelland, 1988), so assuming a respiratory rate of 20 breaths per minute, this creates a minute volume of 400 ml/min/kg. Using a modified Ayres T-piece would therefore require an oxygen flow rate of approximately 0.8–1.2 l/min/kg bodyweight.

Anaesthetic induction

Induction of anaesthesia is simplest via a mask. The bird should be carefully wrapped in a towel with the head exposed. Restraint should be gentle enough to avoid impeding ventilation, but firm enough to prevent flapping or retraction of the head from the mask. Standard facemasks are usually adequate (see Figure 22.1), but for smaller birds syringe cases can be cut and adapted. To avoid infection risks, plastic disposable drinking cups can be used. The mask is placed over the head of the bird (Figure 22.2) and, if required, cotton wool should be placed between the mask and neck of the bird to prevent the escape of anaesthetic gas. Brief pre-oxygenation is recommended (15–20 seconds) and then delivery of the inhalational agent can

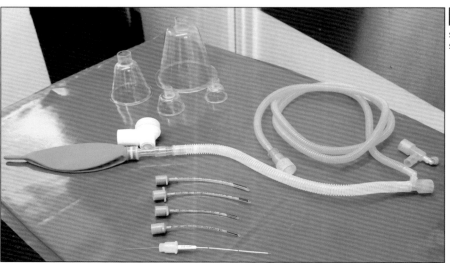

22.1 Equipment used for anaesthesia in poultry. Modified T-piece breathing system, non-cuffed endotracheal tubes and a selection of masks.

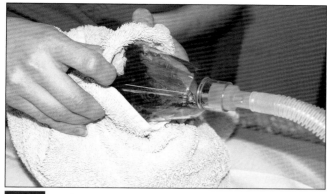

22.2   Mask induction of anaesthesia.

begin, using 5% isoflurane or 8% sevoflurane. Incremental induction (starting at 1% and increasing by 0.5% every 10–15 seconds) prolongs the anaesthetic induction and increases stress and is not recommended by the author. The use of an anaesthetic chamber is not advised as the patient will flap and thrash unacceptably and potentially damage itself. Occasionally, a *diving response* can occur where, upon application of a mask, the bird becomes bradycardic and apnoeic. This is more a feature of water-fowl and is actually a stress response due to stimulation of the trigeminal receptors in the beak and nares. Reducing the concentration of volatile agent used or switching to injectable anaesthesia will overcome this problem.

Endotracheal intubation

Placement of an ET tube is recommended in all but the shortest procedures. Even very small backyard birds can be endotracheally intubated using intravenous cannulae, although these should be monitored for obstruction with respiratory secretions. Intubation is straightforward because the glottis lies at the base of the tongue (Figure 22.3). Pulling the tongue forward with plastic forceps allows easy visualization of the tracheal opening and placement of a 2.0–4.0 mm ET tube (depending on the size of the bird). Some species of waterfowl have a bony protuberance from the ventral floor of the glottis making endotracheal intubation trickier and requiring a smaller tube than expected. Non-cuffed ET tubes (see Figure 22.1) should be used as birds have complete tracheal rings.

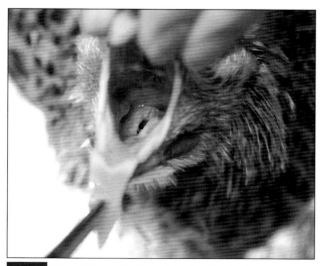

22.3   View of the glottis for endotracheal intubation.

Over inflation of a cuff is likely to lead to tracheal injury and possible stricture formation.

The ET tube can be secured in place by attaching tape or tying a bandage to the ET tube, crossing it over under-neath the beak and then tying behind the head of the bird (Figure 22.4). Great care should be taken not to cause excessive movement of the ET tube within the trachea whilst moving the bird as this can also result in significant tracheal injury. Endotracheal intubation facilitates inter-mittent positive pressure ventilation should it be indicated, protects the airway from reflux and reduces exposure of personnel to anaesthetic waste gases. It should be remem-bered that birds can still vocalize when intubated because of the presence of the syrinx at the tracheal bifurcation. Furthermore, vocalization can occur on both inhalation and exhalation, and can be induced by mechanical ventilation. The mucosal membranes of the trachea produce viscous mucus, so after 15–20 minutes thick secretions can block the ET tube or airway. These secretions should be removed via a urinary catheter using suction.

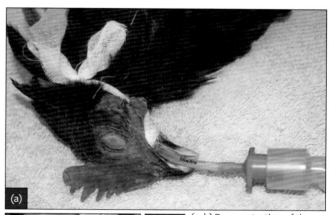

22.4   (a, b) Demonstration of the endotracheal tube tied in place with a bandage.

Anaesthetic maintenance

Following induction and endotracheal intubation, anaes-thesia can be maintained with isoflurane at 1.5–2.5% or sevoflurane at 3–5% delivered in 100% oxygen. Anaesthetic depth will need to be altered depending on the stimulus present, remembering that the increased efficiency of the avian respiratory system will allow changes in depth (both lighter and deeper) to occur more rapidly. Careful observa-tion and monitoring of breathing, withdrawal reflexes and corneal reflex by an attentive anaesthetist are the minimum requirements to ensure adjustments to the anaesthetic depth are made in a timely fashion.

Breathing is primarily achieved by lifting and releasing the sternum through the use of intercostal and pectoral muscles. Lifting of the sternum during inspiration requires strong muscle activity, whereas release during expiration is possible without much effort. Body position can affect ventilation, and in dorsal recumbency the weight of the abdominal viscera compresses the caudal air sacs and can significantly decrease ventilation. Thus, birds should be kept in lateral or sternal recumbency where possible. Interestingly, the volume of the avian respiratory system is 100–200 ml/kg compared with 45 ml/kg in dogs, but gas present in the air capillaries is only 10% compared with 96% in dogs. This lack of significant functional reserve in the lungs reduces the time a bird can remain apnoeic, so prompt action is required if the bird experiences respiratory arrest (see Anaesthetic emergencies below).

Under the depressant effects of anaesthetic drugs, the larger tracheal dead space becomes more relevant. A greater proportion of the minute volume now becomes dead space ventilation with no gaseous exchange, which may lead to hypoventilation and hypercapnia. Therefore, monitoring ventilation with a capnograph (see Monitoring below) is important in avian anaesthesia. Some clinicians routinely ventilate birds using a mechanical positive pressure ventilator to avoid this situation, but the author prefers to allow spontaneous ventilation (as a simple aid to monitoring anaesthetic depth) and will manually ventilate a bird periodically or continuously, as required in individual cases.

Body temperature

Due to their extensive air sac system and high metabolic rate, birds are prone to excessive heat loss and rapid reductions in core temperature under anaesthesia. Normal core body temperature is 39–42°C and monitoring should be undertaken to avoid hypothermia or hyperthermia during anaesthesia (temperatures exceeding 46°C will lead to death). The local environment should be kept warm with no draughts and heat can be provided with radiant heat lamps, warm air blanket systems or covered heat pads (care should be taken not to cause burns). Radiant heat sources are preferable as birds placed on a foam pad or warm water blanket still experience a 3–4°C decrease in core temperature within 20–30 minutes of anaesthetic induction. If it does not interfere with the surgical procedure, the body may be wrapped in bubble wrap or an exposure blanket to conserve heat. In addition, feather plucking of any site and the application of surgical scrub should be kept to the absolute minimum to reduce evaporative heat. Avian skin carries a much smaller bacterial load than mammalian skin, suggesting that exhaustive skin preparation is unnecessary.

Fluid therapy

Fluid therapy is very important during anaesthesia. For procedures longer than 30 minutes, a venous catheter should be placed in the brachial or tarsal vein. Fluids should be warmed to body temperature prior to administration. The author's fluid of choice is Hartmann's solution with added B-complex vitamins, electrolytes, amino acids and dextrose for use as supportive maintenance therapy in conditions of fluid loss at a ratio of 4:1. This should be given at a rate of 10 ml/kg/h, usually with a 10 ml/kg bolus at the start of the procedure. Syringe drivers are useful for the administration of fluids; alternatively, small boluses can be given at regular intervals.

Injectable anaesthesia

The main limitation of injectable anaesthetic protocols is the inability to modify the effects once administered. As with mammals, stress will affect the predictability of any given protocol and maintenance of an appropriate and stable plane of anaesthesia is challenging. These agents are typically metabolized by the liver or kidneys, but the clinician is often unaware of the status of these organs unless a blood sample has been tested prior to anaesthesia. However, there are certain situations where injectable anaesthesia may be preferable. Inhalational equipment may not always be available in the field and surgical procedures that disrupt the air sacs or pneumatic bones expose personnel to a high level of volatile agent if used. Although most drugs can be administered via either the intramuscular or intravenous route, the latter is more reliable and a lower total dose can often be used. Injection sites and techniques are detailed in Chapter 9. Many injectable anaesthetic protocols (Figure 22.5) have been published but doses are often empirical and pharmacokinetic studies are very limited.

Drug	Dose	Route of administration	Comments/uses
Atipamazole	5 times the mg dose of medetomidine	Intramuscular	Antagonizes sedative effects of medetomidine (also antagonizes analgesia)
Diazepam	0.5–1.0 mg/kg	Intramuscular, intravenous	Premedication; sedation; seizure control; intramuscular administration may cause muscle irritation and delayed absorption
Ketamine	20–40 mg/kg	Intramuscular	Not for use as sole agent; insufficient analgesia; poor muscle relaxation; prolonged (3 h) excitation on recovery
Ketamine (K) + diazepam (D)	75 mg/kg (K) + 2.5 mg/kg (D)	Intramuscular, intravenous	Protocols used where diazepam is given intravenously either 5 minutes before or 10 minutes after the ketamine is given intramuscularly. Recovery in 90–100 minutes
Ketamine (K) + medetomidine (M)	3–10 mg/kg (K) + 0.1–0.2 mg/kg (M)	Intramuscular	Short-term anaesthesia; can be antagonized
Ketamine (K) + xylazine (X)	10–25 mg/kg (K) + 1–2 mg/kg (X)	Intramuscular, intravenous	Recumbency within 6 mins; good surgical anaesthesia; can be antagonized. Can be improved with the addition of midazolam at 0.3 mg/kg
Medetomidine	0.25–0.34 mg/kg	Oral	Used for sedation; speed of onset is 6–10 mins
Midazolam	0.1–2 mg/kg	Intramuscular, intravenous, intranasal	Premedication at lower dose and sedation at higher doses. Shorter acting than diazepam
Propofol	5–10 mg/kg	Intravenous	Intubation and ventilation with oxygen recommended. Can be maintained with 0.5 mg/kg/min intravenous constant rate infusion
Yohimbine	0.2–2 mg/kg	Intramuscular	Antagonizes sedative effects of xylazine (also antagonizes analgesia)

22.5 Injectable anaesthetic drugs and protocols used in chickens.

Anaesthetic agents

Ketamine: This is a dissociative anaesthetic that has insufficient analgesic properties to be used alone for surgery. It does not cause muscle relaxation and birds become very excitable on recovery. It should rarely be used as a single agent, but preferably combined with alpha-2 agonists or benzodiazepines.

Alpha-2 agonists: The drug used most widely is medetomidine (some protocols include xylazine), which is often combined with ketamine. The alpha-2 agonists provide analgesia, muscle relaxation, contribute to a smooth recovery and can be antagonized. However, they are very depressant to the cardiovascular system and peripheral vasoconstriction can limit some monitoring aids.

Benzodiazepines: Midazolam and diazepam have more recently been used for premedication or combined with other drugs for their properties of muscle relaxation, sedation and anti-convulsion. They have minimal cardiovascular effects but also provide minimal analgesia and cause ataxia on recovery.

Propofol: This is a short-acting, non-barbiturate isopropyl phenol that must be administered intravenously. Induction is rapid with good muscle relaxation, but the duration of action is very short so intubation and inhalational anaesthesia is required or intravenous catheterization for a total intravenous protocol. As with dogs and cats, apnoea will occur with rapid administration. This may be considered in cases where intravenous access is already in place and gaseous induction would be less desirable.

Local anaesthesia

Local anaesthetics block the sodium channels in nerves, interfering with the conduction of impulses. When used pre-emptively the number and frequency of impulses are reduced, thereby reducing the overall upregulation of pain receptors. The use of local anaesthesia is controversial as the safety margins appear to be small in birds, genuine efficacy is difficult to prove and it does not reduce stress during the procedure. Local anaesthetics are absorbed into the bloodstream in the blocked region. This can be rapid in birds, and metabolism prolonged, increasing the potential for toxicity. Regional infiltration with a local line or splash block is the most common method. The skin and subcutaneous space in birds is thin, so a small gauge needle is recommended to make several small injections.

Lidocaine (without adrenaline) and bupivacaine are most commonly used, but neither the time to effect nor duration of action have been demonstrated in birds. The recommended maximum dose of lidocaine is 2–3 mg/kg and commercial preparations may need to be diluted for small chickens, but it is unknown whether a diluted solution remains effective. The safety index is low with doses of 4 mg/kg causing seizures and death. Bupivacaine has a longer duration of activity in mammals (undetermined in birds) and is often used conservatively at 2 mg/kg because of concern that any toxic effects will last longer (Hawkins and Paul-Murphy, 2011). Higher doses have shown to be no more effective or toxic in other birds. Toxic effects include drowsiness, recumbency, fine tremors, ataxia, seizures, stupor, cardiovascular effects and death; these effects can be sudden with inadvertent intravenous administration.

Analgesia

Attempting to provide an overview of clinically relevant evidence-based analgesia in backyard poultry is challenging due to the lack of specific data. There is much diversity across avian species with respect to their response to analgesic medications, and it has even been shown that there is genetic variation in the response to pain on an individual level in different breeds of chickens. To be able to assess pain, or the efficacy of analgesia, the clinician must have a good understanding of normal behaviour for the bird and remember that, as a prey species, they will often effectively mask signs of pain or illness until very severe. In chickens, crouching immobility has been associated with prolonged pain, stress and fear responses. For example, when a noxious stimulus was applied to ulcerated buccal lesions, chickens remained motionless in a crouch-like stance with the head pulled into the body and had significantly fewer alert head movements (Gentle *et al.*, 1987). Changes in grooming patterns can be interpreted in both ways: grooming may decrease with pain, but some feather destructive behaviours are associated with chronic pain. The pharmacokinetics (plasma levels) and pharmacodynamics (response to medication) vary considerably across avian species, so extrapolation is not ideal but there are limited studies. Often experimental studies in parrots and chickens use pain stimuli that may not extrapolate to pain behaviours relevant to clinical pain. Thus, any analgesics used should be critically evaluated on a case-by-case basis when applied clinically. Commonly used analgesics are listed in Figure 22.6. It must be remembered that pre-emptive analgesia can block sensory noxious stimuli from onward transmission to the central nervous system (CNS), thereby reducing overall pain or the need for prolonged analgesia.

Opioids

Opioids are often used to provide perioperative analgesia that may reduce the concentrations of volatile anaesthetics required. Most are used parenterally due to poor oral bioavailability (<10% in some studies). Opioids vary in their receptor specificity (delt, kappa and mu), but there is a lack of published data on receptor distribution density and functionality in birds. Some avian species have been shown to have high numbers of kappa-type receptors, perhaps explaining why birds do not seem to respond as well to mu agonists (i.e. morphine) as they do to more selective kappa agonists (i.e. butorphanol). More research is needed, but there appear to be major differences in the response to opioids across avian species, and in chickens differences between breeds and ages have also been found.

Morphine and fentanyl

Morphine and fentanyl (mu agonists) are not commonly used in available medicine because of confusing and conflicting clinical efficacy data.

Butorphanol

Butorphanol is a mixed agonist/antagonist with low mu receptor and stronger kappa receptor activity that produces less dose-related respiratory depression than mu agonists. Adverse effects such as dysphoria have not been reported in birds. There is some species variability, but a number of studies have shown that preoperative use of butorphanol in birds reduced the amount of isoflurane

Drug	Dose	Route of administration	Comments/uses
Buprenorphine	0.01–0.05 mg/kg q8–12h	Intramuscular	There are doubts about the efficacy of this drug (administered by any route) in chickens. Studies have also shown no effect intra-articularly in chickens up to 1 mg/kg. The dose suggested is anecdotal
Butorphanol	0.2–0.4 mg/kg q12h	Intramuscular	Dose evaluated in chickens; other species frequently require 0.5–2.0 mg/kg q4–6h
Carprofen	1–4 mg/kg	Intramuscular, subcutaneous	Lower doses have been effective for short periods. Dosing interval not clearly established.
Flunixin	1.1 mg/kg	Intravenous	Only evaluated as a one-off dose. Potenially nephrotoxic in many bird species. Good hydration is essential. Minimal justification for use given there are several alternatives
	3 mg/kg	Intramuscular	
Ketoprofen	2–12 mg/kg	Intramuscular	Rapid clearance at low dose; higher doses last for 12 hours in chickens. Other avian species have died using doses of 5 mg/kg
Meloxicam	0.2–2 mg/kg q12–24h	Intramuscular, oral	Variable doses and intervals evaluated. Used by the author at 0.5–1 mg/kg q24h in chickens
Morphine	10–20 mg/kg	Intramuscular	Effective at this dose in quail but no effect in chickens at 1–3 mg/kg intra-articularly and no effect in chicks at 200 mg/kg intravenously
Tramadol	5–11 mg/kg q12h	Oral	No data in chickens

22.6 Analgesic drugs used in chickens.

required for anaesthetic maintenance. Some authors prefer not to administer butorphanol during anaesthesia as it has been shown to prolong recovery in some avian species.

Buprenorphine

Buprenorphine is a complex opiate which is believed to act as a mu agonist with some kappa receptor agonist/antagonist properties, and has a ceiling effect with increased doses. It is unclear whether this analgesic is useful in birds and dose ranges vary widely.

Nalbuphine

Nalbuphine is a kappa receptor agonist and partial mu antagonist used in humans. It has been shown to be effective in parrots at a dose of 12.5 mg/kg i.m. and due to its receptor activity and minor side effects, it may become a promising analgesic in chickens.

Tramadol

Tramadol is a synthetic analogue of codeine with opioid, alpha-adrenergic and serotonergic receptor activity. Tramadol has become popular recently despite minimal evidence of its efficacy. In therapeutic and pharmacokinetic trials in other avian species it shows higher oral bioavailability than in dogs and cats and causes insignificant side effects.

Non-steroidal anti-inflammatory drugs

Non-steroidal anti-inflammatory drugs (NSAIDs) are the most commonly used class of analgesic in veterinary medicine. Their activity has been widely evaluated in mammals and the principles should apply to birds as cyclooxygenase (COX)-1 and COX-2 are known to be important in avian pain. The selection of specific NSAIDs often depends on the ease of administration of different formulations. There is little scientific evidence for a washout period in birds and where there is cause to switch NSAIDs, withholding them for this reason is thought to expose birds to more risk from the effects of pain. There is wide pharmacokinetic variability across avian species, so these analgesics should

be used with care. Potential side effects and risk factors may be similar to those seen in dogs and cats (e.g. gastrointestinal irritation, renal toxicity and coagulation problems); however, the most commonly reported adverse effects are on renal tissue and function. With this in mind, care should be taken when using NSAIDs perioperatively or in any other circumstance when circulation and perfusion may be compromised.

Monitoring

Attentive monitoring by an experienced veterinary nurse is essential in avian anaesthesia to allow early recognition of complications and prompt intervention. Reflexes, breathing rate, heart rate and manual assessment of pulses are the basic requirements to assess anaesthetic depth. The monitoring equipment detailed below can provide useful additional information that will improve anaesthetic safety if used and interpreted with care.

Breathing, heart rate and pulse

The patient should be continuously monitored for changes in breathing, heart rate and pulse, with values recorded at 5-minute intervals to enable rapid detection of trends that may require action. Heart rate can be monitored using an oesophageal stethoscope in the crop or standard stethoscope over the dorsal or lateral cranial body cavity. The pulse can be palpated most easily over the tibiotarsal artery on the cranial aspect of the intertarsal joint or over the radial artery on the underside of the wing at the carpal joint. Normal breathing, heart and pulse rates depend on the size of the bird and should be established prior to anaesthesia. Changes and trends are more important than specific figures.

Reflexes

Pedal reflex

A short sharp pinch of the toe will elicit a withdrawal response. This will be present at light anaesthetic depth but lost at surgical anaesthesia.

Corneal reflex

Touching a clean cotton bud to the surface of the cornea should cause the nictitating membrane to sweep across the surface of the globe (Figure 22.7). The slower the reflex, the deeper the plane of anaesthesia. If absent, then the patient is likely to be too deep under anaesthesia. The reflex can become absent if excessively stimulated (in which case the other eye should be checked) and care should be taken not to cause corneal abrasions.

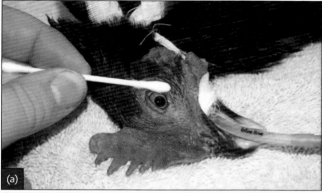

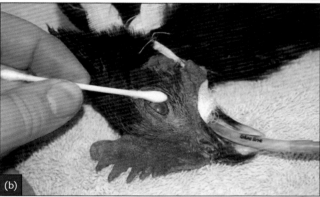

22.7 Corneal reflex. (a) Gently touching the corneal surface with a cotton bud will (b) cause the nictitating membrane to sweep briskly across the globe at a light plane of anaesthesia.

Feather pluck

Feather plucking is very painful to a chicken and the absence of movement when a body contour feather is plucked usually indicates surgical anaesthesia.

Equipment
Capnography

Capnography provides important data regarding respiratory function. Determination of expired CO_2 allows assessment of appropriate ventilation, especially in cases where anaesthesia is prolonged. Spontaneous respiration usually causes a gradual rise in the partial pressure of carbon dioxide (PCO_2). Normal end-tidal CO_2 is 20–40 mmHg and monitoring is especially important if using a ventilator.

Pulse oximeter

The probe can be placed on a skin web or cloacal reflectance probes can be used. Differences in avian haemoglobin mean that only trends of oxygenation should be relied upon rather than specific values.

Temperature probe

Birds are susceptible to hypothermia under anaesthesia, so temperature should be monitored and kept in the region of 40°C. Probes can be inserted into the cloaca for continuous measurement or handheld thermometers can be used at regular intervals.

Non-invasive blood pressure measurement

A standard Doppler transducer can be placed on the ulnar or tibiotarsal artery, which allows simple auditory recognition of pulse rate and intensity. A paediatric cuff and sphygmomanometer placed proximally can be used to obtain non-invasive blood pressure readings (Figure 22.8). These readings represent an estimation of systolic blood pressure and are not reported to be very accurate but will enable early recognition of trends. Normal non-invasive blood pressure should be >90 mmHg and an intravenous bolus of fluids (or a constant rate infusion) should be administered if a bird is hypotensive under anaesthesia. Oscillometric devices have not been shown to be reliable in birds.

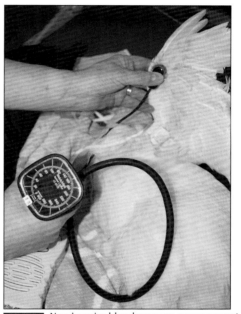

22.8 Non-invasive blood pressure measurement. The Doppler probe is placed over the ulnar artery and the cuff inflated to obtain an estimate of systolic blood pressure.

Air sac cannulation

Due to the unique anatomy of the avian respiratory system, placement of a tube directly into one of the air sacs (usually the caudal thoracic or abdominal air sac) can allow ventilation and maintenance of anaesthesia without endotracheal intubation. This technique may be used where there is tracheal obstruction, where tracheal surgery is due to be carried out, or where the surgeon wishes to operate in the head region without interference by anaesthetic equipment. Some clinicians also use air sac perfusion anaesthesia for ocular surgery as it causes pupil dilation. If a bird presents as an emergency with an upper airway obstruction, placement of an air sac breathing tube will allow the bird to be ventilated whilst the obstruction is treated. If there is evidence of ascites or organomegaly, air sac cannulation may be contraindicated.

Technique

1. With the bird anaesthetized (or using local anaesthesia), place the patient in right (or left) lateral recumbency, pull the leg caudally and palpate the last two ribs. Make a skin incision over the gap between the last two ribs, ventral to the dorsal spinal musculature (Figure 22.9a).
2. Using a pair of artery forceps, carefully make a blunt stab incision through the body wall musculature and into the caudal thoracic air sac in the coelomic cavity (Figure 22.9b). Take care not to damage the internal organs with overzealous introduction of the forceps.
3. For the air sac tube, use ET tubes cut to size, with pre-placed sutures mid-way along in the wall of the tube to secure the tube when inserted. Introduce the tube into the air sac through the incision and use a feather to check for air movement through the tube (Figure 22.9c).
4. Thread a suture needle over each of the loose suture ends and pass the suture material around the cranial and caudal ribs and tie in place (Figure 22.9d).
5. If required, an ET tube connector can be fitted to the end of the tube and anaesthetic gas can be delivered via an attached non-rebreathing system. Be aware that anaesthetic gases will escape from the trachea with air sac perfusion anaesthesia. These tubes are well tolerated in conscious birds and enable ventilation where there is a tracheal obstruction.
6. The tube can be maintained for a few days as needed, with regular suction of accumulated mucus or debris. Sometimes placing 1–2 drops of hyaluronidase down the tube helps maintain patency. If being used for a tracheal obstruction, the tube can be blocked temporarily with a cotton bud or injection cap to assess how the bird copes ventilating via the trachea as normal.

Recovery

Once inhalational anaesthesia is discontinued, poultry should remain on oxygen until reflexes start to reappear. At this point, the ET tube should be carefully removed and the bird gently wrapped in a clean, dry towel to allow continued monitoring of breathing and reflexes. As the bird regains consciousness and begins to move voluntarily, it can be placed in a warm, dimly lit environment, still wrapped in the towel (Figure 22.10). The bird should be placed in sternal recumbency and observations continued until the patient is able to wriggle from the towel and stand normally. Keeping poultry wrapped in a towel during recovery prevents excessive wing flapping and self-trauma whilst they are still disoriented. Once strong enough to struggle free from the towel, birds are much less likely to harm themselves.

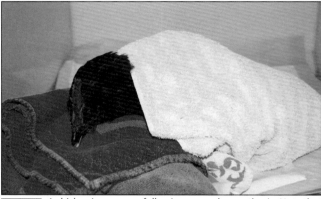

22.10 A chicken in recovery following general anaesthesia. Note that the bird is wrapped in a towel and the head is elevated.

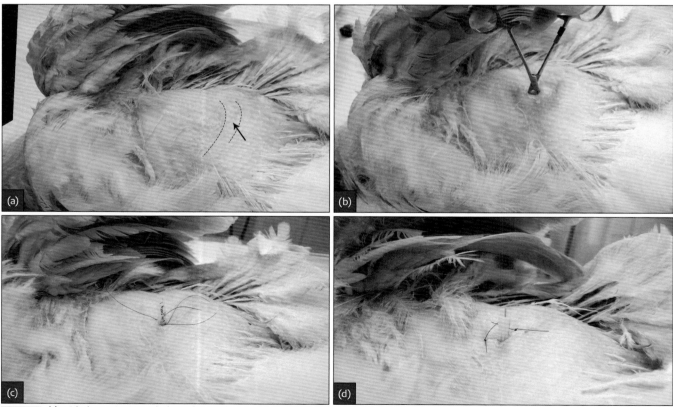

22.9 (a) With the patient in right lateral recumbency, the leg is pulled caudally and wings dorsally to locate the last two ribs (dotted lines). The site for air sac tube placement is the gap between these two ribs (arrowed). (b) Artery forceps are placed bluntly through the muscle layers into the air sac. Opening the forceps creates space to place the endotracheal (ET) tube. (c) A cut down ET tube with pre-placed sutures is placed through the incision. Air flow through the tube can be confirmed using a feather. (d) The tube is secured by passing the suture material around the cranial and caudal ribs.

Anaesthetic emergencies

As with all anaesthetic procedures, following the 'ABCDE' protocol is useful in poultry:

- A = Airway
- B = Breathing
- C = Circulation
- D = Drugs
- E = Equipment failure.

Accurate and continuous monitoring of birds is vital to identify problems early, and rapid intervention is the key to a successful outcome. The most common complications that are identified during the 'ABCDE' assessment and the actions to be taken are listed in Figure 22.11. In all cases, colleagues should be alerted so they can provide assistance, the volatile anaesthetic agent should be turned off (or the injectable agent antagonized) and the patient assessed for the cause of the problem. Patients should be weighed before the procedure to enable accurate emergency drug doses to be administered without delay. Pre-calculated doses should be written down and readily available for all patients, but especially those at high risk (Figure 22.12). Equipment should be checked for failure when the patient is more stable or if the problem remains unidentified. ET tubes can become displaced, blocked or disconnected from the anaesthetic machine. The vaporizer may be empty or faulty, the oxygen supply may have been interrupted or the flowmeter may be broken. There may be leaks in the anaesthetic breathing system or the anaesthetic monitoring devices may have failed, giving an incorrect reading.

Emergency	Cause	Signs	Action
Apnoea	Plane of anaesthesia too deep; toxicity from medications; result of hypoventilation (and marked hypercapnia)	Absence of respiratory movements	• Check anaesthetic level with reflexes • Turn off inhalational agent (or reverse injectable agent) • Place bird in lateral recumbency • Intubate trachea if not already done • Start IPPV (12 breaths per min) • Confirm pulse and heartbeat Most birds will resume breathing; attempts can then be made to return the bird to an appropriate anaesthetic level. If there is no response, doxapram can be administered and repeat after 2 mins if there is still no response. Good prognosis if recognized early
Airway obstruction	Mucus obstructing trachea; blockage in ET tube	Exaggerated respiratory movement or slow/non-existent expiration. Clicking or squeaking can be mistaken for light anaesthetic depth. Cyanosis can be seen in chickens	• Remove ET tube and clear it or replace with another tube • Aspirate mucus from airway with a urinary catheter • Consider air sac cannulation in severe cases Using pre-emptive anticholinergics is controversial. Prognosis good if detected early
Cardiac arrest	Plane of anaesthesia too deep; toxicity from medications; catecholamine-induced arrhythmias	Lack of pulse and audible heartbeat; ECG abnormalities; pallor	With isoflurane and sevoflurane, cardiac arrest usually occurs sometime after respiratory arrest • Turn off inhalational agent (or reverse injectable agent) • Intubate trachea if not already done • Start IPPV (12 breaths per min) • Re-check for pulse and heartbeat • Attempt compressions with intermittent digital pressure on keel • Administer adrenaline, atropine and doxapram as needed depending on response Prognosis is poor to grave at this stage
Hypovolaemia	Loss of blood or other fluid; pre-existing dehydration	Thready pulses; slow capillary refill time	• Replace fluids with warmed isotonic fluids, colloids or whole blood as indicated; administer intravenously or intraosseously Birds may lose up to 30% of their circulating volume before suffering shock. Prognosis fair to good depending on the volume lost. Give 10 ml/kg initially as a bolus, then maintain on surgical rates of 10 ml/kg/h – increase if persistently hypovolaemic
Hypothermia	Inadequate heat retention and failure to reduce losses	Cloacal temperature <37 °C	• Warm the bird with warm air heating, radiant heat lamps or provide warmed fluids
Hyperthermia	Excessive heating measure; failure to consider ambient temperature	Cloacal temperature >40°C	• Remove warming devices • Use cooled, moist towels or fans
Regurgitation	Food in crop or proventriculus	Liquid or food from the mouth	• Place head lower than airway to drain ingesta • Clean oral cavity with cotton buds • Check choana (slit in the roof of mouth) is clear of food • Check ET tube for obstruction Prognosis is fair depending on whether aspiration has occurred

22.11 Avian anaesthetic emergencies. ECG = electrocardiogram; ET = endotracheal; IPPV = intermittent positive pressure ventilation.

Drug	Dose	Route of administration	Comments/uses
Adrenaline	0.5–1.0 mg/kg	Intravenous, intratracheal	Stimulate heart function; treat anaphylactic shock and bronchial spasm
Atropine	0.5 mg/kg	Intramuscular	Increase heart rate and relaxation of bronchial smooth muscle
Calcium gluconate	50–100 mg/kg	Intramuscular	Hypocalcaemic tetany; seizures
Colloid	10–15 ml/kg	Slow intravenous	Volume replacement; hypovolaemic shock
Dextrose	50–100 mg/kg	Slow intravenous	Treatment of hypoglycaemic seizures
Diazepam	0.5–1.0 mg/kg	Intramuscular	Reduction in anxiety and muscle tone; sedation; anti-convulsant
Doxapram	5–20 mg/kg or 1–3 drops on the tongue	Intravenous, intramuscular	Short-acting respiratory stimulant
Naloxone	2 mg slow (total dose)	Intravenous	Opioid antagonist to reverse respiratory depression caused by opioids

22.12 Drugs used in avian anaesthetic emergencies.

References and further reading

Abou-Madi N (2001) Avian anaesthesia. *Veterinary Clinics of North America: Exotic Animal Practice* 4, 147–167

Gentle MJ and Hill FL (1987) Oral lesions in the chicken: behavioural responses following nociceptive stimulation. *Physiology and Behaviour* 40, 781–783

Hall LW, Clarke KW and Trim CM (2001) General pharmacology of inhalational anaesthetics. In: *Veterinary Anaesthesia, 10th edn*, pp. 133–147. WB Saunders, London

Hawkins MG and Paul-Murphey J (2011) Avian analgesia. *Veterinary Clinics of North America: Exotic Animal Practice* 14, 61–80

King AS and McLelland J (1988) *Form and Function in Birds: Volume 4.* Academic Press, London.

Lierz M and Korbel R (2012) Anesthesia and analgesia in birds. *Journal of Exotic Pet Medicine* 21, 44–58

Ludders JW (2001) Inhaled anaesthesia for birds. In: *Recent Advances in Veterinary Anaesthesia and Analgesia: Companion Animals*, ed. RD Gleed and JW Ludders. International Veterinary Information Service, New York

O'Malley BM (2005) Avian anatomy and physiology. In: *Clinical Anatomy and Physiology of Exotic Species*, ed. BM O'Malley, pp. 97–164. Elsevier Saunders, Germany

Chapter 23

Soft tissue surgery

Bob Doneley

Surgical procedures on backyard poultry are becoming increasingly common as the expectations of the bird-owning public rise. In particular, gastrointestinal and reproductive procedures are becoming commonplace, as is the surgical repair of traumatic injuries. Although there are many similarities between surgery in birds and surgery in other species, there are some differences based on the anatomy and physiology of avian patients. This chapter discusses the principles of soft tissue surgery in birds and considers some of the common procedures performed on poultry and waterfowl in general practice.

General principles

Despite the many anatomical and physiological differences between birds and mammals, surgical principles remain constant. With a metabolic rate typically exceeding that of most mammals, birds have a higher susceptibility to anaesthetic and surgical complications associated with pain, hypothermia, hypovolaemia, hypoxia and infection. These complications are addressed by basic surgical principles. In order to maximize surgical success, the following principles must be understood and applied:

*   Minimize haemorrhage
*   Minimize tissue trauma
*   Minimize anaesthetic time
*   Minimize anaesthetic and metabolic complications
*   Provide post-surgical support and analgesia.

    To comply with these principles, the surgeon should:

*   Be familiar with the anatomy and physiology of birds
*   Ensure that the patient is in the best possible condition prior to surgery
*   Develop an anaesthetic and analgesic plan that maximizes patient safety and comfort
*   Ensure that patient support procedures and adequate surgical preparation are in place to minimize infection and maximize patient safety
*   Use instruments, techniques and suture materials that minimize tissue damage, blood loss and inflammatory responses.

Anatomy and physiology

The unique features of avian anatomy and physiology are described in Chapter 2. Of particular relevance to the

surgeon is the function of the respiratory tract and cardiovascular system, the anatomy of the internal organs (especially the reproductive tract) and thermogenesis. These areas should be reviewed, where appropriate, prior to undertaking a surgical procedure.

Patient evaluation

Assessment of the patient begins with a comprehensive physical examination, including evaluation of the weight and body condition of the bird. The crop and coelom must be palpated and the presence of ingesta/fluid in the crop and any evidence of coelomic distension noted (Figure 23.1). Respiratory recovery time can be assessed after handling the bird; a healthy patient should return to breathing normally within 3–5 minutes following capture. Cyanosis, prolonged mouth-breathing and exaggerated sternal lift are indicative of respiratory compromise.

Diagnostic testing should include haematology and biochemistry. Ideally, packed cell volume (PCV), total plasma protein and blood glucose should be measured prior to most routine surgical procedures. A crude estimate of clotting time can be obtained through a pin prick of the basilic vein; clotting should be seen after 1 minute under direct pressure.

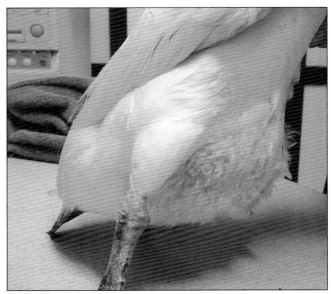

23.1 Coelomic distension in a duck with yolk peritonitis.

If any of the abnormalities listed in Figure 23.2 are detected, appropriate medical therapy should be instituted (e.g. fluid therapy, blood transfusion, tube feeding, diet conversion, weight reduction). Vitamin supplementation may be of use in mildly malnourished birds, but should be given several days prior to the surgery in order to be of benefit. If a coagulopathy is suspected (remember that not all potential coagulopathic conditions (i.e. hepatic lipidosis) will be detected by biochemical screening), vitamin K may be of benefit, but must be administered at least 24 hours before commencing surgery.

In some cases, it may be necessary (and feasible) to delay surgery for several days or months until the patient is more stable and in better body condition. If the patient's medical condition is critical and surgery cannot be postponed, the owner must be informed of the increased risks prior to the procedure.

Physical examination findings
• Respiratory distress or prolonged recovery time • Obesity • Severe emaciation • Concurrent diseases unrelated to the surgical condition (e.g. cardiovascular disease, infectious disease) • Crop full of fluid or ingesta • Coelomic distension
Clinical pathology parameters
• Packed cell volume <20% or >60% • Prolonged bleeding time • Total plasma protein <20 g/l • Glucose <11 mmol/l • Uric acid >700 µmol/l • Aspartate aminotransferase >650 IU/l (in the presence of a normal creatine kinase) • Cholesterol >18 mmol/l

23.2 Medical conditions and clinical pathology parameters which may necessitate postponement of surgery.

Anaesthesia and analgesia

It is generally accepted that birds perceive pain along neurological pathways similar to those in mammals. However, birds may indicate pain in less obvious ways. They appear to respond to painful stimuli in one of two ways: 'fight-or-flight' responses (excessive vocalization, wing flapping), usually associated with acute pain; or 'conservation–withdrawal' responses (immobility, closure of eyes, inappetence, 'fluffing' of feathers), commonly associated with more chronic pain. Care must therefore be taken not to misinterpret lack of movement or vocalization as an indication that the bird is not in pain.

Whilst pain is a response to a noxious stimulus that serves the purpose of alerting an animal to the presence of that stimulus and thereby provoking a response that removes the animal from the stimulus and therefore further injury, it has wider, more far-reaching consequences. Through stimulation of the adrenal glands and the subsequent release of corticosterone, pain has an adverse effect on wound healing and the immune system. Survival and recovery rates of birds in pain are much lower than those receiving effective analgesia. A good analgesic plan is therefore essential when contemplating a surgical procedure. For more information on suitable analgesic drugs and routes of administration, see Chapter 22.

Anaesthesia in birds is complicated by their unique anatomy, their rapid metabolism, their reduced ability to conserve body heat whilst anaesthetized and the fact that few procedures are elective (i.e. most patients are ill). The requirements for ideal avian anaesthetic agents and techniques are:

- Rapid induction and recovery to minimize stress and heat loss
- Rapid metabolism and excretion, avoiding 'hangover' effects that may delay the bird's return to eating and its normal metabolic rate
- Minimal cardiac and respiratory depressant effects, combined with good ventilation
- Operator health and safety.

Anaesthetic agents and techniques are described in detail in Chapter 22.

Planning the surgical procedure

Although prolonged exploratory surgery can be performed in birds, surgical time can be reduced if a good surgical plan is in place. The surgeon should revise the appropriate anatomy (if necessary) and become familiar with the surgical approaches to the area in question. The next step is to determine the extent of the lesion or disease process prior to the procedure. This can be achieved through careful physical examination, radiography, ultrasonography and/or endoscopy. This information is collated and used to plan the procedure. Once the plan has been developed, the surgeon should check that all equipment and materials likely to be used in the procedure are accessible and fully functional prior to anaesthetizing the patient. Finally, there must be a discussion with theatre and nursing staff about the procedure, so that all personnel involved know what is happening and what their role is in the surgery. A verbal rehearsal at this stage often detects and allows correction of preparation errors that could result in a delay during the procedure. A surgical preparation checklist is provided in Figure 23.3.

Patient support

During anaesthesia and surgery the most likely problems that will be encountered are hypothermia, hypovolaemia, hypotension and hypoxia. The anaesthetic, analgesic and surgical plans must take into account these complications. Precautions that can be taken include the provision of thermal support, circulatory support and respiratory support. These supportive measures are discussed in more detail in Chapter 22.

Patient preparation

Preparation of the surgical site is a compromise between achieving an aseptic surgical field and minimizing hypothermia. General guidelines include the following:

- Pluck feathers; do not cut them if at all possible. This encourages new feather growth following surgery, rather than waiting for cut feathers to moult and regrow. Be careful to pluck the feathers along the line of growth, as pulling against the line of growth can tear the skin and damage the feather follicle
- Soak the feathers to be removed with the skin preparation solution prior to plucking to minimize the number of loose, dry feathers that may potentially contaminate the surgical site
- Minimize feather removal by using either water-soluble lubricating jelly (which is easily wiped off following surgery) or adhesive tape to hold back the surrounding feathers

Procedure	Equipment	Completed?
Prior to anaesthesia and surgery	Weight, physical examination findings, pre-anaesthetic blood tests recorded	
	Anaesthetic and surgical procedure plans developed and communicated to all staff	
Anaesthesia	Patient preparation and support: fluids, heating, fasting	
	Premedication and induction: medications, intravenous catheters	
	Maintenance: endotracheal tubes, anaesthetic machine, pharyngeal packing materials, intermittent positive pressure ventilation (IPPV)	
	Monitoring – capnography, electrocardiography, Doppler, temperature probes	
Surgery	Tape, sandbags and ties to position the patient	
	Non-alcoholic preparation solutions	
	Drapes (cloth, paper, plastic)	
	Instrument kits	
	Radiosurgery, laser or other surgical devices	
	Vascular clips	
	Retractors	
	Suture materials	
	Sterile cotton wool buds (Q tips) and swabs	
	Equipment for sample collection (swabs, syringes, formalin)	
Recovery	Analgesia	
	Heated cage	
	Supplemental oxygen	
	Fluid support	

23.3 Checklist for surgical procedures.

- Use chlorhexidine or povidone–iodine to prepare the surgical site. Do not use alcohol-based disinfectants, as evaporative heat loss can be significant, especially in small patients (Figure 23.4).

Draping of the surgical site is usually determined by the preference of the surgeon. Transparent plastic drapes allow visualization of the patient and have heat-retaining characteristics, but unless they are adhesive they can move over the surface of the patient during surgery. If adhesive drapes are not used, placement of towel clamps around large feathers rather than through the skin should be considered. Cloth or paper drapes can also be used, but the view of the patient is compromised. However, the use of anaesthetic monitoring (e.g. capnography, electrocardiography and indirect blood pressure measurements) reduces the requirement for continuous visualization of the patient.

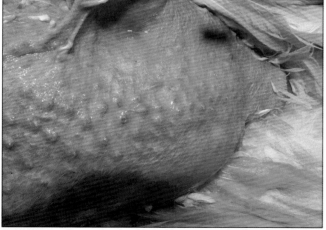

23.4 Swollen coelom in a bird with pyometra that has been plucked and prepared for surgery.

Surgical instruments and equipment

The selection of instruments is dictated by the size of the patient, the procedure being performed and the preference of the surgeon. Surgical dissection should be performed using fine, sharp instruments. Microscopic and ophthalmic instruments are useful for some procedures as they allow delicate and atraumatic handling of the tissues. Long-handled fine instruments may be required in other cases. Sterilized cotton buds (Q tips) or swabs are useful for removing blood and other fluids from the surgical field, as well as manipulating tissues. They can also be used for gentle blunt dissection when required. Radiosurgery, laser surgery and endosurgery may be used for some procedures and can help minimize tissue trauma when utilized correctly (Figure 23.5).

Magnification using either binocular loupes or an operating microscope allows for much finer work than can be achieved with the naked eye. Most units come with in-built illumination that complements and enhances the magnification achieved.

A wide selection of suture materials is available to the surgeon, which are classified depending on their absorption characteristics and whether they are monofilament or braided. It is incumbent on the surgeon to understand how long different tissues take to heal, how long different suture materials maintain their tensile strength and how long it is before the suture material is absorbed (Figure 23.6). These factors need to be taken into consideration when selecting the suture material for a particular procedure (McFadden, 2011). Desirable characteristics of suture material include:

- High tensile strength whilst the tissues heal
- Good knot security
- Resistance to infection
- Minimal inflammatory, immunogenic or carcinogenic reactions.

Parameter	Radiosurgery	Laser surgery (carbon dioxide or diode)
Mechanics of operation	High-frequency radiowaves (3.8–4.0 MHz) are modified by a wave form adaptor and then focused from the active electrode tip to the indifferent plate (antenna). These radiowaves produce alternating electromagnetic fields that generate heat due to resistance in the tissue. This localized heat volatilizes intracellular fluids, causing cell disruption along the path of the electrode. Note, this is not electrosurgery, which uses an electric current to 'burn' tissue	The light emitted from a laser has a wavelength that is absorbed by fluid in the cells, creating a thermal effect. The degree of penetration can be controlled, allowing fine, precise dissection of tissue
Advantages	Offers both haemostasis and minimal tissue damage when used correctly	• Haemostasis – the laser cuts and coagulates blood vessels up to approximately 0.5 mm in diameter. Larger vessels may need to be cauterized or ligated • Analgesia – theoretically, as the laser cuts, it seals nerve endings and axons, reducing the sensation and transmission of pain. However, this is not always the case and some clinicians have reported postoperative pain to be significant • Decreased postoperative swelling – the laser seals lymphatic vessels, decreasing the extravasation of lymphatic fluid into the surgical site postoperatively
Disadvantages	Can result in excessive tissue damage (due to lateral heat), increasing the possibility of dehiscence. The extent of the damage is determined by: • Electrode size – the greater the size, the more lateral heat generated, and the more tissue damage results • The time the tissue is exposed to the electrode – the longer the time, the more lateral heat is generated • The skill and experience of the operator. Training should be undertaken prior to use on a live patient	• Equipment cost • Extensive training needed to become competent • Potential for lateral heat damage when used incorrectly

23.5 Comparison of radiosurgery and laser surgery.

Suture material	Type	Time >50% tensile strength retained (days)	Time to complete resorption (days)	Advantages	Disadvantages
Chromic catgut	Monofilament	<7	60–90	Cheap and readily available	Poor knot security Intense inflammatory reaction Rapid loss of strength
Polyglactin 910 (Vicryl)	Braided	14–21	90–110	Absorbed by hydrolysis High tensile strength	Increased tissue drag Moderate inflammatory reaction Can act as a wick for ascending infections
Polyglycolic acid (Dexon)	Braided	7–14	60		
Polydioxanone (PDS)	Monofilament	21–28	180–210	Absorbed by hydrolysis Minimal inflammatory reaction High tensile strength	Stiff Tendency to kink
Polyglyconate (Maxon)	Monofilament	21–28	180		High degree of tensile memory (coil) when removed from package
Glycomer 631 (Biosyn)	Monofilament	14–21	90–110		
Poliglecaprone 25 (Monocryl)	Monofilament	7–14	90–110		

23.6 Suture material characteristics.
(McFadden, 2011)

Absorbable sutures of biological origin are broken down by phagocytosis, provoking a marked inflammatory response. Chromic catgut is a classic example of a biologically derived suture material. It rapidly loses its tensile strength and is quickly absorbed. Synthetic polymers are absorbed by hydrolysis. Hydrolysis involves breaking down polymers into monomers by direct water cleavage; once broken down, the monomers are absorbed and metabolized by the body. The speed at which this occurs and the time to complete resorption is determined by the composition of the monomers and polymers in the material.

The characteristics of the various suture materials are summarized in Figure 23.6. When these characteristics are taken into account, polydioxanone (PDS) emerges as the suture material of choice for many procedures, especially those involving closure of muscle and other fascia (Figure 23.7). For gastrointestinal surgery (where tissue healing times are faster), polyglactin 910 (Vicryl), glycomer 631 (Biosyn) and poliglecaprone 25 (Monocryl) are suitable choices.

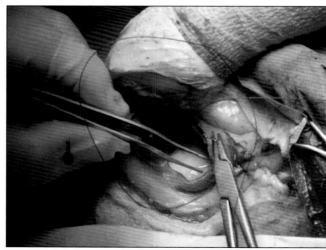

23.7 Polydioxanone (PDS) suture material (3 metric; 2/0 USP) being used to close a coeliotomy incision.

The suture pattern used is determined by the nature of the tissue, the selection of suture material and the preference of the surgeon. Interrupted patterns (simple, cruciate or horizontal mattress) are often preferred by many surgeons for closure of the coelom, whilst continuous patterns (simple, Ford interlocking or inverting/everting/appositional) are often used for ingluviotomy procedures and skin closure.

PRACTICAL TIPS

- Haemostasis of small vessels can be achieved through the use of radiosurgery or laser surgery. Larger vessels should be ligated with suture material or vascular clips
- Inflammatory responses to surgical procedures can be minimized by gentle tissue handling, the correct use of modalities such as radiosurgery and laser surgery (i.e. minimizing lateral heat damage) and the selection of suture material

Coeliotomy

Indications

Coeliotomy is indicated for both the diagnosis and treatment of coelomic conditions detected by physical examination, imaging (radiography, ultrasonography and endoscopy) or laboratory testing (haematology and biochemistry). A list of these conditions is given in Figure 23.8. It is also useful for the diagnosis of cases involving persistent, non-specific clinical signs that prove to be unresponsive to medical management, including weight loss and polyuria. Less invasive entry into the coelomic cavity via rigid endoscopy, whilst allowing high magnification and access for biopsy to most organs, does not permit the breadth of surgical procedures when compared with coeliotomy.

Anaesthetic considerations

Once the coelom has been opened and the air sacs incised, the bird will be able to breathe room air and the anaesthetic plane may lighten. This can be overcome by the use of manual intermittent positive pressure ventilation (IPPV), higher oxygen flow rates and increasing the

Gastrointestinal conditions
• Foreign bodies
• Biopsy of the liver, pancreas and gastrointestinal tract
Reproductive conditions
• Hernia
• Neoplasia (e.g. testicular)
• Orchitis
• Uterine/ovarian cysts
• Salpingitis
• Decreased egg production
• Misshapen eggs
• Egg binding
• Yolk-related peritonitis
Miscellaneous conditions
• Renal biopsy
• Ascites

23.8 Common conditions that may require coeliotomy for diagnosis and treatment.

concentration of anaesthetic agent (e.g. isoflurane). On rare occasions, the use of an intravenous anaesthetic agent to 'top up' the anaesthetic plane may be required. The use of a scavenger system is strongly recommended to remove as much waste anaesthetic gas as possible. Heat loss from an open coelom can be significant and thermal support is essential. A good surgical plan that minimizes the time the coelom is open is mandatory.

Approach

There are two approaches for coeliotomy: a left lateral approach and a ventral midline approach. A left lateral approach is indicated for access to the gonads, left kidney, oviduct, proventriculus and ventriculus. A ventral midline approach is indicated for biopsy of the liver and pancreas, cloacopexy and to access the duodenum, small intestine, oviduct, ovary and testes.

Techniques
Left lateral coeliotomy

1. Place the bird in right lateral recumbency with the cranial end of the body elevated 30–40 degrees to prevent fluid from entering the lungs. Extend the wings dorsally and secure in place. Abduct the left leg and draw it slightly forward.
2. Incise the inguinal skin web between the body wall and left leg and abduct the leg further. Continue this incision from the sixth rib to the level of the left pubic bone (Figure 23.9).
3. Cauterize or ligate the superficial medial femoral artery and vein where they transverse (in a dorsoventral direction) the lateral body wall medial to the coxofemoral joint.
4. Tent the muscles (external, internal abdominal oblique and transverse abdominal muscles) up and make a stab incision with pointed scissors, whilst protecting the viscera. Extend this incision from the pubic bone to the eighth rib. This may require transection of the last two ribs at the level of the uncinate process, which is achieved by passing bipolar forceps around the rib, cauterizing the intercostal blood vessels and then cutting the ribs with scissors (Figure 23.10).
5. Place a retractor (e.g. Lone Star) to allow visualization of the internal organs (Figures 23.11 and 23.12).

Closure:
- Close the muscle and skin layers separately with absorbable sutures in a continuous (small patients) or interrupted (large patients) pattern.
- No attempt to re-join the transected ribs or repair the air sacs is necessary.

Ventral midline coeliotomy

1. Place the bird in dorsal recumbency with the cranial end of the body elevated 30–40 degrees. Extend the legs caudally.
2. Tent and incise the skin in the ventral midline from 2–5 mm distal to the sternum and continue towards the pre-pubic space (Figure 23.13). Avoid incising the peri-cloacal blood vessels distally.
3. To allow greater exposure, extend the incision laterally at the proximal and distal ends to create flaps. This will form a C-shaped incision with a unilateral flap or an I-shaped incision with bilateral flaps. (Note that

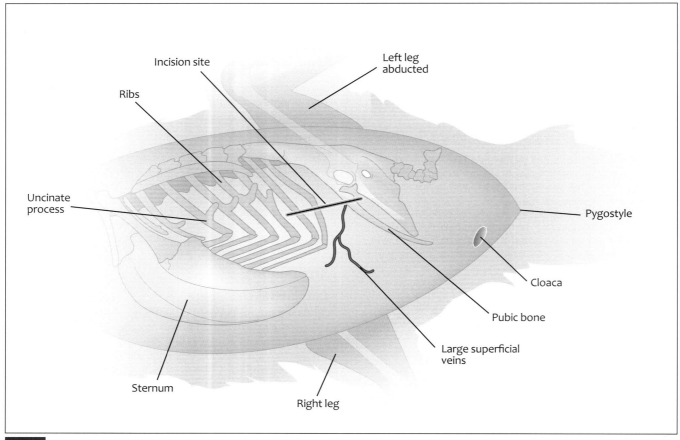

23.9 Landmarks for a left lateral coeliotomy.

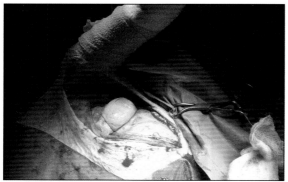

23.10 Initial incision for a left lateral coeliotomy. The procedure, in this case, is being performed to treat yolk peritonitis.

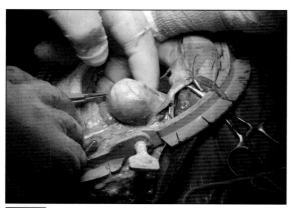

23.11 Placement of a Lone Star retractor.

although lateral flaps increase exposure they also allow increased anaesthetic gas and heat loss through the open coelomic cavity.)

4. Many species have a relatively large superficial vein located subcutaneously on the ventral abdomen. Ligate or cauterize this vessel prior to entering the coelomic cavity.

5. Tent and incise the linea alba in a craniocaudal direction, avoiding iatrogenic damage to the underlying viscera. If a flap incision is used, the coelomic muscles should be carefully transected.

6. Place a retractor (e.g. Lone Star) to allow visualization of the internal organs.

Closure:
- Close the muscle and skin layers separately with absorbable sutures in a continuous or interrupted pattern.
- No attempt to re-join the peritoneum is necessary.

Postoperative care

Birds recover quickly from gaseous anaesthesia. To avoid self-trauma from uncontrolled wing flapping during the excitement phase of recovery, some birds need to be partially restrained in a towel. The bird should be placed in a cage with minimal fixtures with no food or water until upright. Supplemental heat should be provided following surgery until the bird is capable of maintaining thermal homeostasis. There may be some advantage in administering a small amount of glucose or recovery supplement as soon as the bird is able to stand unaided. Once awake,

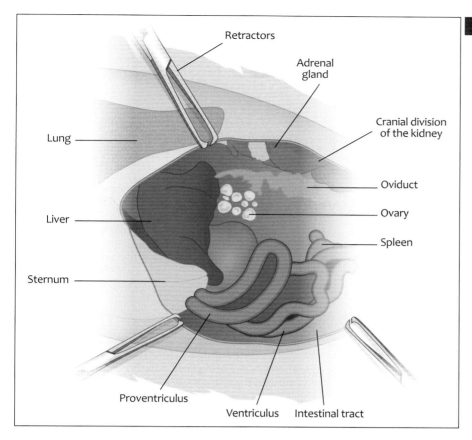

Exposure obtained with a left lateral coeliotomy.

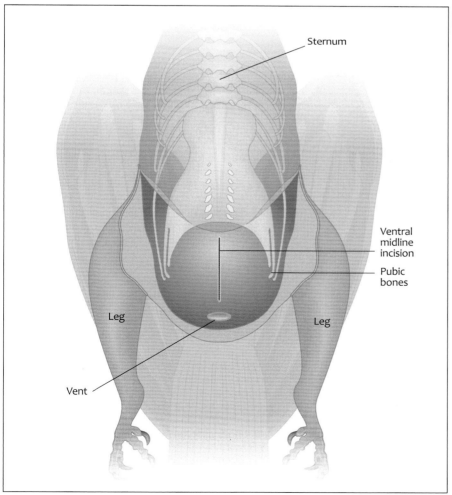

23.13 Landmarks for a ventral midline coeliotomy.

the bird should be closely monitored for signs of distress or haemorrhage for at least 1–2 hours, and regularly monitored for a period of 6–12 months. If mild haemorrhage is present, it can often be contained with a light body pressure bandage (exerting sufficient pressure to minimize or stop the bleeding, but not so tight as to restrict breathing). Analgesia should be provided during the recovery period. Antibiotic therapy may be required if infection is suspected or sterility has been compromised during the procedure. Skin sutures should be removed 12–14 days after surgery, if necessary.

Ingluviotomy

Indications

The indications for ingluviotomy include:

- Biopsy
- Retrieval of foreign objects
- Relieving impaction of the crop with fibrous materials
- Endoscopic access to the proventriculus
- Placement of feeding tubes.

Technique

1. Wherever possible, withhold food or empty the crop prior to surgery.
2. Place the bird in dorsal or lateral recumbency with the head elevated above the level of the crop. Intubate the bird and, if possible, pack the pharynx (e.g. with a gauze swab). (Note that it is feasible to perform an ingluviotomy on a conscious patient using local anaesthesia.)
3. Pluck the feathers and prepare the skin around the surgical site and the drape.
4. Incise the skin over the left lateral wall or ventral midline of the crop, close to the thoracic inlet. Gently blunt dissect the skin edges free of the underlying crop.
5. Select a relatively avascular area of the crop. Tent this area and make an incision into the crop. Extend this incision as required. The crop mucosa will often evert when the crop is opened. Care must be taken to prevent contamination of the subcutaneous tissues with fluids or other ingesta. Stay sutures may be required in some cases.

Closure

- Close the crop with an inverting suture pattern in two layers.
- If unsure whether a good seal has been obtained, pass a feeding tube through the mouth into the crop and gently fill the crop with saline. If there is no leakage, the saline and tube can be withdrawn prior to recovery.
- Flush the subcutaneous tissues thoroughly with sterile saline.
- Close the skin separately in either a continuous or interrupted pattern.

Postoperative care

As a general rule, postoperative recovery and monitoring is as for coeliotomy (see above). Food and water should be withheld for 6–12 hours, after which only fluids and soft foods (soaked poultry mash, chopped vegetables) should be offered for 2–3 days. Gavage feeding with a semi-liquid diet (e.g. parrot hand-rearing formula, soaked and crushed poultry pelleted foods) can be considered in anorectic patients until they are able to eat by themselves (see Chapter 9).

Proventriculotomy

Indications

A proventriculotomy is most commonly used for the retrieval of foreign bodies from the proventriculus or ventriculus that cannot be accessed via the crop. It can also be used to obtain biopsy samples from the proventriculus, although this needs to be considered carefully, weighing up the risks of leakage if the proventricular wall is not fully viable.

Technique

1. Perform a left lateral coeliotomy (as described above).
2. Break down the proventricular suspensory ligaments.
3. Place two stay sutures in the tendinous part of the ventriculus and bring it up into the surgical field. Attach it to the skin. If possible, pack off the rest of the abdomen with saline-soaked gauze swabs.
4. Identify the triangular lobe of the liver overlying the proventricular isthmus and gently reflect with a sterile cotton swab.
5. Make a stab incision into the isthmus and extend it with scissors (Figure 23.14).
6. Use suction to remove any fluid from the proventriculus and ventriculus, and then perform the desired procedure (biopsy, removal of foreign bodies).
7. If necessary, use an endoscope placed in the incision to ensure all foreign objects have been removed.

Closure

- Close the proventricular incision with synthetic monofilament absorbable suture material in two layers: the first layer should be appositional, the second layer should be inverting.
- Tack the liver down over the incision using fine suture material (e.g. 1.5 metric (4/0 USP) polydioxanone) to attach the liver capsule to the serosal surface of the proventriculus.
- Remove the stay sutures and replace the proventriculus into the coelom. Observe for leakage.
- Close the coelom as described above.

Postoperative care

As a general rule, postoperative recovery and monitoring is as for coeliotomy (see above). Food and water should be withheld for 6–12 hours, after which only fluids and soft foods (soaked poultry mash, chopped vegetables) should be offered for 2–3 days. Gavage feeding with a semi-liquid diet (e.g. parrot hand-rearing formula, soaked and crushed poultry pelleted foods) can be considered in anorectic patients until they are able to eat by themselves. Overfeeding should be avoided. Patients should be fed multiple times a day with small amounts of food for 1 week.

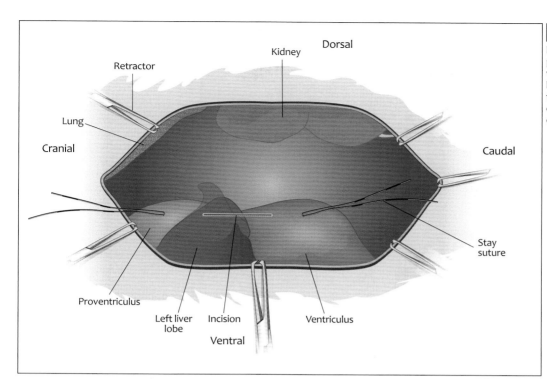

23.14 Proventriculotomy. Stay sutures have been placed in the cranial proventriculus and the ventriculus. The tip of the liver lobe can be reflected to expose the incision site and then tacked down over the incision after closure.

Intestinal surgery

Indications

Although uncommon, intestinal surgery is occasionally required to remove foreign bodies, reduce and/or resect intussusceptions, repair traumatic injuries or iatrogenic surgical damage, or to obtain intestinal biopsy samples (Forbes, 2002). It carries a guarded to poor prognosis in smaller birds, but in poultry the outcome can be good.

Surgical principles

The same principles for intestinal surgery in mammals are applicable to birds: gentle, atraumatic handling of tissues; avoidance of desiccation of exposed tissues; the prevention of spillage of intestinal contents into the coelom; preservation of the intestinal and mesenteric blood supply; and the use of monofilament absorbable suture materials. The only differences lie in the size of the patient.

Surgical instruments and equipment

Microsurgical instrumentation and techniques, combined with adequate magnification and illumination, will give the best results. Microsurgical vascular clamps (e.g. Acland clamps) can be used to occlude the intestines to prevent spillage and contamination. Ring-tipped microsurgical forceps can be used to minimize iatrogenic trauma to the intestines. Counter-balanced scissors and needle holders allow for delicate handling of tissues and suture material. Fine hand control and dexterity are essential; the surgeon should be seated for procedures and utilize forearm support to prevent tremors. When appropriately equipped and trained, the surgeon should be able to perform procedures such as enterotomies, enterectomies, and end-to-end, side-to-side and end-to-side anastomoses.

Approach

A ventral midline approach is most commonly used, although a left lateral approach may provide better access to the rectum and dorsal cloaca (see above).

Technique

Once the affected area of intestine has been identified, it should be exteriorized (if possible) and the coelomic cavity packed off with moistened gauze laparotomy sponges to minimize contamination. The exteriorized intestine must be kept moist by frequent gentle lavage with warmed sterile fluids.

Closure

Intestinal incisions and anastomoses are closed with 0.4–1.5 metric (8/0–4/0 USP) monofilament absorbable sutures in an appositional method using either a simple interrupted or continuous pattern. The method chosen is determined by the size of the intestine and the preference of the surgeon. It is important that no leakage occurs from the site. It should be remembered that in backyard poultry there is no omentum to seal off leaking surgical sites.

Reproductive tract surgery

Salpingohysterectomy

Indications

Salpingohysterectomy can be considered for any oviductal disease that cannot be managed medically. This may include neoplasia, metritis, egg retention or egg binding, yolk peritonitis and ovarian cysts.

Patient evaluation

Reproductive disease rarely occurs in isolation. Generalized peritonitis, underlying liver, lung or kidney disease and ascites all carry a higher risk of surgical complications. An enlarged oviduct in a reproductively active bird occupies the left side of the coelom, making surgery more difficult (Figure 23.15). Thus, if possible, the nutritional status of the patient should be improved, underlying diseases treated and the reproductive cycle 'turned off' through behavioural, social and environmental modification and hormonal therapy (e.g. deslorelin implants) prior to surgery (see Chapter 17).

Approach

In the author's opinion, the left lateral approach gives the best exposure, but other surgeons prefer a ventral midline

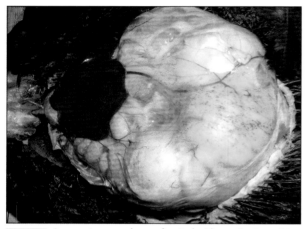

23.15 Any surgeon may be confronted with a patient requiring surgery for yolk peritonitis. In this case the bird was diagnosed with a uterine adenocarcinoma. The enlarged oviduct can be seen on the left side of this bird's coelom.

approach. The approach used will be determined by the clinical condition of the patient and the experience and/or preference of the surgeon.

Technique

Safe removal of the ovary is very difficult and many surgeons opt not to remove it. The blood supply to the ovary is tightly adherent to major blood vessels, making its removal without an operating microscope extremely dangerous. Individual follicles can usually be 'twisted off' starting with the largest. Care should be taken not to retract the ovary away from its blood supply during the procedure. Hormonal implants are usually needed long term to prevent the ovary from ovulating again.

1. Identify and gently retract the infundibulum out through the incision after ligating the large blood vessel running between the infundibulum and the ovary.
2. Break down the ventral suspensory ligament. This ligament is poorly vascularized and serves to coil the oviduct. Breaking it down makes it easier to exteriorize the oviduct during the procedure. Sharp dissection or radiosurgery can be used to break down the ligament.
3. Cauterize or ligate the dorsal suspensory ligament blood vessels as needed (i.e. the cranial, middle and caudal oviductal arteries). This is performed as the dorsal ligament is broken down by sharp dissection and the oviduct exteriorized.
4. Once the oviduct is exteriorized, identify the junction of the oviduct and the cloaca. If necessary, insert a cotton bud or gloved finger into the cloaca to delineate the structure. Place two vascular clips or sutures across the oviduct near this junction and then transect the oviduct proximal to this ligation (Figure 23.16). A common mistake is to not remove the entire

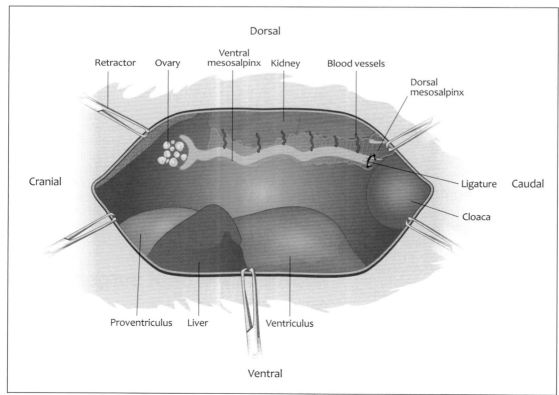

23.16

Landmarks for a salpingohysterectomy. The ovary is located between the cranial division of the kidney and the lung. The oviduct is suspended from the dorsal coelomic wall by the dorsal mesosalpinx, which contains several large and many small blood vessels. The oviduct opens into the cloaca; the site for ligation is indicated by the black ligature.

oviduct. Often a large vaginal stump is left at the cervix and this can act as a nidus for infection or produce sufficient hormonal feedback to encourage ovulation.

5. Remove the oviduct and examine the coelomic cavity for any haemorrhage or blood pooling.

Closure:
- Closure is as described above for coeliotomy.

Postoperative care

Postoperative haemorrhage from ovarian or oviductal vessels is a major and common complication with salpingohysterectomy. Often these vessels are not identified at the time of surgery but bleed once the patient starts to move around. Weakness or obvious blood loss should be investigated with this in mind. Re-entering the coelom, identifying and ligating the bleeding vessels is the most effective way of resolving the problem. If there has been coelomic bleeding or ascites, it is not uncommon for the patient to be mildly dyspnoeic and/or cough up blood or fluids for a few days following surgery. This is due to fluids entering the air sacs and then the lungs. This needs to be monitored carefully and supportive measures (e.g. oxygen cage) provided if necessary. In severe cases it may be necessary to explore the coelom surgically. If there are no complications, postoperative care is similar to that for coeliotomy (see above).

Patient follow-up

Continued ovulation and yolk release with subsequent yolk-related peritonitis has been reported in several birds following salpingohysterectomy. Follow-up surgery may be required, although in many cases hormonal manipulation and anti-inflammatory medications may control this problem.

Orchidectomy

Indications

Orchidectomy (castration or caponization) is indicated in cases of testicular disease, such as orchitis or testicular neoplasia. It can also be useful for some behavioural problems (such as aggression or crowing); however, it should be borne in mind that cocks with these problems usually have very enlarged, vascularized testicles and surgery whilst their libido is high is potentially risky. Behavioural modification and hormonal manipulation may reduce the testicles to a quiescent size, simplifying the surgery and making the procedure safer.

Approach

The testicles can be accessed via one of three approaches: a left lateral approach (Figure 23.17), a bilateral flank approach or a ventral midline coeliotomy with cranial flaps.

Technique

1. Visualize the testicle and gentle retract it ventrally.
2. Place a haemoclip or suture across the dorsal blood vessel (the mesorchium).
3. Free the testicle below the haemoclip or ligature using sharp dissection or radiosurgery. Take care to avoid iatrogenic damage to the adrenal glands, which lie in close proximity to the testicles, as this may result in tachycardia or even cardiac arrest.

Closure:
- Closure is as described above for coeliotomy.

Postoperative care

Postoperative care is as described for coeliotomy (see above).

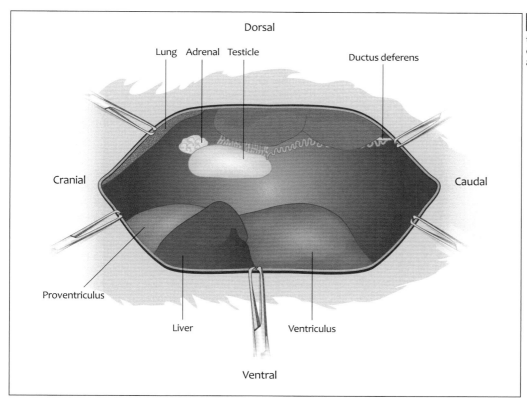

23.17 Landmarks for an orchidectomy. The testicle lies between the cranial division of the kidney and the lung, adjacent to the adrenal gland.

Patient follow-up

Regrowth of testicular remnants is common if not all testicular tissue is removed (which can be quite difficult). Complete removal can be especially difficult if the rete testis extends cranially into the adrenal gland. In some birds, male characteristics are retained, indicating that testosterone may be produced in other tissues.

Omphalectomy

The newly hatched chick receives some nutrients and possibly immunoglobulins from the yolk sac, which is attached to the intestine via the vitello-intestinal duct. Yolk sac contents are drained by both this duct and via absorption by the mesenteric blood vessels that surround the yolk sac. A few hours before hatching the yolk sac is drawn into the coelom and the muscles close over it at the navel. The yolk is resorbed over 10–14 days and only a vestigial remnant remains after 3 weeks.

Occasionally the umbilicus fails to close fully, exposing a portion of the yolk sac. If the exposure is only small, dressing it with iodine and bandaging until closure is complete may be all that is required. Larger exposures may require surgical correction (if economically practical). Affected chicks need to be monitored carefully for omphalitis and yolk sac retention.

Omphalitis (yolk sac infection) is a multifactorial problem seen in chicks <1 week of age. Chicks that have been stressed by incorrect incubator/hatcher temperature and humidity, or chicks that are weak or undersized at hatch, are predisposed to bacterial infection. This infection usually arises due to poor hygiene in the hatcher or brooder, although transovarian and transoviductal infections and shell contamination can also be involved. Many chicks with yolk sac retention subsequently develop omphalitis. The incidence in commercial flocks can be reduced by correcting incubator and hatcher problems and hygiene, and applying an iodine ointment and bandage to the umbilicus of newly hatched chicks. If chicks from a particular hen show a high incidence of omphalitis (without chicks from other hens being affected), then the hen needs to be investigated for the possibility of salpingitis.

Yolk sac retention is a failure of the yolk sac to be resorbed in the absence of infection. This is primarily a management problem and possible causes include faults in the incubator or hatcher, chick nutrition and exercise. Unless secondary omphalitis develops, clinical signs do not become evident until the chick is 2–6 weeks old and the autolysing yolk begins to release potentially toxic substances that are absorbed by the mesenteric blood vessels. These chicks fail to thrive and usually start to lose weight. The yolk sac is often palpable in the abdomen or detectable via ultrasonography.

Technique

As antibiotics do not penetrate the yolk sac, treatment for both omphalitis and yolk sac retention is the surgical excision of the yolk sac. Although a relatively simple procedure, the success rate for omphalectomy is not high due to pre-existing toxaemia and immunosuppression. Where possible, affected chicks should be treated with broad-spectrum antibiotics and fluids for 2–3 days prior to surgery. Assisted feeding may be required if the chick is anorexic or inappetent. During the procedure, intravenous fluid therapy and/or possibly a heterologous blood transfusion can increase the surgical success rate.

1. Place the patient in dorsal recumbency having plucked and prepared the ventral abdomen for surgery.
2. Taking care not to open the yolk sac, make a small circular incision through the skin and coelomic muscles around the umbilicus.
3. Extend the incision rostrally and caudally to expose the yolk sac.
4. Carefully remove the yolk sac from the coelomic cavity.
5. Identify and ligate the vitello-intestinal duct, freeing the yolk sac completely.

Closure

- Close the ventral midline incision in 2–3 layers using 1.5–2 metric (4/0–3/0 USP) monofilament suture material.

Cloacal surgery

Cloacal surgery is indicated for the treatment of cloacal diseases such as cloacal prolapse, neoplasia and cloacoliths.

Ventoplasty

Indications

A ventoplasty is a temporary or permanent narrowing of the vent (cloacal opening), which is indicated for the treatment of cloacal prolapse or atony.

Technique

The initial step in many cases is to assess the prolapse to determine what tissues have prolapsed, whether the tissues are viable and if there are any life-threatening complications.

1. Gently lavage the prolapsed tissues with warmed saline and manually remove any dirt, grass or faecal material.
2. Examine the prolapsed tissues to determine their origin (oviductal *versus* gastrointestinal).
3. Identify and resect (if possible) any necrotic or devitalized tissue.
4. Replace the prolapsed tissue and lavage the cloaca before exploring with an endoscope or manually to confirm replacement.

Closure:

- Mentally divide the vent into three equal lengths.
- Close the outer two lengths with 1–2 simple or vertical mattress sutures. Leave the middle third open for the passage of faeces, urates and urine (Figure 23.18).
- If a permanent narrowing of the vent is required, trim the mucocutaneous borders of the dorsal and ventral vent lips on the outer lengths to create a bleeding surface before suturing. The upper and lower lips will then heal together on both sides, resulting in a permanently narrowed opening in the middle.

WARNING

A purse-string suture is contraindicated in birds, as the vent is a horizontal slit opening in a dorsoventral direction (rather than a circular opening)

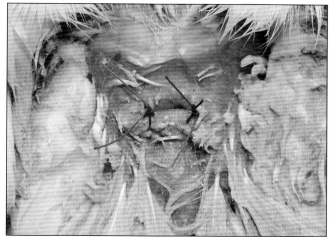

23.18 Temporary ventoplasty. Simple interrupted sutures have been used to close the lateral margins of the slit-like vent. A purse-string suture is contraindicated as it would distort the shape of the vent.

Egg-laying should be taken into consideration when determining whether a temporary or permanent ventoplasty should be performed in female birds. If permanent ventoplasty is chosen, consideration should be given to preventing egg production by performing a salpingohysterectomy. If further egg production is desired, a permanent procedure should not be performed. In these cases, temporary ventoplasty combined with hormonal manipulation (e.g. a deslorelin implant) may be required. The use of sutures that can be untied and retightened to allow the passage of an egg can be helpful in these patients.

Cloacopexy
Indications

Wherever possible, chronic cloacal prolapses should be treated by identifying and correcting the underlying cause. A cloacopexy is a last resort 'salvage' procedure indicated in cases of chronic cloacal prolapse that cannot otherwise be resolved. It involves fixing the cloaca to the ventral body wall and sternum to prevent prolapse.

Technique

1. Perform a ventral midline coeliotomy (as described above).
2. Replace the prolapsed tissue and have an assistant place a gloved finger (large birds) or cotton bud (small birds) into the cloaca to define its extent and lift it up to the body wall.
3. Remove the intra-coelomic fat located ventral to the cloaca by careful sharp and blunt dissection. Simply reflecting the fat may not provide sufficient serosal exposure for suture attachment.
4. Using monofilament non-absorbable suture material, place sutures through the full thickness of the cloacal wall and around the last rib (at the junction of the sternal and vertebral portions) on each side, or through the cartilaginous border of the sternum. Pre-place the sutures and then tie them once they are all in position, thereby anchoring the cloaca in a reduced position with the cloacal wall apposed to the ribs (albeit more cranial than normal).
5. Incise the ventral cloacal serosa to the level of the submucosa and place taking sutures through the body

wall to attach the submucosa to the body wall. Incorporate some of these sutures into the abdominal wall closure.

It should be noted that this technique only attaches the ventral aspect of the cloaca to the ribs and body wall; the dorsal cloaca is not included. If the bird continues to strain, the dorsal cloacal tissues can still prolapse. With time and continued straining, the sutures may break or cut through the attached tissues and prolapse of the cloaca can occur. As with ventoplasty, consideration needs to be given to the performance of this procedure in egg-laying hens.

Cloacotomy
Indications

Cloacotomy (the surgical opening of the cloaca) is an infrequently used technique for the removal of cloacoliths and the debridement and/or excision of cloacal neoplasia.

Technique

1. Place the bird in dorsal recumbency.
2. Insert a gloved finger or moistened cotton bud into the cloaca to outline the structure.
3. Incise through the skin, cloacal sphincter and cloacal mucosa from the vent to the cranial end of the cloaca, taking care not to extend the incision into the coelom. Extreme caution must be exercised in the region of the reproductive and ureteral openings. This opens the ventral wall of the cloaca, exposing the coprodeum, urodeum and proctodeum.

Closure:
- Close the incision in three layers: the mucosa with a continuous suture pattern; the cloacal sphincter with a single mattress suture; and the skin in a separate third layer.

Phallus prolapse

Prolapse of the phallus is not an uncommon problem in sexually mature Anseriformes (Figure 23.19). The cause is probably multifactorial but usually involves frequent sexual behaviour, often complicated by chronic inflammation and infection at the base of the phallus. The result is a prolapsed phallus that may dry out or be traumatized.

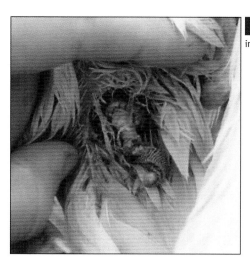

23.19 Phallic prolapse in a drake.

Treatment

Treatment in the early stages involves manual replacement of the phallus into the cloaca, accompanied by systemic non-steroidal anti-inflammatory drugs (e.g. meloxicam), topical antibacterial ointment (e.g. silver sulfadiazine) and sexual 'rest' (i.e. complete removal from contact with female birds). If this is not sufficient to retain the phallus in the cloaca, a temporary ventoplasty (see above) may be necessary for several weeks whilst the phallus becomes quiescent and heals. In persistent cases, especially when the phallus is badly traumatized, amputation may be required. The amputation needs to be complete (i.e. at the base of the phallus) to minimize postoperative complications such as pain, incontinence and cloacitis. The phallus should be clamped at the base, excised and the stump oversewn. If excessive haemorrhage occurs, transfixing sutures can be placed.

Pododermatitis

Pododermatitis (also known as bumblefoot) is an inflamed and often infected lesion on the plantar surface of the foot. Although most commonly seen in raptors, it is often reported in gallinaceous birds as well as other species. It is a disease of captivity and is rare in wild birds.

The plantar surface of the foot is protected by a thick layer of stratified squamous epithelium, which in turn is covered by a layer of keratin. Over the surface of this keratin is a layer of papillae, which are thought to evenly spread the weight bearing requirement of the foot. When this barrier is eroded or breached, an inflammatory response is often provoked and infection can be introduced. These infections are usually associated with *Staphylococcus aureus*, but other bacteria including *Escherichia coli*, *Pasteurella* spp., *Klebsiella* spp., *Clostridium* spp., *Corynebacterium* spp., *Bacillus* spp., *Diplococcus* spp., *Nocardia* spp., *Actinobacillus* spp., *Actinomyces* spp., *Aeromonas* spp., *Proteus* spp. and *Pseudomonas* spp. have been implicated. *Candida* spp. and *Aspergillus* spp. may also be involved in some cases. The inflammation and/or infection may extend into the joints, tendons and bones of the foot.

Contributing factors to the erosion or breach of the keratin barrier include:

* Trauma (e.g. from inappropriate perch design or surface)
* Hypovitaminosis A
* Obesity or heavy bodyweight (e.g. turkeys)
* Long periods of inactivity leading to excessive weight bearing without relief
* Excessive weight bearing on one leg due to a problem with the other leg (e.g. unilateral lameness may lead to pododermatitis in the contralateral leg). In many cases, pododermatitis in one foot will lead to some degree of pododermatitis in the other foot.

Classification

Veterinary surgeons (veterinarians) who treat raptors have developed a classification scheme for pododermatitis, which provides clinicians with a treatment plan and guide to prognosis. This classification scheme has been extended to other species with good results (Figure 23.20).

Class	Description
I	Early devitalization of a prominent plantar area without disruption of the epithelial barrier. It can be subdivided into: • Hyperaemia (bruise) or early ischaemia (a blanched area with compromised capillary perfusion) • Hyperkeratotic reaction (an early callus)
II	Localized inflammation/infection of underlying tissues in direct contact with the devitalized area. No gross swelling. It can be subdivided into: • Puncture wound • Ischaemic necrosis of the epithelium (a penetrating callus or scab)
III	More generalized infection with gross inflammatory swelling of the underlying tissues. The origin may be a puncture wound or ischaemic necrosis; however, by this stage the initial cause is of minor insignificance in comparison with the ongoing pathology. It can be subdivided into: • Serous (acute) – oedema and hyperaemia of the tissues • Fibrotic (chronic) – attempt at encapsulation and confinement • Caseous – accumulation of necrotic debris
IV	Established infection with gross swelling and involvement of deeper vital structures. Radiology and surgical exploration are often required to differentiate types III and IV. Class IV is a chronic condition causing tenosynovitis and occasionally arthritis and osteomyelitis
V	An extension of Class IV, characterized by crippling deformities

23.20 Classification of pododermatitis.

Treatment and prognosis of pododermatitis is determined by the classification of the condition.

* Class I – carries a favourable prognosis as there is no evidence of infection. The lesions generally respond to conservative husbandry changes (e.g. alternative perching surfaces and substrates) and the application of topical emollients (e.g. petroleum jelly). Emollients utilize fats and lipids to establish a protective barrier on the surface of the skin. This oily layer of lipids traps water in the stratum corneum (the outermost layer of the epidermis), thus protecting the skin.
* Class II – carries a good prognosis as the infection is localized (Figure 23.21). The lesions respond well to surgery as the total affected area is easily resected and the epidermal defects are characteristically small, hence the architecture of the weight bearing structures of the plantar aspect of the foot remain intact. This class of lesion will generally not respond to conservative treatment.
* Class III – traditionally carries a good to guarded prognosis as the infection is well established and structural changes have affected the foot (Figure 23.22). Some lesions can be treated as for Class II pododermatitis; however, the majority should be treated by complete surgical removal of all affected tissue, followed by primary intention healing i.e. suturing the surgical wound closed.
* Class IV – carries a guarded to poor prognosis as infection is harboured in and affects deeper vital structures, making surgical debridement difficult or impossible (Figure 23.23). It should be noted that encapsulated infective tissues are often present, which, if not removed, will result in later reoccurrence of pododermatitis.
* Class V – carries a poor to hopeless prognosis and may require euthanasia (Figure 23.24).

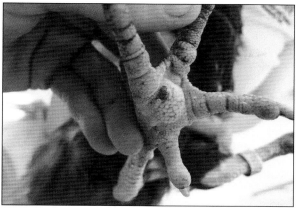

23.21 Class II pododermatitis lesion in a chicken.
(Courtesy of Dr A Chamness)

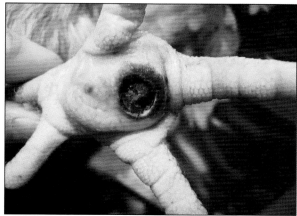

23.22 Class III pododermatitis lesion in a chicken.
(Courtesy of S Silvetti)

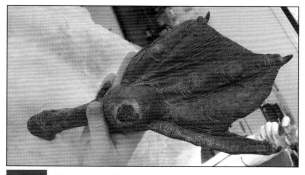

23.23 Class IV pododermatitis lesion in a swan.

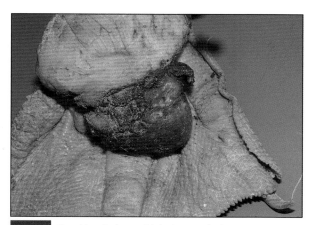

23.24 Class V pododermatitis lesion in a duck.

Treatment

Treatment must include improving the health and nutritional status of the bird, as well as husbandry where appropriate. If surgery is contemplated, culture and sensitivity testing should be performed in advance so that the results are available at the time of surgery. This allows an appropriate antibiotic to be administered at the time of the procedure, rather than several days later when post-surgical fibrotic encapsulation of pathogenic bacteria is already underway. Whilst waiting for the results, broad-spectrum antibiotic coverage and analgesia can be commenced.

Surgery is aimed at debulking the infection, removing all caseous debris and infected/necrotic tissue (via curetting and debriding), and then closing the site (if possible) so that healing by primary intention can occur. Placing antibiotic impregnated polymethylmethacrylate beads into the wound prior to closure can assist with the long-term delivery of antibiotics into the affected area. The beads can be removed once wound healing is complete.

Following surgery, it is important that pressure is relieved from the surgery site. This is achieved through the use of padded bandages or gauze/rubber 'doughnuts', which evenly distribute pressure across the whole foot (Figure 23.25). In addition, these bandages help to keep the surgery site clean and away from potentially contaminated surfaces. Close attention must be paid to the contralateral foot to ensure that it does not subsequently develop pododermatitis (Figure 23.26).

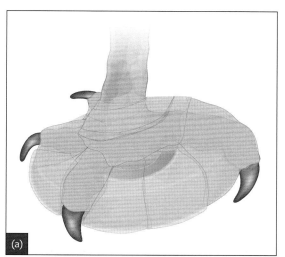

(a)

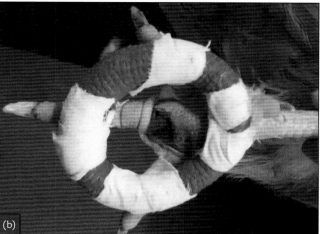

(b)

23.25 (a) Doughnut bandage. (b) Bandage in place in a case of unilateral pododermatitis.

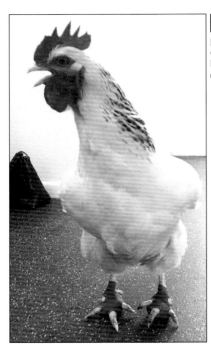

23.26 Chicken with bilateral pododermatitis with doughnut bandages on both feet.
(Courtesy of Dr A Gallagher)

Enucleation

Indications

Enucleation is indicated in cases of severe, irreversible panophthalmitis, perforating corneal ulcers and ocular/orbital neoplasia (Figure 23.27). This procedure is more difficult in birds than in mammals because of the relatively larger globe compared with the size of the orbit, the short optic nerve (excessive traction can result in contralateral blindness) and because the area is highly vascularized.

Technique

The technique described below is for enucleation of the eye; an alternative procedure is evisceration of the globe contents (see Chapter 14 for details of this technique).

1. Suture the eyelids together in a simple continuous pattern, leaving the ends long as stay sutures.

2. Make a circumferential incision through the skin (not the conjunctiva), 2–3 mm from the lid margins. Note that the ligamentous attachments at the medial canthus are firm. Haemorrhage can be expected in this area and at the lateral canthus.
3. Dissect between the palpebral conjunctiva and the bony orbit as it is not feasible to identify and transect each individual muscle. The sutured eyelids can be manipulated to provide traction on the globe.
4. In many large birds, it may be necessary to collapse the globe prior to enucleation. This can be achieved by incising through the cornea, evacuating the globe contents with a syringe and large gauge needle, and then, where necessary, incising the sclera.
5. Where feasible, blindly apply a vascular clip (using an angled applicator) to the optic stalk or ligate it, incorporating the nerve and blood vessels. Take care to apply only minimal traction to the globe at this point to avoid iatrogenic damage to the optic chiasm or the contralateral optic nerve.
6. After the optic stalk has been clipped or ligated, transect it and remove the eye. If it has not been feasible to clip or ligate the stalk, retract the globe using sharp dissection. Haemorrhage is expected at this stage and can usually be controlled by placing a vascular clip directly on to the now visible optic stalk. If this is not feasible, packing the orbit with absorbable gelatine sponges is usually effective.

Closure

- Suture the eyelid margins together in a simple interrupted pattern to close the site.

Submandibular lingual entrapment in waterfowl

This condition occurs when fibrous food becomes trapped beneath the tongue in herbivorous waterfowl, stretching the inter-mandibular space and creating a 'pocket' into which the tongue becomes entrapped (Figure 23.28). This in turn leads to difficulty in the prehension and mastication of food. It is unclear whether neurological deficits contribute to the problem, or whether it is more associated with over-stretched and atrophic glossal muscles.

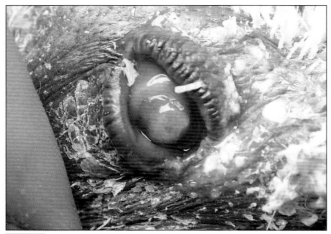

23.27 Corneal ulceration and panophthalmitis requiring enucleation.

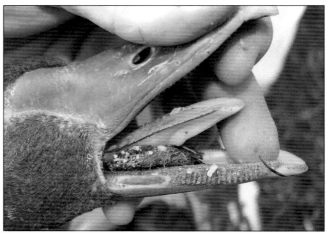

23.28 Submandibular lingual entrapment in a black swan.
(Courtesy of Dr D Brown)

The clinical signs seen with submandibular lingual entrapment include:

- Swelling on the ventral aspect of the intra-mandibular space
- Weight loss
- On physical examination, the tongue is found to be sitting in a pocket within the inter-mandibular space and the bird is unable to reposition it.

Technique

The aim of the procedure is to obliterate the inter-mandibular pocket and reposition the tongue into a normal position.

1. Resect the redundant tissue in the inter-mandibular skin and lingual frenulum.
2. Place bilateral sutures through the basohyoideum (caudal bone of the hyoid apparatus) and the caudal aspect of the mandibular symphysis. Tighten these sutures to draw the tongue forward into a more normal position.

Closure

- Close the skin over the frenulum and inter-mandibular space. If concern exists about the ability of the bird to eat soon after the procedure, place an oesophagostomy tube.

Integumentary surgery

Skin laceration repair

Skin lacerations are not uncommon in backyard poultry, with injuries inflicted by predator attacks, sharp objects and even other birds. Some of these injuries are simple lacerations; others are more complex injuries associated with extensive soft tissue and even bone damage (Figure 23.29).

Avian skin is closely attached to the underlying bone and muscle. Loose skin in most birds can be found on the neck and in the inguinal area, but the skin covering the rest of the body is relatively immobile. This makes undermining and mobilizing skin to close wounds more difficult in birds compared with many mammalian species. Avian skin is also thin and, especially in poultry, has a fatty subcutaneous layer. Subcutaneous sutures do not hold very well and are therefore of limited value. Postoperative swelling is not as severe in birds as it is in mammals, thus sutures can be placed closer together and tied tighter.

Skin laceration repair in birds requires that the surgeon:

- Thoroughly debrides and flushes the wound. In most cases, the use of sterile saline is satisfactory as a flushing solution. Chlorhexidine and povidone–iodine, even when diluted, can be toxic to granulation tissue and should be avoided if possible
- Mobilizes available skin where possible to achieve primary closure without tension on the wound edges
- Avoids the use of drains unless combined with a flushing or irrigation system. Avian heterophils lack lysozymes, meaning that pus is usually caseated and therefore does not drain from a contaminated wound readily.

Wherever possible, wounds should be closed to heal by primary intention. Where primary closure cannot be achieved, either skin grafts or flaps, or healing by second intention is required. The same techniques used in mammals for skin grafts and flaps can be employed in birds (Ferrell, 2002; Stroud et al., 2003). If skin grafts are not utilized, good healing can often be achieved by secondary intention. In these cases, drying out of the underlying subcutis and muscle should be avoided by he use of wet or hydrocolloid dressings. Aggressive postoperative antibiosis and analgesia significantly improves morbidity and mortality rates in these patients.

Spur removal

The spur is a bony, conical projection found on the medial aspect of the distal leg (arising from the tarsometatarsus) of sexually mature male gallinaceous birds (chickens, turkeys, guinea fowl, partridges and pheasants) (Figure 23.30). However, it should be noted that not all species develop spurs, and that they can also be found in some adult hens. The spur, which is used as a weapon by the bird, is an outgrowth of the tarsometatarsus covered with keratin. In male chicks the projection is called a papilla. As the bird matures, the papilla grows larger, hardens and starts to curve.

The aggression displayed by sexually mature birds, where spurs are used to inflict trauma to other birds, animals and even people, is a frequent indication for spur removal or trimming. In chicks, the soft papilla can be trimmed off at the skin using a pair of nail clippers. In older birds, it can be either trimmed down to the bony core (using a rotary tool such as a Dremel) or amputated at the level of the tarsometatarsus. A regional block using lidocaine or bupivacaine can assist with analgesia.

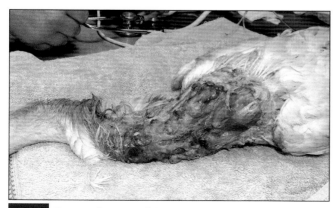

23.29 Dog attacks can result in severe trauma.

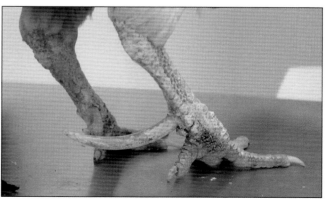

23.30 Spurs on adult roosters can be quite dangerous and removal may be required.

Amputation requires general anaesthesia or, at the least, systemic analgesia and sedation combined with a local anaesthetic block. A bone saw is used to cut the spur at its base from the tarsometatarsus. If possible, the skin edges should be sutured; at worst, the wound should be allowed to heal by secondary intention. Postoperative analgesia and wound dressing to prevent infection may be indicated.

References and further reading

Ferrell ST (2002) Avian integumentary surgery. *Seminars in Avian and Exotic Pet Medicine* **11**, 125–135

Forbes NA (2002) Avian gastrointestinal surgery. *Seminars in Avian and Exotic Pet Medicine* **11**, 196–207

McFadden MS (2011) Suture materials and suture selection for use in exotic pet surgical procedures. *Journal of Exotic Pet Medicine* **20**, 173–181

Stroud PK, Amalsadvala T and Swaim SF (2003) The use of skin flaps and grafts for wound management in raptors. *Journal of Avian Medicine and Surgery* **17**, 78–85

Chapter 24

Orthopaedic surgery

Aidan Raftery and Sergio Silvetti

This Manual covers a wide range of different sized birds, from Bantams weighing <400 g to turkeys that can weigh >15 kg. This presents a challenge in terms of orthopaedic surgery. In addition to the range of surgical skills required, anaesthesia and supportive care are very important for a successful outcome, and a comprehensive plan for analgesia is imperative.

Fractures in poultry are not very common and can sometimes be the result of underlying disease, which needs to be considered when planning corrective management. Developmental diseases are more commonly seen in fast-growing birds, such as meat-producing chickens, turkeys and geese. Genetics, environment and diet composition all play an important role in these conditions.

General principles

Minimal handling is important during the initial examination and during subsequent surgical procedures to maintain the viability of the tissues, minimize postoperative swelling and preserve the blood supply to the affected area. The equipment and techniques used in fracture management will reflect the skills and preferences of the surgeon, but it is important to have alternative fixation devices available at the time of surgery in case the surgical plan has to change during the procedure. The use of small atraumatic instruments and blunt dissection of the tissues is essential to minimize trauma and vascular damage to the soft tissues.

Patient evaluation

History

A full evaluation of any injured bird has to include a complete history (environmental, nutritional, past medical history, behaviour) and information about the trauma (when it happened, how it happened, if the owner was present at the event).

Examination

Without restraining the patient, the following factors should be assessed: symmetry; weight-bearing; the presence of bruising; open wounds; the presence of blood; and any signs of systemic illness. Following the initial assessment, a thorough orthopaedic examination should be performed with gentle restraint of the patient.

Minimum database

A complete blood profile with haematology (packed cell volume), differential white cell count and smear evaluation of cell morphology) and biochemistry is recommended. If any underlying problems are identified, they may affect the surgical plan; for example, some conditions may increase the anaesthetic risk, and some may have predisposed the bird to pathological fractures and therefore influence the surgical repair technique selected.

Diagnostic imaging

Radiography is essential to assess the extent of the injuries sustained by the bird. At least two good quality radiographic views are required for diagnosis (Figure 24.1). It is also important to obtain radiographs of the contralateral normal bone for comparison. Patient positioning is important to achieve diagnostic radiographs, and the reader is referred to Chapter 11 for detailed information on diagnostic imaging.

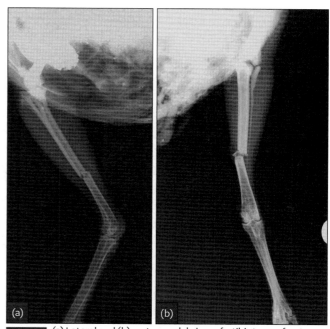

24.1 (a) Lateral and (b) rostrocaudal view of a tibiotarsus fracture in a hen. With simple diaphyseal fractures, as in this case, the preferred technique for fixation is with a type IA or type IIA external skeletal fixator (depending on the size of the bird) or a tie-in procedure.

Bone structure and composition

The bones of birds have a higher content of inorganic substances (hydroxyapatite) and thinner cortex than mammals, which gives them a relatively brittle consistency with an increased risk of comminuted and exposed fractures. The bones of the sternum, humerus, pelvis and the cervical and thoracic vertebrae are pneumatized, which means that there are extensions of the air sacs into these bones. This has to be considered when determining the surgical approach, techniques and prognosis of fracture repair. It should also be remembered that the bones not only provide support to the bird's body but also store calcium for the physiological processes that occur during egg formation. The most important calcium reserve for egg development is the medullary bone.

In mammals, most long bones have one or more epiphyseal or secondary centres of ossification. The tibiotarsus of birds appears to follow a classic mammalian ossification pattern. The ends of the bones grow rapidly and establish secondary centres of ossification (epiphyses). However, the humerus, radius, ulna and femur develop with endochondral ossification. The growth plates of birds are structurally different from mammalian growth plates, but they are controlled by the same physiological processes. Blood vessels arising from the epiphyseal area supply the transitional zone and penetrate the depth of the proliferative zone of the growth cartilage.

Bone healing

The majority of the callus tissue during the healing process is derived from the periosteal surface, and the blood supply to the periosteum from the surrounding soft tissues is very important. The intramedullary circulation appears to be of less importance in avian bone healing than in mammals. Healing is also faster in birds than in mammals. The healing process begins with formation of the blood clot, which is then substituted with mesenchymal cells and woven bone. If the fracture site is stable, the healing process progresses without the formation of cartilage and the remodelling with lamellar bone is complete at 8 weeks. A simple closed fracture can be stable within 3 weeks.

Fracture management

The choice of technique used reflects the fracture site, the nature of the fracture (e.g. simple *versus* compound fractures), the location of the fracture (e.g. metaphysis *versus* diaphysis) and whether a joint is involved. Other important factors include the function of the bone (e.g. the tibiotarsus in a turkey bears a lot more weight than its humerus or the tibiotarsus of a Bantam). Any factors affecting bone strength will influence the repair technique, as will age and any associated soft tissue damage (see Appendix 1).

The principles of fracture management in birds are generally modifications of those for domestic small mammals. However, familiarity with the unique surgical anatomy and surgical approaches used in birds is important to successfully diagnose and treat those cases that require orthopaedic surgery. The goal of accurate anatomical alignment involves restoration of the original length of the bone, axial alignment and rotation orientation, whilst minimizing the trauma to the surrounding tissues and maintaining the blood circulation (periosteal blood supply) will minimize healing time and reduce the incidence of complications. In backyard poultry, an incomplete return to function is sometimes acceptable; restoration of flight is not usually necessary.

Initial stabilization

Fractures of the main bones of the limbs should be immobilized as soon as possible to minimize soft tissue damage and to reduce the risk of the fracture becoming compound and/or open if the bird struggles. Immobilizing the fracture will also reduce pain, making the bird more comfortable. Fractures of the humerus, radius, ulna and carpometacarpus can be bandaged with a figure-of-eight bandage against the body wall. This is a temporary measure as external coaptation may cause rotation and/or displacement at the fracture site. It should also be remembered that as the humerus is pneumatized, subcutaneous emphysema can develop. In addition, if there is an open fracture, any contamination can spread to the air sacs. Pelvic limb fractures of the tibiotarsus and tarsometatarsus are temporarily immobilized by splinting. The femur cannot be effectively splinted due to the surrounding muscles. Further soft tissue damage can be reduced in birds with femoral fractures by restricting movement and care during management. Fractured toes can be supported with ball or ball-type bandages.

Common fracture repair techniques

It is important to have a good knowledge of a variety of fracture fixation techniques and to be ready with alternative surgical repair plans (Figure 24.2). Reassessment of the injury intraoperatively may necessitate a change in the surgical procedure.

Non-surgical management
Cage rest

In some cases, no treatment may be necessary besides analgesia for the initial few days following injury. This would certainly be true for stable fractures of the thoracic limb distal to the radius and ulna in flightless birds. Limitation of movement and restraint in small cages is an acceptable choice for many fractures of the wings and pectoral girdle. Cage rest for 3–4 weeks is often sufficient. However, non-union, malalignment and shortened bone length are common sequelae. In addition, fracture union will not be as rapid as in cases where more rigid fixation is achieved by surgical fixation methods.

External coaptation

The use of bandages and other external splints and casts is common in avian orthopaedics. The best results are obtained with simple minimally displaced fractures. However, this method also carries a high risk of fracture disease (malalignment, delayed union, joint ankylosis, muscle atrophy, shortened bone length, pseudoarthrosis/neoarthrosis). External coaptation is normally indicated as a preliminary technique to stabilize the fracture site prior to surgery. It is also indicated in patients with metabolic bone disease, where the bone is too weak or soft for surgical repair, and in critically ill birds. The position of the bone fragments should be checked radiographically once the external coaptation has been applied for good alignment and to ensure there is no rotation.

Techniques: A figure-of-eight bandage (Figure 24.3) is indicated for fractures of the coracoid/clavicle, transverse

Type of fracture	Treatment options				
	Cage rest	Bandage	Intramedullary pin fixation	External skeletal fixation (ESF)	Plating
Beak		In association with a pharyngostomy tube		Miniature external fixation pins ± interfragmentary cerclage wiring	
Coracoid, scapula and clavicle	Functional healing achieved in most cases	Figure-of-eight bandage extended around the body	Severely displaced fractures can be repaired with an intramedullary pin and external coaptation		
Humerus	In flightless birds, if minimal displacement	Figure-of-eight bandage extended around the body		Tie-in technique or type IA ESF frame	Possible in larger birds
Radius and ulna		Figure-of-eight bandage	Intramedullary pin or Kirschner wire and bandage for 1 week	Tie-in technique or type IA ESF frame	Possible in larger birds (rarely indicated)
Carpometacarpus		Figure-of-eight bandage	Intramedullary pin or Kirschner wire and bandage for 1 week		
Femur			Intramedullary pin or Kirschner wire	Tie-in technique or type IA ESF frame	Possible in larger birds
Tibiotarsus				Type IA or IIA ESF frames or medial tie-in	Possible in larger birds
Tarsometatarsus				Type IA or IIA ESF frame	
Phalanges	Cage rest for closed fractures that are not displaced	Coaptation in a physiological position. Modifications of a ball bandage commonly used			

24.2 Management options for different types of fractures seen in backyard poultry.

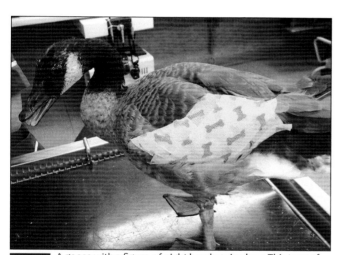

24.3 A goose with a figure-of-eight bandage in place. This type of external fixation is indicated for fractures of the radius and ulna with good alignment or fractures of the carpometacarpus.

proximal humeral fractures, fractures of the radius or ulna that are in good alignment, and fractures of the carpometacarpal bones. To be effective it must immobilize the proximal and distal joints from the fracture. With fractures of the coracoid/clavicle, humerus and elbow, the best results are obtained when the bandage is extended around the body of the bird to bind the wing against the body wall. The bandage must be secure enough that the bird cannot wriggle out of it, but still be able to breathe. In addition, figure-of-eight bandages should not be applied too tight, as this is more likely to result in loss of range of movement

in the joints. These bandages should be removed at least every 7 days under general anaesthesia to perform physical therapy on the affected wing to minimize the risk of propatagial contracture, loss of joint flexibility and muscle contracture. Robert Jones bandages have been used for temporary immobilization of pelvic limb fractures distal to the femur. However, the management of dressings on the pelvic limb to support fractures is difficult. Surgical repair is recommended for these fractures in all but the smallest birds.

Surgical management
Intramedullary pinning

Depending on the size of the bird and the bone involved, Steinmann pins or small Kirschner wires can be used for intramedullary pinning (no more than 50% of medullary cavity). However, it should be noted that intramedullary pinning will damage the network of bony trabeculae in the medullary cavity, which are important in providing extra strength in avian long bones. The use of an intramedullary pin cannot counter the rotational and shearing forces acting at the fracture site. Thus, it is often used in a tie-in configuration with external fixators to improve rotational stability (see below). The intramedullary pin is bent at right angles to the bone where it exits the skin and is incorporated into the external fixation device. The use of stack-pinning, cross-pinning or Rush-pinning with multiple small diameter pins, sometimes combined with cerclage wire and external coaptation, has been recommended in the past; however, where possible, external fixation is the preferred method.

Fractures of the coracoid bone can be immobilized by intramedullary pinning. The fracture is exposed and the pin is passed retrograde out of the shoulder, the fracture is aligned and the pin, after having the sharp end blunted, is passed into the distal portion of the coracoid. The pin is removed from the shoulder when healing is shown to be sufficiently advanced on radiography. Intramedullary pinning can also be used to repair fractures of the ulna and radius, where the pin is inserted in the radius. The ulna may, in some cases, be supported with a figure-of-eight bandage for at least a week following the surgery. However, on occasion, it is necessary to use either intramedullary pinning or external fixation for fractures of the ulna. In anterograde and retrograde insertion, it is recommended that the distal end of the pin is blunted, to avoid migration and perforation of the distal joint. The advantage of intramedullary pinning is that the surgical procedure is much quicker than that for external fixation or bone plating. The disadvantages are that rotational and shearing forces can still act at the fracture site and there is an increased potential to cause articular and periarticular damage, resulting in ankylosis of the joints. Even correctly placed pins that exit near a joint can cause significant tendon or ligament damage, resulting in a partially dysfunctional limb.

Plating

The use of bone plates in backyard poultry orthopaedic surgery is not very common, as the thin bone cortex of the birds does not hold the implant very well. The larger surgical incision required, with its associated increased tissue trauma, delays the healing process and increases the risk of infection. Other factors that make bone plating difficult in birds include the reduced amount of soft tissue covering many of the bones and the relative inflexibility of the skin. Many different plate sizes (titanium plates for use in human fingers, semitubular plates, dynamic compression plates, cuttable plates) and shapes can be used to fit even small bones. The advantage of these plates is that they can be modelled to reproduce the shape of the bone. Self-tapping screws should have a pilot hole predrilled, otherwise there is an increased risk of them fracturing the thin brittle cortex of avian bone. The bones in which a plating technique is sometimes used include the femur and humerus. With these bones there are sufficient overlying soft tissues to cover the bone plate. The use of bone plates, if correctly applied, can stabilize bone fragments almost perfectly. First intention healing is possible and the time for return to normal function of the wing or leg is very short. Removal of the plate is not always indicated. When plates are left in place, there can be a problem of pain from the conduction of cold in the winter.

External fixation

External skeletal fixation (ESF) is the most useful technique in avian orthopaedic surgery. It has the advantage of being minimally invasive with little disruption of the fragments, the soft tissue attachments and the blood supply. If there is an area of shattered bone, stabilization can still be achieved as the area is bridged and normal bone length can be maintained as the fragments heal. If there is contamination at the fracture site, there is no implant providing tracts to potentiate the infection. External fixation facilitates a quick return to function, reducing the incidence of fracture disease, allowing normal joint movement and better, more rapid healing.

Following the general orthopaedic techniques described for small mammals (see the *BSAVA Manual of Canine and Feline Musculoskeletal Disorders*), the best result for stiffness and resistance to bending, torsion forces and axial loading is dependent on the pins (size, number, type, length), configuration of the implants (unilateral, bilateral, mono-biplanar) and the connecting bar material. As a general rule, the size of the pins used should be no more than 25% of the diameter of the bone to be fixed. There should be a minimum of two pins per fragment. To increase the stabilization of the fracture, an increased number of pins can be used, but the stiffness of the implant reaches its maximum with four pins per fragment. To reduce the possibility of early loosening of the pins, the use of positive threaded pins is always advisable (Figure 24.4). These pins can be used directly on the bone, even if predrilling with a smaller diameter drill is the most effective technique.

A common approach that combines the advantages of intramedullary pinning with external fixation is a tie-in configuration in which a small intramedullary pin is inserted in a retrograde or anterograde manner into the medullary cavity, bent at 90 degrees to the shaft of the bone and connected to the stabilizing bar. When using an intramedullary ESF tie-in technique, there should be at least one or two external fixation pins per fragment connecting with the external bar. This technique is indicated for a more stable alignment and to prevent rotation and shearing forces.

Due to the wide variety in size of backyard poultry, a broad selection of connecting bars can be used for ESF frames. The choice of connecting system is also driven by the size of the bird and the relative total weight of the implant. 'Classic' metallic clamps can be used in birds weighing >1 kg to improve stiffness and where the relative weight of the implant is not a problem. The FESSA (Fixateur Externe du Service de Santé des Armees) system is an alternative often used in avian orthopaedics. The FESSA tubular external fixator is made of stainless steel and is available in different diameters (6, 8 or 12 mm) for which pins of up to 2–2.5 mm can be used. A system of screws and holes is used to attach the pins to the tubular connector, replacing the use of metallic clamps.

In small birds, the weight of the fixation frame can be lightened by the use of polymethylmethacrylate (PMMA) connecting bars instead of the heavier metal connecting bars. Latex tubes (Penrose drains) or plastic straws are placed on the free ends of the pins and then PMMA is injected, which when it solidifies makes an effective and light connecting bar. Where necessary, the PMMA bar can be further strengthened by incorporating a reinforcing metal pin in the straw or tube before injecting the PMMA.

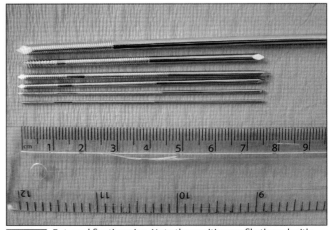

24.4 External fixation pins. Note the positive profile thread with factory roughened central area to enhance the interface between the acrylic frame and the pin.

Many of the smaller external fixation bars have a roughened area that is designed to form a strong join with PMMA. The spatial configuration is dependent upon which bone is fractured. The most commonly used configurations are unilateral (type IA), bilateral (type IIA) and the tie-in configuration. The biplanar configuration (type I) is rarely used because of its weight and bulk. It could be considered in closed comminuted fractures of the tibiotarsus in heavy birds.

ESF provides more stability than the use of intramedullary pins alone. It is a versatile technique which can be used in most birds. Complications are rare and when correctly positioned, external fixation allows a rapid return to function with many birds weight-bearing within hours of surgery. The joints do not have to be immobilized, resulting in a reduced risk of fracture disease. It is the most suitable technique for comminuted fractures with many small fragments.

Fractures of the beak and skull

Fractures of the beak in backyard poultry are not very common (Figure 24.5). They are most commonly caused by predator attacks. Open fractures are more common in this site, with the increased risk of infection leading to malunion. External fixation is frequently used for mandibular fractures. Many small pins can be placed to stabilize the fragments and this allows feeding to continue whilst the fracture heals. Occasionally, depending on the fracture and size of mandible, interfragmentary cerclage wiring or pinning may be used as the sole repair method, using the principles developed for use in mammals.

Skull fractures can be stabilized by bandaging the mouth in a closed position and placing an oesophageal feeding tube for nutritional support until the dressing is removed. Sometimes cerclage wires need to be used to stabilize skull fractures. Mandibular fractures where the bone will not support external fixation pins can be stabilized by the same method. It is important to ensure that the external nares are exposed and that they are patent; if the bird is not able to breathe through the nasal cavities, the mouth can be left slightly open.

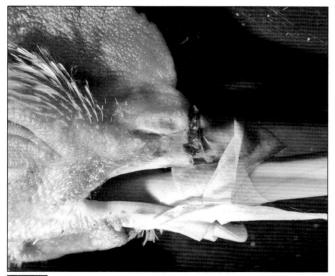

24.5 Fracture of the upper beak.

Fractures of the thoracic limbs
Coracoid, scapula and clavicle

In poultry, coracoid, scapula and clavicle fractures are not commonly diagnosed. Many of these fractures will heal satisfactorily with no treatment. The application of a figure-of-eight bandage, which incorporates a loop around the body to keep the wing immobilized against the body wall, usually results in functional healing. The bandage may have to be left in place for 4–5 weeks; however, as mentioned above the support should be removed at least every 7 days, so that physical therapy can be applied to the wing. The wing is alternately extended and flexed through its full range of movement for approximately 5 minutes. This is usually performed under general anaesthesia so as not to disrupt the fracture site. Radiographic evaluation of the fracture site at 2-week intervals will provide information on healing. Malunions and osteomyelitis can be identified early and decisions can be made as to when the support is no longer required.

Humerus

Most humeral fractures are mid-diaphyseal or distal towards the elbow. Proximal humeral fractures are usually minimally displaced and will respond to a figure-of-eight bandage with a body wrap. Mid-diaphyseal fractures can usually be successfully managed with a type I ESF frame. Larger birds or those with unstable spiral fractures require an ESF tie-in technique. A small intramedullary pin is inserted in a retrograde or anterograde fashion. It is bent at 90 degrees upon exit from the proximal humerus just distal to the shoulder joint, and connected to the connecting bar. At least two (preferably four) external fixation pins (one or two per fragment) are also connected to the bar. The tie-in technique allows good alignment of the fragments and good longitudinal and rotational stability. Fractures located in the distal part of the humerus near the elbow joint can be stabilized with a cross-pin technique, the Rush-pin technique or, if the distal fragment is large enough, a tie-in technique with only one half pin in the distal fragment. Fractures of the humerus have a higher risk of developing fracture disease because contraction of the muscles can cause displacement of the bones.

Radius and ulna

With these bones, coaptation with a figure-of-eight bandage should be satisfactory when only one bone is fractured because the intact bone acts as a natural splint. In cases where both bones are fractured, surgery will provide the best results. In poultry where flight is not important, intramedullary pinning and external fixation of the ulna are the most common approaches (see above). In larger birds, the radius may also need surgical fixation. A figure-of-eight bandage is usually applied for the first 2–3 days post surgery for extra support.

Metacarpals

The metacarpals have minimal soft tissue covering with the result that there is often extensive soft tissue damage and open fractures are common. Tendons are often exposed and the trauma may compromise the blood supply, which can lead to avascular necrosis that necessitates amputation of the distal wing tip. Wounds should be cleaned and, if not too contaminated, sutured closed. External coaptation provides sufficient support for satisfactory healing of most metacarpal fractures in poultry. Figure-of-eight bandaging is the most commonly used pattern.

Fractures of the pelvic limbs

Femur

Fractures of the femur are rarely comminuted because of the protection offered by the overlying muscle layers. Fractures of the femur are often mid-diaphyseal and due to the strong musculature the fragments are often dislocated. In small birds weighing <200 g, intramedullary pinning alone is often a satisfactory technique to immobilize the bone fragments and achieve good healing. However, most poultry species are heavier than this, with the result that the intramedullary pin needs to be tied in with an external fixator. The intramedullary pin (which should be no more than 50% of the diameter of the bone) is inserted retrograde into the proximal fragment. Once the pin exits from the greater trochanter, the fragments are aligned and the pin is inserted into the distal fragment. The intramedullary pin is bent at 90 degrees to the shaft of the bone as it exits through the skin and connected to the external bar. At least two external pins per fragment are also fixed to the bar. Fractures of the trochanter and proximal femur can be repaired with a tension-band wiring technique. Fractures of the distal part of the femur are best repaired using a cross-pinning or Rush-pinning technique. Splinting is inappropriate for fractures of the femur as the bone cannot be immobilized and malunion with fracture disease is the most common outcome.

Tibiotarsus

Tibiotarsal fractures are often diaphyseal and may or may not be comminuted depending on the force of the trauma. These fractures are easily diagnosed as the patient usually suspends the affected leg, and there may be obvious alterations in the shape of the leg. Coaptation with a Robert Jones or Spica splint technique may be an option when only minimal displacement of the fracture is present or in cases of metabolic bone disease; however, tibiotarsal fractures are often oblique and inherently unstable. ESF techniques are the preferred fracture repair method. A type I ESF frame is sufficient in smaller birds weighing up to 1 kg. In larger birds, a uniplanar type II ESF device is preferable. The proximal and distal pins are the first to be inserted, and once the normal length of the bone has been restored, the remaining pins are inserted in both bone fragments. A technique described by Redig (2001) recommends a medial tie-in by inserting the intramedullary pin via a medial approach, avoiding the tibiopatellar ligament, into the tibial plate. The pin is bent at 90 degrees as it exits the skin and connected to the external bar. Two to four external pins placed laterally are also fixed to the bar. With this technique it is possible to remove the intramedullary pin after a couple of weeks to increase loadbearing of the bone.

Tarsometatarsus

Tarsometatarsal fractures present with the same clinical signs as tibiotarsal fractures. In poultry, surgical fixation is required. The preferred technique is fixation using a type I (Figure 24.6) or type II ESF device (as detailed above for

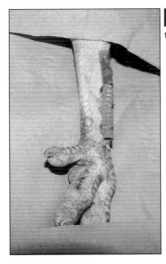

24.6 A type IA external skeletal fixation device being used to fix a tarsometatarsal fracture.

fractures of the tibiotarsus). The tarsometatarsal bone has a peculiar shape (C-shaped) and many tendons running very superficially (the caudal concavity contains the flexor tendon and the extensor tendon runs dorsally), thus a craniomedial approach is the best option for these fractures.

Phalanges

Fractures of the phalanges may go unnoticed because many birds do not show lameness or any other clinical signs. The fibrous sheath of the flexor tendons often acts as an effective splint. Lameness and a deviation, malposition or swelling of one or more digits are clinical signs that trigger veterinary intervention. Occasionally, birds will self-mutilate the affected phalanx. Cage rest is usually sufficient to facilitate the repair of a closed and non-displaced phalangeal fracture. Displaced fractures have to be reduced and stabilized with a ball or shoe bandage.

Ball bandages (Figure 24.7) need to be made from soft material that provides some support but still allows some movement at the joint. The fibrous sheath of the flexor tendon provides good support. Rigid fixation of the toes may cause adhesions to form, resulting in a stiff or rigid toe that may need to be amputated. Dislocated phalangeal joints are common. Usually there is no ligamentous damage and, if caught early, they can be replaced under

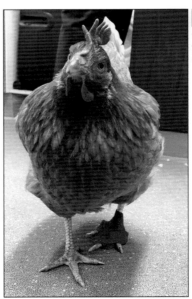

24.7 Ball bandage in a chicken. This technique is used for fractures or dislocations of one or multiple phalanges.

general anaesthesia. In most cases, external support is not required. Occasionally, there is rupture of a collateral ligament. This needs to be repaired using absorbable suture material that provides extended tensile strength, such as polydioxanone; 1.5 metric (4/0 USP) suture material is most commonly used (see Chapter 23).

Amputation

In cases of advanced osteomyelitis or bone tumours, amputation is indicated when the damage suffered is too extensive to attempt any other surgical options. Care must be taken to control bleeding to prevent potentially dangerous haemorrhage. The use of a radiosurgical unit is recommended, especially for the delicate dissection required in the smaller patient. A tourniquet will help to minimize blood loss. A balanced analgesic plan is important for all orthopaedic procedures (see Chapter 22), but particularly for amputations. The use of local anaesthetic (lidocaine and bupivacaine) topically on the nerves at least 1 minute before they are incised and an incisional splash block are important additions to the analgesic plan for amputations.

Wing amputation

As most species of poultry do not need to fly, wing amputation is well tolerated and does not affect the life and/or behaviour of the patient following surgery. Various approaches have been used for wing amputation: distal, mid-wing and proximal. It is preferable to amputate as far distal as possible, to allow the greatest return of normal function of the wing for balance. This is an important consideration in reproductively active male birds. However, in most cases the level of the amputation is dictated by the location of the lesion (Figure 24.8).

The *distal approach* at the level of radiocarpal articulation is used for lesions distal to the carpal joint. Feathers proximal and distal to the carpal joint are removed and the area aseptically prepared. A skin incision is made to preserve enough skin to suture over the stump.

Mid-wing approaches are performed at the level of the elbow joint. Feathers are removed proximal and distal to the elbow joint and the area aseptically prepared. A circular skin incision is made, taking care to ensure that sufficient skin remains to allow closure of the incision. The muscles are transected at the insertion of the elbow joint, and the elbow cartilage is removed with rongeurs. The muscles are then sutured over the stump and the skin closed routinely.

The *proximal approach* is performed at the level of the mid- or proximal humerus, or with a joint disarticulation. The feathers should be removed and the skin aseptically prepared. A circular incision is made, taking care to ensure that sufficient tissue remains to allow closure of the incision. The muscles are transected at the distal insertion and all the vessels ligated or coagulated with the radiosurgical unit. The humerus is transected using a sagittal saw, Gigli wire or other instrument appropriate to the size of the patient. The use of bone cutters or osteotomes is not indicated because of the brittle nature of avian bones. The muscles are then sutured over the stump and the skin incision closed routinely (Figure 24.9). Care should be taken to prevent blood seeping into the air sac from the open humeral end following surgery. Inserting a piece of gelatine or collagen foam into the medullary cavity of the humerus reduces the risk of haemorrhage into the respiratory system. Due to the potential for haemorrhage through the pneumatic portion of the humerus, the patient should be observed carefully.

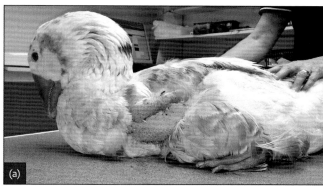
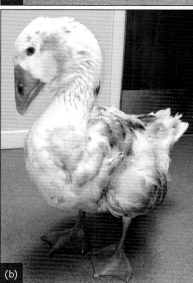

24.9 (a, b) Post surgical appearance of the wing of a goose following amputation.
(Courtesy of G Poland)

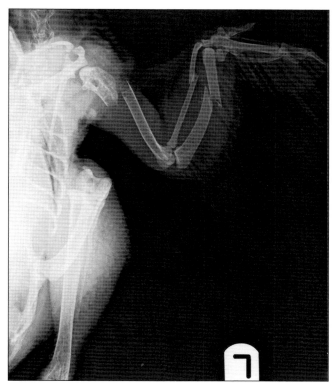

24.8 Wing with multiple fractures and exposure of the humeral distal fragment following a fox attack. The wing had to be amputated.

Digit amputation

This is the only amputation commonly performed on the pelvic limb. Amputation of a digit is best performed through a phalangeal bone. Radiography and manipulation provide information regarding the level at which to amputate. Non-functional toes are a hindrance to the bird and if they cause pain may lead to uneven weight-bearing, resulting in podo-dermatitis in the contralateral foot. The flexor and extensor tendons should be sutured over the cut end of the phalan-geal bone, and the skin closed over the tendons. The skin must not be under tension, otherwise there is an increased chance of wound breakdown.

Leg amputation

Leg amputation is more challenging and pododermatitis of the contralateral foot is an inevitable result in all but the smallest birds. A small percentage of Bantams may avoid developing pododermatitis of the contralateral foot due to their low bodyweight. However, they should be monitored carefully and dressings applied to the affected area as soon as any changes are seen. In addition to developing pododermatitis, aquatic fowl also have difficulty swim-ming following the surgery. Thus, humane euthanasia may be the best plan when the only remaining option is pelvic limb amputation.

In small birds weighing <500 g, a mid-femoral approach is most common. This approach provides an adequate amount of tissue to cover the end of the bone and is easier than a coxofemoral disarticulation. As with humeral amputations, the feathers should be removed and the skin aseptically prepared. The femur is transected using a sagittal saw, Gigli wire or other instrument appro-priate to the size of the patient. The use of bone cutters or osteotomes is not indicated because of the brittle nature of avian bones. A more distal leg amputation can be per-formed through the tibiotarsus or by disarticulation at the stifle joint. The bird will attempt to use the stump for ambulation. A rubber or silicone cap can be fitted over the stump during the day and removed at night for cleaning.

Prosthetic limbs

Research on prosthetic limbs in mammals is progressing and it may be possible to apply the same methods in birds. There are already some reports of the use of pros-thetic limbs in birds in the literature (Rush et al., 2012). A prosthetic limb is more likely to be successful in cases of distal amputation (e.g. mid-shaft or at the tibiotarsus joint).

Fracture disease

Fracture disease is more likely to occur if an inappropriate technique has been used. Severe systemic disease, meta-bolic bone disease, compromised blood supply and micro- or macro-movement of bone fragments are all pos-sible causes of bone disease. Fracture disease is most often encountered when external coaptation is used as the sole fixation technique.

- Malunion: healing of bones in an abnormal position. It can occur with both axial deviations and rotational deformities. Viable and non-viable malunions may be seen and the final result can be pseudo- or neoarthrosis.
- Delayed union: this is present when an adequate period of time has elapsed since the initial injury and bone union has not been achieved.
- Non-union: cessation of all reparative processes of healing without bony union.
- Malalignment: both fragments have <20% contact and have not properly re-aligned.
- Shortened bone length: consequence of malaligned bones in which strong muscle contraction causes overriding of the fracture fragments or where there is loss of bone.
- Joint ankylosis, muscle atrophy and patagium contraction: can be the result of prolonged immobilization.
- Osteomyelitis: can occur due to contamination of exposed fractures (the infection can spread to the air sacs if a pneumatized bone is involved) or during surgery. Caseous dry material occurs in pockets at the fracture site and the bone in the surrounding area usually becomes sclerotic.

Developmental disorders

Angel wing

Angel wing is characterized by outward rotation of the distal part of one or both wings. It is most commonly seen in geese, but has also been reported in ducks. It occurs during the growing phase when the primary feathers are emerging. It is associated with rapid growth rates and high protein diets. If not corrected, it will result in a permanent deformity of the carpometacarpal bones. These birds will be unable to fly. If noticed early, it should be corrected by taping the wing in the correct anatomical position for 3–7 days. The tape must be removed after a maximum of 7 days or it will cause a deformity of the rapidly growing wing. The diet should be reviewed and, if necessary, the protein level decreased.

Vitamin D3, calcium and phosphorus deficiencies

Vitamin D3 deficiencies and calcium and phosphorus defi-ciencies and/or imbalances are very common, especially in ducks and geese (see Chapter 20 for a full discussion). The most common end results of these deficiencies are wing and leg deformities, with the tibiotarsus being the most commonly affected bone. During the early stages, and in order to try and prevent permanent deformity, coap-tation of the wing or taping the leg to a pad made of soft sponge can help to restore the normal anatomy. It is also important to ensure that the bird is receiving the correct level of calcium, phosphorus and vitamin D3. A bird that has finished growing will require corrective osteotomy to restore normal anatomy and function of the limb. There are usually rotational as well as angular deformities that require correction. Due to abnormal weight-bearing on the joints during the growing phase, these will also not be normal, which may compromise a full return to normal function. Following a full evaluation of the limb, including radiography and assessment of joint movement, a surgical plan should be formulated that improves the quality of life for the bird. Usually, the final decision about the degree of rotation and straightening that will benefit the bird, within the limitations of the shape of the articular surface, is made once the bone has been cut.

Chondrodystrophy, valgus/varus deformity and perosis, and slipped tendon syndrome

These are metabolic diseases that result in long bone deformities of the pelvic limbs (see Chapter 18 for further information). Displacement of the gastrocnemius tendon due to the abnormal shape of the bones is common with these conditions (Figure 24.10). In some early cases, it may be possible to surgically replace the gastrocnemius tendon. Corrective osteotomy is often required and the level of success depends on the degree of joint and long bone deformity that has occurred.

An incision is made over the caudolateral aspect of the joint, midway between the lateral condyle of the tibiotarsus and the displaced tendon. The tendon should be freed from any adhesions and returned to its correct position within the trochlear groove. The groove may have to be deepened. The tendon is sutured to the periosteum to prevent re-luxation medially. If it is difficult to get a strong anchor in the periosteum then a tunnel through the lateral ridge of the trochlea can be used to anchor the sutures. In the very early stages, a supportive bandage with or without a splint can help to restore the normal anatomy. A corrective osteotomy is often needed, which requires careful planning (Bennett, 1997). It is also important to correct any dietary deficiencies.

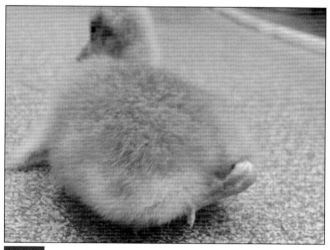

24.10 Luxated gastrocnemius tendon in a gosling.

Dyschondroplasia

This condition is sometimes called tibial dyschondroplasia as the tibiotarsus is the most commonly affected bone. It is seen in chickens, turkeys and ducks (the reader is referred to Chapter 18 for further details). Clinically affected birds usually have an abnormal gait; however, some birds may show no clinical signs. On radiography, when comparing the affected limb with the contralateral limb in unilateral cases, or when comparing an affected bird with a normal bird in bilateral cases, there is an abnormally large area of cartilage at the affected physis. This weakens the bone with the result that pathological fractures occur (Praul *et al.*, 2000). Surgical repair is unlikely to be successful due to the lack of bone strength. However, if the growth rate is reduced and any nutritional deficiencies corrected, external coaptation can be applied to provide some support whilst the bone strengthens. Some cases heal leaving a deformity at the affected area; this often leads to degenerative joint disease as the bird gets older.

Spondylolisthesis

Spondylolisthesis (also known as kinky back) is seen in chickens (mainly broilers) between 3 and 6 weeks old. It is due to ventral rotation of the fourth thoracic vertebra causing compression of the spinal cord (Angel, 2007). Affected birds are unable to stand and are found sitting on their hocks. Diagnosis is confirmed by radiography. There is no treatment.

Crooked neck

Crooked neck (also known as wry neck syndrome) (Figure 24.11), is described mainly in turkeys affected by *Mycoplasma meleagridis* that caused cervical vertebrae osteodystrophy and cervical airsacculitis. It is occasionally seen in other poultry species (chickens and waterfowl) with abnormal flexure of the neck and intense neurological signs; there are multiple causes (embryo toxin exposure, nutritional deficiencies, osteodystrophy, trauma). If treated early, a rigid neck brace/bandage kept on for at least 7 days could help to restore normal shape/function (Crespo and Shivaprasad, 2003).

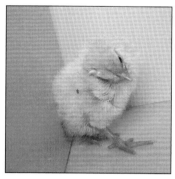

24.11 A chick with wry neck. This condition may have a muscular or skeletal aetiology. Early splinting can be helpful in some cases.

Femoral head necrosis

Femoral head necrosis is one of the most common causes of lameness in chickens. It is mainly seen in broilers >22 days old. Birds present as severely lame. Lesions are seen on radiography or post mortem in the proximal femur or occasionally in the proximal tibiotarsus. It is a form of bacterial osteomyelitis; *Staphylococcus* spp. are the most commonly implicated bacteria. Treatment with antibiotics has a low success rate (Dinev, 2009) (see Chapter 18 for additional information).

Degenerative joint disease

Degenerative joint disease is most commonly seen in older birds as a result of wear and tear. It is also frequently seen as the end result of a previous disease or injury to the affected joint or another joint or bone in the same limb. Increased incidence is associated with increasing weight of the bird. In some cases, the only clinical sign is lameness; swelling of the affected joint(s) is typically seen. Radiography, in conjunction with cytology and culture of joint fluid, can help rule out other causes of periarticular swelling, joint pain and joint effusion. Radiographic signs include increased radiodensity of the subchondral bone, osteolysis and regional periosteal reactions (Figure 24.12).

Non-steroidal anti-inflammatory drugs are the mainstay of treatment and are used to reduce the inflammatory response, swelling and pain associated with degenerative joint disease, as well as to reduce the fibrosis that limits

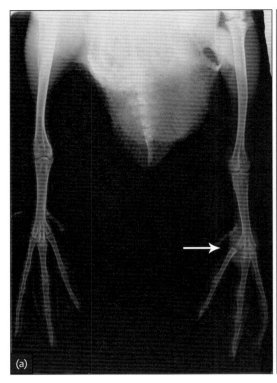
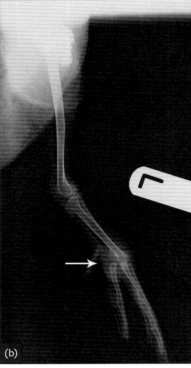

24.12 (a) Ventrodorsal and (b) lateral radiographs showing joint disease in a duck (arrowed). There is evidence of soft tissue oedema, an increased articular space due to joint effusion of the second tarsometatarsal–phalanx joint and a proximal periosteal reaction. The cytological examination revealed a septic arthritis. It is important to obtain radiographs of the contralateral limb for comparison.

normal range of movement. This facilitates more normal ambulation with the result that muscle atrophy is reduced, maintaining joint support and function for a longer period of time. Monosodium urate crystals can be found in cytology samples where gout is an underlying condition. Gout can lead to secondary degenerative joint disease. The cause of the gout must be investigated and treated. Any disease process that results in hyperuricaemia can cause gout.

Pinioning

Pinioning is illegal in farmed birds under The Mutilations (Permitted Procedures) Regulations 2008 (see Chapter 26). However, it is legal in pet and ornamental birds. Pinioning is commonly performed in waterfowl to permanently prevent flight. Under general anaesthesia, the distal parts of one wing are removed from the level of the carpus. A tourniquet is placed around the distal humerus. The skin is incised midway down the carpometacarpus. After dissecting through the soft tissues, the fused carpometacarpal bones are incised just proximal to the skin incision. The soft tissues are used to cover the two bone stumps and sutured in place; the skin is then closed so that it is not under tension. Temporary control of flight can be achieved by annually clipping approximately one-third of the primary feathers on one wing (see Chapter 7).

References and further reading

Arthurs G, Brown G and Pettit R (2018) *BSAVA Manual of Canine and Feline Musculoskeletal Disorders, 2nd edn*. BSAVA Publications, Gloucester

Angel R (2007) Metabolic disorders: limitations to growth of and mineral deposition into the broiler skeleton after hatch and potential implications for leg problems. *Journal of Applied Poultry Research* **16**, 138–149

Bennett A (1997) Orthopaedic surgery. In: *Avian Medicine and Surgery*, ed. RB Altman *et al*., pp. 733–766. WB Saunders, Philadelphia

Cook ME (2000) Skeletal deformities and their causes: introduction. *Poultry Science* **79**, 982–984

Crespo R and Shivaprasad HL (2003) Developmental, metabolic and other non-infectious disorders. In: *Diseases of Poulty, 12th edn*, p.1161. Iowa State Press, Ames

Dinev I (2009) Clinical and morphological investigations on the prevalence of lameness associated with femoral head necrosis in broilers. *British Poultry Science* **50**, 284–290

Flinchum GB (2006) Management of waterfowl. In: *Clinical Avian Medicine*, ed. GJ Harrison and TL Lightfoot, p. 846. Spix Publishing, Florida

Glimcher MJ, Shapiro F, Ellis RD and Eyre DR (1980) Changes in tissue morphology and collagen composition during the repair of cortical bone in the adult chicken. *Journal of Bone and Joint Surgery* **62**, 964–973

Harcourt-Brown NH (1996) Foot and leg problems. In: *BSAVA Manual of Raptors, Pigeons and Waterfowl*, ed. PH Beynon *et al*., pp. 147–168. BSAVA Publications, Cheltenham

Harcourt-Brown NH (2002) Orthopaedic conditions that affect the avian pelvic limb. *Veterinary Clinics of North America: Exotic Animal Practice* **5**, 49–81

Hatt JM (2008) Hard tissue surgery. In: *BSAVA Manual of Raptors, Pigeons and Passerine Birds*, ed. J Chitty and M Lierz, pp. 157–175. BSAVA Publications, Gloucester

Nunamaker DM, Rhinelander FW and Heppenstall RB (1985) Delayed union, non-union and malunion. In: *Textbook of Small Animal Orthopaedics*, ed. CD Newton and DM Nunamaker, pp. 1218–1223. Lippincott Williams and Wilkins, Philadelphia

Olsen JH (1994) Anseriformes. In: *Avian Medicine: principles and applications*, ed. BW Ritchie *et al*., pp, 1237–1326. Zoological Education Newtork, Florida

Praul CA, Ford BC, Gay CV, Pines M and Leach RM (2000) Gene expression and tibial dyschondroplasia. *Poultry Science* **79**, 1009–1013

Redig PT (2001) Effective methods for management of avian fractures and other orthopaedic problems. *Proceedings of the 6th EAAV Conference*, Munich, pp. 26–41

Rush EM, Turner TM, Montgomery R, *et al*. (2012) Implantation of a titanium partial limb prosthesis in a white-naped crane (*Grus vipio*). *Journal of Avian Medicine and Surgery* **26**, 167–175

Tully TN Jr. (2002) Basic avian bone growth and healing. *Veterinary Clinics of North America: Exotic Animal Practice* **5**, 23–30

Van Wettere AJ, Redig PT, Wallace LJ, Bourgeault CA and Bechtold JE (2009) Mechanical evaluation of external skeletal fixator-intramedullary pin tie-in configurations applied to cadaveral humeri from red-tailed hawks (*Buteo jamaicensis*). *Journal of Avian Medicine and Surgery* **23**, 277–285

Wise DR and Jennings AR (1973) The development and morphology of the growth plates of two long bones of the turkey. *Research in Veterinary Science* **14**, 161–166

Chapter 25

Post-mortem examination

Drury Reavill and Robert Schmidt

In avian medicine, the post-mortem examination is a valuable part of the diagnostic work-up. It provides correlations between the clinical signs, the results of ante-mortem diagnostic tests and, on many occasions, the cause of the disease. With chickens, other gallinaceous birds (e.g. turkeys, pheasants and guinea fowl) and waterfowl, the findings in one animal may help others in a collection. This chapter describes the steps in a post-mortem examination and provides a broad overview of possible interpretations of some common lesions. More in-depth information is provided in the relevant chapters.

When considering disease in a flock or group of waterfowl, poultry or other gallinaceous birds, there are, in general, two categories of investigation. The first category is relatively straightforward and involves a post-mortem examination and laboratory confirmation to make a diagnosis of a specific pathological condition. The second category is more complex and involves in-depth investigations as the problem is generally multifactorial with potentially vague clinical signs, which require careful assessment to determine the cause(s) and possible treatment(s).

For a flock with increasing morbidity and/or mortality, it is important to select the appropriate birds to examine. These birds should be representative of the population exhibiting the clinical signs. In diseases that present with high morbidity and mortality, such as some strains of avian influenza (AI) and Newcastle disease (NDV/velogenic viscerotropic Newcastle disease (VVND)/paramyxovirus-1), rapid collection of readily processed diagnostic samples is necessary.

Whilst it is well within the scope of experience and training for a general practitioner to perform a post-mortem, consideration should be given to sending the body to a pathologist for examination, if there is any possibility that the owner may be dissatisfied with the treatment or results. In such cases, it is best to use a pathologist who has training, experience or an interest in avian species.

In cases where a zoonotic or reportable disease is suspected (e.g. chlamydia, mycobacteria, AI, NDV/VVND) and the practice does not have facilities to adequately contain the organisms, the body should be submitted to an appropriate external laboratory. Before submission, the carcass should be cooled by thoroughly soaking the plumage in a mixture of cold water and a small amount of liquid dishwashing detergent. Dry feathers insulate the body, preventing adequate cooling and promoting autolysis.

Embryos, nestlings and small adult birds are subject to rapid autolysis. For the best results, these small birds can be submitted in their entirety in formalin. The body cavity should be carefully opened, to limit any possible exposure to disease agents, along with the skull to ensure fixation of the tissues. It is always best to contact the external laboratory for specific instructions before making a submission.

Equipment

Suggested equipment required for a post-mortem examination includes:

- Disposable gloves
- Any common disinfectant or detergent to wet the body and control dust and feathers
- Appropriate and adequate volume of fixative
- Selection of instruments, including scissors, bone forceps and scalpels
- Sterile swabs or other appropriate culture material and containers for tissue samples to be frozen or used for toxicological tests
- A ruler and/or callipers
- Digital camera
- An adequate work surface and lighting
- Appropriate reference books
- A list of notifiable or reportable diseases and details regarding sample collection for those diseases.

Appropriate precautions (e.g. use of necropsy hood and protective clothes/mask) should also be taken to protect the examiner in cases of suspected zoonotic diseases. Several diseases are zoonotic, including avian influenza (H5N1), avian paramyxovirus, chlamydophilia, *Salmonella*, *Campylobacter jejuni*, *Erysipelothrix rhusiopathiae* and mycobacteria. It is considered important that minimal protection such as gloves and a mask be used for all necropsy examinations. It is important to remember that potential zoonotic diseases do not always have definable or characteristic lesions.

History

As with any examination, obtaining an adequate history is paramount. Often this historical information helps with the development of a differential diagnoses list (Figure 25.1) in the face of a rapidly progressing outbreak with high morbidity and mortality. The age, sex and species of the

Aetiology	Clinical signs and/or lesions	Species	Diagnostic tests and/or control
Ascites syndrome of broilers	Ascites	Chickens	Presence of transudate to modified transudate
Avian cholera (*Pasteurella multocida*)	Arthritis/synovitis; swollen wattles; septicaemia; mottled swollen liver	Chickens, turkeys, waterfowl	PCR, serology
Avian encephalomyelitis (AE)	Lenticular cataract; neurological signs (muscular tremors in chicks); drop in egg production	Chickens, pheasants, turkeys	Serology of paired serum samples using virus neutralization or ELISA
Avian influenza (highly pathogenic)	Swelling of head; swelling, necrosis and haemorrhage of the wattles and comb; subcutaneous ecchymosis; high mortality	Chickens, turkeys, waterfowl	Specific reverse transcription RT-PCR tests
Avian influenza (low pathogenic)	Sinusitis; drop in egg production; sneezing; coughing; ocular and nasal discharge; swollen infraorbital sinuses	Chickens, turkeys, waterfowl	Specific RT-PCR tests
Chlamydophila psittaci	Conjunctivits; sinusitis; green to yellow-green droppings; inactivity; ruffled feathers; weakness; weight loss; pneumonia; hepatomegaly; splenomegaly	All birds	PCR, serology
Duck virus enteritis (herpesvirus)	High mortality; blood-stained vents and nares; penile prolapse; necrotizing and haemorrhagic enteritis	Ducks, geese and swans of all ages	Serology of serum samples using virus neutralization
Duck viral hepatitis	High mortality; enlarged liver with haemorrhagic foci	Ducks (ducklings; not pathogenic for goslings)	History, lesions
Fowlpox	Proliferative skin lesions; laryngotracheitis	Chickens, turkeys, waterfowl	Vaccination
Goose parvovirus (Derzsy's disease)	High mortality in goslings; haemorrhagic nephritis and enteritis; ascites; whitish discoloration of the heart; hydropericardium	Geese (goslings), Muscovy ducks (ducklings)	Clinical signs, histology, virus isolation, PCR, serology
Haemophilus paragallinarum (infectious Coryza)	Sinusitis; drop in egg production	Chickens	Virus isolation, PCR
Infectious bronchitis virus (coronavirus)	Sinusitis; swollen pale kidneys ± urolithiasis; air sacculitis; drop in egg production; abnormal eggs	Chickens	Virus isolation, RNA quantitative RT-PCR tests
Infectious bursal disease (Gumboro disease) (birnavirus)	Watery diarrhoea; soiled vent feathers; vent picking and inflammation of the cloaca; immunosuppression	Chickens	Agar gel immunodiffusion (AGID)
Infectious laryngotracheitis (herpesvirus)	Laryngotracheitis	Chickens, pheasants	ELISA, PCR
Lymphoid leucosis (avian retrovirus)	Bursa of Fabricius enlargement	Chickens	Control
Marek's disease (herpesvirus)	Enlarged peripheral nerves (vagus, brachial and sciatic); diffuse or nodular lymphoid tumours in various organs (liver, spleen, gonads, heart, lungs, kidneys, muscle and proventriculus); enlarged feather follicles	Chickens (>3–4 weeks old)	Biopsy, vaccination
Mycoplasma gallisepticum	Sinusitis; tracheitis; pneumonia; air sacculitis	Chickens, turkeys	PCR, serum rapid plate agglutination (RPA)
Mycotoxins	Ventricular erosions; drop in egg production; fatty liver (ducks)	Chickens, waterfowl	Feed testing
Newcastle disease (NDV/VVND) (avian paramyxovirus-1)	Gasping; coughing; sneezing and rales; neurological signs (tremors, paralysed wings and legs, twisted necks, circling, clonic spasms and complete paralysis); swelling of the tissue of the head and neck; drop in egg production; abnormal eggs	All birds	ELISA
Salmonella pullorum and *S. gallinarium* (fowl typhoid)	High mortality; grey-white nodules in the liver, spleen, lungs, heart, gizzard and intestine; 'cheesy' material in the caeca (caecal cores); synovitis	Chickens, turkeys, guinea fowl, pheasants	Isolation and serotyping

25.1 Clinical signs and/or lesions associated with specific diseases. ELISA = enzyme-linked immunoabsorbent assay; PCR = polymerase chain reaction; RT = reverse transcription.

birds involved are important, as well as the percentage of birds that are showing clinical signs and the number of birds that may have died. For example, duck viral hepatitis (DVH) is a highly contagious disease in young ducklings. This could be mistaken for duck viral enteritis (DVE) which is an acute, highly contagious disease of ducks, geese and swans of all ages. Goose parvovirus, which is a highly contagious and fatal disease of goslings and Muscovy ducks, can be differentiated from DVH as DVH is not pathogenic for goslings or Muscovy ducks. Chickens are most susceptible to a Newcastle disease outbreak, and waterfowl the least susceptible.

Marek's disease primarily infects chickens and is very rarely identified as a natural infection in other gallinaceous birds. Marek's disease is controlled by vaccination, as almost all chicken flocks are infected with

Marek's herpesvirus. This infection results in enlarged nerves and lymphoid tumours in various viscera as well as the skin; however, it does not result in bursal tumours, which helps distinguish it from lymphoid leucosis. Marek's disease can develop in chickens as young as 3 weeks old, whereas lymphoid leucosis is typically seen in chickens >14 weeks of age. Waterfowl schistosomiasis can also be suspected on the basis of history and species of birds affected. This is an intravascular trematode infection for which water birds are the common hosts for the blood flukes. The infection is severe in swans and affected birds develop encephalitis, whereas wild ducks, particularly diving birds, are fairly resistant and may even be the source of the schistosomiasis.

Evaluation of husbandry, including housing, temperature, ventilation, cleanliness, stocking density, substrates and food items offered, is essential. The environment where the animals are kept is important when considering the potential differential diagnoses. For example, rapid die-off of ducks on a pond, particularly a pond that has become stagnant and where there have been no recent additions to the flock, should raise suspicion for a toxic exposure such as botulism. High mortality in a collection of both waterfowl and gallinaceous birds kept outside could suggest an explosive outbreak of AI.

The husbandry history can also help determine the cause of diseases (e.g. exposure to other animals). In turkeys and guinea fowl (uncommonly), histomoniasis can result in significant fatal disease. This particular protozoan parasite, *Histomonas meleagridis*, is transmitted through the embryonated eggs of the caecal nematode *Heterakis gallinarum*, harboured in earthworms. Birds with access to the ground and earthworms can be expected to be exposed to *H. meleagridis*. Many healthy chickens carry infected caecal worms. Thus, mixing bird species, particularly chickens and turkeys, should be discouraged, and may explain the presence of disease in turkeys that are in contact with chickens.

Knowing whether birds are free-range or fed an appropriate commercial diet can also help determine the list of differential diagnoses. Birds fed a diet deficient in vitamin A could develop oral and oesophageal lesions, which may be confused with trichomoniasis or the wet form of fowlpox. For poultry, vaccination history is important, as is documentation of any previously attempted drug treatments. Recent additions to the flock, exposure to wild bird populations and the recent movement of any affected birds (e.g. agricultural fairs, poultry exhibitions, bird shows, breeding) should be recorded. All of this information is vital, from the single pet bird to commercial flocks.

In addition, although the history from an owner may suggest the unexpected death of a healthy bird, there are a few findings that point to an unobserved disease. Some signs of chronic disease include: inadequate muscle mass, poor feather quality, feather loss, exudate and possible plugging of the nares, enlargement of the sinuses, faecal staining at the mucocutaneous junction of the vent and visceral urate deposits.

Procedure

The post-mortem examination steps can vary widely amongst practitioners. There is no right or wrong way to approach the examination; however, it is important to be consistent, so that examination of a body system is not missed or collection of an important sample forgotten. For

this reason, many facilities have developed checklists for post-mortem examinations and keep forms with the necropsy equipment. The following is one possible method for a post-mortem examination.

- **Step 1:** Record the bodyweight of the bird. Evaluate body condition and feather quality. If external parasitism is noted, obtain scrapings of the lesions or remove affected feathers (Figures 25.2 and 25.3). The feathers can be placed in self-sealing bags and the scrapings applied to labelled glass slides. A drop of mineral oil should be placed on to the slide with the scraped material and a coverslip applied before examination. Obtain radiographs to determine whether any bony lesions, fractures or metallic densities are present. Note any external lesions (e.g. on the bottom of the feet) and/or discharges (e.g. stained vent feathers, nasal or ocular discharges) before soaking the plumage thoroughly in a mixture of cold water and a small amount of liquid dishwashing detergent. This allows close examination of the skin (Figure 25.4). The dense and waterproof plumage of most waterfowl will resist wetting, therefore, careful palpation is recommended.

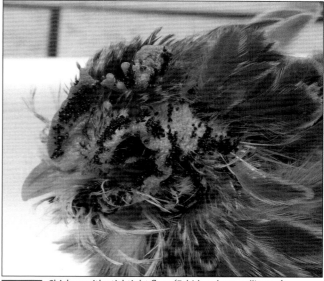

25.2 Chicken with sticktight fleas (*Echidnophaga gallinacea*). (Courtesy of Geoffrey Olsen)

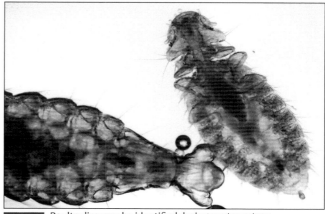

25.3 Poultry lice may be identified during post-mortem examination.

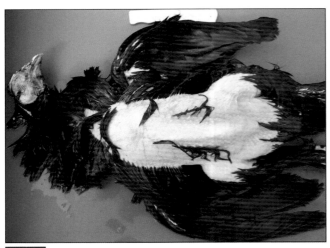

25.4 Wetting of the plumage allows close examination of the skin.

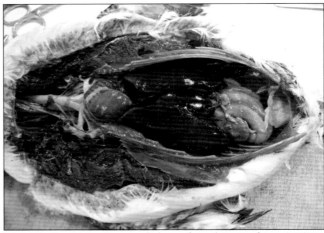

25.6 The skin has been peeled away from the area of examination in this common guillemot.

- **Step 2:** Pull the legs away from the body. Incise the skin between the leg and the abdomen, and keep pulling the leg until the head of the femur is dislocated from the acetabulum. Examine the internal surface of the leg and the femoral head (Figure 25.5). Separate the muscle groups to identify the sciatic nerve and evaluate thickness. The loss of cross-striations and variable swelling of the nerve is abnormal.
- **Step 3:** To control flyaway feathers from adhering to the exposed tissues (particularly in waterfowl), the skin can be peeled away from the ventrum. One method is to make a ventral midline cut with a scalpel and peel the skin laterally (Figure 25.6). In poultry, wetting the feathers provides enough control; however, making a ventral midline incision and peeling back the skin and feathers exposes the musculature for closer examination. Make two incisions through the exposed musculature, or through the skin and underlying muscles, at the level of the thoracic inlet from the crop to the vent (Figure 25.7). Then, make an incision through the thin abdominal soft tissues and, using blunt scissors, cut the ribs along both lateral surfaces. Lift the sternum and make additional cuts through the coracoid bones and clavicle (as needed) to permit removal of the sternum (Figure 25.8).

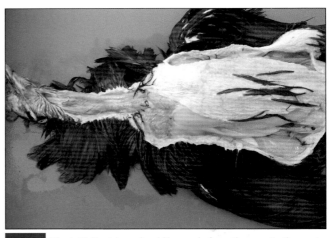

25.7 The initial incisions should be made from the crop to the vent.

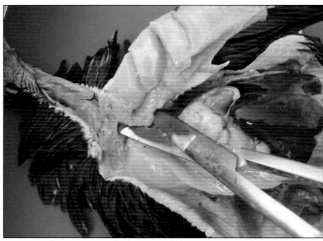

25.8 Cutting through the coracoid bones to lift and remove the sternum.

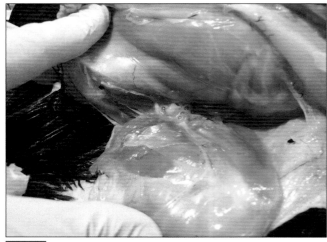

25.5 Examination of the head of the femur.

- **Step 4:** Reflect the skin over the caudal abdomen downwards, revealing the contents of the coelom. Examine the organs *in situ* noting colour, size and position. Check for the presence of ascitic fluid. Any fluid should be collected, quantified and described. The collection tube can be left in an upright position to allow cells or microbes to settle by gravity. Once the post-mortem examination of the bird is complete, a syringe can be used to collect the sediment and multiple slides for cytology can be made. Total protein/solids can be measured with a refractometer.

- **Step 5:** Examine the complex air sac system by carefully moving the abdominal organs from side to side. Note that normal air sacs should be translucent (Figure 25.9).
- **Step 6:** Examine and collect the smaller organs, as well as samples for culture. The thyroid and parathyroid glands should be visible at the thoracic inlet, lying along the ventral aspect of the common carotid artery at the level of the jugular vein and the origin of the vertebral artery (Figure 25.10). If the crop is full or distended, carefully dissect and remove the structure intact to prevent fluids from obscuring the field. The thyroid glands are usually bilaterally symmetrical in size and shape. Lobes of the thymus are usually located within the same area, although they can be found from the thoracic inlet to the angle of the beak (Figure 25.11). Blood samples can be collected via cardiac puncture or by aseptically opening the right ventricle and aspirating the blood remaining in the chamber.

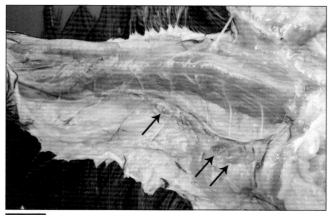

25.11 Location of lobes of the thymus (arrowed).

- **Step 7:** Incise through the air sacs and fascial attachments, and roll the liver, proventriculus and ventriculus laterally, to expose the dorsal surface. The spleen is located at the junction of the proventriculus and ventriculus (Figure 25.12). The shape of the spleen varies depending on the species; it is triangular in ducks and geese, and spherical in many poultry species. The normal size of the spleen is approximately one-third to one-half the size of the proventriculus.
- **Step 8:** Carefully lift the heart, reflecting the apex cranially, to reveal the proventriculus. Transect the cranial proventriculus at the level of the cloaca. Remove *en bloc* the organs from the proventriculus to the cloaca.
- **Step 9:** Incise the proventriculus and ventriculus to examine the mucosa and koilin (Figure 25.13). Grit is frequently present within the ventriculus. Collect any material within the gastric lumen for further examination if it does not appear consistent with normal foodstuffs. The koilin is normally readily peeled from the ventricular mucosa, depending on the degree

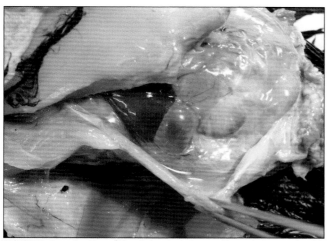

25.9 Examination of the abdominal air sacs. Normal air sacs should be translucent.

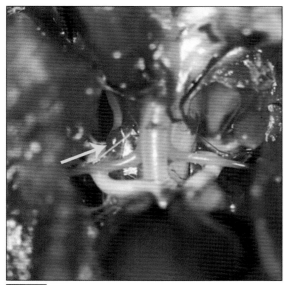

25.10 Location of the thyroid gland (arrowed) in a pheasant.

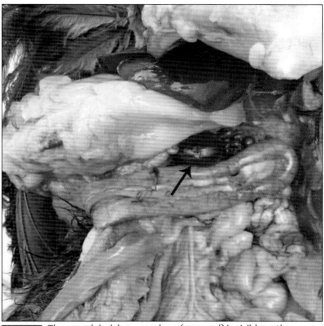

25.12 The round dark brown spleen (arrowed) is visible as the proventriculus and ventriculus are rolled laterally in this chicken.
(Courtesy of Leila Marcucci)

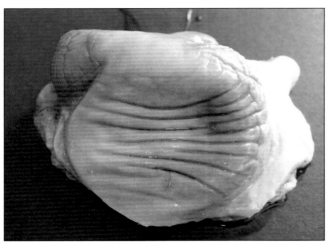

25.13 The ventriculus has been incised to allow examination of the koilin.

of autolysis. It should be elevated as nematodes may be found embedded in the ventricular mucosa. Although the luminal size may limit ease of opening, incise and examine the intestines along their entire length, collecting mucosal scrapings and samples for wet mounts and smears. To assess the mucosa, it may be possible to cut along the entire length of the intestines using fine blunt-nosed scissors. Alternatively, representative cuts can be made, especially in grossly abnormal areas. It is important to evaluate the caecal tonsils, which are located at the base of the caeca. Several diseases can result in lesions within these lymphoid aggregates (e.g. proliferation and necrosis). Most waterfowl have relatively long and slender caeca. The caeca of Galliformes are also generally long and slender, and are similar in appearance to the intestines (Figure 25.14).

In young birds, examine the yolk sac for expected normal resorption. In recently hatched birds, the yolk sac is a thick opaque mass connected to the small intestine by the yolk stalk (ductus vitellinus) and opens on the antimesenteric side of the jejunoileal junction. In chickens, by day 10, the residual yolk has resorbed and the yolk sac has become a sacculum containing a small cavity with no yolk. It persists as Meckel's diverticulum (a lymphoepithelial organ) in the older bird (Figure 25.15).

- **Step 10:** Removal of the gastrointestinal tract exposes the gonads, adrenal glands and kidneys. Examine the gonads (Figure 25.16) and identify the location of the adrenal glands. Carefully remove the kidneys by blunt dissection; the three divisions extend from the lungs to the caudal synsacrum (Figure 25.17). Removal of the

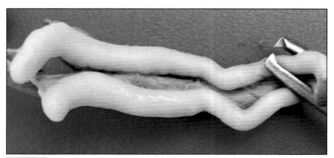

25.14 The caeca from a chicken. This is a fixed specimen.

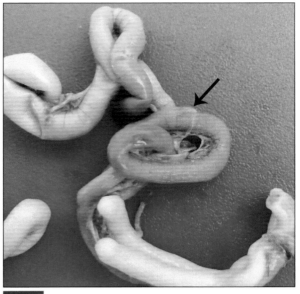

25.15 Location of Meckel's diverticulum (arrowed).

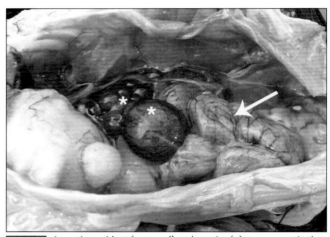

25.16 An active oviduct (arrowed) and ovaries (*) are present in the coelom of this chicken.

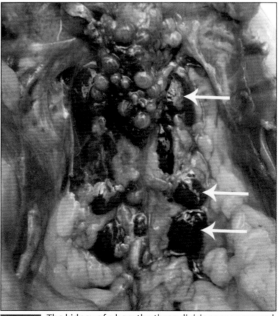

25.17 The kidney of a hen: the three divisions are arrowed. (Courtesy of Leila Marcucci)

kidneys permits examination of the sciatic plexus (Figure 25.18) and determination of any abnormality, such as thickening in association with Marek's disease.

- **Step 11:** In young birds, examine the bursa of Fabricius by lifting the colon and cloaca ventrally out of the coelomic cavity and examining the dorsal surface of the cloaca. The bursa is a firm white structure that involutes in the adult.
- **Step 12:** Removal of the gastrointestinal tract also allows the heart and lungs to be evaluated. In most cases, examine the heart by opening the chambers in the direction of blood flow. The apex of the heart can be collected and held for West Nile virus testing. Use the scalpel handle to loosen the lungs from the thorax. Normal lungs should be pink (Figure 25.19) and float when placed in formalin.
- **Step 13:** Open the beak and from the angle of the jaw make an incision, using scissors, inside the oesophagus and continue down the neck, exposing the pharynx, oesophageal lining and interior crop. Most Galliformes have a complex crop and many ducks and geese have a fusiform or spindle-shaped enlargement of the cervical oesophagus (Figure 25.20).

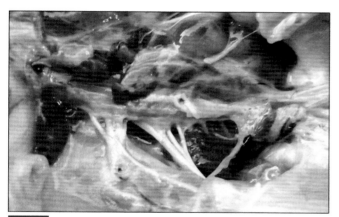

25.18 With the kidney removed, the sciatic plexus can be examined.

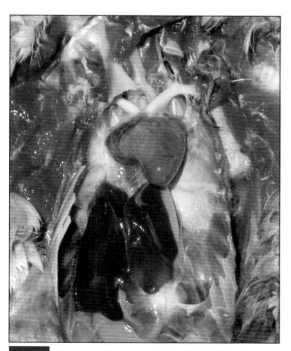

25.19 The normal lungs are pink in this bufflehead.

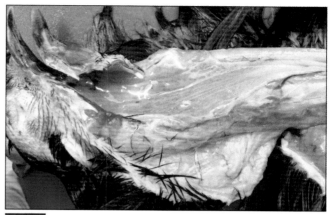

25.20 The cervical oesophagus is open.

- **Step 14:** Incise the trachea along its length and examine. The syringeal bulla is a bony enlargement inside the thoracic inlet found in males of many species of surface feeding ducks, especially domestic mallard ducks (Figure 25.21).
- **Step 15:** Cut through the upper beak with sharp scissors to evaluate the nasal cavities and sinus.
- **Step 16:** Remove and examine the brain. This is especially important if neurological clinical signs have been described. Incise the skin and reflect it laterally to expose the skull. Carefully incise around the calvaria and then lift to expose the cerebrum and cerebellum. The brain can be fixed *in situ* and subsequently removed, or the nerve attachments can be gently cut using blunt scissors and the brain removed.
- **Step 17:** Assess the bone structure at the time of sectioning, including the degree of bend or snap of the long bones. Obtain aspirates from any joint swellings and examine the material by exfoliative cytology (Figure 25.22).

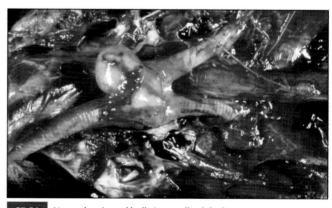

25.21 Normal syringeal bulla in a mallard duck.

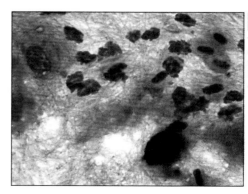

25.22 Urate crystals from a bird with articular gout are readily identifiable by exfoliative cytology.

Sample collection

At the time of the post-mortem examination, a complete set of tissue samples (and in some cases two sets, if the animal is an endangered species of gallinaceous bird or waterfowl and a set of samples needs to be submitted, for example, to the Species Survival Plans (SSP) pathologist) should be collected and preserved in formalin for histopathology. It should be remembered that formalin penetrates tissue at a rate of approximately 1 mm per hour, and can only penetrate a maximum of 5 mm into solid tissues, with some exceptions (e.g. brain tissue). Thus, the ideal biopsy sample size is about 1 cm x 1 cm x 1 cm. Densely cellular tissues, such as the spleen, can take longer for adequate fixation and may need to be sectioned for best preservation.

Cytological preparations (impression smears) of blood, body fluids, bone marrow or tissues can be valuable and provide a rapid diagnosis in some cases, so that therapy of other birds in the flock can be initiated whilst pending the results of the more comprehensive necropsy. *Plasmodium*, *Haemoproteus*, *Toxoplasma* and *Leucocytozoon* are often readily identified from impression smears of the liver and spleen. An impression smear can also quickly differentiate tumours from mycobacterial or other bacterial granulomas. Smears can be made from blood samples obtained from the heart during post-mortem examination and evaluated for parasites. If cytology preparations are to be sent to an external laboratory, they should be kept separate from formalin-fixed tissues as formalin fumes can cause artefactual changes to unfixed cytology slides.

Representative tissue samples (e.g. lung, liver, kidney and intestine) can be collected and frozen for molecular diagnostics or genetic testing. Depending on the clinical signs and suspected infectious diseases, swabs for bacterial, fungal and mycoplasmal culture should be available. Aseptic collection of samples from multiple organs, including the liver, spleen, kidneys and lung, should also be considered for culture. All young birds should have samples collected to culture for *Salmonella*. Samples for culture (bacterial and fungal), viral polymerase chain reaction (PCR) and chlamydophilia testing should be collected soon after opening the body cavity in order to reduce contamination. Toxicological testing and measuring tissue micronutrients may require additional tissue samples, including fat, kidney, liver, brain, stomach contents and eye, to be placed in properly labelled glass and/or foil containers and frozen until examination.

Technique for collecting samples for culture

1. Sear the surface of the organ with a heated spatula.
2. Make a stab incision into the tissue using a sterile scalpel blade.
3. Insert a sterile swab into the stab incision to collect a sample.

Evaluation and interpretation

Each organ and/or tissue should be evaluated and described as the necropsy proceeds. Changes should be described using parameters such as size, shape, colour, consistency and smell.

- **Size** – use of metric measurements is preferable (do not use comparisons to fruit, vegetables or other foodstuffs as some people may not understand the reference). Tissue loss may result in symmetrical or asymmetrical changes in organ size and weight. An abnormal excess of tissue can be due to hypertrophy, hyperplasia or neoplasia and may be symmetrical or asymmetrical.
- **Shape** – round, elliptical, rhomboid.
- **Texture** – granular, smooth, rough.
- **Consistency** – watery, firm, hard, fluctuant. The consistency of an organ can be affected by the post-mortem conditions, as well as ante-mortem changes including cellular infiltrations and connective tissue proliferation. The cut surface can be described as solid, cystic or mucoid.
- **Colour** – redundancy such as 'brown in colour' should be avoided. Colour changes can occur ante-mortem or post-mortem. Examples include:
  - Red – haemorrhage if it is a focal lesion. If the lesion is more diffuse, congestion and hyperaemia should be considered
  - White – generally, this suggests inflammation, necrosis, calcium, fibrous connective tissues, urates, lipid or bone
  - Yellow – inflammation, fat and fibrin can have a yellowish colour. A fatty liver will be friable with a yellow-orange colour
  - Green – bile pigments, haemosiderin and algal/fungal infections appear green
  - Black – melanin, blood, necrosis, exogenous carbon and hydrogen sulphide (from the gastrointestinal tract) impart a black colour to tissues.

Describing the pattern of the lesions present is also helpful and a good practice to cultivate. Patterns can provide clues as to the underlying cause.

- **Diffuse** – this term describes lesions that affect an entire area or organ equally (e.g. the diffuse interstitial pneumonia caused by a systemic viral infection such as AI or the diffuse enlarged yellow friable liver in fatty liver haemorrhagic syndrome (FLHS) in chickens). If the entire organ is not uniformly affected, better terms to describe the lesions may be disseminated or generalized (e.g. the multifocal 'target' lesions throughout the liver in turkeys with *Histomonas meleagridis* or the white gritty lesions in the kidney of the urate tophi).
- **Locally or focally extensive** – focally extensive refers to a large area of the organ being affected. For example, gangrenous dermatitis, which is characterized by gangrenous necrosis of the skin over the wings, thighs, breast and head of chickens. This is a common sequela in immunocompromised young chicks with infectious bursal disease or chick anaemia virus. The causative bacteria enter through skin lesions due to trauma, wet litter, picking or treading wounds.
- **Multifocal to coalescing** – this term describes either discrete multifocal lesions or multifocal lesions that appear occasionally to coalesce. These often represent either lesions that are caused by blood-borne pathogens or metastatic neoplasia. Staphylococcal septicaemia associated with severe pododermatitis produces irregular pale multifocal to coalescing lesions in the liver. *Mycobacterium* can also produce multifocal to coalescing yellow caseous nodules in the liver, spleen and intestine.
- **Segmental** – this term is generally reserved for tubular organs (e.g. gastrointestinal tract or trachea). The descriptor can be used to describe the lesions of

site-specific coccidial infections, such as *Eimeria necatrix*, that produce a mid-jejunum catarrhal (thick, gelatinous fluid containing mucus and epithelial debris) enteritis in chickens.

Non-specific interpretation of findings

Enlargement

Enlargement means that something has been added to the tissue or organ. The general causes of enlargement are fluid (oedema or blood), cells (inflammatory, neoplastic or hyperplastic) and gas (usually bacterial in origin). Mild to moderate enlargement of the liver, spleen and kidney can occur with organ congestion. In the gallbladder, if an obstruction cannot be identified, the enlargement may be due to a physiological failure to empty. This is often associated with anorexia.

Petechial haemorrhage

Haemorrhage of the epicardium, myocardium and endocardium can be induced by euthanasia.

Pseudohaemorrhage within the skull

What can appear to be haemorrhage within the bones of the skull is a common gross finding due to vascular congestion. Once the overlying bone has been removed, the cerebrum should be examined closely. Calvarium blood is only significant if there are lesions recognized in the underlying tissues of the brain.

Melanosis

A dark grey to black pigmentation of various tissues is due to the deposition of melanin. Pigmented ovaries and testes are seen in some species. Other areas of normal serosal or mucosal pigmentation include the thyroid gland, cerebrum, crop and oral mucosa.

Pseudomelanosis

Areas of grey to black discoloration may occur post-mortem due to hydrogen sulphide release from bacterial decomposition of blood. This reaction can occur rapidly in the gastrointestinal tract and discoloration may be seen on areas of the kidneys, liver or spleen where they were in contact with the gut, as well as in the gastrointestinal tract wall itself.

Pulmonary congestion and oedema

Pulmonary congestion and oedema is most commonly an artefact, resulting from blood pooling in the lungs. It manifests as a mottled reddened lung that is heavier than normal. On examination the lung is full with blood. This occurs during dissection when blood spilled into the coelom flows back from the air sacs into the lungs via the secondary bronchi. Inhalational anaesthetic agents can also cause severe pulmonary congestion, which mimics exposure to noxious gases such as those released from overheated polytetrafluorethylene or elevated ammonia in enclosed housing.

Gastrointestinal tract dilatation

Any degree of autolysis results in dilatation of the gastrointestinal tract. However, it should be noted that this can be a normal finding in young birds still being handfed.

Koilin sloughing from the ventriculus

The koilin sloughing from the ventriculus is a common lesion of autolysis and occurs shortly after death.

Reddened intestines with reddened content

After death, blood may leak into the intestines and stain the ingesta. As blood breaks down, its colour changes to green.

Enhanced lobular or reticular pattern of the liver

Many diseases cause exaggeration of the normal lobular pattern of the liver. Each lobule has an alternating red and yellow area, which is visible on the capsular and cut surfaces of the liver (Figure 25.23). This pattern is common in hepatitis, passive hepatic congestion, mild hepatic lipidosis and some haematopoietic tumours.

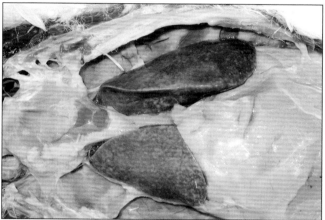

25.23 The enhanced lobular or reticular pattern can be appreciated in this liver from a goose.

Euthanasia solution injection sites

Some euthanasia solutions (such as sodium pentobarbital) may produce artefactual changes in the heart and lungs when given as a bolus intravascular injection. At death the solution causes the blood clots forming in the cardiac chambers to become brown and friable. This change can extend into the cardiac tissues, resulting in brown, dry issues that may be slightly gritty, and if extending to the epicardium can resemble visceral gout. This material may have a medicinal (ethanol) odour.

Specific interpretation of findings

Figure 25.24 provides details of the clinical signs and causes for a number of diseases encountered in backyard poultry.

External features and integument

There are a number of diseases that can manifest skin lesions. Scaly lesions on the legs are generally due to *Knemidocoptes mutans* in chickens (Figure 25.25), whereas small subcutaneous nodules can be caused by cyst mites (*Laminosioptes cysticola*) (Figure 25.26). Rarely, fungal infectious agents such as *Microsporum gallinae* can be identified in superficial lesions, presenting as white crusts on the comb and skin.

Several bacterial infections can result in extensive skin lesions, leading to various degrees of dermatitis, necrosis,

System	Clinical signs and/or lesions	Aetiology	Species
Systemic	Ascites	Ascites syndrome of broilers	Chickens
		Sodium toxicity	Chickens
		Parvovirus	Geese
		Spontaneous cardiomyopathy of young turkeys	Turkeys
	High morbidity and mortality	Newcastle disease (NDV/VVND)	Chickens are most susceptible and waterfowl least susceptible
		Avian influenza	Chickens, turkeys
		Duck virus enteritis (herpesvirus)	Ducks, geese and swans of all ages
		Duck hepatitis	Ducklings (2 weeks old)
		Salmonella pullorum and *S. gallinarum* (fowl typhoid)	Chickens, turkeys, guinea fowl, pheasants
Skin	Skin mass and/or lump	Marek's disease	Chickens
	Skin mass and/or lump; non-feathered regions	Cutaneous fowlpox	Chickens, turkeys, waterfowl
	Folliculitis	*Staphylococcus*	Chickens
	Proliferative skin lesions	Fowlpox	Chickens, turkeys
	Swollen wattles; septicaemia	Avian cholera (*Pasteurella multocida*)	Wide host range
	Swollen wattles and comb	Avian influenza	Chickens, turkeys
		Avian cholera	Chickens
	Swollen tissues of the head and neck	Newcastle disease (NDV/VVND)	All
	Subcutaneous haemorrhage on the beak	Lead toxicity	Waterfowl
	Swellings/ulcerations on the plantar surface of the feet	Bumblefoot	Poultry, waterfowl
	Proliferative plaques on the web of the feet	Pox virus	Waterfowl
Musculoskeletal	Arthritis/synovitis; septicaemia	Avian cholera (*Pasteurella multocida*)	Chickens
Cardiovascular	Fibrinous pericarditis	*Pasteurella anatipester*	Waterfowl
	White to yellow thickening of the great vessels	Atherosclerosis	Waterfowl
	Dissecting aneurysm	Unknown	Turkeys (usually fast growing tom turkeys), rarely chickens
Respiratory	Sinusitis	*Haemophilus paragallinarum* (infectious coryza)	Chickens
	Sinusitis; air sacculitis	Infectious bronchitis virus	Chickens
	Sinusitis; tracheitis; pneumonia; air sacculitis	*Mycoplasma gallisepticum*	Chickens, turkeys
	Haemorrhagic laryngotracheitis	Infectious laryngotracheitis (herpesvirus)	Chickens
	Laryngotracheitis; yellow-grey plaques in the mucosa	Fowlpox	Chickens, turkeys
	Gasping; coughing; sneezing; rales	Newcastle disease (NDV/VVND)	All
	Sinus swelling	*Chlamydophila psittaci*	All
	Rhinitis; sinusitis; conjunctivitis; excessive urates in the urinary tract	Vitamin A deficiency	All
	Water in the air sacs and lungs	Drowning	Waterfowl
Gastrointestinal	Swollen liver with mottled appearance; septicaemia	Avian cholera (*Pasteurella multocida*)	Chickens, turkeys, waterfowl
	Swollen liver with pale to yellow appearance; bile duct proliferation	Mycotoxins, aflatoxin	Ducks
	Swollen liver with pale liver	Amylodosis	Poultry, waterfowl
	Hepatomegaly with necrotic foci	Duck viral hepatitis	Ducks
	Hepatomegaly	*Chlamydophila psittaci*	All
	Pendulous crop		Chickens, turkeys, quail
	Ulcerative enteritis	*Clostridium colinum*	Chickens, turkeys, quail
	Fibrinous pseudomembrane in the oral cavity; catarrhal enteritis	Goose parvovirus (Derzsy's disease)	Waterfowl
Urinary	Swollen kidney ± urolithiasis	Infectious bronchitis virus	Chickens

25.24 Possible aetiology for clinical signs and lesions encountered in backyard poultry. (continues)

System	Clinical signs and/or lesions	Aetiology	Species
Reproductive	Drop in egg production	Avian encephalomyelitis	Chickens, turkeys, pheasants
	Drop in egg production	*Haemophilus paragallinarum* (infectious coryza)	Chickens
	Drop in egg production; eggs are misshapen with wrinkled shells	Infectious bronchitis virus	Chickens
	Drop in egg production; abnormal eggs (colour, shape or surface and have watery albumin)	Newcastle disease (NDV/VVND)	Chickens
	Drop in egg production	Mycotoxins	Chickens
Immune	Enlarged bursa of Fabricius	Lymphoid leucosis	Chickens
	Enlarged (acute) or atrophic (chronic) bursa of Fabricius; common sequela to gangrenous dermatitis in poults	Infectious bursal disease (Gumboro disease)	Chickens
	Splenomegaly	*Clostridium colinum*	Chickens, turkeys
	Splenomegaly	*Chlamydophila psittaci*	All
Nervous	Tremors of head and neck; paresis; paralysis; muscle tremors in chicks	Avian encephalomyelitis	Chickens, turkeys, pheasants
	Tremors; paralysed wings and legs; torticollis; circling; clonic spasms; complete paralysis; diarrhoea	Newcastle disease (NDV/VVND)	All
	Torticollis; stupor; paresis; paralysis; septicaemia	Listeria monocytogenes	Chickens, turkeys, geese, ducks
	Paresis to paralysis; flaccid head and neck	Botulism, toxins of *Clostridium botulinum* type A	Chickens, waterfowl
Eyes	Conjunctivitis	*Chlamydophila psittaci*	All (particularly turkeys)
	Lenticular cataract	Avian encephalomyelitis virus	Chickens, turkeys, pheasants

25.24 (continued) Possible aetiology for clinical signs and lesions encountered in backyard poultry.

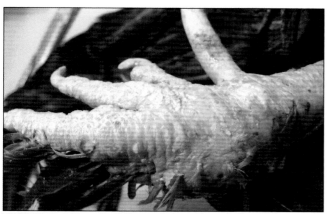

25.25 Variable epithelial hyperplasia and hyperkeratosis due to scaly leg mites (*Knemidocoptes mutans*) in a chicken.

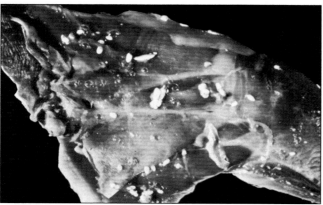

25.26 Subcutaneous mites (*Laminosioptes cysticola*) may be found at post-mortem examination.

cellulitis and folliculitis (Figure 25.27). Culture of samples collected from these lesions will reveal a bacterial aetiology. Plantar pododermatitis is an ulceration of the metatarsal and digital footpads affecting Galliformes and waterfowl (Figure 25.28). These lesions also generally have bacterial involvement. Severe irregular swelling of the wattles can suggest chronic avian cholera caused by *Pasteurella multocida*.

Several viral infections also result in skin lesions. AI is another differential diagnosis for swollen wattles and is associated with high mortality. With Marek's disease, cellular proliferations in the feather follicles and gross nodules develop (Figure 25.29). Proliferative skin lesions primarily on the non-feathered areas are typical for fowlpox (Figure 25.30).

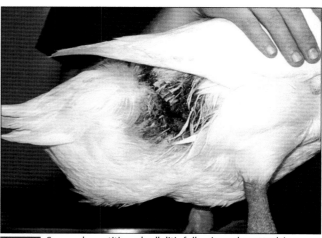

25.27 Severe dermatitis and cellulitis following a dog attack in a duck.

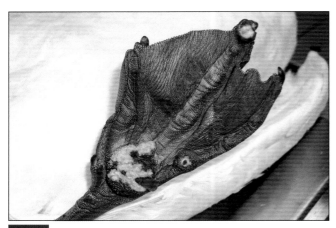

25.28 Severe pododermatitis in a mute swan.

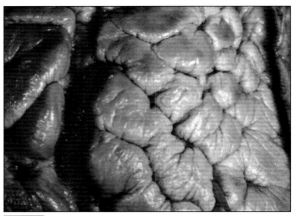

25.31 Thickened skin in a chicken with xanthomatosis.

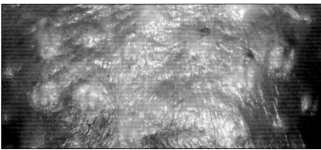

25.29 Multifocal nodular swellings of the skin due to Marek's disease. Many lesions involve the feather follicles (the feathers have been removed in this case).

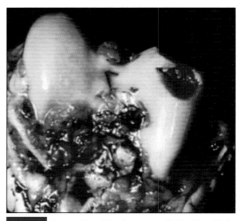

25.32 Synovitis of the intertarsal joint (hock) due to *Mycoplasma*.

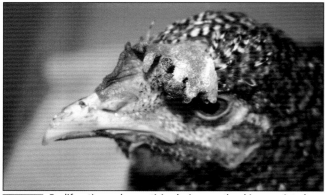

25.30 Proliferative and necrotizing lesions on the skin associated with fowlpox infection.
(Courtesy of Greg Rich)

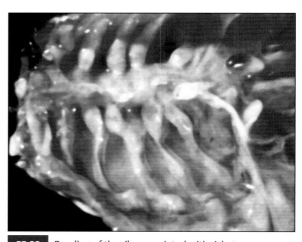

25.33 Beading of the ribs associated with rickets.

Although xanthomatosis is not as common in poultry today, it has been suggested that it occurs due to hydrocarbon toxicity. Affected skin becomes thickened and rugous (Figure 25.31).

Musculoskeletal system

Avian cholera *(Pasteurella multocida)* in chickens develops as a purulent arthritis and/or synovitis with yellow inspissated exudate. Synovitis is frequently caused by *Mycoplasma synoviae* in chickens (Figure 25.32). Beading of the rib heads and increased flexibility of the long bones is typical for dietary deficiency of calcium and vitamin D3 (Figure 25.33). A plug of cartilage extending from the growth plate into the metaphysis of the proximal tibiotarsus is characteristic of dyschondroplasia in chickens. Multiple factors are associated with this syndrome.

Dyschondroplastic lesions are masses of avascular cartilage extending from the growth plate in the metaphysis and are attributed to the failure of chondrocytes to differentiate. The most common neoplastic condition involving the bone in chickens is osteopetrosis due to the leucosis/sarcoma group of viruses. There is marked diaphyseal swelling of the long bones due to excessive growth of subperiosteal bone (Figure 25.34). Grossly yellow-white foci and streaks due to schizonts of *Sarcocystis* can be seen in the skeletal muscle mass of ducks and other birds (Figure 25.35). Vitamin E deficiency can result in

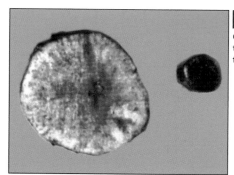

25.34 Osteopetrosis (note: the normal bone is on the right).

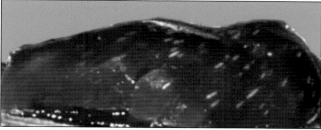

25.35 Sarcosporidial schizonts causing numerous foci and streaks in the skeletal muscle of a duck.

large areas of skeletal muscle degeneration. If there is haemorrhage into the muscle, it will be dark red-purple and localization of infection can lead to grey-yellow or white foci.

Body cavities and fluids

A transudate to modified transudate fluid accumulating in the ventral and dorsal hepatic cavities can suggest ascites syndrome in broilers. Spontaneous cardiomyopathy in young turkeys, a condition of unknown aetiology, is associated with ascites, hydropericardium and a rounded heart. Young chicks with sodium intoxication develop ascites, subcutaneous oedema and hydropericardium. Many acute systemic viral infections may also be associated with ascites and hydropericardium. Knowing the species susceptibility, age and other lesions helps to identify the aetiology. The exposed serosal surfaces of the liver, heart and intestines should be examined for discoloration, exudates and depositions such as urates. Petechiae on serosal membranes is typical for Newcastle disease. Release of yolk into the peritoneal cavity can result in the accumulation of a grey-yellow exudate on serosal surfaces and free exudate in the coelomic cavity, and is an indicator of yolk peritonitis.

Cardiovascular system

Dilatation of the right ventricle is typical of round heart disease in turkeys. Rupture and dissecting aneurysm of the aorta (Figure 25.36) is a frequent lesion in young tom turkeys and has been seen in waterfowl. The common sequela of *Escherichia coli* septicaemia in chickens is pericarditis. Fibrinous pericarditis and epicarditis is characteristically seen in ducks with *Riemerella* (*Pasteurella*) *anatipestifer* infection. Listeriosis can result in severe necrotizing myocarditis. A pale rounded heart is typical for goose parvovirus in goslings and Muscovy ducklings. Visceral gout (urate deposition) leads to a grey-white thickening of the pericardium and epicardium and must be differentiated from infectious disease.

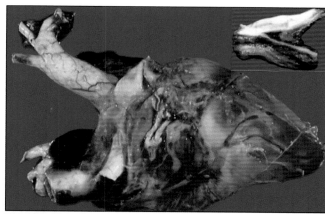

25.36 Dissecting aneurysm with periarterial haemorrhage. Inset: close-up view of the dissection.

Respiratory system

Periocular sinus: Diseases associated with sinusitis include *Haemophilus paragallinarum* (infectious coryza), infectious bronchitis virus, *Chlamydophila* and *Pasteurella multocida*. The swellings can close the eye and exudate is present in the external nares (Figure 25.37). Avian influenza, *Chlamydophila* and cryptosporidiosis all distend the infraorbital sinuses and cause conjunctivitis in turkeys. *Mycoplasma gallisepticum* produces massive volumes of mucoid exudate in the infraorbital sinuses of turkeys.

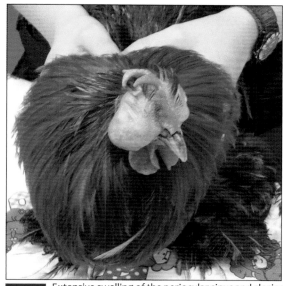

25.37 Extensive swelling of the periocular sinus and closing of the eye.
(Courtesy of Geoffrey Olsen)

Trachea: Infectious bronchitis virus (a coronavirus of chickens) can produce mucoid exudate in the trachea and bronchi. Caseous plugs may also be found in the trachea of young birds with infectious bronchitis virus. There should be a high index of suspicion for this virus if there is a rapidly developing infection with a high morbidity. The wet form of fowlpox is associated with fibrinonecrotic plaques in the larynx, trachea and oesophagus. Infectious laryngotracheitis in chickens and other birds is caused by herpesvirus. Severe haemorrhage and a fibrinopurulent exudate may be seen (Figure 25.38). *Mycoplasma gallisepticum*, a common pathogen of chickens and turkeys, can also present with tracheitis, as well as sinusitis, pneumonia and air sacculitis.

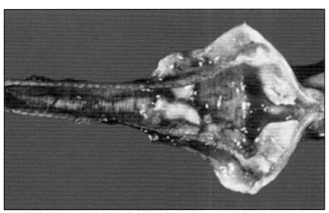

25.38 Haemorrhage and tracheal exudate in a chicken with infectious laryngotracheitis.

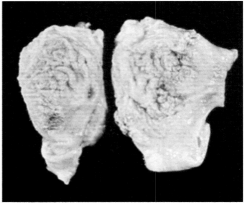

25.40 Candidiasis (thrush) in the crop of a chicken. Note the proliferative mucosa.

Lung: Multiple nodules are typical for fungal pneumonia. Pulmonary oedema can develop with goose parvovirus in goslings and Muscovy ducks. A variety of bacterial and parasitic diseases can lead to lung lesions, with sequestered necrotic lung lesions typical for avian cholera in poultry.

Air sacs: Many infections (infectious bronchitis virus, lower virulence Newcastle disease) can involve the air sacs, resulting in thickening with or without exudates. Air sacculitis in turkeys is typical for both *Riemerella antipesifer* and *Chlamydophila* infection. The air sacs can be swabbed for cytological preparations.

Gastrointestinal system

Oral cavity: Exudative oral ulcers can be caused by toxins such as T-2 myotoxin (trichothecenes) and quaternary ammonium. Fibrinous pseudomembrane covering the tongue and oral cavity is a common presentation of goose parvovirus in goslings and Muscovy ducklings. Similar lesions are typical for the diphtheritic form of fowlpox (Figure 25.39). Differential diagnoses for caseous, necrotic foci of the oral cavity, oesophagus and crop include *Trichomonas* infection and vitamin A deficiency.

Oesophagus and crop: Fibrinoexudative plaques on the oesophageal mucosa are typical of duck virus enteritis in ducklings. The diphtheritic form of fowlpox is associated with fibrinonecrotic plaques in the upper gastrointestinal and respiratory tracts (see above). In all birds, *Candida* may colonize the superficial mucosal epithelium resulting in a proliferative ingluvitis (Figure 25.40). *Capillaria* spp.

infections produce thickening of the crop and oesophageal mucosa in many gallinaceous birds. Vitamin A deficiency results in focal white pustules in the nasal passages, mouth, oesophagus, pharynx and crop. Pendulous crop (a syndrome seen in chickens, turkeys and quail) is characterized by a crop distended with fluid and/or impacted food material.

Proventriculus and ventriculus: Mycotoxins can produce ventricular erosions, as can lead toxicity in waterfowl. The presence of intraluminal wood shavings in turkeys is characteristic of starved poults. In chickens, proventricular and intestinal mucosal haemorrhage (Figure 25.41) is suggestive of Newcastle disease, infectious bursal disease or chicken infectious anaemia (circovirus), whilst ventricular erosions are due to adenoviral infection. Nematodes can be found within gastric secretions not only within the lumen but also under the koilin and within the proventricular glands.

Small and large intestine: A number of protozoan and metazoan parasites can be found in the intestines. Wet mount and direct slide preparations can be used to identify coccidia, *Cochlosoma anatis*, *Histomonas*, spironucleosis and trichomonads. Fresh samples are preferred (wet mount) in order to see movement, which helps to identify many protozoa (Figure 25.42). Spironucleosis (*Hexamita*) is typically located within the duodenum. The intestines appear pearl grey and enlarged with coccidial infections. Ascarid worms should be visible grossly within the lumen of the intestine (Figure 25.43). Some nematodes are readily identified by examining the eggs on faecal flotation (e.g. *Capillaria* spp., which have characteristic bipolar caps on the eggs).

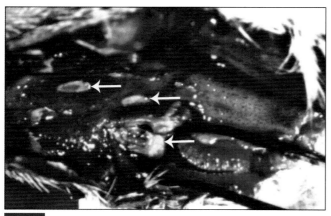

25.39 Fowlpox lesions in the oral cavity (arrowed).

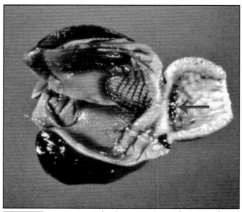

25.41 Proventricular haemorrhage (arrowed) which can be seen in birds with Newcastle disease or chicken infectious anaemia.

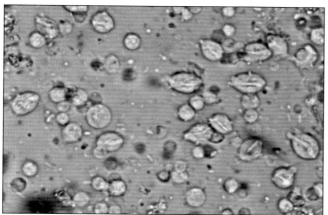

25.42 | A wet mount cytology preparation of *Trichomonas* from the intestine of a quail.

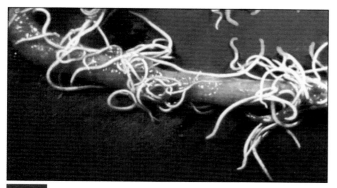

25.43 | Ascarids in the small intestine.

Several viral infections are associated with intestinal lesions (usually necrosis and haemorrhage). As in the proventriculus, haemorrhage of the intestinal mucosa is suggestive of Newcastle disease. Duck virus enteritis (duck plague) leads to haemorrhage and fibrinonecrotic debris (Figure 25.44). In goslings, haemorrhagic enteritis is typically seen with goose parvovirus and in turkeys is due to a type II adenovirus. There are many bacterial infections associated with intestinal lesions. *Clostridium perfringens* is the cause of necrotic enteritis in chickens, turkeys and geese. Ulcerative enteritis (Figure 25.45) is caused by *Clostridium colinum* in chickens and other gallinaceous birds; cytology readily identifies the Gram-positive spore-forming bacteria with characteristically slightly curved rods. *Salmonella pullorum* is often the cause of severe

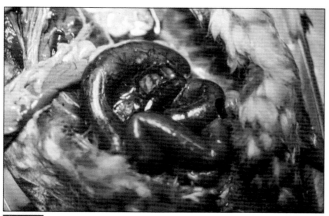

25.44 | Severe haemorrhage due to duck virus enteritis infection.

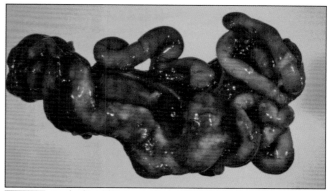

25.45 | Multifocal necrotizing ulcerative enteritis due to *Clostridium colunum* in a Bobwhite quail.

enteritis in older chickens. *Mycobacterium* infection causes thickening of the intestinal wall due to granulomatous inflammation.

Necrotic haemorrhagic areas in the caecal tonsils is typical for Newcastle disease. *Heterakis isolonche* produces characteristic nodules in the walls of the caeca of pheasants. *Histomonas meleagridis* causes severe typhlitis (Figure 25.46) and organisms may be seen on wet mounts from the caecum. Caecal coccidiosis causes severe gross lesions that must be differentiated from *Histomonas* infection. In young chickens, *Salmonella pullorum* causes a severe typhlitis with a purulent exudate accumulation.

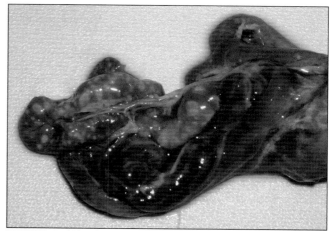

25.46 | Marked typhlitis in a turkey with *Histomonas meleagridis* infection.

Liver

Septicaemia can result in a mottled appearance with variable hepatic enlargement. The possible causes of septicaemia include *Chlamydophila*, *Pasteurella multocida* (Figure 25.47) and other bacteria. Peri-hepatitis is a feature of *Riemerella* (*Pasteurella*) *anatipestifer* infection.

In turkeys, liver granulomas are caused by *Eubacterium tortuosum*; mycobacteria also cause granulomas in all bird species. A greenish discoloration of the liver in turkeys is seen as part of the turkey osteomyelitis complex and is associated with many different opportunistic organisms, particularly *Staphylococcus aureus* and *Escherichia coli*. A similar greenish discoloration is typical with lead toxicity in waterfowl.

Histomonas meleagridis in turkeys can be recognized by circular necrotic foci (Figure 25.48) and confirmed by a wet smear of the liver lesions and identification of protozoa

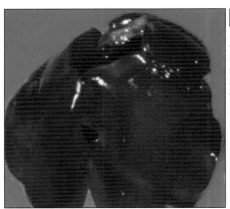

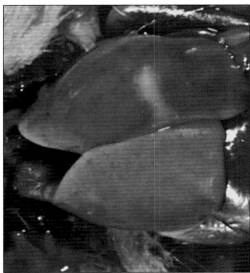

25.47 Slightly enlarged liver with multiple yellow-white foci indicative of septicaemia due to *Pasteurella* (fowl cholera).

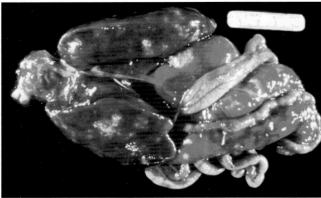

25.48 Necrotic foci in the liver and caeca of a turkey associated with histomoniasis.

25.50 Enlarged liver with a mottled appearance in a duck with duck viral hepatitis.

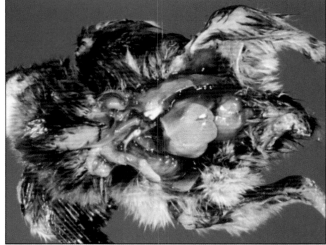

25.51 Enlarged yellow liver, typical for hepatic lipidosis, in a Palawan pheasant.

with a single flagellum. White spots in the liver of turkeys can represent aberrant migration tracts of *Ascaridia dissimilis* larvae.

Retroviruses cause disease in several Galliformes. Lymphoid leucosis results in liver enlargement and a mottled appearance in chickens (Figure 25.49). An enlarged liver in turkeys is the most common clinical sign of reticuloendotheliosis. Marek's disease is a common cause of hepatic enlargement in chickens, and in ducks the liver can be enlarged with haemorrhagic foci in cases of duck virus hepatitis (Figure 25.50).

An enlarged pale liver can also be caused by toxic exposure from the ingestion of aflatoxin, especially in ducks. A fatty liver due to many causes appears large, pale and friable (Figure 25.51).

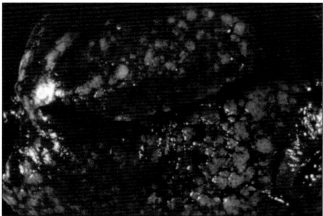

25.49 Enlarged liver with a mottled appearance in a chicken with lymphoid leucosis.

Kidneys

The kidneys may appear pale as a result of many diseases. Nephropathogenic strains of infectious bronchitis virus (coronavirus of chickens) can produce swollen, pale kidneys with the tubules and ureters distended by urates and uroliths. Renal gout, characterized by white gritty streaks to disseminated foci, can occur secondary to chronic vitamin A deficiency. The development of urolithiasis has been associated with some myotoxins, a high calcium diet, infectious bronchitis and water deprivation. Nephroblastoma is a common tumour in chickens and is caused by the avian leucosis virus. Grossly, these tumours destroy the normal renal architecture and may have solid and cystic regions. Polycystic kidneys have been identified in chickens.

Reproductive tract

Duck virus enteritis (duck plague) commonly results in penile prolapse. Cystic testes in young chicks should raise suspicion for sodium toxicity. Hypoplasia of the oviduct in a mature chicken suggests that the bird was exposed to infectious bronchitis virus as a chick. A cystic right oviduct is a common incidental finding in chickens during necropsy. Ovarian carcinoma is seen sporadically and these tumours may implant on serosal surfaces. Older hens may have enlarged, discoloured and friable oviducts, which may be impacted with yellow caseous material.

Immune system

Thymus: Oedema around the thymus is reported in cases of Newcastle disease. Atrophy of the thymus occurs with chicken infectious anaemia.

Spleen: Enlargement of the spleen can be due to haemorrhage, oedema or cellular infiltrates (neoplastic and inflammatory). Several diseases, including infection with *Chlamydophila*, *Salmonella*, avian spirochetosis (*Borrelia anserina*) and mycobacteria, result in an enlarged spleen with grey or yellow foci (Figure 25.52). Several adenoviral infections in Galliformes are associated with splenomegaly.

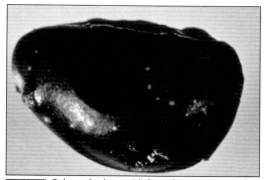

25.52 Enlarged spleen with foci of necrosis and inflammation scattered throughout the parenchyma. This appearance is typically seen with bacterial septicaemia.

Bursa of Fabricius: Enlargement of the bursa with multiple nodules is suggestive of lymphoid leucosis (a retrovirus of chickens). Atrophy of the bursa is expected with Marek's disease and chronic infectious bursal disease in chickens. If there is any doubt about the degree of atrophy or involution, comparison with a normal age-matched control is necessary.

Nervous system

Some important agents that cause neurological disease may not leave gross or, in some cases, even histological lesions. These diseases include Newcastle disease, botulism and avian encephalomyelitis. Botulism (limberneck), caused by ingestion of preformed toxins of *Clostridium botulinum* type A, is characterized by cervical paralysis and is generally seen in waterfowl resident on small ponds. Avian encephalomyelitis is caused by a picornavirus and results in central nervous system signs (e.g. epidemic tremor) in affected birds less than 3 weeks old. Susceptible species include chickens, Japanese Quail, turkeys, pheasants and pigeons. Haemorrhage and oedema may be seen in the cerebellum of chickens with nutritional encephalomalacia (vitamin E deficiency).

Enlarged peripheral nerves (vagus, brachial and sciatic) are seen with Marek's disease. A cytological touch preparation from these nerves or from any lymphoid visceral tumours will contain predominately lymphocytes, confirming the diagnosis of Marek's disease. Riboflavin deficiency results in 'curled toe paralysis', which is the clinical manifestation of a peripheral neuropathy.

Endocrine system

In chickens with rickets the parathyroid glands may be enlarged. Goitre and neoplasia can result in enlarged thyroid glands, but this is infrequently seen in poultry.

Sensory organs

Eyes: High atmospheric levels of ammonia in densely housed poultry result in corneal erosions and keratitis. Numerous bacteria, including *Escherichia coli*, *Pseudomonas aeruginosa* and *Salmonella* spp., can be associated with infectious keratitis in any avian species. Irregularity and loss of normal iris pigmentation is typically seen in chickens with Marek's disease (Figure 25.53).

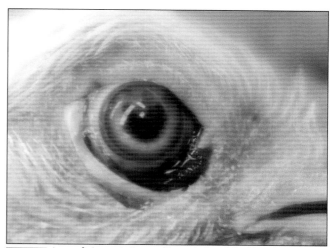

25.53 Loss of pigmentation and irregularity of the iris is due to Marek's disease.

Summary

The post-mortem examination is usually the final step in obtaining an answer as to the cause of disease. However, the complete examination requires careful collection of the history, signalment and other clinical findings for proper interpretation. Where possible, clinical signs should be noted and blood samples collected prior to euthanasia. The method of euthanasia should also be noted as part of the clinical information provided to the pathologist, as all methods can result in lesions that may be misinterpreted. In addition, it should be remembered that when a notifiable disease has been identified, the relevant authorities need to be informed. Notifiable diseases vary from country to country and region to region. In California, for example, the current diseases in poultry and waterfowl that are required to be reported include Newcastle disease, highly pathogenic avian influenza, *Chlamydophila*, turkey rhinotracheitis (avian metapneumovirus) and pullorum disease (fowl typhoid caused by *Salmonella gallinarum* and *S. pullorum*). The regulations for the UK can be found in Chapter 26.

References and further reading

Abdul-Aziz TA (2010) *Multiple choice questions in poultry medicine*. Raleigh, North Carolina

Beynon PH, Forbes NA and Harcourt-Brown NH (1996) *BSAVA Manual of Raptors, Pigeons and Waterfowl*. BSAVA Publications, Cheltenham

Boucher M, ehmler TJ and Bermudez AJ (2000) Polytetrafluoroethylene gas intoxication in broiler chickens. *Avian Diseases* **44**, 449–453

Charlton BR (2006) *Avian Disease Manual*. American Association of Avian Pathologists, College Station, Texas

Grieves JL, Dick EJ, Schlabritz-Loutsevich NE, Butler SD, Leland MM *et al.* (2008) Barbiturate euthanasia solution-induced tissue artefact in non-human primates. *Journal of Medical Primatology* **37**, 154–161

Jordan FTW and Pattison M (1996) *Poultry Diseases, 4th edn*. WB Saunders, Philadelphia

Kahn CM and Line S (2010) *The Merck Veterinary Manual, 10th edn*. Merck Sharp & Dohme Corp., Whitehouse Station, New Jersey

McLelland J (1991) *Color Atlas of Avian Anatomy*. WB Saunders, Philadelphia

Pandiri AKR, Cortes AL, Lee LF and Gimeno IM (2008) Marek's disease virus infection in the eye: chronological study of the lesions, virus replication and vaccine-induced protection. *Avian Diseases* **52**, 572–582

Randall CJ (1985) *A Colour Atlas of Diseases of Domestic Fowl and Turkeys*. Iowa State University Press, Ames

Saif YM, Fadly AM, Glisson JR, McDougald LR, Nolan LK and Swayne DE (2008) *Diseases of Poultry, 12th edn*. Wiley-Blackwell, Ames

Stephens RS, Myers G, Eppinger M and Bavoil PM (2009) Divergence without difference: phylogenetics and taxonomy of *Chlamydia* resolved. *FEMS Immunology and Medical Microbiology* **55**, 115–119

Chapter 26

Legal issues

Guy Poland

The veterinary profession is highly regulated in most countries of the world. Regulation aims to protect veterinary patients, their owners and the public as a whole. In practising veterinary medicine, legislation relating to professional conduct, medicines control, animal welfare, disease control, food safety and human health and safety must be adhered to. Practitioners must have a good working knowledge of such legislation. The treatment of poultry, however, offers an additional challenge to companion animal veterinary surgeons (veterinarians) who may not be as familiar with rules relating to food safety as their farm animal colleagues. Additionally, it is beneficial for veterinary surgeons to be able to advise their clients of relevant legislation that may apply to the keeping of their flocks.

This chapter will make specific reference to legislation in the United Kingdom of Great Britain (UK). Similar laws will be applicable in other countries, particularly within the European Union, where there is a move to unify the laws of member states. The legislation specific to other countries is beyond the scope of this book, and so it is the responsibility of clinicians outside the UK to be familiar with their local rules. For users within the UK, this information is provided as a guide only and is not exhaustive. There may be some differences in regulation between the countries of the UK. In the interests of simplicity, regulations quoted will be those in force in England. Legislation primarily concerned with commercial operations will not be covered. Knowledge of legislation regarding general veterinary practice will be assumed. Acts and regulations quoted are those that are current at the time of writing and are liable to change. Where there is doubt, relevant legal advice should be sought.

Legal definitions

In the UK, legislation may take the form of Acts, Regulations and Orders. Acts of Parliament are primary legislation brought in to law by parliament. Regulations and Orders (collectively known as Statutory Instruments) are pieces of secondary or delegated legislation passed by a Minister (or in some cases, a Privy Council) under the authority of an Act of Parliament. At the time of writing, European Union (EU) Regulations and Decisions are directly applicable to all member states and reference to EU Regulations is frequently made in UK regulations. The UK government is in the process of amending the legislation to operate outside of the EU, although initially there will not be a change to the substance of the legislation. This chapter will reference EU regulations to reflect the current position, and in the interests of simplicity, reference will not be made to the 'EU Exit' regulations.

Codes are not legally binding; they provide guidance for best practice. Adherence to a code does not confer protection from prosecution, but may contribute to a defence.

Definition of a 'food-producing animal'

Any animal with the potential to be a food-producing animal must be treated as such with regard to the use of veterinary medicinal products (VMPs). A traditional definition of poultry is a group of species of birds that have been domesticated in order to produce eggs or meat for human consumption, or for the production of feathers. Unfortunately, there is no single legal definition of poultry or farmed birds and it will vary slightly from one piece of legislation to another. The Avian Influenza (Preventive Measures) (England) Regulations 2006 state that 'poultry' means all birds that are reared or kept in captivity for the production of meat or eggs for consumption, the production of other commercial products, for restocking supplies of game or for the purposes of any breeding programme for the production of these categories of birds. These same regulations require that chickens (including bantams), turkeys, ducks, geese, partridges, quail, pheasants, pigeons (reared for meat), guinea fowl, ostriches, emus, rheas and cassowaries be entered into a register of poultry holdings (see below). Elsewhere, emus, rheas and cassowaries are defined, for legal purposes, as ratites. The remainder of this list includes all of the species/groups of poultry covered by this manual, and consideration of the purpose for keeping the species is only made for pigeons, which are covered elsewhere in the BSAVA Manual of Raptors, Pigeons and Passerine Birds. It would seem sensible to use this list as a definition of poultry species/groups and therefore, by implication, of food-producing species/groups of bird.

Flock registration

Under The Avian Influenza (Preventive Measures) Regulations 2006, it is required that any premises at which a flock of 50 or more poultry birds is kept is registered in the

GB Poultry Register. This includes flocks of mixed poultry types, not just of a single species. The premises must be registered regardless of whether the flock is kept there for only part of the year. Keepers of smaller numbers of poultry are encouraged to register on a voluntary basis. Registrants will be required to provide the following information:

- The keeper's name
- The premises address for the holding
- The premises County Parish Holding (CPH) number (if registered; this can be obtained from the Rural Payments Agency (RPA))
- The number of poultry usually on the premises (this is the number usually present when the premises are stocked)
- The type of poultry housing
- The reason for rearing poultry
- Answers to risk assessment questions, such as whether the poultry have access to the open air and whether there are bodies of water close by that may attract wild birds.

Keepers must notify the authorities of any changes to the information above within 1 month of the changes happening.

The GB Poultry Register is intended to help with national veterinary surveillance and to help manage any potential disease outbreak by allowing resources to be targeted where they are needed most.

Separately, under The Control of Salmonella in Poultry Order 2007, occupiers of a holding on which one or more breeding flocks or laying flocks of at least 250 poultry of any single species are kept, or who have the capacity to incubate 1000 or more eggs, are required to register in the Hatcheries register and must comply with measures to control *Salmonella* infection.

Environmental legislation

As with all livestock, poultry keeping has the potential to impact on the immediate, local and surrounding environment. Poultry keepers must pay attention to the effects of ammonia, nutrients from manure, litter and slurry, effluent discharges, dust, odour and noise, all of which are subject to various pieces of legislation (Figure 26.1).

Record keeping for the supply and receipt of veterinary medicinal products

The Veterinary Medicines Regulations 2013 require that for any supply or receipt of VMPs classified as prescription-only medicine – veterinarian (POM-V) or prescription-only medicine – veterinarian, pharmacist or suitably qualified person (POM-VPS) for food-producing animals, the following records should be kept for at least 5 years:

- Transaction date
- Name of the veterinary medicinal product
- Batch number
- Quantity
- Name and address of the supplier or recipient
- Name and address of the person who wrote the prescription and a copy of the prescription (if there is a written prescription).

Records may be by means of documentation accompanying the transaction, or by means of records stored elsewhere so long as these records are made as soon as is reasonably possible.

Record keeping responsibilities of the poultry keeper

The Veterinary Medicines Regulations 2013 require that the food-producing animal keeper must, for a period of at least 5 years following the administration or other disposal of the product, irrespective of whether or not the animal concerned is no longer in that keeper's possession or is alive during that period:

- Keep proof of purchase of all veterinary medicinal products acquired for the animal (or, if they were not bought, documentary evidence of how they were acquired)
- When a veterinary medicinal product is bought or otherwise acquired for a food-producing animal the keeper must, at the time, record:

Legislation/Code	Coverage	Implementation authority
Environmental Protection Act 1990	Dust, steam, smell or efflua being prejudicial to health or a nuisance	Local Authority Environmental Health Department
Pollution Prevention and Control Act 1999	Emissions into air, water and soil	Environment Agency
A Code of Good Agricultural Practice for farmers, growers and land managers (CoGAP)	Emissions into air, water and soil	Not applicable. Available online from Defra and in print from The Stationery Office
Water Resources Act 1991	Water pollution	Environment Agency
The Protection of Water Against Agricultural Nitrate Pollution (England and Wales) (Amendment) Regulations 2006	Nitrate pollution of water	Environment Agency
The Animal By-Products (Enforcement) (England) Regulations 2013	Disposal of carcasses	Local Authority
Highways Act 1980	Deposition of material (e.g. slurry or solid manure) on to a highway causing interruption, injury, danger or nuisance	Local Authority
Waste Management (England and Wales) Regulations 2006	Disposal of agricultural waste such as pesticide containers, silage wrap, bags and sheets, tyres, batteries, old machinery and oil, to protect the environment and human health	Environment Agency

26.1 Environmental legislation relevant to poultry keeping.

- Name of the product and the batch number
- Date of acquisition
- Quantity acquired
- Name and address of the supplier.
- At the time of administration (unless the administration is by a veterinary surgeon in which case the record must be in accordance with regulation 18) the keeper must record:
  - Name of the product
  - Date of administration
  - Quantity administered
  - Withdrawal period
  - Identification of the animals treated.
- When disposing of any or all of the veterinary medicinal product other than by treating an animal must record:
  - Date of disposal
  - Quantity of product involved
  - How and where it was disposed of.

A veterinary surgeon who administers a veterinary medicinal product to a food-producing animal must either enter the following information personally in the keeper's records or give it to the keeper in writing (in which case the keeper must enter the following into those records):

- Name of the veterinary surgeon
- Name of the product and the batch number
- Date of administration of the product
- Amount of product administered
- Identification of the animals treated
- Withdrawal period.

The prescribing cascade

The principles of the cascade

Under The Veterinary Medicines Regulations 2013, drugs prescribed for the treatment of animals must be selected according to the prescribing cascade. The prescribing cascade allows veterinary surgeons to legally prescribe unauthorized drugs under certain conditions and aims to ensure that:

- The safest drug is used
- The most efficacious drug is used
- Consumers are protected from unsafe levels of veterinary medicinal residues in food products
- Drug companies are fairly rewarded for their investment in research and development.

There are differences in how the prescribing cascade is applied to companion animals and food-producing animals. When treating a horse, which is potentially a food-producing animal, the companion animal interpretation of the cascade may be used so long as the owner signs a declaration to ensure that the horse will not be slaughtered for human consumption. Unfortunately, no such allowance exists for the treatment of poultry, and so the prescribing cascade must be followed as it would be for a food-producing animal.

Applying the cascade

The prescribing cascade for food-producing animals is laid out below in the form of a dichotomous key:

1. Is there a veterinary medicine authorized in the UK to treat the specific condition in the species being treated?
   Yes: Go to question 3.
   No: Go to question 2.
2. Is there a veterinary medicine authorized in the UK for use in another animal species or for a different condition in the same species which could be used to treat this condition?
   Yes: Go to question 3.
   No: Go to question 5.
3. Is the veterinary medicine authorized for use in animals intended for human consumption and, if a laying bird, for use in birds producing eggs for human consumption?
   Yes: **Use this veterinary medicine, stating the given withdrawal times.**
   No: Go to question 4
4. Is there an alternative veterinary medicine fulfilling the criteria in questions 1 and 3 or 2 and 3?
   Yes: **Use that veterinary medicine.**
   No: Go to question 8.
5. Is there a suitable medicine authorized in the UK for human use?
   Yes: Go to question 8.
   No: Go to question 6.
   or is there a veterinary medicinal product (VMP) not authorized in the UK but authorized in another Member State (MS) for use in a food-producing species, for which an import certificate has been issued by the Veterinary Medicines Directorate (VMD)?
   Yes: Go to question 7.
   No: Go to question 6.
6. Is there a medicine that can be prepared extemporaneously by a veterinary surgeon, a pharmacist or a person holding an appropriate manufacturer's authorization? In exceptional circumstances, medicines may be imported from Third countries through the VMD's import scheme.
   Yes: Go to question 8.
   No: **No medical treatment for this condition may be used.**
7. Is a withdrawal period stated on the EU product literature?
   Yes: **Use this drug in strict accordance with the EU authorization, stating the withdrawal periods given.**
   No: Go to question 8.
8. Is the pharmacologically active substance listed in the Table of Allowed Substances in Commission Regulation EU (European Union) No. 37/2010?
   Yes: Go to question 9.
   No: **You cannot prescribe this drug. Seek an alternative.**
9. Are you able to recommend an appropriate drug withdrawal time for meat and, if appropriate, eggs for this drug?
   Yes: Go to question 10.
   No: **You cannot prescribe this drug. Seek an alternative.**
10. Is your appropriate recommended withdrawal time shorter than 28 days for meat and 7 days for eggs:
    Yes: **Prescribe this drug, but state the statutory minimum meat withdrawal time of 28 days and (if appropriate) the statutory minimum egg withdrawal time of 7 days.**
    No: **Prescribe this drug and state your appropriate recommended meat and (if appropriate) egg withdrawal times.**

In addition, specific to medicated feeds: If there is no suitable VMP, a veterinary surgeon may prescribe (a) a

VMP authorized for another species or for another condition in the same species and (b) include more than one VMP for incorporation into the feedingstuff **provided that all VMPs prescribed (even under the cascade) are authorized for inclusion in feedingstuffs (a premix –** see 'medicated feed stuffs' below). Other relevant conditions of the cascade should still be applied, for example standard withdrawal periods.

Maximum residue levels and Commission Regulation EU (European Union) No. 37/2010

Commission Regulation EU (European Union) No. 37/2010, referred to in question 8 above, can be found online (see 'Useful websites'). Table 1 lists allowed substances, including substances for which a maximum residue limit has been established, substances where it is not necessary for a residue limit to be established, and substances for which a provisional maximum residue limit has been established. Table 2 lists prohibited substances for which a maximum residue limit could not be established because residues of those substances, at whatever limit, constitute a hazard to human health.

The list of prohibited substances includes:

- *Aristolochia* spp. and preparations thereof
- Chloramphenicol
- Chloroform
- Chlorpromazine
- Colchicine
- Dapsone
- Dimetridazole
- Metronidazole
- Nitrofurans (including furazolidone)
- Ronidazole.

Human homeopathic products may be used under the rules of the cascade, but only if the pharmacologically active substances are listed in Table 1 Allowed Substances of Commission Regulation EU (European Union) No. 37/2010. In this case, the statutory withdrawal period must be applied.

Record keeping under the cascade

There are specific record-keeping requirements when medicines are prescribed under the cascade. These records must be retained for at least 5 years and be made available on request. The VMD guidance notes state that 'if the client or other records already have this information no additional separate records are needed as long as the information is accessible on request', but recommends that the veterinary surgeon also keeps a record of the identification of the individual animals being treated. The information recorded must include the following:

- Date of examination
- Owner's name and address
- The identification and number of animals treated
- Result of the veterinary surgeon's clinical assessment
- Trade name of the product(s) prescribed, if applicable
- Manufacturer's batch number if there is one
- Name and quantity of the active substance
- Doses administered or supplied
- Duration of treatment
- Withdrawal period.

Labelling under the cascade

Drugs prescribed under the cascade also require additional labelling. Labels must include the following information:

- Name and address of the pharmacy, veterinary surgery or approved premises supplying the VMP
- Name of the veterinary surgeon who has prescribed the product
- Name and address of the animal owner
- Identification (including the species) of the animal or group of animals
- Date of supply
- Expiry date of the product, if applicable
- Name or description of the product, which should include at least the name and quantity of active ingredient
- Dosage and administration instructions
- Any species storage precautions
- Any necessary warnings for the user, target species, administration or disposal of the product
- Withdrawal period
- 'Keep out of reach of children' and 'For animal use only'.

If some of this information is included on the original packaging, and the original packaging is included, then it need not be repeated on the label. Where there is too much information to put on the label, a separate sheet must be provided.

Informed consent under the cascade

It is not a legal requirement under the Veterinary Medicines Regulations to obtain informed consent from the owner of an animal to be treated under the cascade, but it is required as part of the Royal College of Veterinary Surgeons (RCVS) Code of Professional Conduct, to which practitioners should refer for further information.

Difficulties applying the cascade

The VMD and RCVS Code of Professional Conduct provide guidance as to the use of the cascade, particularly the VMD in *The Cascade: Prescribing unauthorised medicines* (see 'Useful websites'). The correct implementation, however, is still open to interpretation and in the case of ambiguity it would be ultimately up to a court of law to decide if the cascade has been correctly applied. In the opinion of the author, the following areas offer particular difficulty to the prescribing clinician.

The market authorization 'Do not use' clause

In the datasheets of several veterinary medicines that are authorized for use in poultry, there are statements in the contraindications and warnings section similar to 'Do not use in laying birds' or 'Not authorized for use in birds producing eggs for human consumption'. This clearly prohibits the *authorized use* of the drug in laying birds, but it is not clear whether this would prohibit the cascade use of the product in laying birds.

MRLs listed for a substance for food stuffs other than poultry meat and eggs

Many substances listed in Table 1 of Commission Regulation EU (European Union) No. 37/2010 state an MRL in foodstuffs other than poultry meat or eggs. The guidance notes suggest that inclusion in the table is sufficient to confer eligibility for its use under the cascade. It is not explicit, however, as to whether an MRL for poultry meat or eggs is specifically required.

'Not for use in animals from which eggs are produced for human consumption'

Table 1 (Allowed substances) of the Commission Regulation EU (European Union) No. 37/2010 contains a column with the heading 'Other Provisions'. Under a number of substances, there is a comment similar to 'Not for use in animals from which eggs are produced for human consumption'. The use of such a substance in egg-laying animals would therefore appear to contravene Commission Regulation EU (European Union) No. 37/2010. The guidance notes for use of the cascade, however, seem to contradict this provision by stating that a substance need only be listed in table 1 to be eligible for use under the cascade in any food-producing animal.

Determining an appropriate withdrawal time

This is less a matter of interpretation of the cascade and more a problem of implementing it. It is the responsibility of the prescribing veterinarian to provide an appropriate withdrawal time for meat and (if appropriate) eggs. What this means is that the veterinarian must state a period of time sufficiently long enough to ensure that the concentration of drug that is in the foodstuff has fallen below the allowed maximum residue level. Unfortunately, arbitrary time periods are of little use without scientific knowledge of the pharmacokinetics of the substance in question. Whilst drug companies may be a good source of information on the unauthorised use of drugs, studies regarding residue levels of substances are relatively few and those that are available may be hard for the clinician to obtain. This problem may be great enough to render lower tiers of the cascade useless in many cases and, since poultry should always be treated as food producing animals, it may be impossible to treat many cases legally.

Medicated feedingstuffs

Medicated feedingstuffs (MFS) are feeds containing VMPs or specified feed additives (SFAs). A premixture is a mixture of a VMP or SFA with feedingstuffs material, intended for further mixing with feedingstuffs before being fed to animals.

SFAs are categories of feed additives, which require inspection and appropriate approval by the VMD for their manufacture and supply. These are either prophylactic coccidiostats or additives indicated for growth. They do not, however, require a prescription to supply feedingstuffs containing them or to be used by the keeper of animals.

MFS containing VMPs may only be supplied to a keeper of animals on receipt of a medicated feedingstuffs prescription (MFSp). This must be done by a veterinary surgeon if the VMP is classified POM-V. If the VMP is classified POM-VPS it may be also be prescribed by a pharmacist or suitably qualified person (SQP). MFSps must:

- Not be valid for more than 3 months
- Be written, in ink or other indelible format, or it may be produced and sent electronically
- Be sufficient for only one course of treatment

- Contain the following:
  - Name and address of the person prescribing the product
  - Qualifications enabling the person to prescribe the product
  - Name and address of the owner or keeper of the animal
  - Species of animal, identification and number of the animal
  - Premises at which the animals are kept if this is different from the address of the owner or keeper
  - Date of the prescription
  - Signature or other authentication of the person prescribing the product
  - Name and amount of the product prescribed
  - Dosage and administration instructions
  - Any necessary warnings
  - Withdrawal period
  - Manufacturer or the distributor of the feedingstuffs (who must be approved for the purpose)
  - A statement that, if the validity exceeds one month, not more than 31 day's supply may be provided at any time. It is the veterinary surgeon's responsibility to specify how much should be provided for each 31-day supply
  - The name, type and quantity of feedingstuffs to be used
  - Inclusion rate of the VMP and the resulting inclusion rate of the active substance
  - Any special instructions for the keeper
  - The percentage of the prescribed feedingstuffs to be added to the daily ration
  - If it is prescribed under the cascade, a statement to that effect.

More than one VMP may be included on the same MFSp if they are to be mixed into the same feed. The longest withdrawal period must then be used. A copy of the MFSp must be supplied to the manufacturer or distributor, the keeper of the animals to be treated and a copy retained by the veterinary surgeon.

In order to supply MFS or premixtures containing VMPs or SFAs, businesses must be approved as a Category 8 distributor by the VMD's Inspections & Investigations Team (IIT). Users of premixtures containing VMPs must be approved as a manufacturer of medicated feeding stuffs. This applies to anybody mixing premix into feed including end users and feed manufacturers. The vast majority of veterinary practices will not be approved as Category 8 distributors and therefore will not be able to supply MFS or premixtures. There are, however, two important derogations related to domestic premises. Here, animals kept on domestic premises must be non-food producing, or food producing kept for private consumption by the keeper. Private consumption means that the birds, or meat or eggs from these birds cannot be sold, including farm-gate sales. These derogations are:

1. In addition to an approved manufacturer or Category 8 distributor, a veterinary surgeon, or pharmacist in a registered practice or a suitably qualified person (SQP) in an approved retail premises, is able to obtain and supply premixtures or feedingstuffs containing VMPs to end users who are domestic keepers.

   Whilst this is permissible, the veterinary surgeon, pharmacist or SQP must treat the premixture or feed as if it was a POM-VPS medicine, which means they must orally prescribe it, advising the customer on its safe administration and on any warnings, contraindications etc.

The VMD advise that suppliers obtain written confirmation from the keeper that they do not sell birds, meat or eggs.

2. Under the derogation, the domestic keeper is able to manufacture medicated feed using a VMP or premixtures containing a VMP without being approved as a manufacturer under the appropriate Category.

Welfare requirements

The Animal Welfare Act 2006 consolidated many pieces of animal welfare legislation and it covers most aspects of poultry welfare, although several other pieces of legislation also apply (such as The Protection of Animals Acts 1911 to 1964, The Animals Act 1971 and The Agriculture (Miscellaneous Provisions) Act 1976). A comprehensive review of this legislation will not be made here, but certain poultry specific issues will be emphasized and attention drawn to the responsibilities of poultry owners.

The Animal Welfare Act 2006 is concerned with domesticated animals only (protection to wild animals is offered by the Wild Mammals (Protection) Act 1996 and Wildlife and Countryside Act 1981) and covers prevention of harm and promotion of welfare. Of particular note to owners of backyard poultry are the following points:

- It is an offence to act or fail to act so as to cause an animal to suffer unnecessarily
- It is an offence to carry out or allow a prohibited procedure
- It is an offence to cause, allow, publicize or profit from an animal fight
- It is an offence not to take reasonable steps to ensure the needs of animals are met, namely:
  - A suitable environment
  - A suitable diet
  - An ability to exhibit normal behaviour patterns
  - Housing with or without other animals as appropriate
  - Protection from pain, suffering, injury and disease.
- Whilst it is not an offence to not follow a recommended code of practice from an appropriate national authority, failure to do so will tend to establish liability in the case of a prosecution.

Defra has published the following codes of practice relating to poultry:

- Code of practice for the welfare of laying hens and pullets
- Code of practice for the welfare of meat chickens and meat breeding chickens
- Broiler (meat) chickens: welfare recommendations
- Poultry: welfare recommendations
- Ducks (mallard and Pekin): welfare recommendations
- Turkeys: welfare recommendations.

The code of practice for the welfare of laying hens and pullets covers 'single or multiple laying hens kept on a smallholding (hobby/backyard flock), as well as commercial laying hen producers'. Owners of laying birds should therefore be directed to this code and are advised to adhere to it. The other codes are oriented more towards commercial producers, but contain a wealth of useful information and should be adhered to where appropriate. Readers should refer to the codes for further details.

Surgical procedures

The Animal Welfare Act 2006 Section 5 defines a number of offences related to carrying out prohibited procedures, which are procedures that involve 'interference with the sensitive tissues or bone structure of the animal, otherwise than for the purpose of its medical treatment'. The Mutilations (Permitted Procedures) (England) Regulations 2007, The Mutilations (Permitted Procedures) (England) (Amendment) Regulations 2008 and The Mutilations (Permitted Procedures) (Amendment) Regulations 2010 define procedures that may be carried out in poultry without being required for medical reasons. The definition of poultry in these regulations includes domestic fowl, turkeys, geese, ducks, guinea fowl and pheasants. In being excluded from these regulations, any other procedure involving interference with sensitive tissues or bone structure, for example the devoicing of cockerels, is not permitted. 'Farmed birds' in the regulations 'means, in relation to an animal, bred or kept for the production of food, wool or skin or for other farming purposes'. It is not clear under which circumstances backyard poultry might not be covered under this definition. Except for in the case of beak trimming (discussed below), none of these procedures may be performed on conventionally reared meat chickens or on birds that are laying hens or that are intended to become laying hens unless they are kept on establishments with fewer than 350 such birds.

Identification procedures

Microchipping and other methods of identification involving a mutilation required by law are permitted.

Neck tagging and web notching

This may only be carried out on farmed ducks and only where performed within 36 hours of hatching for the purposes of a breed improvement programme.

Web tagging and wing tagging

These may only be carried out on farmed birds for the purposes of breed improvement programmes or testing for the presence of disease. When carried out in non-farmed birds, they may only be done for conservation purposes (including education and captive breeding programmes) or for research.

Castration, ovidectomy and vasectomy

These may not be carried out on farmed birds and may only be carried out as part of a conservation breeding programme and only under anaesthetic.

Implantation of a subcutaneous contraceptive

This may not be carried out on farmed birds and may only be carried out as part of a conservation breeding programme.

Beak trimming of poultry

Beak trimming (debeaking) is permitted as a preventive measure in laying birds (in establishments with 350 or more birds), and in response to feather pecking or cannibalism in broiler birds. It must not be carried out in birds over 10 days old and infrared technology must be used. Trimming may be carried out in laying birds over 10 days old and without infrared technology when it is required as an emergency measure to control an outbreak of feather pecking or cannibalism. It should be noted that this is not the same as trimming overgrown beaks, which is not the subject of current regulation. It is likely that future legislation will prohibit debeaking as a preventive measure in all fowl.

Desnooding

Where the turkey is aged not more than 21 days, the procedure may be carried out either by manual pinching-out or with a suitable instrument.

De-toeing of domestic fowl and turkeys

This procedure may not be carried out on a bird that is aged 3 days or over unless a veterinary surgeon considers that it is necessary that it be carried out. An anaesthetic must be administered where the bird is aged 3 days or over.

Dubbing

This procedure may not be carried out on a bird that is aged 3 days or over unless a veterinary surgeon considers that it is necessary that it be carried out. An anaesthetic must be administered where the bird is aged 3 days or over.

Laparoscopy

An anaesthetic must be administered.

Wing pinioning

This may not be carried out on farmed birds. An anaesthetic must be administered where the bird is aged 10 days or over.

Administration of medical treatment and performance of surgical procedures

The Veterinary Surgeons Act (1966) restricts the giving of medical treatment to and the performance of surgical procedures on animals to veterinary surgeons except for under certain circumstances. Schedule 3 of the act, The Veterinary Surgery (Exemptions) Order 2015, The Veterinary Surgery (Blood Sampling) Order 1983 (as amended) and The Veterinary Surgery (Wing and Web Tagging) Order 2009 exempt the following procedures in poultry from the requirement to be performed by a veterinary surgeon:

- Administration of medical treatment by the owner of the animal or by a person engaged or employed in caring for animals so used
- Emergency first aid treatment for the purpose of saving life or relieving pain or suffering
- Wing tagging
- Web tagging.

And by somebody 18 years of age or older:

- Administration of vaccines
- Blood sampling by a trained person
- In fowl, beak-trimming of not more than a one-third part of both its upper and lower beaks, or one-third of its upper beak only, measured from the tip towards the entrance to the nostrils, if the removal is carried out as

a single operation, and the arrest by cauterization of any subsequent haemorrhage from the beak. Laying hens are excluded from this exemption.
- Desnooding of a turkey poult before it has reached 21 days' old
- Removing of the comb and/or dependent party of the wattle of fowl before it has reached 72 hours old.

These procedures may only be performed using an instrument specifically designed or commonly used for the purpose, which is in a fit state of repair.

Feeding

The manufacture and sale of animal feeds are controlled by several regulations not covered in this text. The Food Standards Agency is responsible for regulation of animal feedstuffs.

The Animal By-Products (Enforcement) (England) Regulations 2013 prohibit the feeding of catering waste to farm animals. For the purpose of the regulations, catering waste includes any food that has originated from a household kitchen, and farm animals include any pet animals that belong to a farmed species such as poultry species. It is permitted to feed vegetable material originating from outside the kitchen, which has not entered the kitchen, and which has not come into contact with material of animal origin (e.g. plants grown in the garden). Birds must be excluded from any compost heap containing food waste.

Transportation

The Welfare of Animals (Transport) (England) Order 2006 SI 2006/3260 Art 4 makes it an offence to transport any animal in a way which causes, or is likely to cause, injury or unnecessary suffering to that animal. It requires that animals must be transported 'under conditions (in particular with regard to space, ventilation, temperature and security) and with such supply of liquid and oxygen, as are appropriate for the species concerned'. The order refers to Council Regulation (EC) No. 1/2005, which lays out numerous requirements that apply when vertebrate animals are transported as part of a commercial activity. Certain backyard poultry may be subject to other parts of the order and this council regulation (e.g. if they are selling their birds at a show) and in such cases the reader should refer to the Defra guidance on *Welfare of animals during transport* or seek further advice from the Animal and Plant Health Agency (APHA) (see 'Useful websites').

Poultry movements are not routinely subject to standstill periods in the UK.

Transport of Animals (Cleansing and Disinfection) (England) (No. 3) Order 2003 SI 2003/1724 specifies that transportation equipment must be cleansed and disinfected as soon as possible (within 24 hours at most) following transportation of poultry. The order does not apply when:

a. transport is not of a commercial nature
b. an individual animal is accompanied by a person having responsibility for the animal during transport
c. a pet animal accompanies their owner on a private journey.

The order does not define 'pet' or 'commercial nature'.

The sale of poultry meat and eggs

Under The Food Safety Act 1990 (as amended), live poultry are defined as a food source, and eggs and slaughtered poultry are defined as food. The act exists to ensure that food businesses take 'all reasonable precautions' to prevent food safety incidents and therefore applies where food is sold. The definition of 'sale' in the act is broad and may not involve the transfer of money (e.g. when the product is offered as a prize). Keepers of backyard poultry must consider whether they fall under this definition when they distribute eggs and/or meat from their poultry.

The General Food Regulations 2004 (as amended) state that:

a. Unsafe food must not be placed on the market
b. Consumers must not be misled
c. Food must be traceable
d. Businesses must act where food is found not to meet food safety requirements.

The body charged with developing policy and enforcing food safety legislation is the Food Standards Agency (FSA) established as a result of The Food Standards Act 1999.

Regulation (EC) 853/2004 (as amended) lays down specific hygiene rules for products of animal origin. However, poultry producers who slaughter less than 10,000 birds per annum on the farm and sell the meat directly to the final consumer or to local retail establishments directly supplying the final consumer are exempt from its scope. It is therefore acceptable for poultry meat to be sold 'over the farm gate' in small numbers without inspection so long as The General Food Regulations 2004 (as amended) are adhered to as well as the requirements of Schedule 5 to the Food Hygiene (England) Regulations 2013 (as amended). These require the producer to ensure that the meat bears a label or other marking clearly indicating the name and address of the farm where the bird from which it is derived was slaughtered. Additionally, the producer is required to keep a record in adequate form to show the number of birds received into, and the amounts of fresh meat dispatched from, his premises during each week. The producer must retain the record for a period of 1 year and make the record available to an authorized officer on request. Such producers are also exempt from The Poultrymeat (England) Regulations 2011, which regulate the sale of poultry meat under terms such as 'free range'.

If keepers of backyard poultry wish to consign birds to a slaughterhouse they must ensure that food chain information (FCI) as required by Regulation (EC) 853/2004 is provided to the slaughterhouse operator at least 24 hours in advance of the birds. The Food Standards Agency has produced a model form for FCI that can be used for poultry. This can be accessed via their website (see 'Useful websites').

The Animals and Animal Products (Examination for Residues and Maximum Residue Limits) Regulations 1997 as amended prohibit:

a. The sale of certain substances for administration to food producing animals
b. The possession of certain substances that might be administered to food-producing animals
c. The administration of certain substances (including all substances not listed in Table 1 of Commission Regulation EU (European Union) No. 37/2010 or those that are contained within Table 2) to food-producing animals

d. The possession or slaughter of animals to whom beta-agonists or hormonal substances have been administered
e. The sale, or supply for slaughter, for human consumption, of animals to which unauthorized substances have been administered, that contain substances above the maximum residue limit or where the withdrawal period has not expired (note that it is permitted to sell the animals for purposes other than slaughter so long as the buyer is informed that the animals are within the withdrawal period)
f. The sale of animal products derived from an animal if the sale or slaughter of the animal is prohibited under the condition above (e).

This act clearly has important implications for the use of veterinary medicines in poultry. A full discussion of this is given earlier in this chapter under 'the prescribing cascade'.

Poultry must be slaughtered in accordance with The Welfare of Animals (Slaughter or Killing) Regulations (as amended) and Council Regulation (EC) No. 1099/2009 (although the slaughter of poultry for private domestic consumption is not covered by the latter regulations). Avoidable excitement, pain and suffering during movement, lairage, restraint, stunning and killing must be prevented. Slaughtermen must be licensed. In the context of poultry, the licensing requirements do not apply to any person who:

- For emergency reasons relating to the welfare of any animal has to slaughter or kill that animal immediately
- Slaughters or kills any animal elsewhere than in a slaughterhouse or knacker's yard, provided that he is the owner of the animal and the slaughter or killing is for his private consumption
- Slaughters or kills any animal other than for a commercial purpose
- Kills by means of a free bullet any animal in the field
- Kills a bird by means of dislocation of the neck or decapitation on premises forming part of an agricultural holding on which the bird was reared
- Kills surplus chicks or embryos in hatchery waste in accordance with Schedule 11 of the regulations.

Egg producers are required to register with the local Egg Marketing Inspectorate (EMI: part of the APHA). Registration is required to ensure that welfare rules, The Eggs and Chicks Regulations and The Egg Marketing Standards Regulations 1995 (as amended) are complied with. Producers are exempt if they:

a. Have less than 350 birds and their eggs are only sold directly to the individual consumer at the farm gate or by door-to-door sales; or
b. Have less than 50 birds and their eggs are only sold directly to the individual consumer at the farm gate, by door-to-door sales or at local public markets.

It is quite possible that owners of birds falling within the scope of this manual will be subject to this requirement, for example if they sell some of their eggs to shops or restaurants. In such cases, the keeper should seek further guidance from Defra and the APHA.

Eggs from exempt producers are classed as ungraded. Under The Ungraded Eggs (Hygiene) Regulations 1990, eggs with cracks visible to the naked eye must not be sold. In other circumstances, eggs are graded as Class A or Class B. Class A eggs may be sold to consumers whereas Class B eggs must be treated and may only be made into egg products.

Under The Food Labelling Regulations 1996 SI 1996/1499 (as amended) any eggs sold at local public markets, even from producers not registered with the EMI, must include the following information:

- Name of the food
- The producer's name and address
- Best before date (maximum 28 days from lay)
- Advice to consumers to keep eggs chilled.

Notifiable diseases

The Animal Health Act 1981 (as amended) requires that any person with an animal suspected of being infected with a notifiable disease must isolate the animal and report the fact to a police constable or the veterinary authorities through the Defra Rural Services Helpline (telephone 03000 200 301) as soon as possible. Currently, the diseases affecting poultry that are notifiable in the UK are avian influenza and Newcastle disease. Equine viral encephalitis is also a notifiable disease that might be seen in poultry (see Chapter 18). Everybody present at the affected premises should remain on site and await instruction from the APHA duty veterinary surgeon.

Disposal of waste and carcasses

The disposal of waste and carcasses is covered by The Animal By-Products (Enforcement) (England) Regulations 2013. Animal by-products are categorized into three bands (this list is not exhaustive) (Figure 26.2):

Animal by-products must be disposed of in a prescribed manner by a licensed operator. Therefore, dead poultry may not be buried. There is a derogation allowing for the burial of pets. A pet is defined in this context as 'any animal belonging to species normally nourished and kept, but not consumed, by humans for purposes other than farming'. Therefore, this derogation does not apply to any poultry. The regulations state that fallen stock should be collected, identified and transported without 'undue delay'. Prior to disposal, animal by-products must be

stored so that animals and birds do not have access to it. A record must be kept of any stock sent for disposal. Most veterinary practices will have an arrangement for animal by-products to be collected by a licensed operator and this would be a route by which poultry owners could dispose of their dead birds. Keepers are not required to register to transport their own animals to a place of disposal, but carcasses must be transported in a suitable sealed container.

There is a derogation allowing for the burial of animal by-products resulting from surgical intervention on healthy animals.

Summary

Key points affecting veterinary surgeons:

- All poultry should be treated as food-producing animals for prescribing purposes
- Drugs must **not** be prescribed if:
  - They are prohibited in food producing animals
  - They are not included in Table 1 of EU regulation No. 37/2010
  - An appropriate withdrawal period cannot be determined.
- Drugs prescribed under the cascade require additional labelling and record keeping
- There is some ambiguity involving the correct interpretation of the prescribing cascade
- Medicated feedingstuffs containing a VMP or SFA and premixtures containing a VMP or SFA cannot be manufactured or supplied by establishments without inspection and appropriate approval by the VMD
- There is a derogation for the requirement to be a Category 8 distributor to supply premixtures or feedingstuffs containing a VMP if the supplier is a veterinary surgeon, a pharmacist or an SQP and only if the end user is a domestic keeper which means that birds, or meat or eggs from these birds, cannot be sold
- It is not permitted to devoice a cockerel unless it is for medical reasons
- 'Farmed birds' cannot be pinioned, castrated, ovidectomised or vasectomized unless it is for medical reasons
- Non-farmed birds may only castrated, ovidectomized or vasectomized as part of a conservation breeding programme
- Pinioning may only be carried out by a veterinary surgeon and an anaesthetic must be used if the bird is aged 10 days or over
- It is permitted, with restrictions, to debeak (beak trim), desnood, de-toe or dub a poultry bird
- Dead poultry carcasses and body parts may be disposed of as Category 2 animal by-product waste.

Key points affecting poultry owners:

- Owners of laying hens and pullets should read and adhere to the Code of Practice for the welfare of laying hens and pullets published by Defra
- Any poultry flock of 50 or more birds must be registered in the GB Poultry Register
- Attention must be paid to the environmental effects of keeping poultry

Category	Waste types (with reference to poultry)
1 (Highest risk)	Pet or zoo animal carcasses Wild animal carcasses expected of having zoonotic infection
2 (High risk)	Eggs which are contaminated with excessive VMP residues Carcasses of animals not killed for human consumption, including for disease control (fallen stock) Dead-in-shell poultry
3 (Low risk)	Eggs (including shells) Carcasses or body parts slaughtered and fit for human consumption but not intended for human consumption Animal by-products from poultry slaughtered on farm which do not show any signs of communicable disease Feathers from healthy live animals Day old chicks killed for commercial reasons

26.2 Categories of animal by-products.

- Withdrawal periods must be adhered to
- There is a derogation for the requirement to be an appropriately approved manufacturer to manufacture medicated feedingstuffs using a VMP or a premixture containing a VMP if the manufacturer is a domestic keeper
- Owners may only mix drugs into food themselves if they do not sell the treated birds or meat or eggs from them
- Unnecessary suffering must be prevented
- Reasonable steps must be taken to ensure that the birds' needs are met
- Kitchen scraps must not be fed to birds and birds must be excluded from compost heaps containing kitchen waste
- Small numbers of birds slaughtered on site may be sold over the farm gate without inspection, but general food regulations still apply
- Birds must be slaughtered humanely
- Eggs may only be sold without inspection if less than 350 birds are kept and the eggs are sold over the farm gate or door to door **or** less than 50 birds are kept and eggs are sold at local public markets
- It is illegal to sell eggs with cracked shells
- Eggs sold at markets require appropriate labelling
- Dead chickens must be disposed of as fallen stock by licensed operators.

References and further reading

Chitty J and Lierz M (2008) *BSAVA Manual of Raptors, Pigeons and Passerine Birds*. BSAVA Publications, Gloucester

Useful websites

Animal and Plant Health Agency
https://www.gov.uk/government/organisations/animal-and-plant-health-agency

Poultry: on-farm welfare codes of recommendations and guidance
https://www.gov.uk/government/publications/poultry-on-farm-welfare

Department for Environment, Food and Rural Affairs (Defra)
http://www.defra.gov.uk

Environment Agency
http://www.environment-agency.gov.uk

Food Standards Agency
http://www.food.gov.uk
- *Meat Industry Guide – Acceptance and Slaughter of Animals*
  https://www.food.gov.uk/sites/default/files/media/document/chapter11-acceptanceslaughter-animals-final-version-2_1.pdf

Legislation.gov.uk
http://www.legislation.gov.uk
- *The Cascade: Prescribing unauthorised medicines*
  https://www.gov.uk/guidance/the-cascade-prescribing-unauthorised-medicines
- *Welfare of animals during transport*
  https://www.gov.uk/government/publications/welfare-of-animals-during-transport

Royal College of Veterinary Surgeons
http://www.rcvs.org.uk

UK Local Authorities
https://www.gov.uk/find-your-local-council

Veterinary Medicines Directorate
http://www.vmd.defra.gov.uk

Problem-based approaches

Pale and anaemic hen

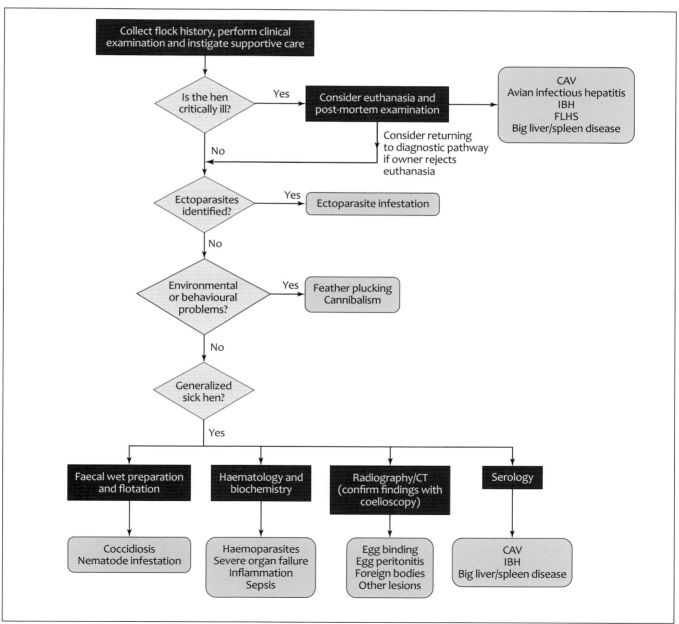

CAV = chicken anaemia virus; CT = computed tomography; FLHS = fatty liver haemorrhagic syndrome; IBH = inclusion body hepatitis.

Scouring bird

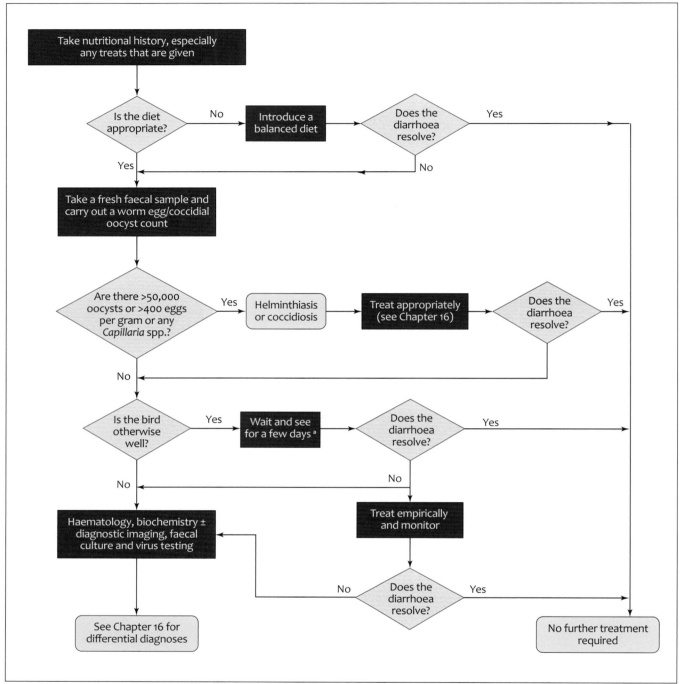

Take nutritional history, especially any treats that are given

↓

Is the diet appropriate? — No → Introduce a balanced diet → Does the diarrhoea resolve? — Yes →

Yes ↓ / No ↓

Take a fresh faecal sample and carry out a worm egg/coccidial oocyst count

↓

Are there >50,000 oocysts or >400 eggs per gram or any *Capillaria* spp.? — Yes → Helminthiasis or coccidiosis → Treat appropriately (see Chapter 16) → Does the diarrhoea resolve? — Yes →

No ↓

Is the bird otherwise well? — Yes → Wait and see for a few days [a] → Does the diarrhoea resolve? — Yes →

No ↓ / No ↓

Treat empirically and monitor

Haematology, biochemistry ± diagnostic imaging, faecal culture and virus testing

Does the diarrhoea resolve? — No → / — Yes →

See Chapter 16 for differential diagnoses

No further treatment required

[a] Free-ranging birds regularly have loose droppings that resolve spontaneously without treatment.

Inappetent bird

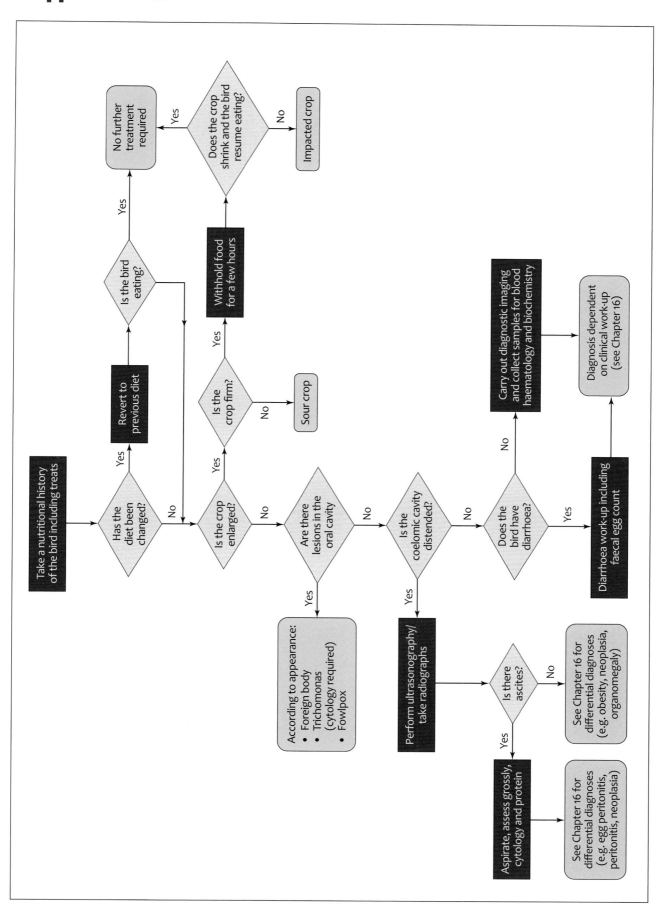

Off-lay hen

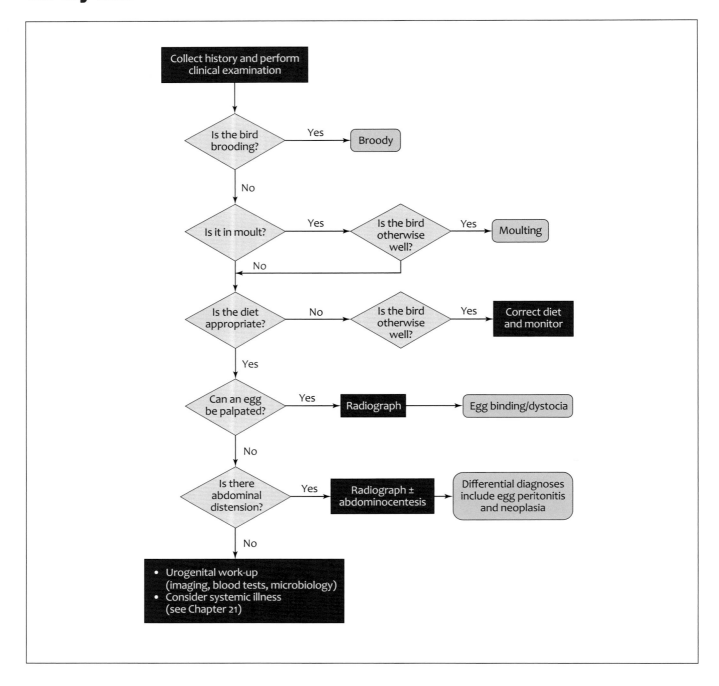

Ill thrifting or slow growing chicks

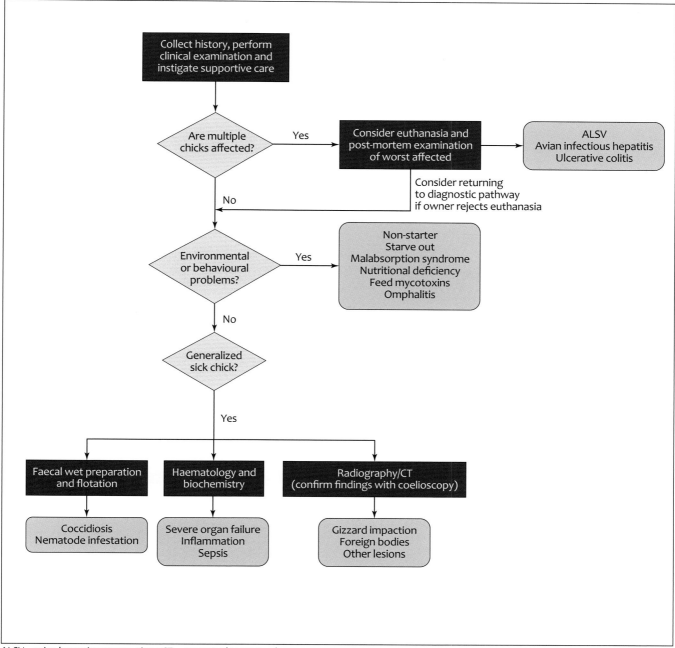

ALSV = avian leucosis sarcoma virus; CT = computed tomography.

Lame bird

Leg deformity

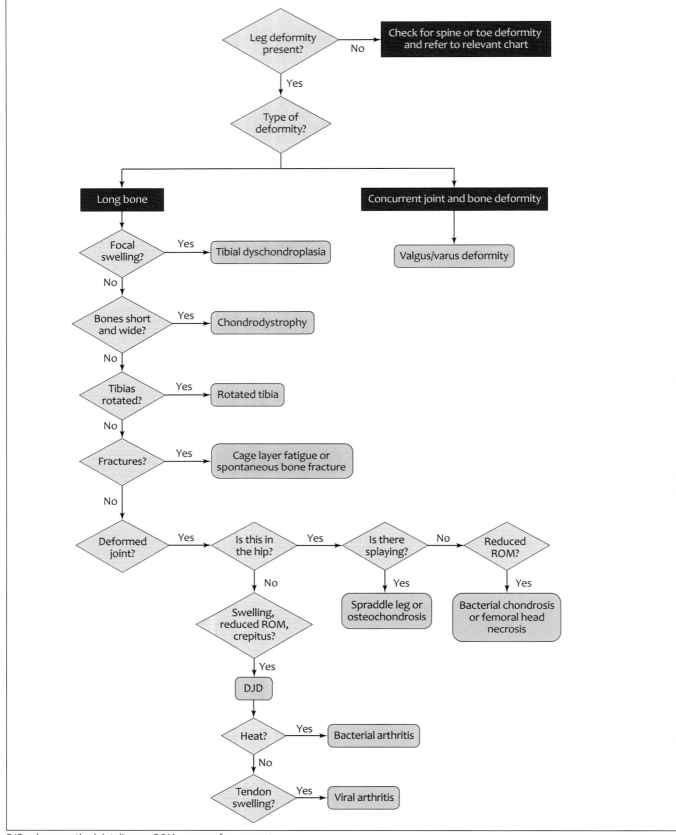

DJD = degenerative joint disease; ROM = range of movement.

Spinal deformity

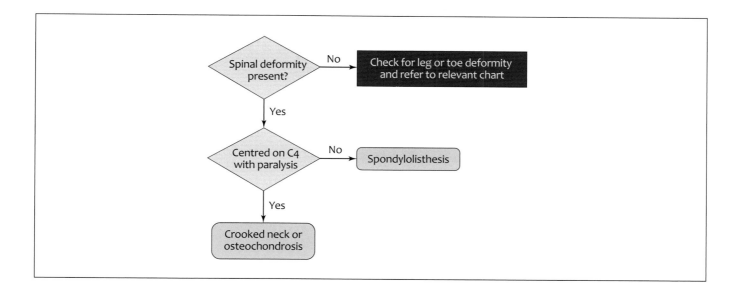

Toe deformity

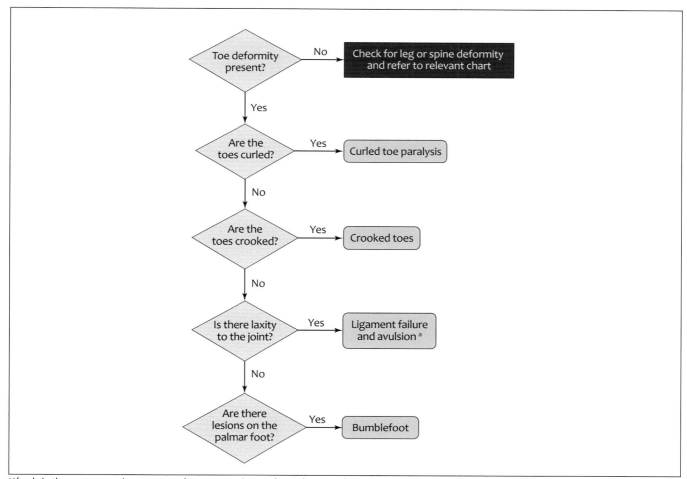

a If only in the gastrocnemius, a ruptured gastrocnemius tendon is diagnosed.

Neurological chicken

Tremors

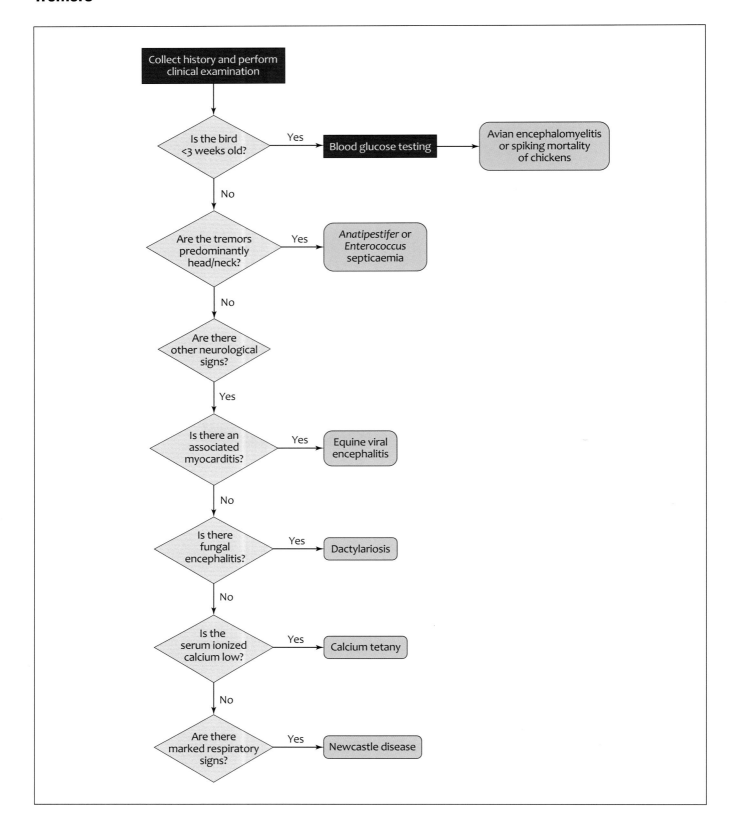

No tremors

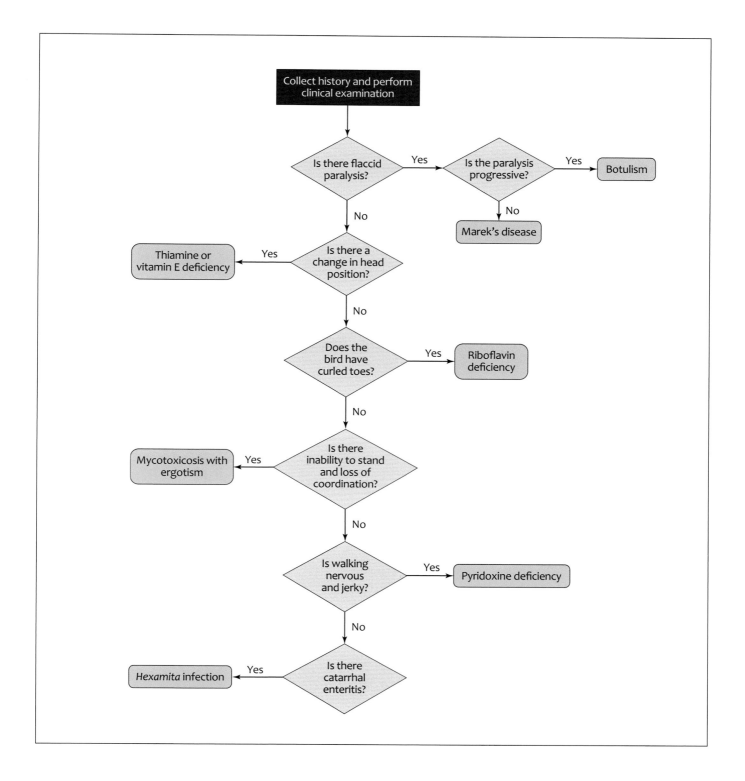

Treatment options for fractured bones

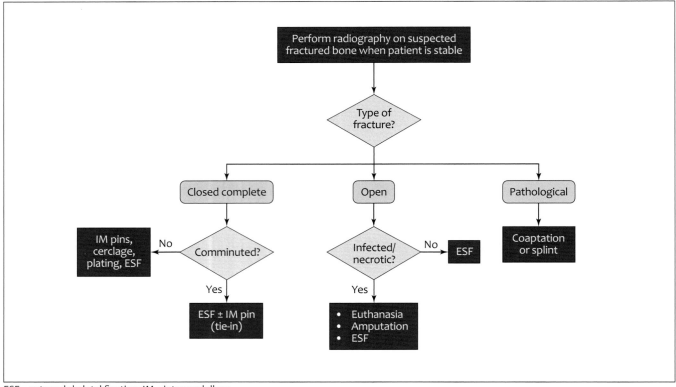

ESF = external skeletal fixation; IM = intramedullary.

Formulary

Guy Poland

Introduction

The following factors should determine drug selection:

- Efficacy
- Safety (for the patient)
- Interaction with other substances
- Residue in meat and eggs
- Likelihood of inducing drug resistance
- Safety (for the operator).

Additionally, preference should be given to drugs licensed for a particular indication. In the UK, a strict protocol for drug selection involving unlicensed preparations applies, known as the 'prescribing cascade' (see Chapter 26 for further guidance). Readers should be familiar with Commission Regulation EU (European Union) No. 37/2010 (also see Chapter 26), which is concerned with drug residues. In the UK, the statutory minimum withdrawal time for meat is 28 days and for eggs is 7 days.

This formulary lists the drugs that have been described for use in poultry in the earlier chapters of this book. They are listed alphabetically by therapeutic class. Both drugs licensed for use in poultry and unlicensed drugs are included. Reference to the product datasheet **must always** be made prior to using any drug and, unless it is clinically justified not to do so, the protocol described on the datasheet (also known as the label in the US) should be followed. Reference to licensed preparations and eligibility for use in poultry described is applicable in the UK only and practitioners elsewhere must familiarize themselves with local regulations. Although the formulary aims to be comprehensive, other preparations not described may be available. Some drugs are included in the formulary even though their use is not recommended; this is because it is important to state this when their use is likely to be considered by practitioners. Vaccines are not included here but are discussed in Chapter 7 and in disease accounts in other chapters.

Drugs

Anaesthesia-related drugs

Drug	Legal status (EU)*	Dose	Indications	Comments
Adrenaline [epinephrine]	Allowed substance (all species); no MRL required	0.5–1 mg/kg i.v., intratracheal	Cardiac resuscitation, treat anaphylactic shock and bronchial spasm	Cardiac route is not recommended
Aspirin [acetylsalicylic acid]	Allowed substance (all species); not for use in animals from which eggs are produced for human consumption	100–200 mg/kg i.m. once	Prevention of arterial thromboembolism; control of mild to moderate pain	Consider NSAIDs (e.g. meloxicam) for control of pain
Atipamezole	Not listed	2.5–5 times the dose of medetomidine or dexmedetomidine on an mg basis i.m. or s.c.	Reversal of sedation due to alpha-2 adrenoreceptor agonists such as medetomidine, dexmedetomidine and xylazine	Reversal of sedation may be sudden following i.v. route, so i.m. route may be preferred unless in the case of an emergency. Dose may be halved if given an hour or more after the administration of the alpha-2 adrenoreceptor agonist. Dose may be repeated in the case of slow recovery

Names in [ ] are alternative non-proprietary names or constituent ingredients. *Please refer to EU 2010/37; all species refers to all food-producing species. Reference to species other than poultry is made only when poultry is not explicitly listed. **Maximum residue limit (MRL) has been added or amended subsequent to the publication of EU 2010/37. NSAIDs = non-steroidal anti-inflammatory drugs. (continues)

Drug	Legal status (EU)*	Dose	Indications	Comments
Atropine	Allowed substance (all species); no MRL required	0.1–0.5 mg/kg i.m. or i.v. once	Prevention and correction of bradycardia and bradyarrhythmias; organophosphate poisoning	Ophthalmic use is ineffective in birds
Bupivacaine	Not listed	2 mg/kg s.c. infusion	Perineural nerve blocks, regional and epidural local anaesthesia	Do not administer intravenously. Do not use in combination with adrenaline where local vasoconstriction is undesirable
Buprenorphine	Not listed	0.01–0.05 mg/kg q8–12h i.m.	Management of mild to moderate perioperative pain; as a sedative or premedicant in combination with alpha-2 adrenoreceptor agonists or acepromazine	Not shown to be effective intra-articularly in chickens up to 1 mg/kg
Butorphanol	Allowed substance (Equidae)	0.2–0.4 mg/kg q12h i.m.	Management of mild perioperative pain; as a sedative or premedicant in combination with alpha-2 adrenoreceptor agonists or acepromazine	Dose evaluated in chickens: other species frequently require 0.5–2 mg/kg q4–6h
Diazepam	Not listed	0.5–1.0 mg/kg i.m., i.v.	Anticonvulsant, anxiolytic and skeletal muscle relaxant; short-term management of feather plucking; as a premedicant or sedation	Intramuscular administration may cause muscle irritation and delayed absorption
Doxapram	Allowed substance (all species); no MRL required	5–20 mg/kg i.v., i.m. or 1–3 drops on tongue	Stimulate respiration during and after anaesthesia	
Fentanyl	Not listed	**DO NOT USE**		
Halothane	Not listed	**DO NOT USE**		
Isoflurane	Allowed substance (Equidae, porcine); no MRL required**	Up to 5% for induction; 1.3–2.5% for maintenance	Induction and maintenance of general anaesthesia	Other anaesthetic agents and opioid analgesics will reduce the dose of isoflurane required. Not metabolized by the liver
Ketamine	Allowed substance (all species); no MRL required	20–40 mg/kg i.m.	Provision of chemical restraint or dissociative anaesthesia	Not for use alone due to insufficient analgesia, poor muscle relaxation and prolonged excitation on recovery for up to 3 hours: largely superseded by gaseous anaesthesia
Lidocaine [lignocaine]	Allowed substance (Equidae); no MRL required; for local-regional anaesthesia only	2–3 mg/kg as local infusion: may require dilution	Provision of local or regional analgesia using perineural, infiltration, local i.v. or epidural techniques	Narrow therapeutic index
Medetomidine	Not listed	0.25–0.34 mg/kg orally	For sedation or premedication use alone or in combination with opioids	Speed of onset 6–10 minutes
Midazolam	Not listed	0.1–2 mg/kg i.m., i.v.	For sedation and as part of a premedication regimen	
Morphine	Not listed	**NOT RECOMMENDED**		
Naloxone	Not listed	2 mg slow i.v. (total dose)	Reversal of the effects of opioid overdose	
Nitrous oxide	Not listed	Inspired concentrations of 50–70%	For use with oxygen as a carrier for volatile anaesthetic agents	
Propofol	Not listed	5–10 mg/kg by slow i.v. to effect for induction of anaesthesia; 0.5 mg/kg/min i.v. constant rate infusion for maintenance	Induction of anaesthesia (and maintenance by constant rate infusion)	Intubation and ventilation with oxygen recommended
Sevoflurane	Not listed	2.0–5.0% for maintenance. Higher concentrations required for induction	Induction and maintenance of general anaesthesia	Other anaesthetic agents and opioid analgesics will reduce the dose of sevoflurane required
Tramadol	Not listed	5–11 mg/kg q12h orally	Management of mild to moderate acute pain and as an adjuvant analgesic in the management of chronic pain	No data found in chickens

(continued) Names in [ ] are alternative non-proprietary names or constituent ingredients. *Please refer to EU 2010/37; all species refers to all food-producing species. Reference to species other than poultry is made only when poultry is not explicitly listed. **Maximum residue limit (MRL) has been added or amended subsequent to the publication of EU 2010/37. NSAIDs = non-steroidal anti-inflammatory drugs. (continues) ▶

Drug	Legal status (EU)*	Dose	Indications	Comments
Xylazine	Allowed substance (bovine, Equidae); no MRL required	See sedative combinations	Sedation or premedication alone or in combination with opioid analgesics. Some references advise do not use	
Yohimbine	Not listed	0.2–2mg/kg i.m.	Reversal of sedation due xylazine	Excitation and death have been reported in guinea fowl at doses over 1 mg/kg

(continued) Names in [ ] are alternative non-proprietary names or constituent ingredients. *Please refer to EU 2010/37; all species refers to all food-producing species. Reference to species other than poultry is made only when poultry is not explicitly listed. **Maximum residue limit (MRL) has been added or amended subsequent to the publication of EU 2010/37. NSAIDs = non-steroidal anti-inflammatory drugs.

Antifungal drugs

Drug	Legal status (EU)*	Dose	Indications	Comments
Itraconazole	Not listed	5–10 mg/kg orally q12–24h	Treatment of fungal infections including candidiasis and aspergillosis	Itraconazole has a narrow therapeutic index in birds
Miconazole	Not listed	Apply topically	Treatment of fungal skin infections	
Nystatin	Not listed	300,000 IU/kg orally q12–24h for 7–14 days	Treatment of fungal infections, particularly *Candida albicans*	Nystatin is not absorbed from the gastrointestinal tract
Voriconazole	Not listed	10 mg/kg orally, i.v. q12h	Treatment of fungal infections including aspergillosis	

*Please refer to EU 2010/37; all species refers to all food-producing species.

Anti-inflammatory drugs

Drug	Legal status (EU)*	Dose	Indications	Comments
Carprofen	Allowed substance (bovine, Equidae)	1–4 mg/kg i.m., s.c.; 40 mg/kg orally in feed	Control of postoperative pain and inflammation following surgery and reduction of chronic inflammation	Use with caution perioperatively and during renal dysfunction and do not use in birds with dehydration, hypervolaemia or hypotension. Lower doses have been effective for short periods. Dosing interval not clearly established. In feed dose required to achieve mammalian therapeutic plasma concentrations (8.3 µg/ml) but analgesia has been shown at lower plasma concentrations (0.28 µg/ml)
Flunixin	Allowed substance (bovine, porcine, Equidae)	1.1 mg/kg i.v.; 3 mg/kg i.m.		Intramuscular administration of flunixin meglumine in birds can result in tissue necrosis at the injection site. Potential nephrotoxicity has been reported in birds: consider alternatives
Ketoprofen	Allowed substance (bovine, porcine, Equidae)	2–12 mg/kg i.m.	Relief of acute pain and management of chronic pain	Not recommend for preoperative use. Rapid clearance at low dose, higher doses last for 12h in chickens. Other avian species have died using 5 mg/kg
Meloxicam	Allowed substance (bovine, caprine, porcine, rabbit, Equidae)	0.2–2 mg/kg q12–24h i.m., orally	Control of postoperative pain and inflammation following surgery and reduction of acute and chronic musculoskeletal pain and inflammation	Use with caution in birds with renal disease. Do not use in birds with dehydration, hypotension, hypovolaemia, gastrointestinal disease or blood clotting disorders. Souza *et al.* (2018) discuss drug residues in eggs following the administration of meloxicam to chickens

*Please refer to EU 2010/37; all species refers to all food-producing species. Reference to species other than poultry is made only when poultry is not explicitly listed.

Antimicrobial drugs

Drug	Legal status (EU)*	Dose	Indications	Comments
Amoxicillin (**Amatib; Amoxinsol; Solamocta; Stabox; Vetremox**)	Allowed substance (all species); not for use in animals from which eggs are produced for human consumption	Follow label of approved preparation, orally via water or feed	Treatment of beta-lactam sensitive bacterial infections	Time-dependent bactericidal action. Morbid animals may have a decreased water and or food intake, which may lead to unreliable dosing when added to water or food
Apramycin (**Apravet**)	Allowed substance (chicken); MRL not required; not for use in animals from which eggs are produced for human consumption	Follow label of approved preparation, orally via drinking water	Treatment of colibacillosis caused by *Escherichia coli* susceptible to apramycin	

Names in [ ] are alternative non-proprietary names or constituent ingredients. Names in ( ) are commercial formulations. Those in bold are approved in poultry species in the UK at the time of writing. *Please refer to EU 2010/37; all species refers to all food-producing species. Reference to species other than poultry is made only when poultry is not explicitly listed. ** Maximum residue limit (MRL) has been added or amended subsequent to the publication of EU 2010/37. (continues)

▶

Drug	Legal status (EU)*	Dose	Indications	Comments
Azithromycin	Not listed	40 mg/kg q24h for 15 days (owl reference)	Infections caused by Gram-positive and some Gram-negative bacterial, mycobacterial, and obligate anaerobic bacterial infections. Useful in respiratory, soft tissue and non-tubercular mycobacterial diseases, and chlamydophilosis	Doses are empirical and subject to change as experience with the drug is gained
Bacitracin, zinc	Bacitracin: allowed substance (bovine, rabbit)	Follow label if an approved formulation exists in feed	Topical treatment of bacterial infections.	Use as a growth promoter is not permitted in the EU
Chlortetracycline (**Aurofac; Chlorsol**)	Allowed substance (all species)	Follow label of approved preparation, orally via drinking water or feed	Treatment and control of respiratory and systemic infections associated with organisms sensitive to chlortetracycline	
Co-amoxiclav	Amoxicillin: allowed substance (all species); not or use in animals from which eggs are produced for human consumption Clavulanic acid: Allowed substance (bovine, porcine)	125 mg/kg orally q8h	Treatment of infections due to Gram-positive and Gram-negative aerobic bacteria and many obligate anaerobes	Bactericidal
Colistin (**Coliplus**)	Allowed substance (all species)	Follow label of approved preparation, orally via drinking water	Treatment and metaphylaxis of gastrointestinal infections caused by non-invasive *Escherichia coli* susceptible to colistin	Colistin possesses virtually no activity against Gram-positive bacteria and fungi. Colistin is poorly absorbed from the gastrointestinal tract. In contrast to very low concentration of colistin in serum and tissues, high and persistent amounts are present within the different sections of the gastrointestinal tract
Doxycycline	Allowed substance (all species); not for use in animals from which eggs are produced for human consumption**	Follow label of approved preparation, orally via drinking water	Treatment of infections due to susceptible bacteria including *Mycoplasma* and *Chlamydophila*, and rickettsial infections. Injection is very irritant to birds	Bacteriostatic
Enrofloxacin (**Baytril; Enroxil; Lanflox; Spectron**)	Allowed substance (poultry); not for use in animals from which eggs are produced for human consumption	Follow label of approved preparation, orally via drinking water	Treatment of susceptible bacteria. Active against *Mycoplasma* and many Gram-positive and Gram-negative bacteria. Relatively ineffective against obligate anaerobes	Where possible, should be reserved for second line treatment and in response to culture and sensitivity. The intramuscular formulation has an extremely alkaline pH so repeat injection by this route should be avoided. Prohibited drug in USA. Cornejo *et al.* (2012), Gorla *et al.* (1997), Lolo *et al.* (2005) and others describe drug residues in the eggs of laying hens following the administration of enrofloxacin
Erythromycin	Allowed substance (all species)	30 mg/kg for 4–5 days in drinking water	Treatment of infections due to susceptible bacteria. It is active against Gram-positive cocci (there are some resistant staphylococcal species), Gram-positive bacilli and some Gram-negative bacilli. It is also active against some strains of *Actinomyces*, *Nocardia*, *Chlamydophila* and *Rickettsia*	May be bactericidal or bacteriostatic. Approved formulation no longer available in the UK
Furaltadone	**Prohibited from use in food-producing animals**	Prohibited		

(continued) Names in [ ] are alternative non-proprietary names or constituent ingredients. Names in ( ) are commercial formulations. Those in bold are approved in poultry species in the UK at the time of writing. *Please refer to EU 2010/37; all species refers to all food-producing species. Reference to species other than poultry is made only when poultry is not explicitly listed. ** Maximum residue limit (MRL) has been added or amended subsequent to the publication of EU 2010/37. (continues) ▶

Drug	Legal status (EU)*	Dose	Indications	Comments
Lincomycin-spectinomycin (**Linco-Spectin**)	Lincomycin: Allowed substance (all species) Spectinomycin: Allowed substance (all species); not for use in animals from which eggs are produced for human consumption	Follow label of approved preparation, orally via drinking water	Treatment of chronic respiratory disease due *Mycoplasma gallisepticum* and *Escherichia coli*	
Metronidazole	**Prohibited from use in food producing animals**	**DO NOT USE**	Treatment of anaerobic infections, giardiasis and other protozol infections	
Monensin (**Coxidin**; **Elancoban**)	Allowed substance (bovine)	Follow label of approved preparation, orally via feed	For the prevention of coccidiosis	Do not give to guinea fowl: ingestion of monensin by guinea fowl can be fatal
Paramomycin [aminosidine]	Allowed substance (all species); not or use in animals from which eggs are produced for human consumption	No dose found	Prevention of histomoniasis	
Penicillin G [benzylpenicillin]	Benzylpenicillin: allowed substance (all species); not for use in animals from which eggs are produced for human consumption	No useful dose found	Treatment of infections susceptible to penicillin such as *Streptococcus* and *Clostridium*	
Phenoxymethyl penicillin (**Phenocillin**)	Allowed substance (poultry)	Follow label of approved preparation, orally via drinking water	Treatment and metaphylaxis of nectrotic enteritis caused by *Clostridium perfringens*	
Sulfadiazine [sulphadiazine], Trimethoprim (**Trimediazine**)	Sulfadiazine as sulfonamides: allowed substance (all species); not for use in animals from which eggs are produced for human consumption; Trimethoprim: allowed substance (all species); not for use in animals from which eggs are produced for human consumption	Follow label of approved preparation, orally via feed	For use in the treatment of diseases caused by bacteria sensitive to potentiated sulphonamides including *Salmonella* infection and pasteurellosis	
Tiamulin (**Denagard; Tialin; Vetmulin**)	Allowed substance (chicken, turkey)	Follow label of approved preparation, orally via drinking water	Treatment and prevention of mycoplasmosis	
Tilmicosin (**Pulmotil; Tilmovet**)	Allowed substance (poultry); not for use in animals from which eggs are produced for human consumption	Follow label of approved preparation, orally via drinking water	Treatment and prevention of mycoplasmosis	
Tylosin (**Pharmasin; Tylan**)	Allowed substance (all species)	Follow label of approved preparation, orally via drinking water	Treatment and prevention of mycoplasmosis. Treatment and prevention of necrotic enteritis caused by *Clostridium perfringens*	
Tylvalosin (**Aivlosin**)	Allowed substance (poultry); not for use in animals from which eggs are produced for human consumption	Follow label of approved preparation, orally via drinking water	Treatment and prevention of mycoplasmosis in chickens and *Ornithobacterium rhinotracheale* in turkeys	

(continued) Names in [ ] are alternative non-proprietary names or constituent ingredients. Names in ( ) are commercial formulations. Those in bold are approved in poultry species in the UK at the time of writing. *Please refer to EU 2010/37; all species refers to all food-producing species. Reference to species other than poultry is made only when poultry is not explicitly listed. ** Maximum residue limit (MRL) has been added or amended subsequent to the publication of EU 2010/37.

Topical antiseptic drugs

Drug	Legal status (EU)*	Dose	Indications	Comments
F10 [cypermethrin; benzalkonium chloride and polyhexanide]	Cypermethrin: Allowed substance (all ruminants, Salmonidae) Benzalkonium chloride: Allowed substance (all species) Polyhexanide: Not listed	Follow label	As a topical anti-septic and as an ectoparasitic agent and fly repellent	Manufacturer's note: do not use in animals for human consumption
Silver sulfadiazine (Flamazine)	Not listed	Use topically	Topical antibacterial and antifungal particularly active against Gram-negative organisms	

Names in [ ] are alternative non-proprietary names or constituent ingredients. Names in ( ) are commercial formulations. *Please refer to EU 2010/37; all species refers to all food-producing species. Reference to species other than poultry is made only when poultry is not explicitly listed.

Antiparasitic drugs

Drug	Legal status (EU)*	Dose	Indications	Comments
Amprolium (Coxoid)	Allowed substance (poultry); no MRL required; for oral use only	Follow label of approved preparation, orally via water or feed	For the treatment of intestinal coccidiosis caused by Eimeria spp. susceptible to amprolium	Coccidiostatic. Consider using other approved coccidiostat
Fenbendazole (Gallifen; Panacur; AquaSol)	Allowed substance (poultry)**	Follow label of approved preparation, orally via drinking water or feed	Treatment of gastrointestinal nematodes in chickens infected with Heterakis gallinarum or Ascaridia galli	Approved doses are not appropriate for the treatment of infections due to Capillaria spp.
Fipronil	Not listed	DO NOT USE	Control of fleas, ticks and lice	Fipronil is highly lipid bound, so may persist in tissues for prolonged periods (Stafford et al., 2018). Fipronil has a potential use in treating ornamental pheasants
Flubendazole (Flimabo; Flubenvet)	Allowed substance (poultry)	Follow label of approved preparation, orally via drinking water or feed	Treatment of nematode related disease including Ascaridia galli, Heterakis gallinarum and Capillaria spp.	
Ivermectin	Allowed substance (all mammalian species)	0.2 mg/kg orally, s.c., i.m. once; can be repeated after 10–14 days	Prevention and treatment of internal and external parasites	
Lasalocid (Avatec)	Allowed substance (poultry)	Follow label of approved preparation orally in feed	To aid the prevention of coccidiosis	
Melarsomine	Not listed	0.25 mg/kg i.m. q24h for 4 days	Anthelmintic	Approved for heartworm treatment in dogs
Praziquantel	Allowed substance (Equidae, ovine): no MRL required	5–10 mg/kg: recommended dosing intervals vary from once (± repeat in 7–10 days) to once daily for 14 days	Treatment of infections due to trematodes and cestodes	
Pyrethrum powders	Pyrethrum extract: Allowed substance (all food producing animals); no MRL required; for topical use only	Follow manufacturer's instructions		
Pyrimethamine	Not listed	0.25–0.5 mg/kg orally q12h for 4–30 days	Treatment of atoxoplasmosis, sarcocystosis and leucocytozoonosis	
Salinomycin (Sacox)	Not listed; salinomycin is, however, approved for using in broilers and chickens being reared for laying	Follow label of approved preparation, orally via feed	As a coccidiostat	
Sulfadimethoxine	As sulfonamides: allowed substance (all species); not for use in animals from which eggs are produced for human consumption	2 g/l drinking water for 5 days	Treatment and control of coccidiosis	Available in UK only as Coxi Plus for racing pigeons. Dose presented is label dose in that species: consider alternative
Toltrazuril (Baycox)	Allowed substance (poultry); not for use in animals from which eggs are produced for human consumption	Follow label of approved preparation, orally via drinking water	Treatment of coccidiosis	2.5% solution is very alkaline: do not gavage

Names in ( ) are commercial formulations. Those in bold are approved in poultry species in the UK at the time of writing. *Please refer to EU 2010/37; all species refers to all food-producing species. Reference to species other than poultry is made only when poultry is not explicitly listed. **Maximum residue limit (MRL) has been added or amended subsequent to the publication of EU 2010/37.

Supportive drugs

Drug	Legal status (EU)*	Dose	Indications	Comments
Aniseed based electrolyte solutions (Anisi aetheroleum)	Allowed substance (all species); no MRL required	Follow manufacturer's instructions		Supportive treatment
Calcium borogluconate/ calcium gluconate	Allowed substance (all species); no MRL required	50–100 mg/kg i.m., s.c. gluconate	Management of hypocalcaemia and hyperkalaemic cardiotoxicity associated with urinary obstruction; hyopcalcaemic tetany and seizures; medical treatment of egg binding	Rapid administration may cause hypotension, cardiac arrhythmias and cardiac arrest. Use with caution in dehydrated birds
Dextrose [glucose]	Not listed	50–100 mg/kg slow i.v.	Treatment of hypoglycaemic seizures	
Duphalyte [dexpanthenol, nicotinamide, potassium chloride, pyridoxine hydrochloride, riboflavin sodium phosphate and thiamine hydrochloride]	Not listed, but product approved in cattle and pigs with zero withdrawal	Up to 10 ml/kg/day slow i.v.	Supportive nutrition in birds unable to receive enteral nutrition	
Hartmann's solution [sodium lactate, sodium chloride, potassium chloride, calcium chloride]	Sodium lactate: Not listed Sodium chloride: Allowed substance (all species); no MRL required Potassium chloride: not listed Calcium chloride: : Allowed substance (all species); no MRL required Product approved in cattle with zero withdrawal			
Oregano	Not listed	Follow manufacturer's instructions, orally in drinking water or feed		Promotes gut health
Solulyte	Nutritional supplement		Rehydration and energy support	

Names in [ ] are alternative non-proprietary names or constituent ingredients. Names in ( ) are commercial formulations. *Please refer to EU 2010/37; all species refers to all food-producing species. Reference to species other than poultry is made only when poultry is not explicitly listed.

Steroid drugs

Drug	Legal status (EU)*	Dose	Indications	Comments
Dexamethasone	Allowed substance (bovine, caprine, porcine, Equidae)	2–4 mg/ kg i.m.	Anti-inflammatory	Use of even low doses of dexamethasone in birds is associated with a high risk of immunosuppression and other effects such as diabetes mellitus like syndrome
Methylprednisolone	Allowed substance (bovine, Equidae)**	2–4 mg/ kg i.m.	Treatment of shock, endotoxaemia and spinal compression.	May cause profound immunosuppression

*Please refer to EU 2010/37; all species refers to all food-producing species. Reference to species other than poultry is made only when poultry is not explicitly listed. ** Maximum residue limit (MRL) has been added or amended subsequent to the publication of EU 2010/37.

Radiographic contrast agents

Drug	Legal status (EU)*	Dose	Indications	Comments
Barium sulphate	Not listed	20 mg/kg of a 25–45% suspension orally	As a radiographic contrast agent during gastrointestinal studies	Do not use in dehydrated birds. Do not use if there is a risk of gastrointestinal perforation. Can also be used for retrograde examination of the cloaca and rectum
Iohexol	Not listed	10 mg/kg body weight of a 250 mg iodine/ml solution for retrograde gastrointestinal studies; 2 mg/kg slow i.v. of a 300–400 mg iodine/ml solution for urographical examinations; 0.1–1 ml of a 200–250 mg iodine/ml solution directly into the paranasal sinus	As a radiographic contrast agent during retrograde gastrointestinal studies; urography; sinography. Please refer to Chapter 11	Do not use in dehydrated birds. The use of lower concentration solutions for urography will render the examination non-diagnostic
Iopamidol	Not listed	10 mg/kg body weight of a 250 mg iodine/ml solution for retrograde gastrointestinal studies; 2 mg/kg slow i.v. of a 300–400 mg iodine/ml solution for urographical examinations; 2–4 mg/kg slow i.v. of a 370 mg iodine/ml for angiography; 0.1–1 ml of a 200–250 mg iodine/ml solution directly into the paranasal sinus	As a radiographic contrast agent during retrograde gastrointestinal studies; urography; angiography; sinography. Please refer to Chapter 11	Do not use in dehydrated birds. The use of lower concentration solutions for urography will render the examination non-diagnostic

*Please refer to EU 2010/37; all species refers to all food-producing species. Reference to species other than poultry is made only when poultry is not explicitly listed.

Miscellaneous drugs

Drug	Legal status (EU)*	Dose	Indications	Comments
Deslorelin (Suprelorin)	Allowed substance (Equidae); no MRL required	4.6 mg s.c. implant	May be useful in the treatment of egg peritonitis; prior to surgery of the reproductive tract	
Vitamin K	Not listed	0.2–2.5 mg/kg i.m., orally q6–12h until stable, then q24h	For the treatment of poisoning due to cumarin and derivative rodenticides	Use a narrow gauge needle to minimise the risk of haemorrhage
(Intrasite)	Not listed	Apply topically to wounds	Management of wounds	
Allopurinol	Not listed	10 mg/kg orally q24h	Treatment of the clinical signs of hyperuricaemia and articular gout	Doses of 50 mg/kg and 100 mg/kg have been reported as toxic and causing renal failure in red-tailed hawks

Names in ( ) are commercial formulations. *Please refer to EU 2010/37; all species refers to all food-producing species. Reference to species other than poultry is made only when poultry is not explicitly listed.

Drugs with egg maximum residue limit set

Drug	Egg maximum residue limit (MRL) (µg/kg)
Chlortetracycline	200
Colistin	300
Erythromycin	150
Fenbendazole	1300
Flubendazole*	400
Fluralaner*	1300
Lasalocid	150
Lincomycin	50
Neomycin	500
Oxytetracycline	200
Phoxim	60
Phenoxymethylpenicillin*	25
Piperazine	2000
Tetracycline	200
Tiamulin	1000
Tylosin	200
Tylvalosin*	200

*Added or amended subsequent to the publication of EU No 37/2010.

Prohibited substances

The following substances must **not** be used in food producing animals in the EU:

- *Aristolochia* spp. and preparations thereof
- Chloramphenicol
- Chloroform
- Chlorpromazine
- Colchicine
- Dapsone
- Dimetridazole
- Metronidazole
- Nitrofurans (including furazolidone)
- Ronidazole.

References and further reading

Carpenter JW and Marion CJ (2018) *Exotic Animal Formulary, 5th edn*. Elsevier Saunders, Philadelphia

Cornejo J, Lapierre L, Iragüen D *et al.* (2012) Study of enrofloxacin and flumequine residues depletion in eggs of laying hens after oral administration. *Journal of Veterinary Pharmacology and Therapy* 35, 67–72

Gorla N, Chiostri E, Ugnia L *et al.* (1997) HPLC residues of enrofloxacin and ciprofloxacin in eggs of laying hens. *International Journal of Antimicrobial Agents* 8, 253–256

Lolo M, Pedreira S, Fente C *et al.* (2005) Study of enrofloxacin depletion in the eggs of laying hens using diphasic dialysis extraction/purification and determinative HPLC-MS analysis. *Journal of Agriculture and Food Chemistry* 20, 2849–2852

Meredith A (2015) *BSAVA Small Animal Formulary, 9th edn – Part B: Exotic Pets*. BSAVA Publications, Gloucester

Souza MJ, Bailey J, White M *et al.* (2018) Pharmacokinetics and egg residues of meloxicam after multiple day oral dosing in domestic chickens. *Journal of Avian Medicine and Surgery* 32, 8–12

Stafford EG, Tell LA, Lin Z *et al.* (2018) Consequences of fipronil exposure in egg-laying hens. *Journal of the American Veterinary Medical Association* 253, 57–60

Useful websites

Australian Pesticides and Veterinary Medicines Authority
https://apvma.gov.au

Commission Regulation (EU) No. 37/2010
https://eur-lex.europa.eu/legal-content/EN/TXT/?uri=celex%3A32010R0037

European Medicines Agency (EMA)
https://www.ema.europa.eu/en

National Office of Animal Health (NOAH) Compendium
http://www.noahcompendium.co.uk/

Preventing Illegal Antibiotic Residues in Beef Products
https://animalagriculture.org/Resources/Documents/1.%20Main%20documents/Antibiotic_Residue_Fact_Sheet_ARMS_072115-07.pdf

Responsible Use of Medicines in Agriculture (RUMA)
https://www.ruma.org.uk

US Food & Drug Administration (FDA)
https://www.fda.gov/animal-veterinary
- Extralabel Use and Antimicrobials
  https://www.fda.gov/animal-veterinary/antimicrobial-resistance/extralabel-use-and-antimicrobials

Veterinary Medicines Directorate
https://www.gov.uk/government/organisations/veterinary-medicines-directorate

Sedative combinations

Drug	Dose	Route	Indications
Ketamine + diazepam	K: 75 mg/kg + D: 2.5 mg/kg	i.m., i.v.	Protocols used where diazepam is given i.v. either 5 min before or 10 min after the ketamine is given i.m. Recovery in 90–100 mins
Ketamine + medetomidine	K: 3–10 mg/kg + M: 0.1–0.2 mg/kg	i.m.	Short-term anaesthesia, can be antagonized
Ketamine + xylazine	K: 10–25 mg/kg + X: 1–2 mg/kg	i.m., i.v.	Recumbency within 6 mins, good surgical anaesthesia, can be antagonized. Can be improved by adding 0.3 mg/kg midazolam

Veterinary acupuncture points

Christine Eckerman-Ross

Introduction

This appendix is designed to aid practitioners who have already trained in veterinary acupuncture but who would like further information about the use of acupuncture in avian patients. One of the benefits of using acupuncture in poultry is that conditions can be treated, where appropriate, without consideration for drug withdrawal periods.

Whilst acupuncture can be a very rewarding addition to avian practice, there are special considerations to address before beginning this therapy. It is important that a thorough clinical examination is carried out in avian patients prior to acupuncture to ensure that the bird is healthy enough to cope with the stress that handling during acupuncture might cause. This is particularly important in birds as they often hide signs of illness until they are extremely compromised.

It is also important to consider the numerous anatomical and physiological variations of birds including vertebral formula, fusion of skeletal elements and pneumatized bones, thick skin and scales on the legs and feet, common outflow for gastrointestinal, urinary and reproductive tract (cloaca), air sacs, superficial location of structures and thin skin. The practitioner is strongly encouraged to consult references and become familiar with these variations before attempting acupuncture (O'Malley, 2005; Ness, 2006).

Dry needle acupuncture, with or without needle retention, is commonly employed. In birds that do not tolerate dry needling, aquapuncture is very commonly used. Special attention needs to be given to anatomy, depth of needle insertion, length of time for the overall treatment, and volume of solution used for aquapuncture. Electroacupuncture and moxa are not commonly used in avian patients due to their generally *Yang* nature. The smoke from burning moxa may also be irritating to birds' respiratory tracts. Laser and LACER (low energy photon therapy) are also frequently employed. The advantage of these techniques is increased safety in areas of thin skin such as over the abdomen, or where structures are superficially located, as on the extremities. Disadvantages include the length of time and restraint needed to complete the treatment, and the potential for stimulating several points at once due to probe size (Partington, 1992; West, 2011ab).

Acupuncture points used in birds (Figures A3.1, A3.2 and A3.3) include traditional points with mammalian counterparts, avian-specific points, and points transposed from mammals and not found in the Chinese literature. Some of the more commonly employed points are described in Figure A3.4 below. Figure A3.5 presents the avian *Shu* points, and a brief discussion of avian conditions that respond well to acupuncture is included in Figure A3.6.

Acknowledgements

The author thanks Chang Wei-Tang and Wang Teng-Wei for translating texts published in Chinese.

References and further reading

Eckermann-Ross C (2011) TCVM approaches to feather damaging behavior in pet and aviary birds. *Application of Traditional Chinese Veterinary Medicine in Exotic Animals: Proceedings of the 13th Annual International TCVM Conference*, ed. H Xie and L Trevisanello, pp. 139–149. Jing Tang Publishing, Reddick

Ferguson B (2002) Basic avian acupuncture. *Exotic DVM* **4**, 31–33

McCluggage M (2001) Acupuncture for the avian patient. In: *Veterinary Acupuncture – Ancient Art to Modern Medicine, 2nd edn*, ed. AM Schoen, pp. 307–332. Mosby, Inc., St Louis

Ness RD (2006) Integrative therapies. In: *Clinical Avian Medicine Volume 1*, ed. GJ Harrison and TL Lightfoot, pp. 344–348. Spix Publishing Inc., Palm Beach

O'Malley B (2005) Clinical anatomy and physiology of exotic species. In: *Structure and Function of Mammals, Birds, Reptiles and Amphibians*, pp. 97–112. Elsevier, Toronto

Partington M (1992) Avian acupuncture. *Problems in Veterinary Medicine* **4**, 212–222

West C (2011a) TCVM for avian species: Introduction, general overview, acupuncture point locations, indications and techniques. In: *Application of Traditional Chinese Veterinary Medicine in Exotic Animals: Proceedings of the 13th Annual International TCVM Conference*, ed. H Xie and L Trevisanello, pp. 53–72. Jing Tang Publishing, Reddick

West C (2011b) TCVM for avian species: Introduction to syndromes, case examples and conclusion. In: *Application of Traditional Chinese Veterinary Medicine in Exotic Animals: Proceedings of the 13th Annual International TCVM Conference*, ed. H Xie and L Trevisanello, pp. 87–138. Jing Tang Publishing, Reddick

Yu C (1995) *Traditional Chinese Veterinary Acupuncture and Moxibustion*. China Agricultural Press, Beijing

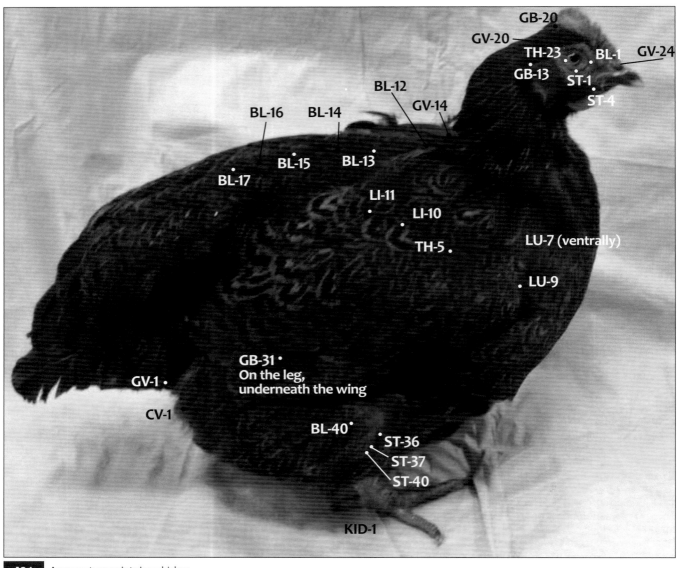

A3.1　Acupuncture points in a chicken.

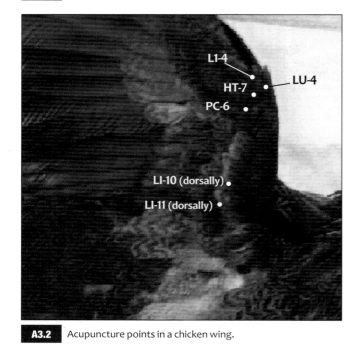

A3.2　Acupuncture points in a chicken wing.

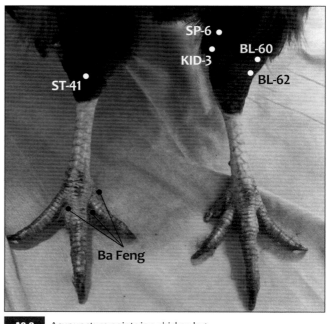

A3.3　Acupuncture points in a chicken leg.

Acupuncture point	Location	Indications
LU-7 (*Lie-que*, Broken Sequence)	On the ventrum of the wing, on cranial margin of distal radius, proximal to tuberculum aponeurosis	Respiratory problems, sinusitis, neck problems, grooming abnormalities, chronic diarrhoea, local point
LU-9 (*Tai yuan*, Greater Abyss)	On dorsal surface of wing proximal to the alula, in the depression in the alular-carpometacarpal joint	Clear phlegm, chronic respiratory diseases
LI-10 (*Shou san li*, Arm 3 Miles)	On the dorsum of the wing, 1/6 of the distance between the humero-radial joint and the alular-carpometacarpal joint, at the anteriolateral edge of the radius, between the bellies of the extensor carpi radialis and the supinator muscles	Weakness of wings, general weakness, diarrhoea
LI-11 (*Qu chi*, Crooked Pond)	On the dorsal surface of the wing in the angle formed by the humerus and radius, immediately caudal to the cranial margin of the brachialis muscle	Bi syndrome, trauma, weakness, aggression, diarrhoea, to relieve heat, to benefit immune function, local point
ST-36 (*Zu san li*, 3 Miles of the Foot)	Lateral to the tibiotarsal crest, in the belly of the cranial tibial muscle	Crop stasis, regurgitation, general debilitation, diarrhoea, Bi syndrome, grooming abnormalities
ST-37 (*Shang ju xu*, Upper Great Emptiness)	On the craniolateral aspect of the tibiotarsus, 1/3 of the way between the stifle and the lateral condyle of the tibiotarsus, in the cranial tibial muscle	Diarrhoea, general infection, to drain damp, to tonify the blood
ST-40 (*Feng long*, Abundant Bulge)	On the craniolateral aspect of the tibiotarsus, ½ way between the stifle and the lateral epicondyle	Respiratory problems, aggression, grooming abnormalities
SP-6 (*San yin jiao*, Three Yin Crossing)	At the caudal border of the tibiotarsus, cranial to the medial epicondyle, ¼ of the way from the epicondyle to the stifle.	Egg binding, infertility, cloacal prolapse, behavioural problems and grooming abnormalities, general infections
SP-9 (*Yin ling quan*, Yin Mound Spring)	On the caudal margin of the mid-tibiotarsus, immediately distal to the head of the fibula	Diarrhoea
HT-7 (*Shen men*, Mind Door)	On the ventrum of the wing, immediately proximal to the carpal joint, in the depression on the radial side of the joined tendons of the flexor carpi ulnaris muscles	Behaviour problems, grooming abnormalities
BL-40 (avian *Xi wan*, Knee Bend)	In the centre of the popliteal fossa	Pododermatitis, leg and foot pain, gastrointestinal (GI) stasis
BL-60 (*Kun lun*, Mountains)	On the lateral aspect of the ankle, immediately proximal to the cartilage tibialis, in the depression between the tibiotarsus and the tendon of the gastrocnemius	Pain, trauma, egg binding
KI-1 (avian *Jiaodi*, Foot Base)	At the distal aspect of the central pad on the plantar surface of the foot	Pododermatitis, to benefit kidneys, to restore consciousness following trauma
KI-3 (*Tai xi*, Greater Stream)	On the medial aspect of the ankle joint, immediately proximal to the cartilage tibialis, in the depression between the tibiotarsus and the tendon of the gastrocnemius	Infertility, egg binding
KI-6 (*Zhao hai*, Shining Sea)	On the medial aspect of the tibiotarsal-tarsometatarsal joint, at the depression on the lower border of the medial malleolus	Infertility, egg binding, to tonify kidney *Yin*, grooming abnormalities, behaviour problems
PC-6 (*Nei guan*, Inner Gate)	On the ventral surface of the wing, in the interosseous space between the radius and ulna, ¼ the distance from the ventral condyle of the ulna to the olecranon, between the flexor carpi ulnaris and extensor carpi longus digiti majoris muscles	Behaviour problems, aggressive behavior, wing problems, egg binding and infertility, regurgitation and GI problems
TH-5 (*Wai guan*, Outer Gate)	On the dorsum of the wing, in the interosseous space between the radius and ulna, ¼ the distance form the ventral condyle of the ulna to the olecranon	Wing problems, behaviour problems, grooming abnormalities
TH-23 (avian *Yan jiao*, Eye Correct)	In the fossa at the posterior margin of the lateral canthus of the eye	Conjunctivitis, depression (traditional)
GB-13 (*Benshen*, Mind Root)	Lateral to TH-23, 3 cun lateral to the midline	Behaviour problems, grooming abnormalities
GB-31 (avian *Kua wai*, Outside thigh)	On the lateral aspect of the leg	Pruritus, grooming abnormalities, to resolve Blood stagnation
GB-34 (*Yin ling quan*, Yang Hill Spring)	On the lateral aspect of the tibiotarsus, in the proximal interosseous foramen, craniodistal to the head of the fibula	Arthritis, muscle/tendon problems, Liver *Qi* stagnation, behaviour problems
LIV-2 (*Xing jian*, Moving Between)	On the medial surface of the foot, distal to the metatarsophalangeal joint of the second digit, midway between the dorsal and medial aspect of the bone	Conjunctivitis, sinusitis/rhinitis, aggression, grooming abnormalities, infertility
CV-1 (*Hui yin*, Yin Meeting)	On the ventral midline, dorsal proximal to the cloaca and distal to the tip of the pubis	Egg binding, cloacal prolapse, diarrhoea
CV-4 (*Guan yuan*, Origin Pass)	On the ventral midline, ¼ of the distance from the cloaca to the distal edge of the keel	Egg binding, cloacal prolapse, conjunctivitis, rhinitis
CV-6 (*Qi hai*, Sea of *Qi*)	On the ventral midline, 1/3 of the distance form the cloaca to the distal edge of the keel	Crop stasis, cloacal prolapse, infertility

A3.4 Commonly used avian acupuncture points, locations and indications. (continues) ▶

Acupuncture point	Location	Indications
CV-12 (*Zhong wan*, Middle Stomach)	On the ventral midline, at the midpoint between the cloaca and the distal edge of the keel	Crop stasis, regurgitation
GV-1 (*Hou hai*, Rear Sea)	On the midline in the supracloacal fossa	Cloacal prolapse, diarrhoea
GV-14 (Avian *Bei ji*, Back Body of the Spine)	On the dorsal midline, in the fossa formed between the spinous processes of the last cervical and first thoracic vertebrae	Respiratory problems, to relieve heat, local point
GV-20 (avian *Guan ji*, Crown Base)	On the dorsum of the head in the midline depression, at the junction of the frontal and parietal bones	Calm Shen, grooming abnormalities, aggression, heat stroke
GV-24 (*Shenting du*, Mind Courtyard)	On the dorsal midline of the skull, above the cere, approximately at a line drawn between the medial canthus of the eyes	Calming, epilepsy, traditionally used for twisted legs
Ba feng (avian *Jiao pan*, Foot Divide)	In the interphlangeal space between the first and second, second and third, and third and fourth phalanges, on the dorsal surface of the foot	Pododermatitis, local pain, foot problems, twisted legs

A3.4 (continued) Commonly used avian acupuncture points, locations and indications.

Acupuncture Point	Location	Indications
BL-11 (Avian *Xin Shu*)	Caudal to the transverse process and medial to the caudal spicule of the last cervical vertebra	Association point for the heart. Behaviour problems, *Shen* disturbance
BL-12 (Avian *Feng Shu*/*Feng men*, Wind Gate)	Caudal to the transverse process and medial to the caudal spicule of the first thoracic vertebra	Association point for the lungs, respiratory disease, neck problems
BL-13 (Avian *Wei Shu*)	Caudal to the transverse process and medial to the caudal spicule of the second thoracic vertebra	Association point for the stomach (crop, proventriculus and ventriculus). GI problems, crop stasis
BL-14 (Avian *Pi Shu*)	Caudal to the transverse process and medial to the caudal spicule of the third thoracic vertebra	Association point for the spleen. To resolve dampness, GI problems
BL-15 (Avian *Xiao chang Shu*)	Caudal to the transverse process and medial to the caudal spicule of the fourth thoracic vertebra	Association point for the small intestine, abdominal pain, diarrhoea
BL-16 (Avian *Gan Shu*)	Caudal to the transverse process and medial to the caudal spicule of the fifth thoracic vertebra	Association point for the liver. To resolve Liver *Qi* stagnation, behaviour problems
BL-17 (Avian *Da chang Shu*)	Caudal to the transverse process and medial to the caudal spicule of the sixth thoracic vertebra	Association point for the large intestine. GI problems, uropygial gland problems

A3.5 Avian *Shu* points.

Medical diagnosis (TCVM Diagnosis)	Relevant acupuncture Points	Treatment goals
Crop stasis	BL-13, BL-16, St-36, SP-6, CV-6, GV-1	Strengthen GI tract and promote motility
Egg stasis	SP-6, ST-36, GV-20, PC-6, KI-3, KI-6	Strengthen body, calm patient, prevent recurrent problems
Decreased egg production/ egg binding	ST-40, LIV-3, GB-34, ST-36, BL-40, SP-6, SP-9, KI-3, KI-6, CV-1, CV-4, CV-6, GV-20	Calm, strengthen body and reproductive tract, resolve stasis
Sinusitis/rhinitis	LI-4, LI-11, *Yin Tang*, *Biting*, LI-20, LU-9, ST-40, BL-12	Stimulate the lungs, clear heat and cold, remove phlegm and stagnation, boost *Wei Qi*
Respiratory problems	GV-14, LU-7, LU-9, ST-40, GV-1	Stimulate lungs, clear heat and cold, boost *Wei Qi*
Conjunctivitis	BL-1, BL-2, ST1, GB-2, GB-20, SP-6, LI-4, LIV-2, ST-36, CV-17	Resolve fever, pain and infection, strengthen immune system, treat channel-specific problems
Arthritis	LI-11, GB-34, ST-36, BL-60, LIV-2, local points	Relieve pain and stagnation, tonify *Qi* and blood
General infection	LI-11, ST-36, ST-37, SP-6, points specific to affected organ	Resolve fever, stimulate immune system, relieve pain
Trauma	PC-6, PC-9, ST-36, LI-11, BL-60, GV-26, KI-1, local points	Resolve pain and stagnation, tonify *Qi* and blood, calm or stimulate Shen as indicated, anchor *Yang*
Grooming abnormalities/ feather picking	ST-36, ST-40, SP-6, HT-7, PC-6, GB-13, LIV-2, GV-20	Calm *Shen*, resolve stagnation, soothe Liver *Qi*, resolve pruritus
Aggressive behaviour	ST-40, LI-11, HT-7, PC-6, TH-5, LIV-2, GV-20	Calm Shen, resolve stagnation
Diarrhea	ST-36, ST-37, SP-9, CV-1, GV-1, LU-7, LI-10, LI-11	Tonify *Qi*, strengthen spleen and stomach, resolve damp
Cloacal prolapse	SP-6, CV-1, CV-4, CV-6, GV-1	Tonify *Yang*, tonify Spleen *Qi*
Pododermatitis	BL-40, BL-60, KI-1, Ba feng	Resolve pain and stagnation
Heat stroke	GV-20	Calming, relieve heat

A3.6 Common conditions responsive to acupuncture.

Breed guide

Victoria Roberts

All pure breeds of chicken are classified as either Hard Feather or Soft Feather; these classifications are further subdivided in the UK into Game, Asian Hardfeather, Soft Feather Heavy, Soft Feather Light, True Bantam and Rare breeds. A True Bantam does not have a large counterpart; what most people refer to as Bantams are technically miniature versions (one-quarter of the size) of the large fowl. The term Rare covers any breed not sustaining sufficient numbers to warrant having its own Breed Club in the UK (see below for details of International Societies). This covers both the genuinely rare breeds and certain recent imports, and is administered by the Rare Poultry Society, which has done much to keep several breeds in existence and holds the Standards for breeds sometimes seen in this country or that have been recently imported. Domestic ducks and geese have several societies, the main ones being the British Waterfowl Association and the Domestic Waterfowl Club. Waterfowl are also classified as heavy and light breeds. All Breed Club details can be found on the Poultry Club of Great Britain website (www.poultryclub.org).

A poultry keeper may in all innocence, and merely passing on acquired information, inadvertently call a breed by the wrong name or assume that because a bird looks similar to a breed that the individual is a pure breed. The only way to overcome this problem is to introduce a system for permanent identification of pedigree bloodlines (other domestic breeds from cattle to pigeons have used tags, tattoos or rings with great success for many years).

The *British Poultry Standards* (Roberts, 2009) has the complete Standards for all pure breeds available in the UK. Light breeds are the best layers; heavy breeds tend to be more docile; and the feather-legged breeds tend to be lazy. All of them produce meat, the heavy breeds produce it in places we have come to expect from broilers, but take about 6 months to do this.

Heavy breeds

Dark brown eggs are the favourite of many, and the two breeds that lay these are the Marans (two-tone grey banding across the feathers known as 'cuckoo') and the Welsummer (typical orange and black farmyard storybook cockerel colour). The egg of the Welsummer is slightly redder, more of a flower-pot colour than that of the Marans, which is dark brown. A light brown egg is laid by the Barnevelder, which has a mahogany plumage with double black lacing on each feather.

Of the British heavy breeds, one of the most popular is the Buff Orpington, which were owned by Her Majesty the Queen Mother. There are several other colours, but none are noted for their egg production. The Sussex is a good egg layer, the most popular colour being Light (white with black points) Rhode Island Red, Australorp, Plymouth Rock and Wyandotte are also good layers of tinted (slightly brown) eggs. The Croad Langshan lays a plum-coloured egg. The heavier breeds include the Dorking (with five toes) and the Indian Game, which is very broad and heavy indeed. The remaining type of heavy breeds are those with feathered legs such as the Cochin, Brahma, and Faverolles. Old English Game and the reachy Modern Game are particularly hardy and colourful. The Frizzle looks strange with its backward-curling feathers but is a decent layer.

Light breeds

There is great variation in colours and types with many being imports. Virtually all of these lay white or light-coloured eggs. The White Leghorn still out-produces most breeds, but there are several other colours. Other Mediterranean breeds are the Ancona (white spots on black), Minorca (black) and Andalusian (blue laced). British breeds include the Derbyshire Redcap, Old English Pheasant Fowl, Hamburg (pencilled or spangled), Scots Dumpy (short legs) and Scots Grey, all of which should have good utility attributes. Within the light breeds are the crested breeds including the Poland, the Araucana (blue/green eggs) and that fluffiest of birds, the Silkie.

Large fowl, Bantams and True Bantams

There are miniatures of certain large fowl, which should be one-quarter the size of the large, usually referred to as Bantams. True Bantams do not have a large fowl counterpart and are primarily for ornamental and aesthetic purposes, but are excellent for young children and those without much space available for poultry.

Selected breed guide

Chickens

Hard Feather

Old English Game (Figure A4.1): Known since at least Roman times. The banning of cockfighting encouraged the development of the exhibition type of this breed. There are two types, the Carlisle (exhibition) and the Oxford (more athletic). With over 30 colours standardized, there is plenty of choice for the breeder, but the chicks have a tendency to be aggressive, at least to other breeds, as do the females who make excellent mothers. There is a club for each type.

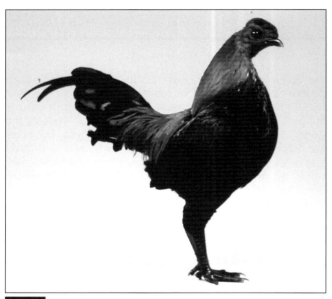

A4.1 Brown-red Old English Game male.

Shamo (Figure A4.2): A Japanese bird of Malayoid type, originally imported to Japan from Thailand in the 17th century – the name being a corruption of Siam, the old name for Thailand. In Japan it was developed into a fighting bird of unmatched courage and ferocity. Its feathers are sparse but strong and shiny, and its powerful bone structure and well muscled body and legs, coupled with its erect posture, make it an impressive and striking bird. It is quite docile with people, however, and comes in several colours.

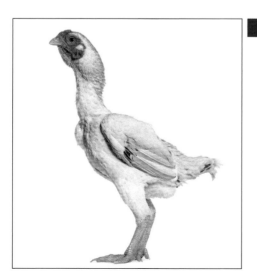

A4.2 Shamo female.

Heavy breed

Light Sussex (Figure A4.3): At the first poultry show of 1845 the classification included Old Sussex or Kent fowls, Surrey fowls and Dorkings. The oldest variety of the Sussex is the Speckled, Whites came a few years later, as sports from Lights. The Light is the most widely kept in this country today among standard as well as commercial breeders. It is one of our most popular breeds for producing table birds. At the time when sex-linkage held considerable popularity the light Sussex was one of the most popular breeds of the day, the females being in considerable demand for mating to gold males.

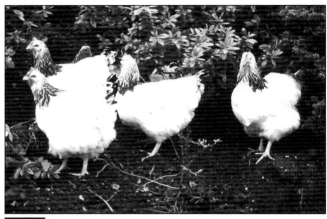

A4.3 Light Sussex females.

Dorking (Figure A4.4): Its purely British ancestry makes the Dorking one of the oldest of domesticated fowls in lineage. A Roman writer described birds of Dorking type with five toes, and no doubt such birds were found in England by the Romans under Julius Caesar. Today, there are five colours, they are reasonable layers and produce a good carcass.

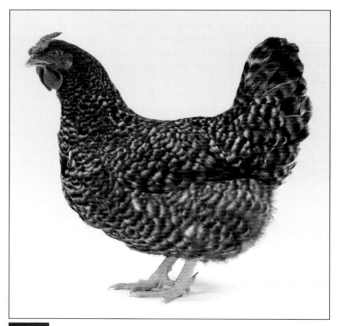

A4.4 Cuckoo Dorking female.

Welsummer (Figure A4.5): Named after the village of Welsum, stock was imported into this country from the Netherlands in 1928. The breed is known in particular for its large terracotta-coloured egg, which remains its special feature, some being mottled with brown spots. The Welsummer has distinctive markings and colours, and is classified in the light-breed exhibition category in the UK, although it has a good body size and is in the medium class in the Netherlands. Judges and breeders work to a standard that values indications of productiveness, so that laying merits can be combined with aesthetics.

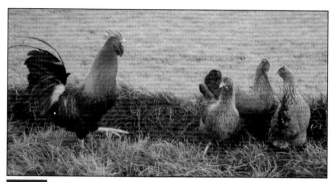

A4.5 Welsummer flock.

Orpington (Figure A4.6): An English breed named after the village in Kent where the originator, William Cook, had his farm. He introduced the Black variety in 1886, the White in 1889 and the Buff in 1894. Within 5 years of the original black Orpington being introduced exhibition breeders were crossing other breeds to increase size, but this crossing at once turned a dual-purpose breed into one solely for show purposes, and it has remained so until today. A late introduction, the Jubilee Orpington, is gaining in popularity.

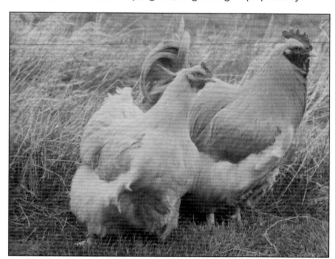

A4.6 Buff Orpington pair.

Laced Wyandotte (Figure A4.7): The first variety of the Wyandotte family was the Silver Laced, which originated in America, where it was standardized in 1883. The variety was introduced into England at the time, and English breeders immediately perfected the lacings and open ground colouring. The White came as a sport from the Silver Laced; the Buff followed by crossing Buff Cochin with the Silver Laced. It is clear that whilst the family of the Wyandotte is large, every variety is a made from various blending of breeds, but with around 15 colours, it remains a popular breed.

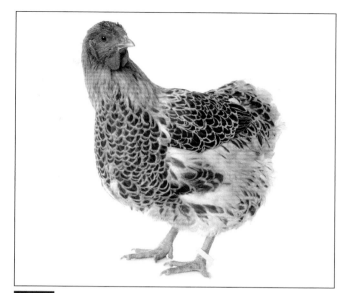

A4.7 Buff Laced Wyandotte female.

Light breed

Leghorn (Figure A4.8): Italy was the original home of the Leghorn, but the first specimens of the White variety reached the UK from America around 1870, and the Brown was introduced 2 years or so later. These early specimens were very light in weight and so UK breeders started to increase the body weight of the Whites by crossing. In the postwar years, the utility and commercial breeders established a type of their own, and that is the one which is now favoured. In commercial circles, the White Leghorn has figured prominently in the establishment of high egg-producing hybrids.

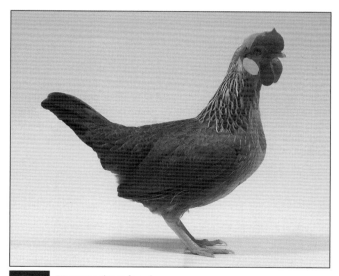

A4.8 Brown Leghorn female.

Silkie (Figure A4.9): Silkie fowls have been mentioned by authorities for several hundred years, although some think they originated in India, whilst others consider China or Japan as the country of origin. Despite their light weight, the Silkie is not regarded as a bantam in the UK, but as a large fowl light breed, and as such it must be exhibited. Its persistent broodiness is a breed characteristic and, either pure or crossed, the breed provides reliable broodies for the eggs of large fowl or bantams.

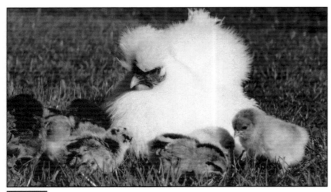

A4.9   White Silkie female.

Hamburgh (Figure A4.10): The Silver Spangled Hamburgh was bred in Yorkshire and Lancashire 300 years ago as Pheasants and Mooneys. In its heyday, the Hamburgh was a grand layer and must have played its part in the making of other laying breeds. However, its breeders directed it down purely exhibition roads, until today the larger version is in few hands; the Bantam version is more popular.

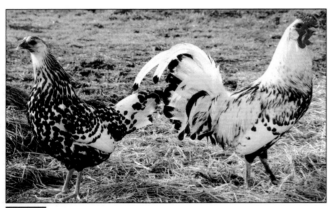

A4.10   Silver Spangled Hamburgh pair.

Scots Grey (Figure A4.11): A light, non-sitting breed originating in Scotland, it has not been bred extensively outside that country where, even if it is less popular today, it will doubtless be maintained by keen breeders. It has been bred there for over 200 years, there is one colour (barred: well defined light and dark grey horizontal stripes) and it comes in large and bantam sizes.

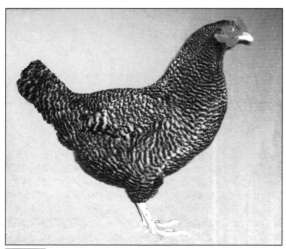

A4.11   Scots Grey female.

Rare

Norfolk Grey (Figure A4.12): This breed was introduced by Mr Myhill of Norwich under the name of Black Marias. They were first shown at the 1920 Dairy Show and were mainly the result of a cross breed between Silver Birchen Game and Duckwing Leghorns. They appear regularly at shows and are plentiful in their county of origin, being a dual purpose bird providing meat and eggs.

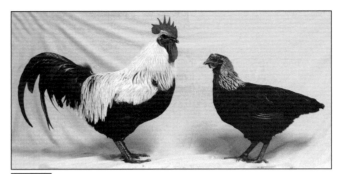

A4.12   Norfolk Grey pair.

Old English Pheasant Fowl (Figure A4.13): This breed was given its name around 1914, previous to which it had been called the Yorkshire Pheasant, Golden Pheasant and also the Old-fashioned Pheasant. That it is a very old English breed is certain. Some Northern breeders retained their strains as Yorkshire Pheasant Fowls until the present tag of 'Old English' was brought officially into use. It has a meaty breast for a light breed, and has always been popular with both farmers and exhibitors.

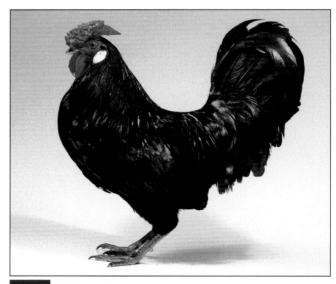

A4.13   Old English Pheasant Fowl male.

Transylvanian Naked Neck (Figure A4.14): Transylvania has been part of Romania since 1918, but was once part of the Ottoman Turkish Empire, and then part of the Austro-Hungarian Empire. Naked Neck chickens have been recorded in many parts of Europe and the Middle East, so it is difficult to be sure about their origin. They are active foragers and productive birds, and their bare necks and reduced plumage are not a problem, especially in warm climates. Indeed, the speed with which cockerels can be hand plucked and ready for cooking has no doubt ensured

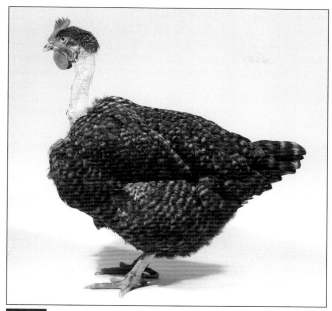

A4.14 Cuckoo Transylvanian Naked Neck female.

their popularity among smallholders. There are now several naked-necked broiler hybrids, a good example of how even the most unexpected old breed can be useful in today's poultry industry.

True Bantams

Dutch (Figure A4.15): The Dutch bantam in its country of origin has been around for a long time, though in the Netherlands a club was only formed on 1 December 1946. The breed first appeared in the UK around the late 1960s, and a club was formed in 1982. Since then the breed has gone from strength to strength, with 13 colours standardized, though in the Netherlands many more varieties have appeared and been exported.

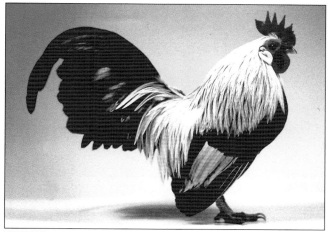

A4.15 Silver Dutch male.

Sebright (Figure A4.16): This breed is a genuine bantam and one of the oldest British varieties. It has no counterpart in large breeds, but has played a part in the production of other laced fowl, notably Wyandottes. There are two colours, gold and silver, both being popular on the show bench. It is a breed for the more experienced poultry keeper with the males having hen-shaped feathering affecting fertility.

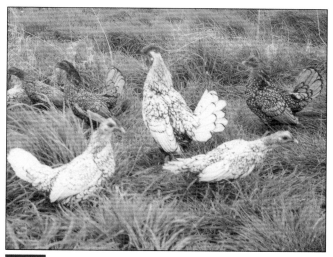

A4.16 Silver and gold Sebright flock.

Japanese (Figure A4.17): These True Bantams are of great antiquity, and without counterparts in the large breeds. They are the shortest legged of all varieties and are standardized in three feather forms: plain or normal feather, frizzle feather (where the ends of all feathers are to curl back and point towards the head) and silkie feather, which refers to the feather construction. Looking more like a table decoration than a chicken, these very small birds have a dedicated following.

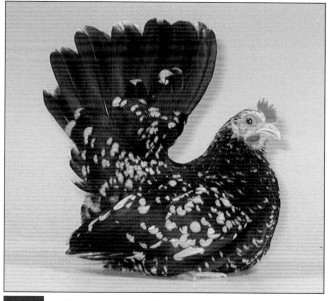

A4.17 Mottled Japanese female.

Turkeys
Bronze (Figure A4.18)

This is the closest in colouring to the Eastern Wild turkey. It is the most popular variety of turkey and a good Bronze is difficult to beat at exhibitions. The Bronze was further developed in England and reintroduced to the Americas where it became extremely popular. There are far fewer Standard Bronzes than Broad-breasted (meat) Bronzes and the meat version (the waddling walk gives this away) is not allowed to enter shows.

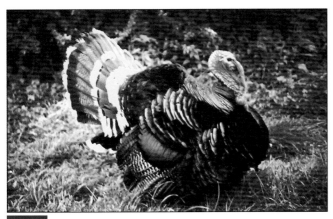

A4.18 Bronze turkey male.

Buff (Figure A4.19)

Classed as light, the Buff turkey is named for the rich cinnamon colour of its body feathers. The breed was recognized by the American Poultry Association in 1874 but very few now exist in America and there is no longer a standard for it there. The breed was extremely popular in Britain at the turn of the last century with its own Buff Turkey Club in the early 1900s. It is difficult to maintain the correct markings.

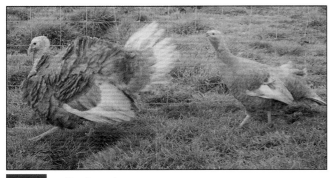

A4.19 Buff turkey pair.

Ducks
Khaki Campbell (Figure A4.20)

One of the first, and certainly the most successful, of the utility breeds developed in the 20th century from the Indian Runner, the Khaki Campbell largely took over as the top egg-laying duck. The colour of farmyard mud, from which it gets the first part of its name, the Khaki Campbell proved to be exceedingly agile, very fertile and extremely prolific, laying a white egg.

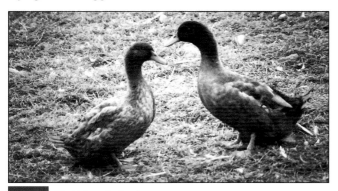

A4.20 Khaki Campbell pair.

Indian Runner (Figure A4.21)

The era of the high egg-laying breeds of ducks started with the introduction of the Indian Runner into the UK from Malaya. A ship's captain brought home Fawns, Fawn-and-Whites and Whites, distributing them among his friends in Dumfriesshire and Cumberland. They proved prolific layers, and there was a class of Fawn Runners at the Dumfries show in 1876. There are now 11 colours, laying a blue egg.

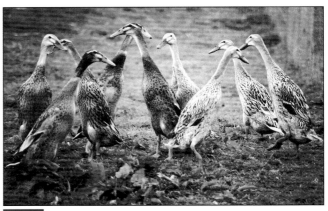

A4.21 Trout Indian Runner duck flock.

Saxony (Figure A4.22)

This single colour, dual purpose breed was bred by Albert Franz at Chemnitz. It was first exhibited at Chemnitz-Altendorf at the first Saxony County Show of 1934. However, the breed stock was almost entirely destroyed during the Second World War and in 1952 Franz was forced to begin a revival using small surviving flocks and reintroducing some of the other breeds employed earlier in 1930. The Saxony duck was recognized in Great Britain in 1982.

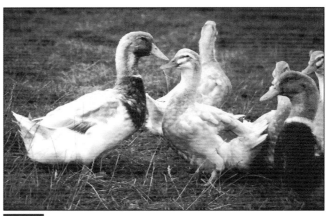

A4.22 Saxony flock.

Cayuga (Figure A4.23)

This breed takes its name from Lake Cayuga in New York State, and is thought to be descended from the wild black duck (*Anas rubripes*). The Cayuga was first recorded in North America between 1830 and 1850. It was first standardized in America in 1874 and in Britain in 1901. It has a black plumage with brilliant green iridescence. The drakes tend to retain their black plumage but the females develop patches of white as they get older, therefore they are only exhibited as young birds. The egg shells have a black outer pigment that fades during lay.

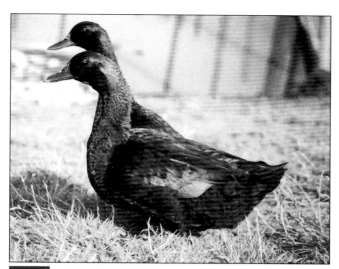

A4.23   Cayuga pair.

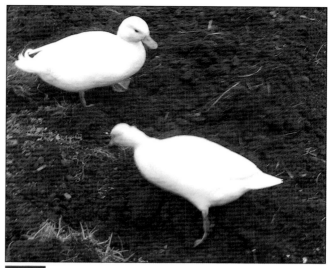

A4.25   White Call duck pair.

Pekin (Figure A4.24)

This duck was imported from China into Great Britain and America between 1872 and 1874. Crossed with other breeds, it had a large impact on the commercial table bird market. The present upright exhibition strain is often referred to as the 'German' Pekin due to the first importation in to the UK from that country in the 1980s, largely to distinguish it from the American Pekin (more horizontal in carriage). This is a variety that continues to thrive as an exhibition breed and also as basic stock for commercial breeding. In addition, it provided genetic material for several modern breeds, including the Saxony.

Geese
Brecon Buff (Figure A4.26)

As the name suggests, this breed has its origins in the hills of Breconshire, Wales. The overall buff colour, unique among British geese, attracted Rhys Llewellyn who is credited with collecting and developing this breed in the late 1920s and working with them, until they were breeding true. It is a hardy, active breed, but as with many poultry breeds, sunshine fades the feather colouring until the next moult restores it.

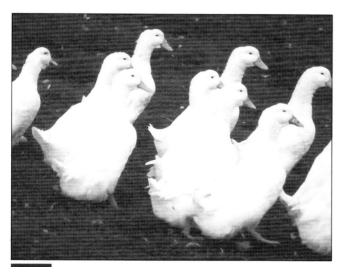

A4.24   Pekin duck flock.

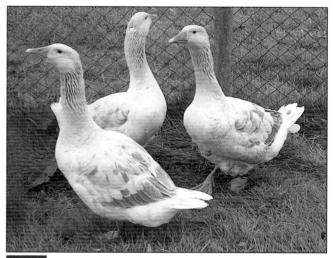

A4.26   Brecon Buff geese.

Call (Figure A4.25)

Whilst known as Call ducks nowadays, these small ducks have been referred to as Decoys or Coys in the past in the Netherlands and other European countries; wildfowlers in Britain also deployed tame or semi-tame ducks to entice their wild relatives. The Call duck is very popular exhibition duck with at least 14 colours. The spare drakes are excellent at slug control in vegetable gardens but the females can be noisy except when broody, when they make good mothers.

Chinese (Figure A4.27)

The Chinese is an elegant, fine, small goose, active and good at foraging. Although it shares the same wild ancestor as the African (the swan goose), which can be seen in the similarity of colour and marking, in shape and size, the two breeds are very different. Chinese geese have been present in Britain since at least the early 18th century. There are two colours, White and Grey (like its ancestor). They lay well, are very noisy and have a reputation for being good 'watch dogs'; they are famous for guarding some whisky distilleries in Scotland.

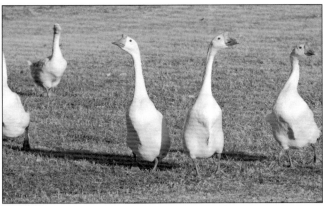

A4.27   White Chinese goose flock.

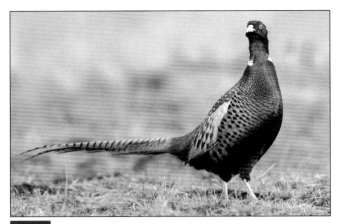

A4.29   Common pheasant.

African (Figure A4.28)

Amongst the largest and heaviest of the domestic breeds of geese with a very deep voice, this relatively docile goose has the swan goose as its ancestor and retains the wild colour. They are distinguished from the Western breeds of geese (greylag descendants) and have a prominent 'knob' rising up from the base of the beak and smooth, and velvet-looking feathering on their necks. The African also has a soft dewlap which hangs below its beak. Both knob and dewlap increase in size as the bird gets older.

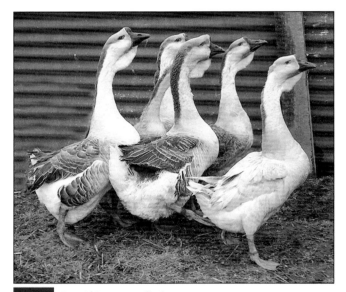

A4.28   Grey African geese flock.

Pheasants, peafowl, guinea fowl and quail

Any of the ornamentals which are not indigenous must be kept in a covered area to avoid release in the UK. Around 45 different pheasant species are available but as these are wild species, colour mutations only occasionally appear and they are not used for exhibition.

Common pheasant (Figure A4.29)

The Common or Ringnecked pheasant is intensively reared in large numbers by game farms all over Europe, the UK and in parts of North America to be released for shooting.

Golden pheasant (Figure A4.30)

Originally from China, probably the most colourful of the ornamental pheasants, small and easy to keep. The male gets his magnificent plumage in his second year and the hens will rear their own chicks.

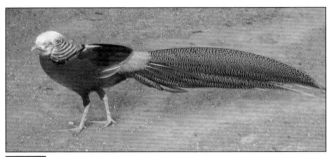

A4.30   Golden pheasant.

Himalayan Monal (Figure A4.31)

A spectacular and large pheasant from India which enjoys digging. They have a docile nature and the hens will rear their own.

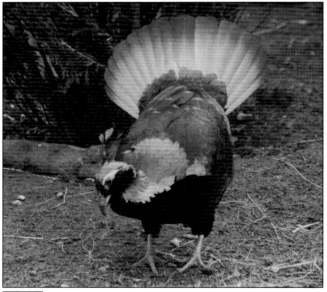

A4.31   Himalayan Monal.

Temminck's Tragopan (Figure A4.32)

A forest pheasant from Asia. A medium-sized bird that is tame and confiding and males have extraordinary blue display skin under their chin in the spring. The hens may rear their own, they prefer to nest in a suspended basket.

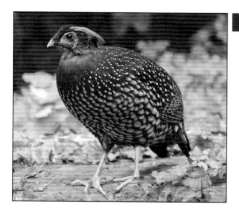

A4.32 Temminck's Tragopan.

Peacock (Figure A4.33)

The familiar Indian Blue is only one colour available; there are also black-shouldered and pure white varieties. The noise of the male can be disturbing in the spring. The Green peacock is a separate species and is not hardy and is therefore more appropriate for the specialist keeper.

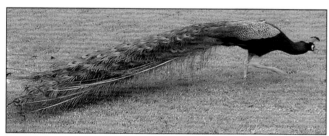

A4.33 Indian Blue peacock.

Guinea fowl (Figure A4.34)

One of several African guinea fowl species, but the only one domesticated, providing mainly meat. The eggs have very thick shells and take 28 days to incubate. Very noisy and good guards, but not fox-proof.

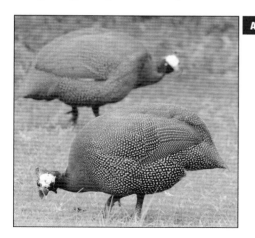

A4.34 Guinea fowl.

References and further reading

Roberts V (2009) *British Poultry Standards, 6th edn.* Wiley Blackwell, Oxford

Useful websites

Area	Poultry Association	Website
International	International Waterfowl Breeders	https://officialiwba.weebly.com/
UK	Poultry Club of Great Britain	http://www.poultryclub.org/breedclubs
USA	American Poultry Association	http://www.amerpoultryassn.com/
USA	The American Livestock Breeds Conservancy	http://www.albc-usa.org/cpl/wtchlist.html
Australia	Rare Breeds Trust of Australia	http://rarebreedstrust.com.au
Germany	Bund Deutscher Rassegeflügelzüchter	http://www.bdrg.de/
Germany (Bavaria)	Verband Bayerischer Rassegeflügelzüchter	http://www.rassegefluegel-bayern.de/
Switzerland	Kleintiere Schweiz	http://www.kleintiere-schweiz.ch/
Italy	Federazione Italiana Associazioni Avicole	http://www.fiav.info/
Italy	Associazione Italiana Razze Autoctone a Rischio di Estinzione	http://www.associazionerare.it/
Denmark	Danmarks Fjerkræavlerforening for Raceavl	http://www.racefjerkrae.dk/
Sweden	Svenska Lanthönsklubben	http://www.kackel.se/
Norway	Norsk Rasefjærfeforbund	http://www.nrff.no/

Index

Tablets, administration of medication 76
Tactile sense organs 22
Tail feathers (rectrices) 8, 11
Tapeworms 101, *104*, 183
Tarsometatarsal bones 11, 12, 215, *283*, *286*
Taste buds 22
Telephone triage 59
Temminck's Tragopan pheasant breed 349
Temperature, environmental
　brooding areas 35–6
　hospitalization 49
　transportation 47, 48
　see also Body temperature
Tenosynovitis 193–4, 221
Terminology see Definitions and Terminology
Territoriality 25
Testicles 20–1, 132
　see also Castration
Tetracycline, maximum residue levels *336*
Thermoregulation 6
　see also Body temperature
Thiamine 39, *226*, 234, *326*
Thoracic fractures 285–6
Thoracic girdle 11
Threadworm see *Capillaria* infection
Thrombocytes 88, *89*, 90, *91*, 93
Thrombograms, haematology 94, *95*
Thrush 179–81
Thymus gland 21, *295*, 307
Thyroid gland *132*, *134*, *295*
Tiamulin *333*
　maximum residue levels *336*
Tibial dyschondroplasia see Dyschondroplasia
Tibiotarsus 11, 12, *281*, *282*, *283*, 286
Tick-related anaemia *240*, 246
Ticks 92
Tidal volume, chickens 254
Toes 11, 12
　amputations 288
　de-toeing, legal issues 315
　developmental abnormalities 215, 224, *325*
　fractures *283*, 286–7
　see also Curled toe paralysis
Toltrazuril 186, *334*
Tongue, clinical examination 66
Tonovet rebound tonometry *152*
Topical antiseptics *334*
Total red blood cell count (TRBC) 92, *93*
Total white blood cell count (TWBC) 93
Touch sense organs 22
Toxic plants 40
Toxoplasmosis, eye disorders 156–7
Trace elements 39–40
Trachea 15
　anaesthesia 252
　endoscopy *132*, *134*
　parasitology *103*
　post-mortem findings 303
　sample collection *86*
　tracheobronchoscopy 128
Tracheitis, endoscopy *164*
Tramadol 258, *330*
Tranquilizers, premedication 253
Transient paralysis see Marek's disease
Transport of Animals (Cleansing and Disinfection) (England) (No. 3) Order (2003) 315
Transportation 47–8, 315
Transylvanian Naked Neck breed 344–5
Trauma
　acupuncture *340*
　beak 147–8
　eyes 157
　feather loss 141
Treadle feeders 29
Treats, food 32
Trematodes 183
Tremor, problem-based approaches *326*

Triage, telephone 59
Trichomoniasis/*Trichomonas* spp. 186–7, *321*
　clinical pathology 101
　differential diagnoses 179, 187, 188
　post-mortem findings *305*
Trichophyton megnini infection (favus) 146, *240*, 247
Tuberculosis *189*, 194
Turkey(s), information specific to 3
　avian metapneumovirus infection *165*
　behaviour 25
　biological and physiological parameters *62*
　caruncles *7*
　chlamydiosis *198*
　chondrodystrophy *222*
　clinical examination *63*, 67
　clinical pathology *90*
　coccidiosis *185*
　courtship displays 26
　desnooding 315
　diarrhoea *189*
　egg laying 20
　feather disorders *142*
　fibrinopurulent sinusitis *168*
　food requirements *37*
　haemorrhagic enteritis *190*
　handling 46
　housing 30
　incubation times *35*
　medication contraindications 186
　models of keeping/regimes 25
　myopathies 225
　parasitology *103*, *183*
　radiography *114*
　reference values, physiological *99*
　reproductive system 19
　respiratory system 15–16
　selected breeds 345–6
　sexing 82
　sexual dimorphism *80*, *81*
　shaky leg syndrome 225
　small intestine 17
　snood 6, *7*
　systemic disease *240*
　terminology *36*
　transportation 48
　vertebrae 10
　vocal signalling 25
　wing clipping 53
Turkey coryza 156, *161*, 172–3
Turkey haemorrhagic enteritis 244–5
Turkey viral hepatitis *240*, 245
Tylosin *333*
　maximum residue levels *336*
Tylvalosin *333*
　maximum residue levels *336*
Typhoid *189*, 195–6, 245

Ulcerative colitis *240*, *323*
Ulcerative duodenitis, quail *247*
Ulcerative enteritis 195
　diarrhoea *189*
　differential diagnoses 186, 190, 245
　post-mortem findings *305*
　systemic infections 246–7
Ulna 11, 68, *282*, *283*, 285
Ultrasonography 105, 119–23
Ultraviolet (UV) rays, pathogen destruction 28
Ungraded Eggs (Hygiene) Regulations (1990) 316
Unretracted yolk sacs 214–15
Upper respiratory tract 15
Urates/urine 19
Uric acid, serum chemistry profiles *100*
Urinary system 18–19
Urography, imaging 113
Uropygial gland 6, 149
Uterine adenocarcinoma 210
Uveitis 154